Sports Nutrition

A Practice Manual for Professionals

5th Edition

Christine A. Rosenbloom, PhD, RD, CSSD, Editor in Chief

Ellen J. Coleman, MA, MPH, RD, CSSD, Assistant Editor

Sports, Cardiovascular, and Wellness Nutrition Dietetic Practice Group

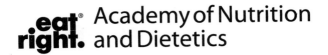

eat right.® Academy of Nutrition and Dietetics

Diana Faulhaber, Publisher
Elizabeth Nishiura, Production Manager

For more information about the Academy of Nutrition and Dietetics, visit www.eatright.org

10 9 8 7 6 5 4 3 2

ISBN: 978-0-88091-452-9

CONTENTS

ACKNOWLEDGMENTS

The 5th edition of *Sports Nutrition: A Practice Manual for Professionals* builds on the previous editions to bring health and sports professionals the latest research with practical applications for athletes of all ages. We would like to extend a special thanks to the following individuals:

- Marie Dunford, 4th edition editor, for her advice and support to create a seamless transition from the last edition to the new edition.
- SCAN leadership, especially Gale Welter, Hope Barkoukis, Michele Macedonio, Tara Coghlin-Dickson, and Enette Larson-Meyer who saw the value in supporting the manual and for their encouragement over the long process of creating the manual.
- The authors who generously contributed their time, talent, and expertise to bring their unique perspective to each chapter.
- The reviewers who provided critical and crucial suggestions to strengthen the chapters.
- The Academy of Nutrition and Dietetics publications team, especially Elizabeth Nishiura and Diana Faulhaber for their guidance.
- The many athletes we have had the privilege of working with over the years, who continue to inspire us and motivate us to provide evidence-based nutrition guidelines to help them achieve their goals.

Christine A. Rosenbloom, PhD, RD, CSSD, Editor in Chief
Ellen J. Coleman, MA, MPH, RD, CSSD, Assistant Editor

CONTRIBUTORS

Katherine A. Beals, PhD, RD, FACSM, CSSD
Associate professor, University of Utah
Salt Lake City, UT

Erica Bland, BSN, RN
Memorial Sloan Kettering Cancer Center
New York, NY

Maria G. Boosalis, PhD, MPH, RD
Professor emeritus, University of Kentucky
Consultant, Nutrition, Health & Wellness
Minneapolis, MN

Nicholas A. Burd, PhD
Department of Kinesiology
McMaster University
Hamilton, ON, Canada

Louise M. Burke, OAM, PhD, APD, FACSM
Head of Sports Nutrition
Australian Institute of Sport
Canberra, Australia

Ellen J. Coleman, MA, MPH, RD, CSSD
Sports dietitian
The SPORT Clinic
Riverside, CA

Nancy DiMarco, PhD, RD, CSSD, FACSM
Professor, Department of Nutrition and Food Sciences
Texas Woman's University
Denton, TX

Marie Dunford, PhD, RD
Nutrition educator
Kingsburg, CA

Charlotte Hayes, MMSc, MS, RD, CDE, ACSM-CES
Diabetes nutrition and exercise specialist
Atlanta, GA

Mark Kern, PhD, RD, CSSD
Professor, Department of Exercise and Nutritional
    Sciences
San Diego State University
San Diego, CA

Jennifer Ketterly, MS, RD, CSSD
Director of Sports Nutrition
University of Georgia
Athens, GA

D. Enette Larson-Meyer, PhD, RD, CSSD, FACSM
Associate professor and director of Nutrition and
    Exercise Laboratory
University of Wyoming
Laramie, WY

Michele A. Macedonio, MS, RD, CSSD
Nutrition consultant, sports dietitian
Nutrition Strategies
Loveland, OH

Caroline Mandel, MS, RD, CSSD
Sports dietitian
University of Michigan
Ann Arbor, MI

Ronald J. Maughan, PhD
Professor, School of Sport, Exercise and Health
    Sciences
Loughborough University
Loughborough, UK

Christopher Melby, DrPH
Professor and department head, Department of Food
    Science and Human Nutrition
Colorado State University
Fort Collins, CO

Christopher M. Modlesky, PhD
Associate professor, Department of Kinesiology and
    Applied Physiology
University of Delaware
Newark, DE

Michelle F. Mottola, PhD, FACSM
Director, R. Samuel McLaughlin Foundation Exercise
    and Pregnancy Lab
University of Western Ontario
London, ON, Canada

Bob Murray, PhD, FACSM
Managing principal
Sports Science Insights, LLC
Crystal Lake, IL

Pamela M. Nisevich Bede, MS, RD, CSSD
Nutrition consultant, Swim, Bike, Run, Eat!
Senior Scientist, Abbott Nutrition
Beavercreek, Ohio

Stuart M. Phillips, PhD, FACN, FACSM
Professor and associate chair, Department of
    Kinesiology
McMaster University
Hamilton, ON, Canada

Janet Walberg Rankin, PhD, FACSM
Professor, Human Nutrition, Food, and Exercise
Virginia Tech
Blacksburg, VA

MAJ Reva Rogers, MHA, RD, CSSD, CSCS
US Army

Christine A. Rosenbloom, PhD, RD, CSSD
Professor emerita, Division of Nutrition
Georgia State University
Atlanta, GA

Susan M. Shirreffs, PhD
School of Sport, Exercise and Health Sciences
Loughborough University
Loughborough, UK

LTC Lori Sigrist, PhD, RD, CSSD, CSCS
US Army

Patti Steinmuller, MS, RD, CSSD
Sports nutrition educator
Gallatin Gateway, MT

Stella Lucia Volpe, PhD, RD, FACSM
Professor and chair, Department of Nutrition Sciences
Drexel University
Philadelphia, PA

Lt Col Dana Whelan, USAF, MS, MA, RD, CHES
US Air Force

CDR Kim A. Zuzelski, MPH, MS, RD, CSSD, CDE
US Navy

REVIEWERS

Hope Barkoukis, PhD, RD
Case Western Reserve University
Cleveland, OH

Dawn Jackson Blatner, RD, CSSD
Sports dietitian, Chicago Cubs
Private practice dietitian
Chicago, IL

Charlotte Caperton-Kilburn, MS, RD, CSSD
NFL Performance
Charleston, SC

Karen Reznik Dolins, EdD, RD, CSSD
Nutrition and Exercise Physiology, Teacher's College,
    Columbia University
Private practice
New York, NY

Suzanne Girard Eberle, MS, RD, CSSD
Private practice, Eat, Drink, Win!
Portland, OR

Stephanie Perkins Giegerich, MS, RD
Corporate Sports Unlimited
Atlanta, GA

Francis Holway, MSc
Club Atlético River Plate
Buenos Aires, Argentina

Diane King, MS, RD, CSSD, ATC
Children's HealthCare of Atlanta Sports Medicine
Suwanee, GA

Kris Osterberg, MS, RD, CSSD
Virginia Polytechnic Institute and State University
Blacksburg, VA

Monique Ryan, MS, RD, CSSD
Personal Nutrition Designs, LLC
Evanston, IL

Susan M. Shirreffs, PhD
School of Sport, Exercise and Health Sciences
Loughborough University
Loughborough, UK

James Stevens, MS, RD
Front Range Community College
Fort Collins, CO

Marissa Wertheimer
Graduate student
University of Georgia
Athens, GA

FOREWORD

This 5th edition of *Sports Nutrition: A Practice Manual for Professionals* contains 22 chapters that comprehensively examine the many theoretical and applied aspects of the continually growing discipline of sports nutrition. The authors are nationally and internationally recognized experts, many of whom are fellows in professional societies such as the American College of Sports Medicine. As a result, this edition will appeal broadly to not only registered dietitians but also athletic trainers, strength and conditioning coaches, fitness trainers, sports medicine professionals, graduate students, and coaches at all levels.

The theoretical and applied aspects of sports nutrition are developed in the four sections of this book: Sports Nutrition Basics; Sports Nutrition Assessment and Energy Balance; Sports Nutrition Across the Life Cycle and for Special Populations; and Sports-Specific Nutrition Guidelines. This edition includes a more global perspective than previous editions, as several chapters are written by internationally recognized experts.

This book provides sports dietitians and other professionals with an invaluable look behind the scenes at what it takes to work successfully with athletes at all levels: children, adolescents, recreational, collegiate, professional, and masters athletes. It also includes insight into how to advise elite athletes, which is based on long-term work conducted at the Australian Institute of Sport. Furthermore, the appendixes list relevant sports nutrition position stands from professional organizations as well as many useful Web sites. Therefore, this book serves as a reference that helps in career building for practitioners of sports nutrition, strength and conditioning, and fitness.

Well known for their ability to translate science into practice-based recommendations, the editors are also practicing sports dietitians, who have balanced the chapters with a combination of research and practical advice for the reader.

I plan to use this book as the textbook for the graduate course I teach in sports nutrition at the University of Texas at Austin. I'm sure that my students will benefit from the wealth of practical information that serves to reinforce and "flesh out" the theoretical concepts. I recommend that this book be part of the professional library for all who work in sports nutrition and fitness. I keep my copy close at hand and refer to it regularly.

Edward F. Coyle, PhD, FACSM
Professor
The University of Texas at Austin
Director, Human Performance Laboratory

PREFACE

Sound nutrition is essential for high-quality sport training and competition. The 5th edition of *Sports Nutrition: A Practice Manual for Professionals* is a joint venture between the Academy of Nutrition and Dietetics (formerly American Dietetic Association) and the Sports, Cardiovascular and Wellness Nutrition (SCAN) dietetic practice group. All five editions of this manual have been edited by SCAN members, and many of the authors are SCAN members, who bring both research and application to the information provided in this book. We are pleased with the 5th edition and hope that you will find this updated edition useful.

Overview of the 5th Edition

The 5th edition of *Sports Nutrition: A Practice Manual for Professionals* is organized in four sections and designed to be a complete reference manual that can be used in its entirety as a textbook for sports nutrition classes. Additionally, this book is a "go to" source for specific evidenced-based information on different sports nutrition topics, such as ergogenic aids, carbohydrate requirements to fuel sport, or working with college athletes. Each chapter includes enough information to make it stand alone as a reference without unnecessarily repeating information that is provided in detail in elsewhere in the book.

Section 1 covers sports nutrition basics. It begins with an overview of nutrition in exercise (Chapter 1) followed by chapters on macro and micro-nutrients as well as fluids and electrolytes for an active population (Chapters 2 through 6). Research advances in the understanding of the role of carbohydrate, protein, fat, vitamins, minerals, and water have been included to provide the most up-to-date information available to guide the professional who works with athletes. Chapter 7 concludes this section by providing a detailed review of dietary supplements that discusses the pros and cons of using supplements and offers a "bottom line" regarding the safety and efficacy for each supplement.

Section 2 covers nutrition assessment and energy balance in athletes. Conducting a comprehensive nutrition assessment (Chapter 8) and choosing the best body composition analysis method (Chapter 9) set the stage for providing quality nutrition care for athletes. Experts take you step-by-step through the process to understand the pros and cons of various assessment techniques. Athletes often expend substantial time and resources to achieve and maintain a desirable body weight and body composition. The chapters on energy balance and weight management (Chapters 10 and 11) provide evidenced- and research-based rationales for various strategies that affect body weight and body composition and dispel myths about gaining muscle mass and losing body fat. Practical advice is given with real-world case studies to guide the professional who works with athletes.

In Section 3 we cover nutrition across the life span. Chapters 12 through 15 address working with children and adolescent athletes, college athletes, masters athletes, and elite athletes. In addition, this section includes chapters on the nutritional concerns of unique athletic populations, such as vegetarian athletes, pregnant athletes, athletes at risk for disordered eating, and athletes with diabetes (Chapters 16 through 19). All of the chapters in this section are authored by expert practitioners, who bring a unique understanding of the subject and provide practical information on applying the research.

Section 4 applies sports nutrition basics to athletes engaged in specific sporting events: from very high–intensity, short-duration sports, like track and field events (Chapter 20) to intermittent, high-intensity or "stop-and-go" sports, like football and soccer (Chapter 21), to the endurance and ultra-endurance events like road cycling, marathon running, or the Ironman triathlon (Chapter 22). Each chapter provides an overview on energy systems used in the sport and gives practical advice for fueling and hydrating athletes engaged in specific sports.

The "At A Glance" section provides quick summaries of nutrition priorities for 18 sports. These brief descriptions of the sports and general nutrition guidelines can help provide the basis for an individualized meal plan or a team nutrition seminar.

New features of the 5th edition include controversial issues or "hot topics" sprinkled in among the chapters. How does prescription medication affect masters athletes who are drug tested? Is beet root juice or beta-alanine the hot new dietary supplement? Should athletes "train low, compete high"? These and many more hot issues are covered in this manual.

About SCAN

SCAN was founded in 1981 and has more than 6,500 members. The e-learning activities, resource materials, and products found on the Web site (www.scandpg.org) promote the mission of SCAN: "to empower members to be the nation's food and nutrition leaders through excellence and expertise in nutrition for sports and physical activity, cardiovascular health, wellness, and disordered eating and eating disorders." Within SCAN, three subunits have unique perspectives and provide resources (available on SCAN's Web site) for the sports dietitian as well as other professionals working with active people:

- The *Sports Dietetics-USA (SD-USA)* subunit advocates for registered dietitians (RDs) who work with athletes, fitness enthusiasts, recreational athletes, as well as firefighters, police, and the men and women of the military who perform physically and demanding work under extreme conditions. (Appendix D describes the varied roles of sports dietitians in the military.) Resources on the SCAN Web site available to professionals working with athletes and active people include sports nutrition fact sheets; reasons to hire a Board Certified Specialist in Sports Dietetics (CSSD); reasons to consult with a CSSD; a video titled *Sports Nutrition: Who Delivers?*; a job description for a sports dietitian; and *SD-USA Score* e-newsletter.
- The *Wellness and Cardiovascular RDs* subunit provides resources to professionals who work with active people in corporate wellness or other positions where people are engaged in physical activity. Information from this subunit can provide resources for athletes who are transitioning from competitive sports to help them stay in good physical condition. Resources are also helpful for the athlete who has high blood pressure, high cholesterol levels, or at risk for developing cardiovascular disease. Resources include *Wellness/CV Connection* e-newsletter and Wellness/CV forums.
- The *Disordered Eating and Eating Disorder* subunit "promotes nutrition practices that aid in the prevention of harmful eating behaviors, the promotion of recovery from disordered eating and

eating disorders, and the development of lifelong health attitudes and behaviors related to food, body weight and physical activity." Resources include feature articles on topics such as orthorexia nervosa, night eating syndrome, eating disorders in adolescent athletes, and addiction and eating behaviors.

About Sports Dietitians

What Is a Sports Dietitian?

Sports dietitians are RDs who apply evidence- and research-based nutrition knowledge in exercise and sports to practical situations. They assess, educate, and counsel athletes and active individuals, and they design, implement, and manage safe and effective nutrition strategies that enhance lifelong health, fitness, and athletic performance. Because providing safe, accurate, timely sports nutrition information and practical application is critical to the health, well-being, and performance of athletes, qualified sports dietitians are invaluable consultants to athletes, coaches, and trainers.

What Is a Board Certified Specialist in Sports Dietetics (CSSD)?

In 2004 SD-USA assisted the Commission on Dietetic Registration (CDR), the credentialing agency of the Academy of Nutrition and Dietetics, in establishing a new certification: Board Certified as a Specialist in Sports Dietetics (CSSD). A sports dietitian who holds the credential of CSSD has the following qualifications:

- Worked as an RD for a minimum of 2 years in the field of sports nutrition to assess, educate, and counsel athlete and active individuals.
- Documented 1,500 hours of specialty practice experience.
- Passed a specialist examination and recertified every 5 years.

For more information on acquiring the CSSD credential, visit the CDR Web site (www.cdrnet.org). The SCAN Web site also provides information on the credential and has a directory of sports dietitians who hold board certification as a CSSD (click "Find a SCAN RD" on the Home page).

*   *   *   *   *

I hope you find this manual a useful addition to your bookshelf and that it contains helpful tools to provide nutrition counseling to athletes, coaches, and trainers. We have selected world-renowned experts as contributors to bring you research- and evidence-based information with a real-world application.

Christine A. Rosenbloom, PhD, RD, CSSD, Editor in Chief

Section 1

Sports Nutrition Basics

A thorough understanding of exercise physiology and the way that nutrients support training and competition is essential for the registered dietitian working with active people. Because of the importance of this topic, the first section of *Sports Nutrition* examines the critical role of macro-and micronutrients in exercise performance.

The physiology of exercise includes more than just energy production; athletic success depends on proper nutrition for growth and development and for an effective immune system function (Chapter 1). Our knowledge of the interrelated roles of dietary carbohydrate, protein, and fat has increased tremendously in the past decade, and this new information is incorporated into Chapters 2, 3, and 4. Micronutrients are covered in detail in Chapter 5, which presents the most current research on how vitamins and minerals affect sports performance. The most essential nutrient for athletes, water, is explained in both scientific and practical terms in the chapter on hydration, electrolytes, and exercise (Chapter 6). Lastly, this section concludes with a comprehensive look at dietary supplements and ergogenic aids that athletes use in the hope of improving performance (Chapter 7). More than 40 substances are critically evaluated and this research- and evidenced-based information will help the sports dietitian provide sound advice to athletes about using these supplements.

Chapter 1

PHYSIOLOGY OF EXERCISE

RONALD J. MAUGHAN, PHD, AND SUSAN M. SHIRREFFS, PHD

Introduction

The human body is an amazing machine. It can survive the harshest conditions even though the surrounding environment may be hostile. In extremes, such as the depths of the oceans or the surface of the moon, artificial life support systems are necessary to protect the body from the environment. However, it can endure without survival equipment in such conditions as the extreme heat of a sauna or the hypoxia encountered on the summit of Mount Everest. This survival is achieved by limiting the disturbances to the internal environment of the body through mechanisms that maintain homeostasis. The human body has evolved to cope with conditions far beyond those that are normally encountered, and, realistically in the activities of daily life, we use only a small part of our functional capabilities. However, participation in sports, unlike daily life, often demands that athletes stress their bodies to their limits. This chapter will review the science of exercise and provide the reader with an understanding of how the body maintains homeostasis when exercise places a high demand on organ systems, such as the cardiorespiratory and musculoskeletal systems. Both acute and chronic responses to muscle stress are discussed as well as the energy systems used to fuel exercise.

Maintaining Homeostasis

All life requires the continuous expenditure of energy. Even at rest, the average human body consumes between 200 and 300 mL of oxygen each minute. This oxygen is used in the chemical reactions that provide the energy necessary to maintain physiological function: energy is required to maintain chemical gradients across membranes, for biosynthetic reactions, for the work of the heart and respiratory muscles, and for all other aspects of basal metabolism. While lying or sitting at rest in a comfortable environment, we do no external work and so a very large fraction of this energy appears as heat, allowing us to maintain body temperature at a higher level than that of our surroundings. During exercise, the muscles require additional energy to generate force or to do work, the heart has to work harder to increase blood supply, the respiratory muscles face an increased demand for moving air in and out of the lungs, and so the metabolic rate must increase accordingly, with a corresponding increase in the rate of heat production. In sustained exercise, an increased rate of energy turnover, and therefore of heat production, must be maintained for the entire

3

duration of the exercise and for some time afterwards. Depending on the task and on the fitness level of the individual, this may be from 5 to 20 times the resting metabolic rate. In very high–intensity activity, the demand for energy may be more than 100 times the resting level, although such intense efforts can be sustained for only very short periods of time. In spite of these large changes, the internal environment of the body changes rather little because effective buffering systems work to limit any change.

All exercise imposes an increased energy demand on the muscles; if the muscles are unable to meet that demand, the exercise task cannot be performed. When the exercise intensity is high or the duration is prolonged, there may be difficulty in supplying energy at the required rate and fatigue ensues. The limiting factor will depend on the nature of the activity and on the physiological characteristics of the individual, but exercise cannot continue past the point at which the body can keep its internal environment within a set of rather narrow limits. An increase of body temperature of more than 1 to 2 degrees or a decrease in tissue pH of more than approximately 0.3 to 0.5 units is usually enough to bring exercise to an end.

For simple activities such as running or swimming, the rate at which energy is required is a function of speed, and the time for which a given speed can be maintained before the fatigue process intervenes is inversely related to the speed. In most sports situations, the exercise intensity, and hence the energy demand, is not constant; games such as soccer or tennis involve brief periods of high-intensity effort interspersed with variable periods of rest or low-intensity exercise. Even in sports such as running or cycling, the energy demand will vary with changes in pace or in other factors such as wind resistance or the topography of the course. Muscles can be trained to meet these varying demands, but there is a limit beyond which further adaptation is not possible. Given the wide range of the requirements placed on muscle, it is not surprising that several different strategies are used to meet the demands.

Acute Responses to Exercise

Muscle

The interaction of the overlapping actin and myosin filaments that make up most of the bulk of skeletal muscle fibers allows muscle to generate force and to shorten. Other proteins are involved in the control of the interaction of these filaments. These proteins include troponin, which is activated by the release of calcium ions into the cell sarcoplasm, and tropomyosin, which blocks the myosin binding sites on the actin molecules when the muscle is in a relaxed state. Myosin functions as an ATPase enzyme, breaking down adenosine triphosphate (ATP) to make energy available to power muscle activity. The unit of contraction is the sarcomere. The maximum force that a muscle can generate is closely related to its physiological cross-sectional area, namely, to the number of sarcomeres in parallel, and the peak velocity of shortening is proportional to muscle fiber length, that is, to the number of sarcomeres in series (1). The strength of a joint, however, is determined by several biomechanical parameters, including the distance between muscle insertions and pivot points, and muscle size. Muscles are normally arranged in opposition so that as one group of muscles contracts, another group relaxes or lengthens. Antagonism in the transmission of nerve impulses to the muscles means that it is impossible to stimulate the contraction of two antagonistic muscles at any one time.

A single nerve and the group of fibers it innervates are referred to as a motor unit. A single motor nerve forms synapses, which are chemical junctions for the transmission of impulses, with many individual muscle fibers, and all these fibers will respond when the nerve is activated unless they are fatigued or otherwise prevented from responding. The extent of activation is determined by the demand placed on the muscle in terms of the force to be generated or the speed of movement. Not all of the motor units are used in most tasks, only enough to generate the force necessary within an active muscle; therefore, there will be some "resting" fibers. The higher the force required, the greater the number of individual muscle fibers that must be activated. The motor units with the lowest activation threshold (ie, the first to be recruited) are those with a low speed of contraction and a high fatigue resistance. This makes sense because these fibers will be used most often in daily tasks. As the weight to be moved is increased or the power output increases (ie, an increased speed in running, cycling, etc), progressively more motor units are recruited. At very high forces, all the fibers are likely to be active. In prolonged exercise, some of the fibers that were recruited in the early stages may become fatigued and will cease to contribute to work performance and will be replaced by others. Box 1.1 describes the various muscle fiber types.

Energetics

All the body's cells require a constant input of energy to maintain homeostasis. Cellular ionic and chemical gradients must be maintained; synthetic reactions proceed in order to manufacture essential compounds that the body requires, such as enzymes, hormones, and neurotransmitters; and other energy-demanding processes must be supported. The ultimate energy source for all of these reactions is the chemical energy made available by the oxidation of the foods that we eat and in the process by which they are converted to degradation products, primarily carbon dioxide and water. The immediate source of energy is the hydrolysis of the terminal phosphate bond in the high energy phosphate compound ATP, releasing a phosphate group, adenosine diphosphate (ADP) and energy, as shown in Figure 1.1. ATP is a large molecule and it is stored in cells in only very small amounts, so the challenge is to regenerate the cellular ATP content as fast as it is

---

BOX 1.1   Muscle Fiber Types

Human muscle fibers can be classified in several ways, depending on their maximum speed of contraction, their biochemical characteristics, and their resistance to fatigue. Contraction occurs by interaction of actin and myosin filaments within the fibers, and the speed of contraction is determined largely by the ATPase activity of myosin. The faster ATP can be hydrolyzed to release energy, the faster contraction can occur. Three main fiber types are generally recognized in skeletal muscle:

- **Type I** slow oxidative (also called slow-twitch or fatigue-resistant fibers) are dark red because of their high myoglobin content and high density of blood capillaries, contain many mitochondria and thus have a high oxidative capacity, have a slow peak contraction velocity, and are relatively fatigue-resistant. They occur in higher numbers in postural muscle. Elite endurance athletes have higher than normal numbers of these fibers.
- **Type IIa** fast oxidative (also called fast-twitch A or fatigue-resistant fibers) also have a high myoglobin content and high density of blood capillaries, contain many mitochondria and thus have a high oxidative capacity, but they can hydrolyze ATP at a high rate and so have a fast peak contraction velocity. They are resistant to fatigue, but less so than the Type I fibers.
- **Type IIX** fast glycolytic (also called fast-twitch B or fatiguable fibers) have a low myoglobin content, low capillary density, and few mitochondria. These fibers can hydrolyze ATP at a high rate and so have a fast peak contraction velocity. They have a high activity of glycolytic enzymes and contain a large amount of glycogen. They are useful when high power outputs are needed, but they fatigue rapidly. The muscles of elite sprinters have high proportions of these fibers.

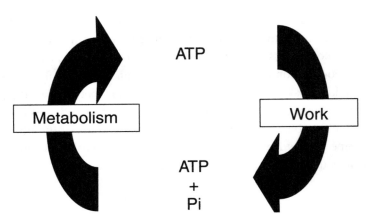

FIGURE 1.1   Energy is made available to cells by the hydrolysis of adenosine triphosphate (ATP) to adenosine diphosphate (ADP) and inorganic phosphate (Pi). The cell's metabolic pathways must invest energy to regenerate ATP and can use a variety of different metabolic pathways to do so.

being used. In some cells, ATP is used at a more or less constant rate, but other tissues, such as muscle, have a relatively low energy demand while resting and an extremely high rate of ATP demand when active. It is the sum of all these ATP-consuming reactions that determines the total energy turnover or metabolic rate.

The regeneration of ATP from ADP requires an input of energy, and there are three main ways in which this is achieved; each offers some advantages (in terms of the peak power that can be achieved) and disadvantages (in terms of capacity, or the amount of work that can be done) to the cell, as shown in Table 1.1. These metabolic pathways are identified as being *anaerobic* if energy is generated without the involvement of oxygen or *aerobic* if oxygen is involved. Muscle cells contain large amounts of creatine, and indeed approximately 95% of the total amount of creatine in the body is found in muscle, which explains why meat is a good source of creatine in the diet. Degradation to creatinine, which is excreted in the urine, occurs at a rate of about 1.6% per day (2 g/d). The non-vegetarian diet provides approximately 1 g of creatine per day. The remainder of the requirement can be synthesized from the amino acids methionine, arginine, and glycine that are obtained from dietary sources.

Approximately two-thirds of the creatine that is stored in skeletal muscle is in the form of creatine phosphate (CP), and the phosphate group can be transferred from CP to ADP to form free creatine and ATP, as shown here in a reaction catalyzed by creatine kinase:

$$ATP \Rightarrow ADP + Pi$$

$$CP + ADP \Rightarrow ATP + Cr$$

In low-intensity exercise, little CP is used. Most of the energy comes from aerobic metabolism. In very high–intensity exercise, the muscle CP concentration decreases to very low levels within 30 to 60 seconds, but this allows the ATP concentration to be maintained.

This is not a full description of the reaction taking place as it ignores the role of the creatine kinase reaction in intracellular buffering during high-intensity exercise. A proton is absorbed during this reaction, and this can help buffer the protons released by the formation of lactate when high rates of anaerobic glycolysis occur:

$$CP^{2+} + ADP^{3-} + H^+ \Rightarrow ATP^{4-} + C$$

TABLE 1.1 Capacity and Power of Three Energy-Supplying Metabolic Processes in Human Skeletal Muscle[a]

Metabolic Process	Capacity, J/kg	Power, W/kg
ATP/CP hydrolysis	400	800
Lactate formation	1,000	325
Oxidative metabolism	Essentially unlimited	200

Abbreviations: ATP, adenosine triphosphate; CP, creatine phosphate.
[a]*Capacity* is defined as the amount of work that can be done and *power* is the rate at which work can be done. These values are expressed per kg of muscle. They are approximations only and will be greatly influenced by training status and other factors.

It is important also to recognize that the majority of the energy used during exercise is generated by oxidative phosphorylation in mitochondria, but ATP utilization during muscle contraction occurs in the cytoplasm. CP shuttles phosphate groups across the mitochondrial membrane, thus serving as a spatial buffer to distribute energy through the cell. The muscle creatine (and therefore creatine phosphate) content can be increased by supplementing the diet with creatine for a few days (at doses of 10 to 20 g/d) or weeks (at 3 to 5 g/d), leading to increases in performance of high-intensity efforts. Creatine as an ergogenic aid is discussed in more detail in Chapter 7.

Two key elements in producing energy are the power (rate of work) that can be achieved and the capacity (amount of work) of the system. CP hydrolysis can support high power outputs because the resynthesis of ATP by this mechanism is very fast, but it has a low capacity, so fatigue soon intervenes, as shown in Tables 1.1 and 1.2. The second source of energy is the breakdown of stored carbohydrate (primarily glycogen stored in the muscle cells) to pyruvate by glycolysis and further conversion of this pyruvate to lactate (often referred to as lactic acid even though it is dissociated at physiological pH). Glycolysis converts one 6-carbon glucose molecule to two 3-carbon molecules, allowing some of the energy liberated to be conserved as ATP. The breakdown of glycogen to pyruvate is accompanied by conversion of nicotinamide adenine dinucleotide (NAD), an essential cofactor within the pathway, to its reduced form (NADH). Conversion of pyruvate to lactate allows regeneration of NAD and thus allows glycolysis to continue. For each glucose molecule converted to lactate, three ATP molecules are formed if glycogen is the starting point. Two are formed if glucose is the substrate. Muscle pH decreases as lactate accumulates and this has a variety of effects on the muscle. In spite of the negative effects of a decreasing pH, the energy made available by anaerobic glycolysis allows a higher intensity of exercise than would otherwise be possible. These pathways are anaerobic—no molecular oxygen is involved in the process of regenerating ATP.

Alternatively, pyruvate is oxidized to CO_2 and H_2O. As shown in Table 1.1, this is a much slower process, but it generates more energy and has a virtually unlimited capacity. Endogenous fuel stores for

TABLE 1.2 Typical VO_{2max} Values for Different Subject Groups[a]

Subject Group	VO_{2max} Range, mL/kg/min
Functionally impaired	15–25
Typical sedentary	30–40
Recreationally active	40–60
Elite endurance athlete	65–85

[a]Values for men are typically somewhat larger (perhaps by 5% to 15%) than those for women.

oxidation (glycogen in muscle and liver, plus triglyceride in muscle and adipose tissues) are large and can be replenished by ingestion of foods containing these substrates during exercise. Complete oxidation of one molecule of glucose to carbon dioxide and water leads to the formation of 38 molecules of ATP. Oxidation of one molecule of palmitic acid, as an example of a typical fatty acid, results in the generation of 127 molecules of ATP. In endurance exercise, aerobic metabolism predominates. Anaerobic metabolism makes a substantial contribution only at the beginning of exercise, at periods when the energy demand is transiently increased (eg, running or cycling uphill or in an intermediate sprint, or in a finishing sprint). Team games consist of multiple short sprints, when anaerobic energy supply is important, but aerobic recovery must follow each sprint. The capacity of oxidative metabolism is essentially unlimited as the system can be continually refueled even during exercise.

The power that can be generated by aerobic metabolism varies greatly between individuals and is usually characterized by the maximum rate of oxygen consumption (VO_{2max}) that can be achieved. This will vary greatly among individuals and is influenced by many factors, including genetic endowment, age, sex, and training and health status (see Table 1.2).

Endurance activities require a high rate of aerobic metabolism, and this is achieved by having a high maximal aerobic capacity and by working at a high fraction of that capacity. If the oxygen supply is limited, it is important to make effective use of the available oxygen. In this regard, carbohydrate is a better fuel than fat; per liter of oxygen, 5 kcal (21.1 kJ) are available when carbohydrate is the fuel, whereas oxidation of fat generates 4.6 kcal (19.5 kJ). Although this difference may seem small, it is important when competing at the limits of what is humanly possible.

The various options open to the muscle for providing energy do not operate independently; they are fully integrated to ensure that, to the extent possible, the energy demand is met with the smallest threat to the cell's homeostasis. Even in a 100-meter sprint some of the energy is provided by oxidative metabolism. The marathon runner who accelerates in midrace will almost certainly generate some ATP from anaerobic metabolism. Table 1.3 shows the relative contributions of anaerobic and aerobic energy supply in races over different distances; these values are only approximations but indicate how the balance of energy supply shifts as the duration of exercise increases.

Metabolic

The metabolic response to exercise is dictated largely by the biochemical characteristics of the muscle fibers and their recruitment pattern. In low-intensity work, only a few motor units are activated and these will involve type 1 fibers. These fibers have a high oxidative capacity, a relatively low glycolytic capacity,

TABLE 1.3 Approximate Contributions of Anaerobic and Aerobic Energy Supply to Total Energy Demand in Races of Varying Distances[a]

Distance	Duration, min:sec	Anaerobic Contribution, %	Aerobic Contribution, %
100 m	0:9.58	90	10
400 m	0:43.18	70	30
800 m	1:41.01	40	60
1,500 m	3:26.00	20	80
5,000 m	12:37.35	5	95
10,000 m	26:17.53	3	97
42.2 km	123:38	1	99

[a]The times given for each distance are the men's world records for these events as of October 2011.

and a good supply of oxygen. This has some important implications for the choice of substrate used. Most of the energy required by these fibers is derived from the oxidation of fatty acids, either from the plasma or from the intracellular fat stores. Carbohydrate breakdown makes only a small contribution to the energy needs of these fibers. As progressively more motor units are recruited, those with a lower capacity for fat oxidation and a greater reliance on carbohydrate as a fuel begin to be activated. Eventually, a point is reached at which, even though the oxidative type 1 fibers are still contributing, some of the fibers being recruited are breaking glycogen down to pyruvate faster than it can be oxidized in the mitochondria. Some of this excess pyruvate is converted to lactate to regenerate the coenzyme NAD within the cytoplasm of the cells, thus allowing glycolysis to continue. Some of this lactate diffuses out of the muscle cells and a progressive increase in the blood lactate concentration is observed.

The pattern of substrate use is dictated primarily by the exercise intensity. It is not fixed, however, and will change over time as well as be modulated by a number of factors, including prior diet and exercise, fitness level, and environmental conditions. Increasing the muscle glycogen content by feeding a high-carbohydrate diet for a few days before exercise will lead to an increased rate of glycolysis at rest and during exercise. Blood lactate will be elevated and carbohydrate oxidation also increased. Likewise, feeding a high-fat, low-carbohydrate diet will shift metabolism in favor of fat oxidation. Increasing aerobic fitness levels as a result of endurance training has several cardiovascular and metabolic effects, but one of the key adaptations is to increase the oxidative capacity of the muscle, and, in particular, to increase the ability to oxidize fatty acids. This results in a marked shift in the pattern of substrate use in favor of fat oxidation.

Respiratory

An individual's maximum oxygen uptake (VO_{2max}) is a key element of performance in exercise lasting more than a few minutes. This represents the highest rate of aerobic energy production that can be achieved—the energy required for any power output in excess of this must come entirely from anaerobic metabolism. The importance of the VO_{2max} for endurance athletes such as marathon runners lies in the fact that endurance capacity is largely a function of the fraction of VO_{2max} that is required; the higher the fraction of aerobic capacity that must be used, the shorter the time for which a given pace can be sustained. Improving performance requires either an increase in VO_{2max}, an increase in the fraction of VO_{2max} that can be sustained for the duration of the race, or a decrease in the energy cost of running. In practice, all of these can be achieved with suitable training. Interestingly, there is some recent information that feeding high doses of nitrate can reduce the oxygen cost of submaximal exercise (see Box 1.2) (2,3), and more recent data suggest that this same effect can be achieved by feeding beetroot juice, which has a high nitrate content.

The factors that limit VO_{2max} have been the subject of much debate over the years, in part because the limitation may vary in different types of exercise, in different environments, and in different individuals. The lungs are not usually considered to limit performance at sea level in the absence of lung disease, and attention has focused primarily on whether the limitation lies in the delivery of oxygen by the cardiovascular system or the ability to utilize oxygen by the working muscles. However, the oxygen content of the inspired air decreases at altitude, leading to a fall in arterial oxygen saturation, decreased oxygen transport and a fall in VO_{2max}. Performance in endurance events is generally reduced at altitudes higher than approximately 1,500 meters. Some highly trained runners show arterial desaturation in maximal exercise even at sea level (see Table 1.4). This is reversed, and VO_{2max} increased, by breathing air with an increased O_2 content. This effect is not normally seen in trained but nonelite runners, suggesting a pulmonary limitation in elite runners (4).

Studies of the responses to training of the inspiratory muscles also provide some support for the idea that there may be a pulmonary limitation. One study measured the effects of 4 weeks of inspiratory muscle

BOX 1.2   Beetroot Juice: The Next Ergogenic Aid?

Only about 20% of the energy turnover is used to do useful work, with the remainder appearing as heat, so a small increase in the efficiency of muscle contraction may be of major significance for exercise performance. Athletes may see a small increase in efficiency—as measured by a reduction in the oxygen cost of a standardized exercise test—in response to prolonged intensive training. There is some interesting information to suggest that acute ingestion of large doses of nitrate may allow the muscle to become more efficient. After supplementation of the diet for 3 days with 0.1 mmol of sodium nitrate per kg of body mass, there was a significant reduction in the oxygen cost of submaximal cycling exercise, corresponding to an increase in mechanical efficiency from 19.7%±1.6% to 21.1%±1.3% (2). This was followed by another study in which volunteers were fed a placebo or 500 mL of beetroot juice per day for 6 days (the beetroot juice contained 11.2±0.6 mmol of nitrate) (3). This study confirmed the reduction in the oxygen cost of submaximal exercise and also showed that during strenuous exercise, the time to exhaustion was extended after ingestion of the beetroot juice (675±203 seconds) relative to the placebo trial (583±145 seconds). Further studies are required to confirm these findings and to establish the underlying mechanisms, but already the use of beetroot juice has become popular with middle-distance and endurance athletes.

training for 30 min/d on cycle ergometer endurance time at 77% of VO_{2max} (5). In untrained subjects, endurance time at the same power output was increased from 26.8 minutes before training to 40.2 minutes after training; in trained subjects, who worked at a higher absolute power output, endurance time was increased from 22.8 minutes to 31.5 minutes. This is an enormous increase in exercise capacity in subjects who were already well trained, but it has not been reproduced in all of the studies that have followed (6).

Cardiovascular

The cardiovascular system fulfils several important functions; it delivers oxygen and nutrients to all tissues and removes waste products, it controls heat flux within the body, and it circulates hormones from the sites of their production to the sites of their action. The idea that limitations to oxygen delivery are imposed by the cardiovascular system has strong experimental support and the limitation may lie at any one or more of several stages. The key element seems to be the maximum cardiac output that can be achieved, as this is closely related to both VO_{2max} and endurance performance. Cardiac output is the product of heart rate, the number of times the heart beats each minute, and stroke volume (the volume of blood ejected by the left

TABLE 1.4 Effects of Maximal Exercise on Maximum Rate of Oxygen Consumption (VO_{2max}) and Oxygen Saturation (SaO_2) of Arterial Blood in Athletes Breathing Normal Room Air vs Air Enriched with Oxygen

Level of Training	21% Oxygen		26% Oxygen	
	VO_{2max}	$\% SaO_2$	VO_{2max}	$\% SaO_2$
Moderately trained	57 ± 2	96 ± 0	57 ± 2	96 ± 0
Elite	70 ± 2	91 ± 1	75 ± 1	96 ± 0

ventricle with each beat). The stroke volume is determined primarily by the dimensions of the heart; a large left ventricle is one of the defining characteristics of a successful endurance athlete. In contrast, the maximum heart rate is little different between trained and untrained individuals. The low resting heart rate of the highly trained endurance athlete (typically about 30 to 50 beats per minute) compared to the sedentary person (typically about 70 beats per minute) reflects the larger stroke volume at rest. A high blood volume will also benefit the endurance athlete by helping to maintain the central venous pressure and thus maintain stroke volume.

The oxygen carrying capacity of the blood is also important, and this will be influenced by the hemoglobin (Hb) concentration and the total blood volume. Almost all of the oxygen in the blood is transported bound to hemoglobin and each gram of hemoglobin can bind 1.34 mL of oxygen; this means that for the average male with a Hb concentration of about 150 g/L, the arterial blood contains approximately 200 mL of oxygen per liter of blood when it leaves the lungs. For the average female, with a somewhat lower Hb concentration of about 130 g/L, the oxygen content is approximately 175 mL of oxygen per liter of blood. This difference accounts in part for the generally higher aerobic capacity of males. It also explains the various strategies used by athletes to increase the hemoglobin content of the blood. These strategies include altitude training, the use of agents such as erythropoietin (EPO) that stimulate the formation of new red blood cells, and the use of blood transfusions prior to competition. These latter strategies are prohibited by the World Anti-Doping Agency, but their use is nonetheless well documented. Oxygen delivery to the muscles depends in part on the density of the capillary network within the muscles. An increase in the number of capillaries, or a reduction in the size of the muscle fibers, means less distance for oxygen to diffuse from the capillary to the mitochondria within the muscle where it is used.

Thermoregulatory

Body core temperature must remain with narrow limits, but approximately 80% of the energy available from the catabolism of nutrients appears as heat. This is useful for the maintenance of body temperature in cold environments, but presents a challenge in prolonged hard exercise in hot environments, where heat is generated at high rates but heat loss to the environment is more difficult. Heat stress during exercise poses a major challenge to the cardiovascular system. In addition to continuing to supply blood to the working muscles, the brain, and other tissues, there is a greatly increased demand for blood flow to the skin to allow for removal of heat. This requires an increased cardiac output, but also means that a large part of the blood volume is distributed to the skin so the central blood volume is decreased. This in turn may reduce the return of blood to the heart and result in a decrease in stroke volume; if the heart rate cannot increase to compensate, cardiac output will fall. If this happens, there must be either a reduced blood flow to the muscles, and hence a reduced supply of oxygen and substrate, or a reduced blood flow to the skin, which will reduce heat loss and accelerate the development of hyperthermia. It seems likely that the temperature of the brain is the most relevant parameter, but there seems to be no set temperature at which exercise must be terminated, and fatigue may occur across a wide range of core temperatures.

Evaporation of sweat from the skin surface promotes heat loss and limits the increase in core temperature, but sweating leads to a loss of body water and electrolytes, especially sodium. If sufficiently severe, dehydration and hyperthermia will both impair physical and cognitive function, but low levels of dehydration (a loss of less than about 1% to 2% of body mass) are probably of little significance in most exercise tasks (7). Some of the adverse effects of sweat loss can be offset by ingesting sufficient fluid during exercise to limit the development of hypohydration to less than about 2% to 3% of body mass (8). Losses of fluid are not as well tolerated in hot environments and apparently also at higher altitudes, but there seem to be large differences in the effects of dehydration on the components of exercise performance.

Fatigue

Whatever the conditions and no matter what the training status, exercise will inevitably lead to fatigue if the exercise is sufficiently intense or prolonged. Fatigue may be defined as a reduced or impaired capacity to generate force or to perform work. The nature of the fatigue process is not well understood, and it is unlikely that any single factor is directly responsible for fatigue. There are some interventions that can enhance performance and, by implication, affect specific aspects of the fatigue process. In very high–intensity exercise that leads to fatigue within 1 to 2 minutes, there is a rapid decrease in the intracellular concentration of CP as high-energy phosphate groups are transferred to ADP to maintain the muscle ATP concentration. ATP concentration will decrease only slightly, but increasing concentrations of ADP may impair contractility. Increasing the pre-exercise muscle CP content by feeding creatine supplements for a few days can lead to higher power outputs and a delay in fatigue, suggesting that the decrease in the contribution of CP to energy supply is a factor in fatigue. In exercise that causes fatigue within about 1 to 10 minutes, the very high rates of anaerobic glycolysis that occur lead to a marked acidosis within the muscle cells as the high rate of hydrogen ion formation overwhelms the buffer capacity of the muscle. Increasing either the intracellular buffer capacity (by feeding beta-alanine, which leads to an increase in the cellular concentration of carnosine) or the extracellular buffer (by ingestion of bicarbonate or citrate) can allow greater amounts of lactate to be formed before the pH within the cell becomes limiting. These substances are discussed in more detail in Chapter 7.

In prolonged exercise, it is more difficult to identify a single factor that might be responsible for fatigue. We know that performance in cycling tests lasting about 1 to 3 hours can be improved by increasing muscle glycogen stores and is impaired if exercise begins in a glycogen-depleted state. Feeding carbohydrate during this type of exercise can also delay fatigue, and these findings suggest that there is a metabolic component to fatigue. We also know that performance of this type of exercise is progressively impaired as the ambient temperature increases above approximately 50°F (10°C). When the temperature is high there seems to still be an adequate amount of glycogen remaining in the muscle, suggesting that glycogen depletion is unlikely to be the cause of fatigue in prolonged exercise in the heat, even though this may be the case in cool environments. Nevertheless, feeding a high-carbohydrate diet in the days prior to exercise can improve endurance performance in the heat even when glycogen availability should not be limiting, so there may well be other factors involved (9). Pre-exercise cooling, either by immersion in cold water or by ingestion of cold drinks, can improve endurance performance in warm environments, apparently by delaying the time until a critical elevation of core temperature occurs. A key mechanism by which acclimatization improves performance in the heat also seems to involve a reduction of the basal pre-exercise core temperature.

From studies of muscle fatigue done in the 19th century, it was generally concluded that fatigue was in part a local phenomenon occurring within the active muscle but that there was also a primary role for the brain in terminating exercise, or at least reducing the intensity, before irreversible damage was caused. Fundamental to this conclusion was the observation that direct electrical stimulation of the muscle or its motor nerve could still produce a strong contraction even when voluntary activation of the muscle was impossible. Technical developments that allowed the collection and analysis of samples from muscle are perhaps responsible for the focus on muscle fatigue that developed in the 20th century; it continues to be much harder to study events occurring within the brain. Results of muscle biopsy analysis, for example, showed a clear link between the depletion of muscle glycogen stores and the onset of fatigue, at least in prolonged cycling exercise. More recently there has been a renewed recognition of the role of the brain in fatigue, even though the mechanisms remain uncertain. This has been described as the action of a "central governor" that acts to regulate pace and effort to optimize performance (10). This is reminiscent of the work of Lagrange, who, in 1889, referred to fatigue as a "regulator, warning us that we are exceeding the limits of useful exercise, and that work will soon become dangerous" (11). The danger referred to here is that of irreversible damage to the muscles.

Several pharmacological interventions have been shown to affect exercise performance without any obvious cardiovascular or metabolic effects that could explain this. Amphetamines, for example, can enhance performance. Their actions on neurons in the brain that use dopamine as a neurotransmitter seem likely to be the explanation for this (12). Paroxetine, a drug that acts on neurons that use serotonin as a neurotransmitter, can reduce performance (13). The use of drugs that can override the sensation of fatigue—the regulator to which Lagrange referred—may result in fatal hyperthermia during hard exercise in the heat, as has happened in the case of athletes who have used amphetamines.

Adaptations to Training

The aim of training is to increase functional capacity, and a few basic principles apply to all types of training. Training affects every organ and tissue of the body, but the adaptation is specific to the training stimulus and to the muscles being trained. A well-designed strength-training program will have little effect on endurance, and vice versa. One leg can be specifically trained for strength and the other for endurance, with relatively little crossover. Training is not entirely specific, though, as the effects on the cardiovascular system will be similar whether running or cycling—or indeed skipping or dancing—is performed. The improvement in performance is, or at least should be, proportional to the training load as described by the intensity, duration, and frequency of the training sessions. Within limits, the harder an athlete trains, the greater the improvements in performance that result. Few athletes reach the limit, but a small number of those who do can experience an overtraining syndrome that results in long-term fatigue and loss of performance. The role of adequate rest during training is now increasingly recognized.

Training for Strength, Power, and Endurance

It used to be thought that a primary role of nutrition in the athlete's diet was to support consistent, intensive training by promoting recovery between training sessions. Although it is undoubtedly true that recovery is an important element, there is an increasing recognition that nutrition has a key role in promoting the adaptations that take place in muscle and other tissues in response to each training session. Training provides the stimulus to turn on the genes responsible for the expression of functional proteins: strength training leads to synthesis of more actin and myosin, making muscles bigger and stronger, whereas endurance training leads to synthesis of more oxidative enzymes and of all the other components necessary for endurance performance. A selective stimulation of protein synthesis and degradation must be taking place. The response is modulated by the nutrient, metabolic, and hormonal environment, and this can be modified by intake of protein-containing foods before, during, and after training. There is good evidence that feeding a small amount of protein or essential amino acids (about 20 g of high-quality protein or 10 g of essential amino acids) after a training session can stimulate protein synthesis for up to 24 hours after training. There is a need, though, for more studies with functional outcomes rather than simply measuring protein turnover rates. This is discussed in detail in Chapter 3.

Training should aim to address the factors that limit exercise performance, shifting the barriers to allow better performance. It is clear in the case of strength training that a substantial part of the adaptation that takes place, especially in the early stages, is neural; strength improves after only a few training sessions, before measurable changes in muscle structure have taken place. In the case of endurance training, a large number of adaptations have been identified, both in the central circulation and in the muscles themselves.

The pumping capacity of the heart is increased, primarily by an increase in stroke volume as a result of an increase in left ventricular volume, and this is thought to be the primary mechanism responsible for the increase in VO_{2max} that occurs with endurance training. Blood volume increases, thus increasing the total oxygen carrying capacity. New capillaries grow in the endurance-trained muscle, shortening the diffusion distance for oxygen and nutrients between the circulation and the muscle fibers. Mitochondrial mass increases, and with it the activity of the enzymes involved in the oxidation of carbohydrate and fat. There is an increase in the capacity of the trained muscle to oxidize fat, thus decreasing the reliance of carbohydrate during exercise. Training on a carbohydrate-restricted diet is effective in further increasing the capacity of the muscle to oxidize fat, but seems to be less effective in promoting performance enhancements than is training on a high-carbohydrate diet. Tissues respond to disuse with a reversal of the adaptations caused by training.

Summary

Exercise imposes a considerable stress on the body, largely due to the increased energy demand and the increased rate of heat production. Energy supply must be increased to meet the metabolic demands of the active muscles. The response of the respiratory and cardiovascular systems is coordinated to supply oxygen to the working muscles at the required rate. At low or moderate intensities, oxidative metabolism can meet the energy demand, but at high exercise intensities, some energy is supplied by nonoxidative pathways. Fatigue is a complex, multifactorial phenomenon, and the limitation to exercise will depend on the nature of the exercise, the physiology of the individual, and the environment. The brain plays a key role in susceptibility to fatigue. Acute exercise causes fatigue, but repeated exercise over sustained periods (training) improves fatigue resistance by inducing specific adaptations in all physiological systems.

References

1. Maughan RJ, Watson JS, Weir J. Strength and cross-sectional area of human skeletal muscle. *J Physiol.* 1983; 338:37–49.
2. Larson FK, Ekblom B, Sahlin K, Lundberg JO, Weitzberg E. Effects of dietary nitrate on oxygen cost during exercise. *Acta Physiol.* 2007;191:59–66.
3. Bailey SJ, Winyard P, Vanhatalo A, Blackwell JR, DiMenna FJ, Wilkerson DP, Tarr J, Benjamin N, Jones AM. Dietary nitrate supplementation reduces the O_2 cost of low-intensity exercise and enhances tolerance to high-intensity exercise in humans. *J Appl Physiol.* 2009;107:1144–1155.
4. Powers SK, Lawler J, Dempsey JA, Dodd S, Landry G. Effects of incomplete pulmonary gas exchange on VO2 max. *J Appl Physiol.* 1989;66:2491–2495.
5. Boutellier U, Buchel R, Kundert A, Spengler C. The respiratory system as an exercise limiting factor in normal trained subjects. *Eur J Appl Physiol.* 1992;65:347–353.
6. Esposito F, Limonta E, Alberti G, Veicsteinas A, Ferretti G. Effect of respiratory muscle training on maximum aerobic power in normoxia and hypoxia. *Respir Physiol Neurobiol.* 2010;170:268–272.
7. Judelson DA, Maresh CM, Anderson JM, Armstrong LE, Casa DJ, Kraemer WJ, Volek JS. Hydration and muscular performance—Does fluid balance affect strength, power and high-intensity endurance? *Sports Med.* 2007;37:907–921.
8. Sawka MN, Burke LM, Eichner ER, Maughan RJ, Montain SJ, Stachenfeld NS. Exercise and fluid replacement. *Med Sci Sports Exerc.* 2007;39:377–390.

9. Pitsiladis Y, Maughan RJ. The effects of exercise and diet manipulation on the capacity to perform prolonged exercise in the heat and cold in trained humans. *J Physiol.* 1999;517:919–930.

10. Swart J, Lamberts RP, Lambert MI, Gibson AS, Lambert EV, Skowno J, Noakes TD. Exercising with reserve: evidence that the central nervous system regulates prolonged exercise performance. *Br J Sports Med.* 2009;43:782–788.

11. Lagrange F. *Physiology of Bodily Exercise.* London, UK: Kegan, Paul, Trench; 1889:63.

12. Roelands B, Meeusen R. Alterations in central fatigue by pharmacological manipulations of neurotransmitters in normal and high ambient temperature. *Sports Med.* 2010;40:229–246.

13. Wilson WM, Maughan RJ. A role for serotonin in the genesis of fatigue in man: administration of a 5-hydroxytryptamine reuptake inhibitor (Paroxetine) reduces the capacity to perform prolonged exercise. *Exp Physiol.* 1992;77:921–924.

Chapter 2

CARBOHYDRATE AND EXERCISE

Ellen J. Coleman, MA, MPH, RD, CSSD

Introduction

Adequate carbohydrate stores (muscle and liver glycogen and blood glucose) are critical for optimum performance during both intermittent high-intensity work and prolonged endurance exercise. To gain this optimum performance status, it is important to use nutritional strategies to enhance the availability of carbohydrate before, during, and after exercise.

Consuming carbohydrate before exercise can help performance by "topping off" existing muscle and liver glycogen stores. Consuming carbohydrate during exercise can improve performance by maintaining blood glucose levels and carbohydrate oxidation. Finally, ingesting carbohydrate after glycogen-depleting exercise facilitates rapid glycogen restoration, especially among athletes engaged in daily hard training or tournament activity.

Carbohydrate Availability During Exercise

Muscle glycogen represents the major source of carbohydrate in the body (300 to 400 g or 1,200 to 1,600 kcal), followed by liver glycogen (75 to 100 g or 300 to 400 kcal), and, lastly, blood glucose (25 g or 100 kcal). These amounts vary substantially among individuals, depending on factors such as dietary intake and state of training. Untrained individuals have muscle glycogen stores that are roughly 80 to 90 mmol per kg of wet muscle weight. Endurance athletes have muscle glycogen stores of 130 to 135 mmol per kg of wet muscle weight. Carbohydrate loading increases muscle glycogen stores to 210 to 230 mmol per kg of wet muscle weight (1).

The energy demands of exercise dictate that carbohydrate is the predominant fuel for exercise (2). Muscle glycogen and blood glucose provide about half of the energy for moderate-intensity exercise (65% of VO_{2max}) and two thirds of the energy for high-intensity exercise (85% of VO_{2max}). It is impossible to meet the adenosine triphosphate (ATP) requirements for high-intensity, high–power output exercise when these carbohydrate fuels are depleted (2). The utilization of muscle glycogen is most rapid during the early stages of exercise and is exponentially related to exercise intensity (1,3).

Liver glycogen stores maintain blood glucose levels both at rest and during exercise. At rest, the brain and central nervous system (CNS) utilize most of the blood glucose, and the muscle accounts for less than

20% of blood glucose utilization. During exercise, however, muscle glucose uptake can increase 30-fold, depending on exercise intensity and duration. Initially, the majority of hepatic glucose output comes from glycogenolysis; however, as the exercise duration increases and liver glycogen decreases, the contribution of glucose from gluconeogenesis increases (1,3).

At the beginning of exercise, hepatic glucose output matches the increased muscle glucose uptake so that blood glucose levels remain near resting levels. (3) Although muscle glycogen is the primary source of carbohydrate during exercise intensities between 65% and 75% of VO_{2max}, blood glucose becomes an increasingly important source of carbohydrate as muscle glycogen stores decrease (2). Hypoglycemia occurs when the hepatic glucose output can no longer keep up with muscle glucose uptake during prolonged exercise (3).

Liver glycogen stores can be depleted by a 15-hour fast and can decrease from a typical level of 490 mmol on a mixed diet to 60 mmol on a low-carbohydrate diet. A high-carbohydrate diet can increase liver glycogen content to approximately 900 mmol (1).

Daily Carbohydrate Recommendations

The relationship between muscle glycogen depletion and exhaustion is strongest at moderate- to high-intensity exercise—65% to 85% of VO_{2max} (1). Consuming adequate carbohydrate on a daily basis is necessary to meet the energy requirements of the athlete's training program as well as replenish muscle and liver glycogen between training sessions and competitive events

Although a high-carbohydrate intake (8 to 10 g/kg/d) promotes greater muscle glycogen repletion and improves endurance performance over 24 to 72 hours (4–6), only a handful of studies show that a high-carbohydrate intake enhances training adaptation or performance more than 7 to 28 days (5,7,8). In addition to methodological issues, it is possible that athletes adapt to lower muscle glycogen stores resulting from a moderate carbohydrate intake (5 to 7 g/kg/d) so that their training and competitions are not adversely affected (5).

There is abundant evidence that enhancing carbohydrate availability before and during a single session of exercise improves endurance and performance (1,5). However, further well-controlled studies are necessary to provide clear evidence that carbohydrate-rich diets enhance training adaptations and performance over the longer term. For now, evidence from studies of acute carbohydrate intake and performance remain the best estimate of the chronic carbohydrate needs of athletes (1,5). So, current sports nutrition guidelines recommend strategies to promote carbohydrate availability to promote optimal performance in key training sessions or competitions (5,9,10).

Carbohydrate recommendations for athletes range from 3 to 12 g of carbohydrate per kg body weight per day (9,10). Athletes with very light training programs (low-intensity exercise or skill-based exercise) should consume 3 to 5 g/kg/d (10). These targets may be particularly suitable for athletes with large body mass or a need to reduce energy intake to lose weight (10). Athletes engaged in moderate-intensity training programs for 60 minutes per day should consume 5 to 7 g/kg/d (10). During moderate- to high-intensity endurance exercise for 1 to 3 hours, athletes should consume 6 to 10 g/kg/d (10). Athletes participating in moderate- to high-intensity endurance exercise for 4 to 5 hours per day (eg, biking in the Tour de France) should consume 8 to 12 g/kg/d (5,10–12). These are general recommendations and should be adjusted with consideration of the athlete's total energy needs, specific training needs, and feedback from their training performance (10). Carbohydrate intake should be spread over the day to promote fuel availability for key training sessions— before, during, or after exercise (10). Recommended daily carbohydrate intake is summarized in Box 2.1. Foods that provide approximately 25 g of carbohydrate per serving are shown in Box 2.2.

BOX 2.1   Recommended Daily Carbohydrate Intake for Trained Athletes

Recommended daily carbohydrate intake ranges from 3 to 12 g/kg. Adjust with consideration of the athlete's total energy needs, specific training needs (see chart), and feedback from training performance. Carbohydrate intake should be spread over the day to promote fuel availability for key training sessions—before, during, or after exercise.

Type of Activity	Recommended Carbohydrate Intake, g/kg
Very light training program (low-intensity or skill-based exercise)	3–5
Moderate-intensity training programs, 60 min/d	5–7
Moderate- to high-intensity endurance exercise, 1–3 h/d	6–10
Moderate- to high-intensity exercise, 4–5 h/d	8–12

Athletes should consume sufficient energy as well as carbohydrate. Consumption of a reduced-energy diet impairs endurance performance due to muscle and liver glycogen depletion (9,13). Adequate carbohydrate intake is also important for athletes in high-power activities (eg, wrestling, gymnastics, and dance) who have lost weight due to negative energy balances (13). Weight loss and consumption of low-energy diets are prevalent among athletes in high-power activities. A negative energy balance can harm high-power performance due to impaired acid-base balance, reduced glycolic enzyme levels, selective atrophy of type II muscle fibers, and abnormal sarcoplasmic reticulum function. In practical terms, the athlete cannot sustain high-intensity exercise. However, adequate dietary carbohydrate may ameliorate some of the damaging effects of energy restriction on the muscle (13).

For many athletes, energy and carbohydrate needs are greater during training than during competition. Some athletes involuntarily fail to increase energy intake to meet the energy demands of increased training. Costill et al (14) studied the effects of 10 days of increased training volume at a high intensity on muscle glycogen and swimming performance. Six swimmers self-selected a diet containing 4,700 kcal and 8.2 g carbohydrate per kg per day. Four other swimmers self-selected a diet containing only 3,700 kcal and 5.3 g carbohydrate per kg per day, and these four swimmers could not tolerate the heavier training demands and swam at significantly slower speeds, presumably due to a 20% decrease in muscle glycogen.

Glycemic Index and Glycemic Load

The glycemic index (GI) provides a way to rank carbohydrate-rich foods according to the blood glucose response after these foods are consumed. The GI is calculated by measuring the incremental area under the blood glucose curve after ingestion of a test food providing 50 g carbohydrate compared with a reference food (glucose or white bread). Foods with a low GI cause a slower, sustained release of glucose to the blood, whereas foods with a high GI cause a rapid, short-lived increase in blood glucose (15).

Foods are usually divided into those that have a high GI (glucose, bread, potatoes, breakfast cereal, sport drinks), a moderate GI (sucrose, soft drinks, oats, tropical fruits such as bananas and mangos), or a low GI (fructose, milk, yogurt, lentils, pasta, nuts, and fruits such as apples and oranges). Tables of the GI of a large number of foods have been published (16) and are available at the Glycemic Index Foundation Web site (www.glycemicindex.com).

BOX 2.2   Carbohydrate Content of Selected Foods[a]

Grains
- 2 slices whole-wheat bread
- ½ deli-style bagel
- 2-oz English muffin
- 1 cup oatmeal
- 1 cup ready-to-eat breakfast cereal
- 1 package snack-type cheese crackers (6 to package)
- 2 fig cookie bars
- ½ cup rice
- ½ cup cooked pasta
- 5 cups popcorn
- ½ large soft pretzel
- 17 mini pretzels
- 1 flour tortilla (12-in diameter)
- 1 oz tortilla chips and ¼ cup salsa

Dairy Products and Other Beverages
- 2 cups milk (low-fat or fat-free)
- 1 cup low-fat chocolate milk
- 4.5-oz container fruit-flavored yogurt
- 12 oz sugar-free yogurt
- 1 cup vanilla-flavored soymilk
- 1 package instant hot chocolate (made with water)

Beans and Starchy Vegetables
- ½ cup black beans
- ½ cup baked beans
- ¾ cup kidney beans
- ½ cup lima beans
- 1 cup green peas
- ½ cup corn
- ¾ cup mashed potatoes
- ½ medium baked potato with skin

Sport Drinks, Bars, and Gels
- 2 cups sport drink (6%–8% carbohydrate-containing sport drink)
- 1 energy bar (average of many energy bars)
- 1 carbohydrate gel
- 8 oz (½ can) Boost or Ensure
- 8 oz (½ can) SlimFast

Mixed Dishes
- 1 slice thin-crust pizza with meat or veggie toppings
- ½ slice thick-crust pizza with meat or veggie toppings
- 1 small bean and rice burrito
- ½ cup black beans and rice
- 1½ cups canned chicken noodle soup
- ¾ cup tomato soup
- 1 cup cooked ramen noodles
- ½ 6-in sub sandwich
- ½ cup macaroni and cheese

Fruit and Juice
- 2 cups fresh strawberries
- 1 large orange
- ¾ cup orange juice
- ½ cup cranberry-apple juice
- 1 medium apple

[a]Each portion provides approximately 25 g of carbohydrate.

Some practitioners suggest that manipulating the GI of foods and meals may enhance carbohydrate availability and improve athletic performance. For example, low-GI/carbohydrate-rich foods are recommended before exercise to promote sustained carbohydrate availability. Moderate- to high-GI carbohydrate foods are recommended during exercise to promote carbohydrate oxidation and after exercise to promote glycogen repletion (15).

Although the GI provides a reliable and consistent measure of relative blood glucose response to carbohydrate-rich foods and meals, the concept has practical limitations. The GI is based on equal grams of carbohydrate (50 g), not average serving sizes. The available numbers are largely based on tests using single foods. The blood glucose response to high-GI foods may be blunted when combined with low-GI foods in the meal. The GI can be applied to mixed meals by taking a weighted mean of the GI of the carbohydrate-rich foods that make up the meal, but this is not very practical. Furthermore, low-GI foods such as whole grain bread and legumes may cause gastrointestinal distress if consumed before endurance exercise. Factors other than GI also affect glucose and insulin levels (15).

The glycemic load (GL) considers both GI and the amount of carbohydrate consumed (16). The formula is: GL = GI (expressed as a decimal) multiplied by dietary carbohydrate content (in grams).

The GL of a food is almost always less than its corresponding GI. Using the GI to choose an individual food may be helpful for athletes in certain situations. The GL provides an overview of the daily diet. The GI and GL for selected foods are listed in Table 2.1.

Several energy bars with lower carbohydrate content claim to reduce blood glucose and insulin levels compared to high-GI foods. Although substituting other macronutrients for carbohydrate reduces blood glucose levels in low-, moderate-, or high-carbohydrate energy bars, insulin levels are not uniformly reduced and may actually be higher for some bars when compared with white bread (17).

The GI may be useful in sports by helping to fine-tune food choices, but it should not be used exclusively to provide guidelines for carbohydrate and food intake before, during, and after exercise. Other features of foods such as nutritional content, palatability, portability, cost, gastric comfort, and ease of preparation are also important. Athletes should choose foods according to their nutrition goals and exercise situation (15).

Communicating Carbohydrate Recommendations

Population dietary guidelines generally express goals for macronutrient intake as a percentage of total energy. For example, the Food and Nutrition Board of the Institute of Medicine established an Acceptable Macronutrient Distribution Range (AMDR) for carbohydrate at 45% to 65% of energy intake (18).

However, the *absolute quantity* of carbohydrate, rather than the percentage of energy from carbohydrate, is important for exercise performance. An athlete's estimated carbohydrate requirements should consider the amount of carbohydrate required for optimal glycogen restoration or the amount expended during training. These estimates should also be provided according to the athlete's body weight to account for the size of the athlete's muscle mass. Carbohydrate guidelines based on gram per kilogram of body weight are user-friendly and practical; it is relatively easy for athletes to determine the carbohydrate content of meals and snacks to achieve their daily carbohydrate goals (5).

Another problem with using percentages is that the athlete's energy and carbohydrate requirements are not always matched. Athletes who have large muscle mass and heavy training regimens generally have very high energy requirements and can meet their carbohydrate needs with a lower percentage of energy from carbohydrate. When an athlete consumes 4,000 to 5,000 kcal/d, even a diet providing 50% of energy from carbohydrate will supply 500 to 600 g/d. This translates into 7 to 8 g/kg for a 70-kg athlete, which should be adequate to maintain muscle glycogen stores from day to day (5,9).

TABLE 2.1   Glycemic Index and Glycemic Load for Selected Foods

Food	Glycemic Index	Glycemic Load
Glucose	96	10
Sucrose	60	6
Lactose	46	5
Fructose	23	2
Gatorade	78	12
Power Bar	56	24
Boost	53	23
Ensure	50	19
Coca Cola	63	16
7-grain bread	55	8
White bread	73	10
All bran cereal	38	9
Corn flakes	81	21
Cheerios	74	15
Cream of wheat	74	22
Oatmeal	66	17
Wheat flakes	70	13
Barley	25	11
Corn	53	17
White rice	64	23
Brown rice	55	18
Soda crackers	74	12
Pretzels	83	16
Spaghetti	42	20
Low-fat fruit yogurt	31	9
Fat-free (skim) milk	32	4
Low-fat (1%) chocolate milk	37	9
Cashews	25	3
Peanuts	23	2
Banana	52	12
Apple	38	6
Mango	51	8
Orange	42	5
Orange juice	52	12
Canned baked beans	48	7
Lentils	29	5
Pinto beans	39	10
Soy beans	18	1
Potato	85	26
Sweet potato	61	17
Yam	37	13
Peas	48	3

Source: Data are from Glycemic Index Foundation Web site: www.glycemicindex.com.

Conversely, when a 60-kg athlete consumes fewer than 2,000 kcal/d, even a diet providing 60% of energy from carbohydrate (4 to 5 g/kg/d) may not provide sufficient carbohydrate to maintain optimal carbohydrate stores for daily training. This situation is particularly common in female athletes who restrict energy intake to achieve or maintain a low body weight or percentage of body fat (5,9).

All in all, it is more reliable and practical to recommend that athletes consume an absolute quantity of carbohydrate (5 to 12 g/kg/d) rather than a relative percentage of energy from carbohydrate (45% to 65%). It is also important for athletes to consume adequate energy, protein, and fat.

Muscle Glycogen Supercompensation

Muscle glycogen depletion is a well-recognized limitation to endurance performance (3). Carbohydrate loading (glycogen supercompensation) can increase muscle glycogen stores from resting levels of 100 to 120 mmol/kg to approximately 150 to 250 mmol/kg and improve performance in endurance events exceeding 90 minutes (19–21).

For endurance athletes, carbohydrate loading is an extended period of "fueling up" to prepare for competition (18). The regimen can postpone fatigue and extend the duration of steady-state exercise by about 20% (22). Carbohydrate loading can also improve endurance performance by about 2% to 3% in sports in which a set distance is covered as quickly as possible (22).

The classic study on carbohydrate loading measured muscle glycogen content and compared the exercise time to exhaustion at 75% of VO_{2max} after 3 days of three diets varying in carbohydrate content (20). A low-carbohydrate diet (< 5% of energy from carbohydrate) produced a muscle glycogen content of 38 mmol/kg and supported only 1 hour of exercise. A mixed diet (50% energy from carbohydrate) produced a muscle glycogen content of 106 mmol/kg and enabled the subjects to exercise 115 minutes. However, a high-carbohydrate diet (≥ 82% of energy from carbohydrate) provided 204 mmol of muscle glycogen per kg and enabled the subjects to exercise for 170 minutes.

Carbohydrate loading enables the athlete to maintain high-intensity exercise longer, but will not affect pace for the first hour. In a field study, runners ran a 30-km race after eating a normal diet or high-carbohydrate diet. The high-carbohydrate diet provided muscle glycogen levels of 193 mmol/kg, compared to 94 mmol/kg for the normal diet. All runners covered the 30-km distance faster (by about 8 minutes) when they began the race with high muscle glycogen stores (21).

The "classical" regimen of carbohydrate loading involved a 3-day "depletion" phase of hard training and a low-carbohydrate intake. The athlete finished with a 3-day "loading" phase of tapered training and a high-carbohydrate intake before the event (22).

Later research found that muscle glycogen stores were elevated to the same extent after 3 days of tapered training and a high-carbohydrate intake (10 g/kg/d), whether preceded by a 3-day "depletion" phase or a more typical diet and training regimen. The modified carbohydrate-loading protocol is more practical and avoids the fatigue and extreme diet and training requirements associated with the "depletion" phase of the "classical" regimen (23).

Several studies suggest that endurance athletes can carbohydrate load in as little as 1 day (24,25). A high-carbohydrate diet of 10 g/kg/d significantly increased muscle glycogen from preloading levels of approximately 90 mmol/kg to approximately 180 mmol/kg after 1 day (24). A high-carbohydrate intake of 10.3 g/kg after a 3-minute bout of high-intensity exercise enabled athletes to increase muscle glycogen levels from preloading levels of approximately 109 mmol/kg to 198 mmol/kg in 24 hours (25). These studies suggest that muscle glycogen supercompensation is probably achieved within 36 and 48 hours of the last exercise session, provided the athlete rests and consumes adequate carbohydrate (19).

For most athletes, a carbohydrate-loading regimen will involve 3 days of a high-carbohydrate intake (10 to 12 g/kg/d) along with tapered training. Carbohydrate-loading guidelines are listed in Table 2.2 (19).

Some athletes may have difficulty tolerating carbohydrate-rich foods that are high in fiber. To avoid gastrointestinal distress, the athlete may benefit from consuming low-fiber foods such as pasta, white rice,

TABLE 2.2   Precompetition Carbohydrate-Loading Guidelines

Day	Training	Carbohydrate, g/kg/d
1	Tapered training (eg, 20 min at 70% of VO_{2max})	10–12
2	Tapered training (eg, 20 min at 70% of VO_{2max})	10–12
3	Rest	10–12
4	Competition	—

Source: Data are from reference 19.

pancakes, cereal and fruit bars, sport bars and gels, yogurt, baked goods, and low-fat or fat-free sweets (eg, hard candy). Most athletes need to eat frequently throughout the day to consume adequate carbohydrate and energy. Carbohydrate-rich fluids such as sport drinks, low-fat chocolate milk, liquid meals, high-carbohydrate supplements, yogurt drinks, and fruit smoothies help to augment carbohydrate and energy intake. As with other nutrition strategies, athletes should test their carbohydrate-loading regimen during a prolonged workout or a low-priority race (19).

Carbohydrate loading will only help athletes engaged in intense, continuous endurance exercise lasting more than 90 minutes. Above-normal muscle glycogen stores will not enable athletes to exercise harder during shorter duration exercise (eg, 5- and 10-km runs) and may harm performance due to the associated stiffness and weight gain.

Although some bodybuilders use carbohydrate loading to increase muscle size and enhance appearance, there was no increase in the girths of seven muscle groups after a carbohydrate-loading regimen in resistance-trained bodybuilders (26).

Endurance training promotes muscle glycogen supercompensation by increasing the activity of glycogen synthase—an enzyme responsible for glycogen storage. The athlete must be endurance-trained or the regimen will not be effective. Because glycogen stores are specific to the muscle groups used, the exercise used to deplete the stores must be the same as the athlete's competitive event. Some athletes note a feeling of stiffness and heaviness associated with the increased glycogen storage (additional water is stored with glycogen), but these sensations dissipate with exercise.

The performance benefits of carbohydrate loading may add to the benefits of consuming carbohydrate during exercise. The combination of carbohydrate loading with other dietary strategies that are used to improve endurance performance (eg, pre-exercise meal, consuming carbohydrate during exercise, caffeine ingestion) should be evaluated (19).

High-Carbohydrate Supplements

Athletes who train heavily and have difficulty eating enough food to consume adequate carbohydrate and energy can utilize a high-carbohydrate liquid supplement (27). Most products are 18% to 24% carbohydrate and contain glucose polymers (maltodextrins) to reduce the solution's osmolality and potential for gastrointestinal distress.

High-carbohydrate supplements do not replace regular food but help supply supplemental energy, carbohydrate, and liquid during heavy training or carbohydrate loading. If the athlete has no difficulty eating enough conventional food, these products offer only the advantage of convenience.

High-carbohydrate supplements should be consumed before or after exercise, either with meals or between meals. Although ultra-endurance athletes may also use them during exercise to obtain energy and carbohydrate, these products are too concentrated in carbohydrate to double for use as a fluid-replacement beverage.

The Pre-exercise Meal

Consuming carbohydrate-rich foods and fluids in the 4 hours before exercise helps to (*a*) restore liver glycogen, especially for morning exercise when liver glycogen is depleted from an overnight fast; (*b*) increase muscle glycogen stores if they are not fully restored from the previous exercise session; (*c*) prevent hunger, which may in itself impair performance; and (*d*) give the athlete a psychological boost (19). Including some low-GI foods may be beneficial in promoting a sustained release of glucose into the bloodstream.

Consuming carbohydrate on the morning of an endurance event may help to maintain blood glucose levels during prolonged exercise. When compared to an overnight fast, consuming a meal containing 200 to 300 g of carbohydrate 2 to 4 hours before exercise provides a much more improved endurance performance (28–30).

Research (29,31) suggests that the pre-exercise meal contain 1 to 4 g carbohydrate per kg, consumed 1 to 4 hours before exercise. To avoid potential gastrointestinal distress when blood is diverted from the gut to the exercising muscles, the carbohydrate and energy content of the meal should be reduced the closer to exercise that the meal is consumed. For example, a carbohydrate feeding of 1 g/kg is appropriate 1 hour before exercise, whereas 4 g/kg can be consumed 4 hours before exercise. Recommendations for carbohydrate intake before exercise are summarized in Box 2.3.

If the athlete is unable to eat breakfast prior to early-morning exercise, consuming approximately 30 g of an easily digested carbohydrate-rich food or fluid (eg, banana, carbohydrate gel, or sport drink) 5 minutes before exercise may improve endurance performance (32).

A number of commercially formulated liquid meals satisfy the requirements for pre-exercise food: they are high in carbohydrate, palatable, and provide both energy and fluid. Liquid meals can often be consumed closer to competition than regular meals because of their shorter gastric emptying time. This may help to avoid precompetition nausea for those athletes who are tense and have an associated delay in gastric emptying.

Some were initially designed for hospital patients (eg, Sustacal and Ensure), whereas others were specifically created for and marketed to the athlete (eg, Nutrament, Gatorade Nutrition Shake, and Go!).

BOX 2.3   Recommended Carbohydrate Intake Before Exercise

- Consider both the amount and timing of carbohydrate intake. See chart for general recommendations.
- If unable to eat breakfast prior to early morning exercise, consuming ~30 g of easily digested carbohydrate 5 minutes before exercise may improve performance.
- Experiment with low–, medium–, and high–glycemic index foods during training.

Timing Before Exercise, Hours	Carbohydrate, g/kg
1	1
2	2
3	3
4	4

Liquid meals produce a low stool residue, thereby minimizing immediate weight gain after the meal. This is especially advantageous for athletes who need to "make weight." They are convenient fuel for athletes competing in day-long tournaments, meets, and ultra-endurance events (eg, Ironman triathlon). Liquid meals can also be used for nutritional supplementation during heavy training when energy requirements are extremely elevated.

Carbohydrate in the Hour Before Exercise

Based primarily on the results of *only one* study, athletes have been cautioned not to eat carbohydrates in the hour prior to exercise. In the late 1970s, a study found that consuming 75 g of glucose 30 minutes before cycling at 80% of VO_{2max} caused an initial rapid decrease in blood glucose and reduced exercise time by 19% (33). The authors attributed the impaired endurance to accelerated muscle glycogen depletion, although muscle glycogen was not measured. The high blood insulin levels induced by the pre-exercise carbohydrate feeding were blamed for this chain of events (33). However, subsequent studies have contradicted these findings (19,31,34). Pre-exercise carbohydrate feedings either improve performance by 7% to 20% or have no detrimental effect. In most cases, the decrease in blood glucose observed during the first 20 minutes of exercise is self-correcting with no apparent effects on the athlete (19).

A small number of athletes react negatively to carbohydrate feedings in the hour before exercise and experience symptoms of hypoglycemia and a rapid onset of fatigue. The reason that some athletes have an extreme reaction is not known. Preventive strategies for this group include: consume a low-GI carbohydrate before exercise; consume carbohydrate a few minutes before exercise; or wait until exercising to consume carbohydrate. The exercise-induced increase in the hormones epinephrine, norepinephrine, and growth hormone inhibit the release of insulin and thus counter insulin's effect in reducing blood glucose.

Pre-exercise Carbohydrate and the Glycemic Index

A 1991 study first sparked interest in the use of the GI in sport by manipulating the glycemic response to pre-exercise meals (35). In theory, low-GI foods (beans, milk, and pasta) provide a slow and sustained release of glucose to the blood, without an accompanying insulin surge. Consumption of 1 g carbohydrate per kg from lentils (low GI) 1 hour before cycling at 67% of VO_{2max} increased endurance compared with an equal amount of carbohydrate from potatoes (high GI). Lentils promoted lower postprandial blood glucose and insulin responses and more stable blood glucose levels during exercise compared with potatoes (35).

Most studies have failed to show performance benefits from consuming low-GI meals before exercise (19). A second study by the same researchers found no differences in time to exhaustion between low- and high-GI meals consumed 1 hour before exercise (36). Other investigators found no differences in work output when a low-GI food (lentils) and a high-GI food (potatoes) were consumed 45 minutes before exercise (37).

It is important to consider the overall importance of the pre-exercise meal for maintaining carbohydrate availability because endurance athletes also consume carbohydrate-rich foods and fluids during prolonged exercise (19). A study evaluated the effects of the GI of pre-exercise meals when 1 g of carbohydrate per kg per hour was also consumed during prolonged cycling (38). There were no differences in performance or carbohydrate oxidation between the low-GI meal (pasta), high-GI meal (potatoes), and control trials. Thus, the effects of the pre-exercise meal on performance and metabolism are diminished when carbohydrate is consumed *during* exercise according to sports nutrition guidelines (19,38).

There is no evidence that athletes will universally benefit from low-GI pre-exercise meals, especially when athletes can refuel during exercise. In situations in which an athlete cannot consume carbohydrate during a prolonged event or workout, a low-GI pre-exercise meal may provide a more sustained release of carbohydrate during exercise (19).

Consuming a high-GI carbohydrate (eg, glucose) immediately before anaerobic exercise, such as sprinting or weightlifting, will not provide athletes with a quick burst of energy, allowing them to exercise harder. There is adequate ATP, creatine phosphate, and muscle glycogen already stored for these anaerobic tasks.

Carbohydrate During Exercise

Consuming carbohydrate during exercise lasting at least 1 hour can delay the onset of fatigue and improve endurance capacity by maintaining blood glucose levels and carbohydrate oxidation in the latter stages of exercise (39-43). Carbohydrate feedings supplement the body's limited endogenous stores of carbohydrate (39). Consuming carbohydrate during cycling exercise at 70% of VO_{2max} can delay fatigue by 30 to 60 minutes (40,41). It has also been shown to improve performance during a 40-km run in the heat (42) and a treadmill run at 80% of VO_{2max} (43). Practically speaking, athletes can exercise longer and/or sprint harder at the end of exercise if they have consumed carbohydrate during the event.

Blood glucose becomes an increasingly important source of carbohydrate as muscle glycogen stores decrease (2). During prolonged exercise, ingested carbohydrate can account for up to 30% of the total amount of carbohydrate oxidized (44). Carbohydrate feedings during endurance exercise maintain blood glucose levels at a time when muscle glycogen stores are diminished. Thus, carbohydrate oxidation (and, therefore, ATP production) can continue at a high rate and endurance is enhanced.

The performance benefits of consuming carbohydrate during exercise may be additive to those of a pre-exercise meal. Cyclists who received carbohydrate 3 hours before exercise and during exercise were able to exercise longer (289 minutes) than when receiving carbohydrate either before exercise (236 minutes) or during exercise (266 minutes) (30). Combining carbohydrate feedings improved performance more than either feeding alone. However, the improvement in performance with pre-exercise carbohydrate feedings was less than when smaller quantities of carbohydrate were consumed during exercise. Thus, to obtain a continuous supply of glucose, the athlete should consume carbohydrate during exercise.

Although it makes sense that athletes should consume high-GI carbohydrate feedings to promote carbohydrate oxidation, the glycemic response to carbohydrate feedings during exercise has not been systematically studied. However, most athletes choose carbohydrate-rich foods (sport bars and gels) and fluids (sport drinks) that would be classified as having a moderate to high GI (15).

There is recent evidence that carbohydrate feedings may improve performance during high-intensity, relatively short-duration exercise (> 75%VO_{2max} for about an hour) by positively influencing the central nervous system. Studies have demonstrated that a carbohydrate mouth rinse improves running and cycling performance, possibly by activating areas of the brain associated with motivation and reward (45). Beneficial effects generally occur when exercise is done in the fasted state or several hours after a meal (45).

Carbohydrate During Intermittent High-Intensity Sports

Carbohydrate feedings may also improve performance in stop-and-go sports such as basketball, soccer, football, and tennis that require repeated bouts of high-intensity, short-duration effort (46-49).

Consuming carbohydrate improved performance during intermittent, high-intensity shuttle-running designed to replicate the activity pattern of stop-and-go sports (46). In a later study, the same researchers found that muscle glycogen utilization was reduced by 22% after carbohydrate ingestion (47). Consuming carbohydrate also resulted in a 37% longer run time to fatigue and faster 20-meter sprint time during the fourth quarter of an intermittent, high-intensity shuttle run designed to replicate basketball (48). Carbohydrate ingestion improved endurance capacity in athletes with high pre-exercise muscle glycogen stores during intermittent high-intensity running (49). The authors attributed the improved performance to higher plasma glucose concentration toward the end of exercise that provided a sustained source of carbohydrate for the muscles and central nervous system (49).

These studies establish that the benefits of carbohydrate feedings are not limited to prolonged endurance exercise. Carbohydrate feedings improve performance in stop-and-go sports by (a) selectively sparing glycogen in type II (fast-twitch) muscle fibers; (b) increasing glycogen resynthesis in type II muscle fibers during rest or low-intensity periods; (c) a combination of both; and/or (d) by increasing blood glucose (47,49).

Carbohydrate Dose

The maximum amount of carbohydrate that can be oxidized during exercise from a single carbohydrate source (eg, glucose) is about 1 g per minute or 60 g per hour because the transporter responsible for carbohydrate absorption in the intestine becomes saturated. Consuming more than 1 g/minute from one source does not increase the rate of carbohydrate oxidation and increases the risk of gastrointestinal distress (50).

By consuming multiple carbohydrates that use different intestinal transporters, the total amount of carbohydrate that can be absorbed and oxidized is increased. When glucose and fructose or glucose, fructose, and sucrose are ingested together during exercise at a rate of 2.4 g/min (144 g/h), the rate of exogenous carbohydrate oxidation can reach 1.7 g/min or about 105 g/h (50,51). Drinks containing multiple transportable carbohydrates are also less likely to cause gastrointestinal distress (52,53).

Water absorption is also enhanced when sport drinks include two to three different carbohydrate sources (glucose, sucrose, fructose, or maltodextrins) compared to solutions containing only one carbohydrate source (54). The addition of a second or third carbohydrate activates additional mechanisms for intestinal transport and involves transport by separate pathways that are noncompetitive (54).

In theory, consuming multiple transportable carbohydrates should enhance endurance performance by increasing exogenous carbohydrate oxidation and reducing the reliance on endogenous carbohydrate stores. Ingestion of glucose and fructose (1.8 g/min) improved cycling time-trial performance by 8% compared to an isocaloric amount of glucose after 2 hours of cycling at 55% of maximal work rate. The glucose and fructose promoted better ATP resynthesis compared to glucose, thus allowing the maintenance of a higher power output (55). This was the first study to provide evidence that increased exogenous carbohydrate oxidation improves endurance performance. The series of studies conducted by researchers at the University of Birmingham have shown that consuming 1.8 to 2.4 g of carbohydrate per minute (108 to 144 g/h) from a mixture of carbohydrates increases carbohydrate oxidation up to 75 to 104 g/h (50-53,55,56).

The recommendations for carbohydrate intake during exercise can be absolute (grams per hour) and not based on body weight (10,56). Consuming carbohydrate is neither practical nor necessary during exercise lasting less than 45 minutes (10). Small amounts of carbohydrate from sport drinks or foods may enhance performance during sustained high-intensity exercise lasting 45 to 75 minutes (10). Athletes should consume 30 to 60 g of carbohydrate per hour from carbohydrate-rich fluids or foods during endurance and intermittent, high-intensity exercise lasting 1 to 2.5 hours (10). As the duration of the event increases, so does the amount of carbohydrate required to enhance performance (10). During endurance and ultraendurance exercise lasting 2.5 to 3 hours and longer, athletes should consume up to 80 to 90 g of carbohydrate per hour (10,56). Products providing multiple transportable carbohydrates are necessary to achieve these high rates of carbohydrate oxidation (10,56). Athletes should individually determine a refueling plan that meets their nutritional goals (including hydration) and minimizes gastrointestinal distress (10,39). The carbohydrate content of selected foods is listed in Table 2.3.

TABLE 2.3   Carbohydrate Content of Selected Foods

Food	Portion	Carbohydrate, g
Gatorade/Powerade	1 quart (~1 liter)	60
PowerBar	1 bar	47
Gu gels	2 gels	50
Sport Beans	28	50
Cliff Shot Blok	6	50
Graham crackers	3 large	66
Fig bars	4 bars	42
Banana	1	30

High concentrations of pure fructose should be avoided because of the risk of gastrointestinal upset (39,57). Fructose is absorbed relatively slowly and must be converted to glucose by the liver before it can be oxidized by the muscle. Because the maximum rate of oxidation of ingested fructose is less than for glucose, sucrose, or glucose polymers, ingesting fructose alone does not improve performance (56). However, in combination with other carbohydrate sources, fructose is well tolerated, increases exogenous carbohydrate oxidation, and improves performance (56).

Liquid vs Solid Carbohydrate

Athletes use a variety of fluids, foods, and gels during training and competition. Liquid and solid carbohydrates are equally effective in increasing blood glucose and improving performance (58–62), although each has certain advantages.

Sport drinks and other fluids containing carbohydrate encourage the consumption of water needed to maintain normal hydration during exercise. Carbohydrate ingestion and fluid replacement independently improve performance, and their beneficial effects are additive (63). The sodium in sport drinks helps to replace sweat sodium losses and stimulate thirst (64). Sport drinks are a practical way to obtain water, carbohydrate, and sodium during training and competition (65). However, compared with liquids, high-carbohydrate foods, energy bars, and gels can be easily carried by the athlete during exercise and provide both variety and satiety (40,60,66). Recommendations for carbohydrate intake during exercise are summarized in Table 2.4.

TABLE 2.4   Recommended Carbohydrate Intake During Exercise

Type of Activity	Recommended Carbohydrate Intake
Exercise lasting less than 45 minutes	Not necessary or practical
High-intensity exercise lasting 45 to 75 minutes	Small amounts of sport drinks or foods
Endurance and intermittent, high-intensity exercise lasting 1 to 2.5 hours	30–60 g/h
Endurance and ultra-endurance exercise lasting 2.5 to 3 hours and longer	≥ 80–90 g/h

Carbohydrate After Exercise

The restoration of muscle and liver glycogen stores is important for recovery after strenuous training. Athletes commonly engage in prolonged high-intensity workouts once or twice a day with a limited amount of time (6 to 24 hours) to recover before the next exercise session. Using effective refueling strategies after daily training sessions helps to optimize recovery and promote the desired adaptations to training. During competition, especially multiday events such as bicycle stage races, there may be less control over the exercise-recovery ratio. In this case, the goal is to recover as much as possible for the next day's event (5).

When there are fewer than 8 hours between workouts or competitions that deplete muscle glycogen stores, the athlete should start consuming carbohydrate *immediately* after the first exercise session to maximize the effective recovery time between sessions. The athlete should consume 1 to 1.2 g/kg/h for the first 4 hours after glycogen-depleting exercise. Consuming small amounts of carbohydrate frequently (every 15 to 30 minutes) further enhances muscle glycogen synthesis (5,10,67-69). Recovery snacks and meals contribute to the athlete's daily carbohydrate and energy requirements (5,10).

During longer periods of recovery (24 hours), it does not matter how carbohydrate intake is spaced throughout the day as long as the athlete consumes adequate carbohydrate and energy. The type, pattern, and timing of carbohydrate intake can be chosen according to what is practical and enjoyable (5,10,15). Carbohydrate-rich foods with a moderate to high GI should be emphasized in recovery meals/snacks to supply a readily available source of carbohydrate for muscle glycogen synthesis (5,70).

There is no difference in glycogen synthesis when liquid or solid forms of carbohydrate are consumed (71). However, liquid forms of carbohydrate may be appealing when athletes have decreased appetites due to fatigue and/or dehydration (5).

There are several reasons that glycogen repletion occurs faster after exercise: the blood flow to the muscles is much greater immediately after exercise; the muscle cell is more likely to take up glucose; and the muscle cells are more sensitive to the effects of insulin during this time period, which promotes glycogen synthesis.

Glucose and sucrose are twice as effective as fructose in restoring muscle glycogen after exercise (72). Most fructose (which is found in foods like fruits and soft drinks) is converted to liver glycogen, whereas glucose (which is found in starchy foods) seems to bypass the liver and is stored as muscle glycogen. The type of carbohydrate (simple vs complex) does not seem to influence glycogen repletion after exercise (73). Recommendations for carbohydrate intake after exercise are summarized in Box 2.4.

Athletes may have impaired muscle glycogen synthesis after unaccustomed exercise that results in muscle damage and delayed-onset muscle soreness. Such muscle damage seems to decrease both the

---

BOX 2.4   Recommended Carbohydrate Intake After Glycogen-Depleting Exercise

- When exercise sessions are less than 8 hours apart, start consuming carbohydrate immediately after exercise to maximize recovery time.
- Consume 1 to 1.2 g of carbohydrate per kg per hour for the first 4 hours after glycogen-depleting exercise.
- Early refueling may be enhanced by consuming small amounts of carbohydrate more frequently—eg, every 15 to 30 minutes.
- Choose medium– to high–glycemic index foods.
- Add small amount of protein (15–25 g) to first feeding to stimulate muscle protein synthesis/repair.

rate of muscle glycogen synthesis and the total muscle glycogen content (74). Although a diet providing 10 g of carbohydrate per kg will usually replace muscle glycogen stores within 24 hours, the damaging effects of unaccustomed exercise results in substantial delays to muscle glycogen repletion. Also, even the normalization of muscle glycogen stores does not guarantee normal muscle function after unaccustomed exercise (74).

Adding Protein to Postexercise Carbohydrate Feedings

Some practitioners recommend adding protein to the postexercise carbohydrate feeding to enhance glycogen repletion. In 1992 Zawadzki et al (75) reported that adding protein to a carbohydrate drink produced higher muscle glycogen synthesis rates after exercise than the carbohydrate drink alone. However, the study findings were criticized because the two drinks were not isocaloric.

Other researchers have investigated whether the improved glycogen synthesis observed by Zawadzki et al was the result of additional protein or additional energy (74–77). These studies have found that adding protein to the recovery feeding does not enhance muscle glycogen storage when the amount of carbohydrate is at or more than the threshold for maximum glycogen synthesis: 1 to 1.2 g/kg/h (5,76–79). Adding a small amount of protein (~0.3 g/kg/h) to a suboptimal carbohydrate intake (< 1 g/kg/h) can accelerate muscle glycogen restoration (70).

Consuming protein with recovery snacks and meals helps increase net muscle protein balance, promote muscle tissue repair, and enhance adaptations involving synthesis of new proteins (80). The athlete's initial recovery snack/meal should include 15 to 25 g of high-quality protein in addition to carbohydrate (5,10,80). This can be provided by 16 oz of fat-free milk (16 g), two to three large eggs (14–21 g), or 2 to 3 oz of lean red meat (14–21 g).

Controversy: Training with Low Carbohydrate Availability

Some practitioners have suggested that athletes train with low carbohydrate availability to promote performance—"train low." In theory, training with low muscle glycogen stores maximizes the physiological adaptations to endurance training and improves performance (81,82).

Although there are numerous ways to reduce carbohydrate availability for training, the current research is limited to studies of "twice a day" training (starting the second session with low muscle glycogen stores) and withholding carbohydrate during training sessions (81,82).

A 2005 study sparked intense interest in the "train low" concept (83). Untrained men performed knee-kicking exercise with one leg trained in a low-glycogen state and the other leg trained in a high-glycogen state. Both legs were trained equally regarding workload and training amount. After 10 weeks, the increase in maximal power was identical for the two legs. However, there was about a two-fold greater training-induced increase in one-leg time to fatigue in the "train low" leg compared to the "train high" leg. The "train low" leg also had higher resting glycogen content and citrate synthase activity compared to the "train high" leg. These results suggested that training adaptations may be enhanced by low glycogen availability, thereby improving endurance (83). However, this study has several limitations. The subjects were untrained, the training sessions were held at a fixed submaximal intensity, and the type of training and performance trial did not remotely resemble how most competitive athletes train and compete (84).

A study of endurance-trained cyclists/triathletes evaluated the effects of "training low" on training capacity, endurance performance, and substrate metabolism (84). The "train high" group alternated between a steady-state aerobic ride one day (100 minutes at 70% VO_{2peak}) and a high-intensity interval training session the next day. The "train low" group trained twice every other day, with the steady-state aerobic ride followed by the interval session 1 hour later. Only the "train low" group experienced significant increases in resting muscle glycogen concentrations, fat oxidation during steady-state cycling, and activity of the muscle enzymes beta-hydroxyacyl-CoA-dehydrogenase and citrate synthase. At the end of 3 weeks, performance increased significantly in both groups but there was no difference between groups. Despite metabolic and muscle enzyme changes indicating an enhanced training adaptation in the "train low" group, there was no obvious benefit to endurance performance compared to when the subjects undertook training with high muscle glycogen stores (84). Additional research has corroborated these findings (85,86).

In theory, "training low" enhances the training stimulus, increases the ability to utilize fat as an exercise fuel, and reduces the reliance on carbohydrate. Despite creating metabolic and muscle enzyme adaptations that should enhance endurance, there is no clear proof that "training low" improves endurance performance (81,82).

An athlete's diet and the ability to complete strenuous training sessions day after day are highly connected. It is generally assumed that training with high carbohydrate availability allows the athlete to train harder and improves performance. "Training low" may interfere with the intensity and/or volume of endurance training. Thus, experimenting with "training low" is most suitable in the beginning of a training cycle when it is least likely to harm performance. High carbohydrate availability is recommended for high-intensity training sessions and when the athlete is preparing to peak for competition (82,83).

Summary

Carbohydrate is the predominant fuel for moderate- to high-intensity endurance exercise and repeated bouts of moderate- to high-intensity exercise. The strategic moves that occur during both endurance and stop-and-go sports depend on the athlete's ability to work at high intensities, which are in turn fueled by carbohydrate. Because the depletion of endogenous carbohydrate stores (muscle and liver glycogen and blood glucose) can impair athletic performance, fueling strategies should optimize carbohydrate availability before, during, and after exercise.

Athletes with very light training programs (low-intensity exercise or skill-based exercise) should consume 3 to 5 g of carbohydrate per kg per day. Athletes engaged in moderate-intensity training programs for 60 minutes per day should consume 5 to 7 g/kg/d. During moderate- to high-intensity endurance exercise for 1 to 3 hours, athletes should consume 6 to 10 g/kg/d. Athletes participating in moderate- to high-intensity endurance exercise for 4 to 5 hours per day (eg, Tour de France) should consume 8 to 12 g/kg/d.

One to 4 hours prior to exercise, athletes should consume 1 to 4.0 g carbohydrate per kg to "top off" muscle and liver glycogen stores. During exercise lasting fewer than 45 minutes, consuming carbohydrate is neither practical nor necessary. Small amounts of carbohydrate from sport drinks or foods may enhance performance during sustained high-intensity exercise lasting 45 to 75 minutes. Athletes should consume 30 to 60 g of carbohydrate per hour from carbohydrate-rich fluids or foods during endurance and intermittent, high-intensity exercise lasting 1 to 2.5 hours. During endurance and ultra-endurance exercise lasting 2.5 to 3 hours and longer, athletes should consume up to 80 to 90 g of carbohydrate per hour from products providing multiple transportable carbohydrates.

When there are fewer than 8 hours between workouts or competitions that deplete muscle glycogen stores, the athlete should start consuming carbohydrate *immediately* after the first exercise session to maximize the effective recovery time between sessions. The athlete should consume 1 to 1.2 g/kg/h for the first 4 hours after glycogen-depleting exercise. Consuming small amounts of carbohydrate frequently—every 15 to 30 minutes—further enhances muscle glycogen synthesis. During longer periods of recovery (24 hours), it does not matter how carbohydrate intake is spaced throughout the day as long as the athlete consumes adequate carbohydrate and energy.

The athlete's initial recovery snack/meal should include 15 to 25 g of high-quality protein in addition to carbohydrate to increase net muscle protein balance, promote muscle tissue repair, and enhance adaptations involving synthesis of new proteins.

These are general recommendations. They should be adjusted with consideration of the athlete's total energy needs, specific training needs, and feedback from training and competition.

References

1. Jacobs KA, Sherman WM. The efficacy of carbohydrate supplementation and chronic high carbohydrate diets for improving endurance performance. *Int J Sport Nutr*. 1999;9:92–115.
2. Coyle EF. Substrate utilization during exercise in active people. *Am J Clin Nutr*. 1995;61(4 suppl):S968–S979.
3. Hargreaves M. Exercise physiology and metabolism. In: Burke L, Deakin V, eds. *Clinical Sports Nutrition*. 3rd ed. Sydney, Australia: McGraw-Hill; 2006:1–20.
4. Costill DL, Sherman WM, Fink WJ, Maresh C, Whitten M, Miller JM. The role of dietary carbohydrate in muscle glycogen resynthesis after strenuous running. *Am J Clin Nutr*. 1981;34:1831–1836.
5. Burke L. Nutrition for recovery after training and competition. In: Burke L, Deakin V, eds. *Clinical Sports Nutrition*. 3rd ed. Sydney, Australia: McGraw-Hill; 2006:415–453.
6. Fallowfield JL, Williams C. Carbohydrate intake and recovery from prolonged exercise. *Int J Sports Nutr*. 1993;3:150–164.
7. Achten J, Halson SH, Moseley L, Rayson MP, Casey A, Jeukendrup AE. Higher dietary carbohydrate content during intensified running training results in better maintenance of performance and mood state. *J Appl Physiol*. 2004;96:1331–1340.
8. Simonsen JC, Sherman WM, Lamb DR, Dernbach AR, Doyle JA, Strauss R. Dietary carbohydrate, muscle glycogen, and power output during rowing training. *J Appl Physiol*. 1991;70:1500–1505.
9. Rodriguez NR, DiMarco NM, Langley S. Position of the American Dietetic Association, Dietitians of Canada, and the American College of Sports Medicine: nutrition and athletic performance. *J Am Diet Assoc*. 2009;109: 509–527.
10. Burke LM, Hawley JA, Wong S, Jeukendrup AE. Carbohydrates for training and competition. *J Sports Sci*. 2011; (Jun 8):1–11. epub ahead of print.
11. Saris WHM, van Erp-Baart MA, Brouns F, Westerterp KR, ten Hoor F. Study of food intake and energy expenditure during extreme sustained exercise: the Tour de France. *Int J Sport Med*. 1989;10(suppl):S26–S31.
12. Garcia-Roves PM, Terrados N, Fernández SF, Patterson AM. Macronutrient intakes of top level cyclists during continuous competition—change in feeding pattern. *Int J Sport Med*. 1998;19:61–67.
13. Walberg-Rankin J. Dietary carbohydrate as an ergogenic aid for prolonged and brief competitions in sport. *Int J Sport Nutr*. 1995;5(suppl):S13–S28.
14. Costill DL, Flynn MJ, Kirwan JP, Houmard JA, Mitchell JB, Thomas R, Park SH. Effect of repeated days of intensified training on muscle glycogen and swimming performance. *Med Sci Sports Exerc*. 1988;20:249–254.
15. Burke LM, Collier GR, Hargreaves M. The glycemic index—a new tool in sport nutrition? *Int J Sport Nutr*. 1998;8:401–415.
16. Atkinson FS, Foster-Powell K, Brand-Miller JC. International tables of glycemic index and glycemic load values: 2008. *Diabetes Care*. 2008;31:2281–2283.
17. Hertzler SR, Kim Y. Glycemic and insulinemic responses to energy bars of differing macronutrient composition in healthy adults. *Med Sci Monit*. 2003;9:CR84–CR90.
18. Institute of Medicine. *Dietary Reference Intakes for Energy, Carbohydrate, Fiber, Fat, Fatty Acids, Cholesterol, Protein, and Amino Acids (Macronutrients)*. Washington, DC: National Academies Press; 2005.

19. Burke L. Preparation for competition. In: Burke L, Deakin V, eds. *Clinical Sports Nutrition.* 3rd ed. Sydney, Australia: McGraw-Hill; 2006:355–375.
20. Bergstrom J, Hermansen L, Saltin B. Diet, muscle glycogen, and physical performance. *Acta Physiol Scand.* 1967;71:140–150.
21. Karlsson J, Saltin, B. Diet, muscle glycogen, and endurance performance. *J Appl Physiol.* 1971;31:203–206.
22. Hawley JA, Schabort EJ, Noakes TD, Dennis SC. Carbohydrate-loading and exercise performance. An update. *Sports Med.* 1997;24:73--81.
23. Sherman WM, Costill DL, Fink WJ, Miller JM. The effect of exercise and diet manipulation on muscle glycogen and its subsequent use during performance. *Int J Sport Med.* 1981;2:114–118.
24. Bussau VA, Fairchild TJ, Rao A. Steele P, Fournier PA. Carbohydrate loading in human muscle: an improved 1 day protocol. *Eur J Appl Physiol.* 2002;87:290–295.
25. Fairchild TJ, Fletcher S, Steele P, Goodman C, Dawson B, Fournier PA. Rapid carbohydrate loading after a short bout of near maximal-intensity exercise. *Med Sci Sport Exerc.* 2002;34:980–986.
26. Balon TW, Horowitz JF, Fitzsimmons KM. Effects of carbohydrate loading and weight-lifting on muscle girth. *Int J Sport Nutr.* 1992;2:328–334.
27. Brouns F, Saris WH, Stroecken J, Beckers E, Thijssen R, Rehrer NJ, ten Hoor F. Eating, drinking, and cycling: a controlled Tour de France simulation study, part II. Effect of diet manipulation. *Int J Sport Med.*1989;10(suppl): S41–S48.
28. Nuefer PD, Costill DL, Flynn MG, Kirwan JP, Mitchell JB, Houmard J. Improvements in exercise performance: effects of carbohydrate feedings and diet. *J Appl Physiol.* 1987;62:983–988.
29. Sherman WM, Brodowicz G, Wright DA, Allen WK, Simonsen J, Dernbach A. Effects of 4 hour pre-exercise carbohydrate feedings on cycling performance. *Med Sci Sports Exerc.* 1989;12:598–604.
30. Wright DA, Sherman WM, Dernbach AR. Carbohydrate feedings before, during, or in combination improves cycling performance. *J Appl Physiol.* 1991;71:1082–1088.
31. Sherman WM, Peden MC, Wright DA. Carbohydrate feedings 1 hour before exercise improves cycling performance. *Am J Clin Nutr.* 1991;54:866–870.
32. Anantaraman R, Carimines AA, Gaesser GA, Weltman A. Effects of carbohydrate supplementation on performance during 1 hour of high-intensity exercise. *Int J Sport Med.* 1995;16:461–465.
33. Foster C, Costill DL, Fink WJ. Effects of pre-exercise feedings on endurance performance. *Med Sci Sport Exerc.* 1979;11:1–5.
34. Hargreaves M, Costill DL, Fink WJ, King DS, Fielding RA. Effects of pre-exercise carbohydrate feedings on endurance cycling performance. *Med Sci Sports Exerc.* 1987;19:33–36.
35. Thomas DE, Brotherhood JR, Brand JC. Carbohydrate feeding before exercise: effect of glycemic index. *Int J Sport Med.* 1991;12:180–186.
36. Thomas DE, Brotherhood JR, Miller JB. Plasma glucose levels after prolonged strenuous exercise correlate inversely with glycemic response to food consumed before exercise. *Int J Sport Nutr.* 1994;4:361–373.
37. Sparks MJ, Selig SS, Febbraio MA. Pre-exercise carbohydrate ingestion: effect of the glycemic index on endurance exercise performance. *Med Sci Sport Exerc.* 1998;30:844–849.
38. Burke LM, Claassen A, Hawley JA, Noakes TD. Carbohydrate intake during exercise minimizes effect of glycemic index of pre-exercise meal. *J Appl Physiol.* 1998;85:2220–2226.
39. Maughan R. Fluid and carbohydrate during exercise. In: Burke L, Deakin V, eds. *Clinical Sports Nutrition.* 3rd ed. Sydney, Australia: McGraw-Hill; 2006:385–414.
40. Coyle EF, Hagberg JM, Hurley BF, Martin WH, Ehsani AA, Holloszy JO. Carbohydrate feeding during prolonged strenuous exercise can delay fatigue. *J Appl Physiol.* 1983;55:230–235.
41. Coyle EF, Coggan AR, Hemmert WK, Ivy JL. Muscle glycogen utilization during prolonged strenuous exercise when fed carbohydrate. *J Appl Physiol.* 1986;61:165–172.
42. Millard-Stafford ML, Sparling PB, Rosskopf LB, Hinson BT, Dicarlo LJ. Carbohydrate-electrolyte replacement improves distance running performance in the heat. *Med Sci Sports Exerc.* 1992;24:934–940.
43. Wilber RL, Moffatt RJ. Influence of carbohydrate ingestion on blood glucose and performance in runners. *Int J Sport Nutr.* 1994;2:317–327.

44. Hawley JA., Dennis SC, Noakes TD. Oxidation of carbohydrate ingested during prolonged endurance exercise. *Sports Med.* 1992;14:27–42.

45. Chambers ES, Bridge MW, Jones DA. Carbohydrate sensing in the human mouth: effects on exercise performance and brain activity. *J Physiol.* 2009;587:1779–1794.

46. Nicholas CW, Williams C, Lakomy HK, Phillips G, Nowitz A. Influence of ingesting a carbohydrate-electrolyte solution on endurance capacity during intermittent, high-intensity shuttle running. *J Sport Sci.* 1995;13:283–290.

47. Nicholas CW, Tsintzas K, Boobis L, Williams C. Carbohydrate-electrolyte ingestion during intermittent high-intensity running. *Med Sci Sport Exerc.* 1999;31:1280–1286.

48. Welsh RS, Davis JM, Burke JR, Williams HG. Carbohydrates and physical/mental performance during intermittent exercise to fatigue. *Med Sci Sports Exerc.* 2002;34:723–731.

49. Foskett A, Williams C, Boobis L, Tsintzas K. Carbohydrate availability and muscle energy metabolism during intermittent running. *Med Sci Sports Exerc.* 2008;40:96–103.

50. Jentjens RL, Achten J, Jeukendrup AE. High oxidation rates from combined carbohydrates ingested during exercise. *Med Sci Sports Exerc.* 2004;36:1551–1558.

51. Jentjens RL, Jeukendrup AE. High rates of exogenous carbohydrate oxidation from a mixture of glucose and fructose ingested during prolonged cycling exercise. *Br J Nutr.* 2005;93:485–492.

52. Jentjens RL, Moseley L, Waring RH, Harding LK, Jeukendrup AE. Oxidation of combined ingestion of glucose and fructose during exercise. *J Appl Physiol.* 2004;96:1277–1284.

53. Jentjens RL, Underwood K, Achten J, Currell K, Mann CH, Jeukendrup AE. Exogenous carbohydrate oxidation rates are elevated after combined ingestion of glucose and fructose during exercise in the heat. *J Appl Physiol.* 2006;100:807–816.

54. Shi X, Summers RW, Schedl HP, Flanagan SW, Chang R, Gisofi CV. Effects of carbohydrate type and concentration and solution osmolality on water absorption. *Med Sci Sport Exerc.* 1995;27:1607–1615.

55. Currell K, Jeukendrup AE. Superior endurance performance with ingestion of multiple transportable carbohydrates. *Med Sci Sports Exerc.* 2008;40:275–281.

56. Juekendrup AE. Carbohydrate and performance: the role of multiple transportable carbohydrates. *Curr Opin Clin Nutr Metab Care.* 2010;13:452–457.

57. Murray R, Paul GL, Seifert JG, Eddy DE, Halby GA. The effects of glucose, fructose, and sucrose ingestion during exercise. *Med Sci Sports Exerc.* 1989;21:275–282.

58. Roergs RA, McMinn SB, Mermier C, Leabetter G, Ruby B, Quinn C. Blood glucose and glucoregulatory hormone responses to solid and liquid carbohydrate ingestion during exercise. *Int J Sport Nutr.* 1998;8:70–83.

59. Lugo M, Sherman WM, Wimer GS, Garleb K. Metabolic responses when different forms of carbohydrate energy are consumed during cycling. *Int J Sport Nutr.* 1993;3:398–407.

60. Coleman E. Update on carbohydrate: solid versus liquid. *Int J Sport Nutr.* 1994;4:80–88.

61. Pfeiffer B, Stellingwerff T, Zaltas E, Jeukendrup AE. CHO oxidation from a CHO gel compared with a drink during exercise. *Med Sci Sports Exerc.* 2010; 42:2038–2045.

62. Pfeiffer B, Stellingwerff T, Zaltas E, Jeukendrup AE. Oxidation of solid versus liquid CHO sources during exercise. *Med Sci Sports Exerc.* 2010;42:2030–2037.

63. Below PR, Mora-Rodriguez R, Gonzalez-Alonso J, Coyle EF. Fluid and carbohydrate ingestion independently improve performance during 1 hour of intense exercise. *Med Sci Sports Exerc.* 1995;27:200–210.

64. Sawka MN, Burke LM, Eichner ER, Maughan RJ, Montain SJ, Stachenfeld NS. American College of Sports Medicine. Position stand: exercise and fluid replacement. *Med Sci Sports Exerc.* 2007;39:377–390.

65. Coyle EF, Montain SJ. Benefits of fluid replacement with carbohydrate during exercise. *Med Sci Sports Exerc.* 1992;24(9 Suppl):S324–S330.

66. O'Conner H, Cox G. Feeding ultra-endurance athletes: an interview with Dr. Helen O'Connor and Gregory Cox. Interview by Louise M Burke. *Int J Sport Nutr Exerc Metab.* 2002;12:490–494.

67. Ivy JL, Katz AL, Cutler CL, Sherman WM, Coyle EF. Muscle glycogen synthesis after exercise: effect of time of carbohydrate ingestion. *J Appl Physiol.* 1988;6:1480–1485.

68. Ivy JL, Lee MC, Broznick JT, Reed MJ. Muscle glycogen storage after different amounts of carbohydrate ingestion. *J Appl Physiol.* 1988;65:2018–2023.

69. Betts JA, Williams C. Short-term recovery from prolonged exercise: exploring the potential for protein ingestion to accentuate the benefits of carbohydrate supplements. *Sports Med.* 2010;40:941–959.
70. Burke LM, Collier GR, Hargreaves M. Muscle glycogen storage after prolonged exercise: effect of glycemic index. *J Appl Physiol.* 1993;75:1019–1023.
71. Reed MJ, Broznick JT, Lee MC, Ivy JL. Muscle glycogen storage postexercise: effect of mode of carbohydrate administration. *J Appl Physiol.* 1989;75:1019–1023.
72. Blom PCS, Hostmark AT, Vaage O, Kardel KR, Maehlum S. Effect of different post-exercise sugar diets on the rate of muscle glycogen synthesis. *Med Sci Sports Exerc.* 1987;19:471–496.
73. Roberts KM, Noble EG, Hayden DB, Taylor AW. Simple and complex carbohydrate-rich diets and muscle glycogen content of marathon runners. *Eur J Appl Physiol.* 1988;57:70–74.
74. Sherman WM. Recovery from endurance exercise. *Med Sci Sports Exerc.* 1992;24(9 Suppl):S336–S339.
75. Zawadzki K, Yaspelkis B, Ivy J. Carbohydrate-protein complex increases the rate of muscle glycogen storage after exercise. *J Appl Physiol.* 1992;72:1854–1859.
76. Van Loon L, Saris W, Kruijshoop M, Wagenmakers A. Maximizing postexercise muscle glycogen synthesis: carbohydrate supplementation and the application of amino acid or protein hydrolysate mixtures. *Am J Clin Nutr.* 2000;72:106–111.
77. Jentjens R, van Loon L, Mann C, Wagenmakers AJ, Jeukendrup AE. Additional protein and amino acids to carbohydrates does not enhance postexercise muscle glycogen synthesis *J Appl Physiol.* 2001;91:839–846.
78. Van Hall G, Shirreffs S, Calbet J. Muscle glycogen resynthesis during recovery from cycle exercise: no effect of additional protein ingestion. *J Appl Physiol.* 2000;88:1631–1636.
79. Carrithers J, Williamson D, Gallagher P, Godard MP, Schulze KE, Trappe SW. Effects of postexercise carbohydrate-protein feedings on muscle glycogen restoration. *J Appl Physiol.* 2000;88:1976–1982.
80. Phillips SM, Moore DR, Tang JE. A critical examination of dietary protein requirements, benefits and excesses in athletes. *Int J Sport Nutr Exerc Metab.* 2007;17(Suppl):S58–S76.
81. Hawley JA, Burke LM. Carbohydrate availability and training adaptation: effects on cell metabolism. *Exerc Sport Sci Rev.* 2010;38:152–160.
82. Burke LM. Fueling strategies to optimize performance: training high or training low? *Scand J Med Sci Sports.* 2010;20(Suppl 2):48–58.
83. Hansen AK, Fischer CP, Plomgaard P, Andersen JL, Saltin B, Pedersen BK. Skeletal muscle adaptation: training twice every second day vs. training once daily. *J Appl Physiol.* 2005;98:93–99.
84. Yeo WK, Paton CD, Garnham AP, Burke LM, Carey AL, Hawley JA. Skeletal muscle adaptation and performance responses to once a day versus twice every second day endurance training regimens. *J Appl Physiol.* 2008;105:1462–1470.
85. Morton JP, Croft L, Bartlett JD, Maclaren DP, Reilly T, Evans L, McArdle A, Drust B. Reduced carbohydrate availability does not modulate training-induced heat shock protein adaptations but does upregulate oxidative enzyme activity in human skeletal muscle. *J Appl Physiol.* 2009;106:1513–1521.
86. Hulston CJ, Venables MC, Mann CH, Martin C, Philp A, Baar K, Jeukendrup AE. Training with low muscle glycogen enhances fat metabolism in well-trained cyclists. *Med Sci Sports Exerc.* 2010;42:2046–2055.

Chapter 3

PROTEIN AND EXERCISE

Nicholas A. Burd, PhD, and Stuart M. Phillips, PhD, FACN, FACSM

Introduction

The energy for muscle contraction was originally hypothesized to be derived from the "explosive break-down of protein molecules" (1). Indeed, the evaluation of daily dietary protein intake among certain cohorts of athletes (eg, bodybuilders, power and/or strength athletes) suggests that many athletes are still firm believers in the aforementioned thesis, reflected by their excessively high protein intakes (2). However, scientists and sports dietitians generally regard protein intake to be inconsequential with respect to providing energy for muscle contraction. For instance, amino acids provide only a minor portion (~2% to 4%) of energy contribution during prolonged dynamic exercise (3,4). This is despite the capacity of human skeletal muscle to oxidize at least seven amino acids during exercise, including the branched chain amino acids (BCAA)—leucine, valine, and isoleucine—which are the amino acids oxidized to the greatest extent (5). Despite the relatively low use of amino acids as fuel during exercise, exercise does have profound influences on skeletal muscle protein turnover: muscle protein synthesis (MPS) and muscle protein breakdown (MPB). For example, distinct phenotypic adaptations occur in response to divergent exercise training stimuli, such as resistance exercise leading to hypertrophy and aerobic exercise leading to an enhanced oxidative capacity. However, to maximize skeletal muscle adaptation induced by a training stimulus, regardless the mode of exercise, intake of dietary protein is fundamental.

This chapter is a practical reference tool about protein and exercise for the scientist, athlete, and general fitness enthusiast. A general overview of muscle protein turnover with regards to both resistance and endurance exercise is provided. Further details on such topics as protein quality, quantity, and timing of ingestion in relation to both resistance and endurance exercise is provided where relevant. Human studies are emphasized; however, other animal models are examined when there is inadequate human research.

Muscle Protein Turnover

Muscle protein turnover (MPS and MPB) is a synchronous and continuous process in human muscle. During the course of the day, fasted-state losses of muscle protein are counterbalanced by fed-state gains of muscle protein so that over time the muscle net protein balance equation (NPB = MPS – MPB) is zero and skeletal muscle mass remains essentially unchanged (Figure 3.1) (6).

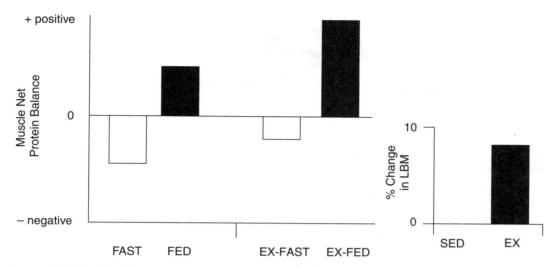

FIGURE 3.1   Muscle net protein balance (NPB) at rest and after feeding and resistance exercise. It is important to note that resistance exercise is fundamentally anabolic such that NPB becomes less negative in the fasted state. The inset illustrates the training-induced changes in lean body mass that manifest from the synergist effect of feeding dietary amino acids and exercise. However, in the absence of an anabolic stimulus, lean body mass remains essentially unchanged, such as in sedentary individuals. **Key**: SED, sedentary; EX, exercise; FAST, fasting for 12 hours; FED, feeding dietary amino acids; EX-FAST, exercise in fasting state; EX-FED, exercise and feeding; LBM, lean body mass.

A detailed description of the regulation of muscle protein turnover is beyond the scope of this chapter; however, a general understanding of the protein pools controlling protein turnover will solidify the concepts presented throughout the chapter. Briefly, consumption of dietary protein is followed by an increase in the concentration of amino acids in the blood, which subsequently are transported into the muscle and ultimately double the rate of MPS (7). It is generally assumed by scientists that the muscle intracellular free amino acid pool functions as a link between the environment and muscle proteins. The amino acid inputs to the muscle intracellular free amino acid pool can come from the blood amino acids during feeding or from the breaking down of muscle proteins during the fasting state. Of course, not all amino acids are used for building muscle proteins. For example, de novo synthesis can occur for certain nonessential amino acids, amino acid use in intermediary metabolism, and oxidation. It is noteworthy that, the muscle aminoacyl-tRNA is really the free amino acid pool leading to MPS. However, because the muscle aminoacyl-tRNA pool is analytically challenging for the scientist to measure in the laboratory, the muscle intracellular free amino acid pool is assumed to be the true precursor pool leading to muscle protein synthesis (8).

Resistance Exercise

Resistance exercise is fundamentally anabolic. For instance, after an isolated bout of resistance exercise, NPB becomes more positive and this effect can last as long as approximately 2 days after the stimulus in untrained subjects (9). Chronic application of resistance exercise (ie, training) results in myofibrillar protein (the predominate protein in skeletal muscle) accretion and an increase in skeletal muscle fiber size and ultimately lean body mass (10,11). Recent research has illustrated that resistance training can have profound effects on muscle protein turnover. For example, resting MPS is chronically elevated in resistance-trained subjects (12–14) whereas MPB is attenuated compared to untrained subjects (15).

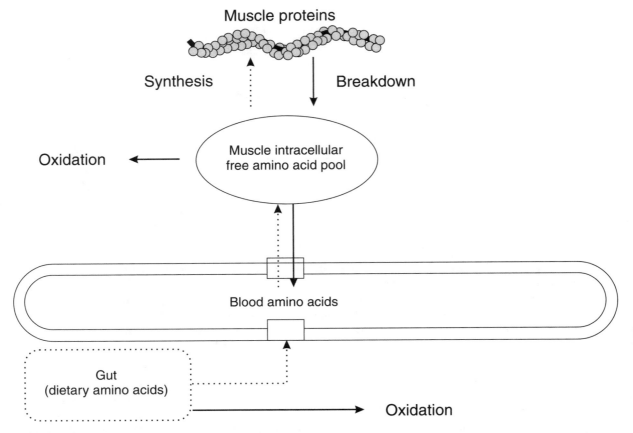

FIGURE 3.2   General overview of the fate of dietary amino acids and protein pools in the body. "Muscle proteins" is a collective term referring to myofibrillar, sarcoplasmic, and mitochondrial proteins. These specific protein subfractions comprise ~60%, ~30%, and ~10% of skeletal muscle, respectively. Solid arrows represent anabolic destinations. Dashed arrows represent catabolic destinations.

Furthermore, resistance training seems to shorten the duration and amplitude of the elevation of MPS after acute resistance exercise (16). The smaller amplitude and duration of the MPS with training suggests an increased need for attention to training-based variables such as load, intensity (ie, effort put forth), and exercise order to maintain a relatively "unique" exercise stimulus. In addition, the importance of timing with regards to feeding dietary protein (ie, essential amino acids; EAAs) close to the completion of the exercise also becomes important in maximizing protein accretion and the subsequent gains in muscle mass. As highlighted in Figure 3.2, postexercise feeding is important in supporting a positive NPB and ultimately eliciting an adaptation (ie, muscle hypertrophy, strength, increases in oxidation capacity). However, as will be discussed in this chapter, certain feeding patterns may be superior to others in inducing positive effects on skeletal muscle.

Endurance Exercise

Studies examining muscle protein turnover utilizing stable isotope methodology after acute aerobic exercise suggests that aerobic exercise can induce increases in MPS, although the response is smaller in both amplitude and duration (13,17–19) compared with resistance exercise (9,14,15,20,21). The training adaptations that occur with aerobic and resistance exercise are markedly different, but aerobic exercise induces considerable increases in oxidative capacity (22) and is generally not associated with substantial amounts of muscle hypertrophy. However, this is not always the case, at least in muscle in the elderly. Specifically, it has been demonstrated that aerobic exercise training can increase thigh muscle volume and single muscle fiber size in older study participants (23). Indeed, resistance training has profound effects on type II fiber area and whole-muscle cross-sectional area (10,11,24,25). Therefore, a logical question would be: if both modes of exercise are inducing increases in MPS, then how is it that these contrasting adaptations occur? Recent data suggest that this can be answered by the types of proteins being synthesized, specifically, mitochondrial (ie, energy-transducing component of skeletal muscle) or myofibrillar (ie, force-producing component of skeletal muscle) in response to aerobic and resistance exercise, respectively (13). Aerobic exercise is generally not associated with prolonged periods of elevations in MPS between training sessions as has been reported with resistance training. Specifically, high-intensity/higher volume resistance exercise can stimulate muscle protein rates for at least 2 days after the acute bout (9). In contrast, MPS is increased for only 2 to 3 hours after the performance of lower intensity aerobic exercise (17,26). However, in an aerobic exercise model that involves unilateral knee extension exercise (which has higher forces per kg of active muscle than cycling or walking), the elevation in MPS is as long-lasting as it is with resistance exercise (19). Thus, a force-MPS relationship that is very likely muscle protein fraction dependent exists. In other words, higher forces elicit increases, which seem to be longer lasting, in myofibrillar protein synthesis, and lower forces elicit increases in mitochondrial and the synthesis of other sarcoplasmic proteins.

Protein Timing: The Clock Is Ticking

Resistance Exercise

Research on maximizing hypertrophy has emphasized the timing of postexercise protein intake. Some of the findings have led to some extreme recommendations, including "peri-workout" nutrition, which describes the concept of feeding protein both pre- and postexercise. Previously, dietary protein recommendations for athletes focused on total daily protein intake, with less emphasis on the timing of protein intake. Considerable research has been devoted to exploring the optimal timing of protein intake to maximize the acute anabolic response and eventual hypertrophy that occurs after resistance training.

Pre-exercise Feeding

In an attempt to determine the optimal time to deliver dietary amino acids to the exercised muscle to optimize anabolism, numerous studies have examined protein ingestion within a short time of resistance exercise (ie, before and/or after) (6). Earlier work demonstrated that administering 6 g of EAA (equivalent to ~15 g of high-quality protein, such as whey) and 35 g sucrose before resistance exercise induced a 160% greater increase in muscle anabolism when compared with a similar drink consumed postexercise. This superior effect was attributed to the pre-exercise supplement promoting an almost 4-fold exercise-induced hyperemia and a subsequent increase in the delivery and uptake of amino acids to the muscle (27). In a subsequent study, Tipton and colleagues examined the influence of intact proteins (ie, whey) fed immediately before or after resistance exercise (28). Both feeding patterns induced similar anabolic responses because there was no stimulation of hyperemia with exercise. However, there were large individual differences in the anabolic responses to pre– and post–resistance exercise feeding, which led the researchers to speculate that "certain" individuals may be more responsive to pre-exercise feeding to induce muscle anabolism (28).

During Exercise

Just as pre– vs post–resistance exercise feeding is controversial, so too is the physiological relevance of feeding during acute resistance exercise (ie, while the muscle is contracting). Indeed, in the fasting state, it has been demonstrated that the energy-consuming process of MPS is not elevated during resistance exercise (20,29,30), and this down-regulation of MPS may be attributed to activation of adenosine monophosphate protein kinase (AMPK), the so-called energy sensor in the muscle cell (20). However, coingestion of carbohydrate (50% glucose and 50% maltodextrin) and casein protein hydrolysate, which in this case would essentially mimic whey (31), during a combined endurance and whole-body resistance exercise session stimulates MPS even when this exercise bout was done when the subjects had eaten before exercise (32). It was speculated that this positive result on MPS during exercise may have been attributed to an enhanced MPS during the rest periods between the exercise sets. What is noteworthy is that this accelerated MPS during exercise did not further augment net muscle protein accretion during the subsequent overnight recovery (32). Therefore, there seems to be little benefit to feeding during the resistance exercise to induce muscle hypertrophy.

After Exercise

Early work by Esmarck and colleagues (33) demonstrated the importance of consuming protein near the time of the exercise bout. Specifically, elderly men (age ~74 years) performed resistance training 3 times a week for 12 weeks and were randomly assigned to receive a high-protein (from nonfat milk and soy) supplement (10 g protein, 7 g carbohydrate, 3 g fat) immediately after or 2 hours after each training session. It was demonstrated that subjects consuming the supplement immediately after each training session had significant increases in thigh muscle mass, whereas delaying protein supplementation by as little as 2 hours after training showed no change in muscle mass (33). Indeed, these data are difficult to reconcile because increases in muscle mass and strength are hallmark adaptations to resistance exercise, regardless of whether a specific nutrition intervention is used in the young or the elderly (25,34–38). Furthermore, in elderly men who habitually consume adequate dietary protein (1.1 ± 0.1 g/kg/d), 10 g of additional protein (ie, casein hydrolysate) supplementation both before and after training had no additional effect on muscle mass and strength gains compared to the nonsupplemented group (39). The importance of a positive energy balance during a resistance training regimen cannot be overestimated, as it has been suggested that an increase of approximately 15% in total energy intake may be necessary to maintain body weight and to support muscle protein accretion during a training period (40). It seems that women (ages 49–74 years) undergoing resistance training for 21 weeks can benefit from appropriate nutrition, guided by nutrition counseling (41). Subjects who were counseled displayed greater increases in thigh muscle mass (~9.5%) as compared to a group without counseling (~6.8%). It is suggested that the main reason for these results is due to increases in energy from protein and the ratio of polyunsaturated to saturated fatty acids.

Resistance-trained men participated in a 12-week training program and were randomly assigned to groups consuming a protein supplement (whey protein, glucose, creatine) either in the morning before breakfast and late evening before bed or pre- and postworkout. The peri-workout nutrition induced superior gains in lean body mass and strength (42). However, in a study using a similar design, there was no difference between the groups consuming the protein supplement (proprietary blend of whey and casein) in the morning/evening or following a peri-workout nutrition protocol after a 10-week resistance training program (43). The authors noted, however, that low energy intakes (~29 kcal/kg/d), regardless of training group, were less than the recommended values for active individuals (43). In another study attempting to delineate the importance of protein timing in relation to resistance training (44), a randomized within-subject crossover design was used. Young men consumed a protein supplement (~40 g casein) twice daily either in the morning and evening (timing of protein intake was not immediately pre- or postworkout) or pre- and postexercise (close to their workout). The group who consumed their supplement in the morning and evening after the training sessions experienced greater increases in fat-free mass than with the other supplement protocol after 8 weeks of resistance training.

Marked differences in study designs, training length, and the type of protein utilized during the training periods in these studies (42–44) preclude the ability to make accurate recommendations about the timing of protein ingestion. However, as a general guideline protein intake close to exercise, and after exercise in particular, seems to offer some benefit in lean mass gains.

Other lines of evidence, in which timing of protein ingestion was not the major manipulated variable, lend support to the conclusion that ingesting protein close to exercise matters in determining lean mass gains. Hartman et al (10) reported lean mass gains in a large cohort (n = 56) of young men after 13 weeks of intense resistance training. To test whether milk was superior to soy or calories from carbohydrate at inducing gains in lean mass, subjects were randomly assigned to consume 500 mL of fat-free milk (18 g protein); an isonitrogenous, isoenergetic fat-free soy drink (18 g protein); or a carbohydrate control (0 g protein) immediately after resistance exercise and again 1 hour after exercise. In this study, milk induced superior increases in type II fiber size and fat- and bone-free mass compared to soy. These data illustrate that the intake of a high-quality protein within the first 2 hours after training is fundamental to maximize the hypertrophic adaptations, but these results also highlight a previously unrecognized benefit of milk proteins vs soy protein. Furthermore, studies show that resistance exercise and feeding are synergistic (6), and that MPS is elevated to the greatest extent within the initial hours after the exercise session (21), so it would seem that eating protein early offers substantial benefits. That is not to say, however, that feeding at a later time does not offer benefits, as illustrated in Figure 3.3. It seems that the synergistic effect of exercise and feeding exists even on the subsequent day after a resistance exercise bout. We studied a group of young subjects who consumed 15 g of whey protein after an acute bout of resistance exercise and demonstrated that the muscle remains more "anabolically sensitive" up to 24 hours (45). The underlying mechanisms that allow this synergism of exercise and feeding to occur the following day are unknown, but may be related to

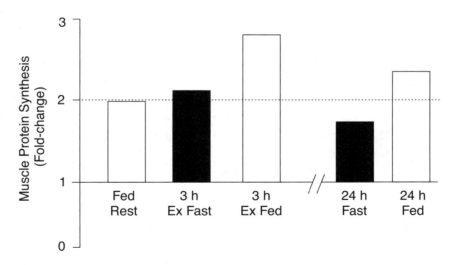

FIGURE 3.3   Fold-change from fasted state resting conditions in muscle protein synthesis after feeding and resistance. Note that the "anabolic sensitizing" effect of resistance exercise is greatest during the immediate acute recovery period; however, this sensitizing effect is still conferred more than 1 day after exercise. The dashed line illustrates the summation of the fed response following exercise.

the anabolic signaling molecules that "turn on" muscle protein synthesis and are more sensitive to feeding. Moreover, it has recently been demonstrated that after consumption of 10 g of EAA that an increase in skeletal muscle amino acid transporters are up-regulated, which may assist in the transport of amino acids into the free amino acid pool (46). It may be that resistance exercise also increases amino acid transport proteins and this phenomenon may last into the days after the exercise bout and ultimately sensitize the muscle to feeding; however, this notion has yet to be investigated.

Endurance Exercise

It has been suggested that feeding protein during endurance exercise may offer some additional performance benefits as compared to feeding carbohydrate alone. For example, it has been demonstrated that consumption of protein (~3.8 g) with carbohydrate (~16 g) given in small doses during 3 hours of intense cycling increased time to exhaustion vs a placebo or carbohydrate only trial in trained male cyclists (47). The beneficial effects of protein supplementation during exercise are not just isolated to this study (48,49); in a well-designed, double-blind, repeated-measures placebo-controlled crossover study, it was reported that there was no additional benefit from the protein coingested with carbohydrate as compared to carbohydrate alone (50). Another study established that in moderately well-trained cyclists coingestion of protein with carbohydrate, as compared with carbohydrate alone, during a 90-minute bout of cycling did not influence the magnitude of glycogen or phosphocreatine utilization or a 20-km time trial performance measured approximately 24 hours after the first exercise bout (51). This finding is in agreement with other data that illustrated no beneficial effect on performance (52,53). Due to the conflicting evidence, it seems that coingestion of protein with carbohydrate during endurance exercise is not beneficial to performance gains. However, as explained in the following paragraphs, protein is fundamental in supporting a positive NPB and the subsequent adaptation to aerobic exercise.

In a recent study, researchers sought to determine the response of whole-body protein turnover in athletes (eg, triathletes, ultramarathon runners, cyclists) who exercise for extended periods of time (ie, > 5 h/d during competition/training) (54). A secondary aim was to investigate whether the addition of protein to carbohydrate ingestion could improve NPB during exercise and recovery compared to carbohydrate alone. Participants performed 2.5 hours of cycling at moderate intensity, followed by 1 hour of treadmill running, followed by another 2.5 hours of cycling (6 hours of total exercise time). Participants were given carbohydrates or carbohydrates and protein before, during, and after exercise. It was established that prolonged exercise did not increase protein breakdown and/or increase protein synthesis as compared to resting situations in these highly trained endurance athletes (55). Furthermore, protein and carbohydrate coingestion improved whole-body NPB by increasing whole-body MPS and decreasing whole-body MPB, resulting in a positive whole body NPB during exercise recovery. These results (55) further illustrate a potential importance of feeding even a small amount of protein during endurance exercise.

In a similar manner as resistance exercise, the importance of protein consumption soon after endurance exercise is most likely equally as important. Hallmark adaptations that occur with aerobic training are increases in capillarization, mitochondrial biogenesis, and increased glucose and fat transporters (56–59). These adaptations all require the "turning over" of proteins and a net addition of new proteins, or in other words, a positive NPB to support optimum adaptation. Providing support for this notion, recent data demonstrated that after a 2-hour bout of cycling, participants who consumed protein (~36 g/h), albeit an excessively high dose, with carbohydrate during postexercise recovery, had enhanced rates of muscle protein synthesis that were greater than after consumption of carbohydrate only after the same exercise bout (60). Unfortunately, only mixed muscle protein synthesis was determined and, as such, it cannot be determined whether the additional protein enhanced the synthesis of myofibrillar or mitochondrial proteins. Of note, the additional protein did not enhance glycogen replenishment during the 4-hour postexercise recovery period (60), but it did facilitate the net synthesis of proteins.

Similar to resistance exercise, aerobic exercise seems to have a nutrient-sensitizing effect on skeletal muscle (61). It was demonstrated on the day after a bout of low-intensity (ie, treadmill walking) aerobic exercise for 45 minutes that the normal muscle protein synthetic response to hyperinsulinamemia in older individuals is restored (61), suggesting a nutrient-sensitizing effect of exercise on skeletal muscle. However, the researchers only examined mixed muscle protein synthesis (ie, the aggregate response of all the proteins in muscle), and therefore it cannot be determined which protein fractions were being affected (ie, myofibrillar, sarcoplasmic, or mitochondrial). Recent data suggest that this response may have been confined to the mitochondrial or sarcoplasmic protein pools. Data reveal that aerobic exercise preferentially stimulates the synthesis of mitochondrial proteins, whereas resistance training stimulates myofibrillar protein synthesis (13). Older subjects performing 12 weeks of training on a cycle ergometer (~60%–80% of heart rate reserve) for 20 minutes had an approximate 12% increase in thigh muscle volume but had a significant decline in myofibrillar concentration (23). These data suggest that other proteins (eg, mitochondrial) were being accrued or possibly that the aerobic exercise enhanced the sensitivity to feeding after each exercise, which over time resulted in protein accretion. Collectively, these data (23,61) suggest that, similar to resistance exercise, aerobic exercise can improve the receptiveness of the protein synthetic machinery to feeding for at least a day after exercise.

From a practical perspective, the caloric demands of aerobic exercise are generally greater than a high-intensity/effort resistance exercise that lasts approximately 30 to 60 minutes in duration, as a single session of aerobic exercise can be sustained for much longer than resistance exercise. Therefore, it is paramount that energy needs are met after aerobic exercise to ensure that the dietary protein is being used for protein synthesis and not being unnecessarily oxidized to meet energy needs (62). Lastly, an individual's diet (ie, daily protein intake) should be assessed before recommendations on supplemental protein are made. The timing of protein intake immediately after exercise seems to be important because this is when protein synthesis is stimulated to the greatest extent; however, the postexercise "window of anabolic opportunity" is greater than what is perhaps commonly believed. The synergistic effect of exercise and feeding on muscle protein synthesis rates still exists, albeit to a lesser extent than feeding immediately after exercise, for at least 24 hours after exercise (45). There is certainly time after exercise to prepare a well-balanced meal that includes high-quality dietary proteins, rather than focusing on supplemental powders or drinks.

Protein Type: "Protein Quality" and Leucine as an Anabolic Trigger

After the consumption of dietary protein, depending on the amount of protein, there is a considerable hyperaminoacidemia compared to fasting levels. Different types of proteins have different digestion kinetics so that the rate of appearance of amino acids in the blood differs substantially based on the type of dietary protein consumed (63-68). In recent years, whey protein, the soluble fraction extracted from milk as a result of cheese manufacturing, has become exceedingly popular within the athletic population as a dietary supplement. Whey protein exists as concentrates (ie, ~80% protein), isolates (usually > 90% protein), and hydrolysates (usually > 90% protein) in powder form. However, for the purpose of this chapter, *whey protein* will be a collective term to describe all three types. Whey protein has a high quality based on its protein digestibility corrected amino acid score (PDCAAS), meaning that its amino acid composition is close or, in most cases, exceeds that of human body proteins, and that it is rapidly and easily digested. Whey protein contains very high concentrations of EAAs, with a surprisingly disproportionate amount of leucine (~14%) of the total amino acid composition. It has been proven that consumption of only the essential amino acids is necessary to stimulate MPS (69), which highlights the importance of consuming a high-quality protein. The importance of leucine as a modulator of muscle protein synthesis (70) has made it a popular supplement among strength-training individuals. This practice is a case of false reasoning. For example, if one assumes that de novo synthesis of nonessential amino acids could keep pace with the stimulatory effect of leucine in its free form on muscle protein synthesis, it would be inevitable that the muscle intracellular free amino acid pool would become depleted of the other EAAs and muscle protein synthesis would be impaired. A superior method of "supplementing" a diet is to simply consume high-quality proteins (containing all the amino acids to build muscle protein) that are rich in leucine (eg, chicken, beef, egg, milk proteins).

An intriguing topic is the essential nature and signaling role of leucine in the stimulation of MPS. For example, could an enriched suboptimal dose of protein be suboptimal simply due to its leucine content? Specifically, if a suboptimal dose of protein is based on the findings that 10 g EAA (~25 g whey) maximizes the anabolic response in young men at rest (71) and exercise sensitizes the muscle to feeding in such a way that 8.6 g EAA maximizes MPS after acute resistance exercise (72), could it be that an approximate 5- to 10-g dose of high-quality protein enriched with leucine equivalent to approximately 25 g whey could also elicit a maximal protein synthetic response? Although this effect currently remains uninvestigated in humans, recent rodent data lend a clue that this may certainly be true (73). The exact explanation behind leucine, as an anabolic signal, remains somewhat elusive. Leucine is insulinogenic, but insulin is not particularly anabolic above levels already present at fasting levels (ie, 5 mcU/mL), and its influence on MPB fully manifests itself at insulin levels of approximately 30 mcU/mL (74), a concentration commonly obtained after a mixed meal. Leucine also may serve as an anabolic mediator by its ability to increase the transport of other amino acids into muscle, where they can accumulate in the muscle free amino acid pool and ultimately be used for protein synthesis (75). A interesting finding from Trappe and colleagues (76) indicating that leucine alone is unable to rescue inactivity-induced atrophy, was that women during bed rest supplemented with a leucine-enriched diet in absence of an exercise stimulus, manifested greater losses of thigh muscle volume as compared to control subjects. It was speculated that leucine acted as an anabolic signaling molecule to "turn on" muscle protein synthesis but also stimulated breakdown, as these processes are linked (77). Thus, the increase in muscle protein turnover without the anabolic stimulus of some form of exercise, let alone resistance exercise, to stimulate the accretion of muscle proteins, meant these amino acids were lost.

Data support the "efficiency" of EAAs, as compared with whey, in stimulating MPS in the elderly (78). A consumption of 15 g EAA induced a superior response in muscle protein synthesis (~1.6-fold increase) as compared to 15 g whey (~1.3-fold increase above rest). These findings are not surprising given that 15 g whey is equivalent to only approximately 6 g EAA, and considering that most high-quality proteins are approximately 40% to 45% EAA, which illustrates that this study is merely a dose-response trial. When these data are considered in combination with other data demonstrating that 20 g of isolated egg protein maximally stimulates the anabolic response after resistance exercise (72), it is easy to see that 15 g EAA vs 6 g EAA are at higher and lower points on the dose-response curve. Therefore, comparing 15 g EAAs (supramaximal dose) to 15 g (suboptimal dose) whey is slightly biased; however, it has been speculated based on these and other data (27,28,78) that feeding a proprietary formula of EAA in free and peptide form before exercise may lead to superior increases in training-induced lean body mass gain (79). This thesis has never been systematically investigated in a training study against other high-quality proteins (ie, whey, dairy milk, etc) whether consumed either pre- or postexercise, and as such these recommendations are currently unsubstantiated.

Tang and colleagues sought to determine the impact of three commonly consumed high-quality proteins (ie, whey, casein, soy) on muscle protein synthesis after recovery from resistance exercise (66). Milk contains two protein fractions, approximately 20% whey and 80% casein, and based on their rate of digestion are commonly referred to as "fast" and "slow" proteins, respectively (66,67). Casein, which is the acid-insoluble fraction of protein, is produced from the solid fraction of milk after exposure to an acidic environment; it is less commonly used in sport drinks and/or bars because of solubility issues and production cost (80). Casein is commonly recommended to be consumed in the late evening (ie, "nighttime" protein), due to its slow digestion (81). The slow and prolonged release of amino acids into systemic circulation is hypothesized to promote a positive balance during the overnight fast/recovery period and thus a greater accretion of muscle proteins; however, this supposition has very little scientific support. Soy, a vegetable protein, contains a single protein fraction and the rate of digestion more closely resembles whey as compared to casein (82). Tang et al's study (66) provided a unique opportunity to compare "fast" animal- and plant-based proteins vs "slow" animal protein and examine the rate of appearance of plasma amino acids in relation to muscle protein synthesis.

It was reported that after a single bout of resistance exercise that consumption of whey protein induces a superior increase in muscle protein synthesis compared with soy or casein (66). Similarly, a rapid increase in the EAAs (leucine, in particular) was shown after whey protein consumption when compared to soy or casein alone. It is interesting to consider that a certain threshold of EAAs, or more likely simply leucine, in the blood must be reached to maximally "turn on" protein synthesis; this leucine "trigger" hypothesis is illustrated in Figure 3.4. A recent report illustrated a graded response relationship between protein dose and rates of MPS (72). It remains to be established, however, if consuming a meal (ie, carbohydrate, fat, and protein) affects the pattern of aminoacidemia and rates of MPS as compared to the same protein dose consumed alone. It has been suggested that there is a direct relationship between the concentration of extracellular amino acids, particularly leucine, and rates of muscle protein synthesis (83).

The superiority of higher quality proteins in inducing maximal responses after resistance exercise is not a novel phenomenon. Wilkinson et al demonstrated that young men who consumed 500 mL of nonfat

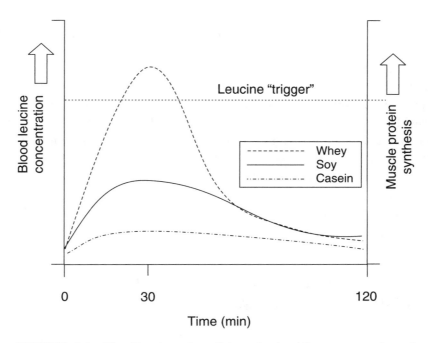

FIGURE 3.4 The "leucine trigger" hypothesis. After consumption of whey protein (which is higher in leucine content than soy or casein), there is a rapid increase in plasma leucine concentration, and this increase corresponds to the extent of stimulation of muscle protein synthesis.

milk elicited a greater anabolic response after strength training than when they consumed an isonitrogenous, isoenergetic, and macronutrient-matched soy beverage (84). A training study confirmed these acute findings in men (10,85). Similarly to these findings, it was found that young men who consume 500 mL milk (~17.5 g protein, ~25.7 g carbohydrate, ~0.4 g fat) within 2 hours after full-body resistance training (5 days/week for 12 weeks) showed the greatest gains in lean body mass and significantly more loss of fat mass as compared to training groups who consumed a soy- or carbohydrate-only product (10). These data (10,84) highlight that examining the acute muscle protein synthetic response can qualitatively predict long-term training adaptations (ie, muscle hypertrophy). The effectiveness of milk in inducing superior training adaptations is not sex-specific, as it has been established that young women who consumed nonfat milk immediately after exercise and an hour later (ie, 2 × 500 mL) had greater increases in bench press strength, greater loss of fat mass, and greater accretion of muscle protein compared to a group who consumed a carbohydrate (isoenergetic, maltodextrin) drink at similar times after whole-body resistance strength training. The women who drank the milk did not gain any weight with strength training, and those in the carbohydrate group had a slight increase in weight. The truly interesting portion of the data is the comparison of the lean mass gains and fat mass losses in both groups, which were far greater in the milk group vs the carbohydrate group. Collectively, these data illustrate that women can clearly benefit by consuming a diet high in healthy low-fat dairy protein, especially when coupled with an anabolic stimulus such as resistance training. This is at odds with the common belief of young women that dairy foods are fattening (85–87).

One typical question related to the beneficial effect of supplementing with milk vs whey after a training period is: would consuming approximately 20 g whey induce superior training adaptations vs consuming, for example, 500 mL of milk? Although this comparison (whey vs milk) has never been investigated, the examination of the current literature would suggest gains in lean body mass and loss of fat mass would be relatively similar (10,42,85,88–90). Of note, however, is that low-fat dairy seems to be exceptionally potent in decreasing fat mass, especially in young women who consume relatively low amounts of dairy (85). This effect may be related to the interplay between calcium and vitamin D on adiopcyte metabolism and inhibition of lipid accretion (91,92).

Finally, it would seem that plant-based proteins (ie, soy) are relatively inferior at eliciting training adaptations as compared to animal proteins (10,93). This supposition leaves a vegetarian athlete at odds with the exact type of protein that should be consumed for optimal recovery from exercise; however, lean mass gains are superior with soy protein consumption than simply consuming carbohydrate alone after exercise (10,93), suggesting that supplementing with soy protein is not entirely without benefit. Of particular interest to a vegetarian athlete may be a plant-based protein, quinoa, whose amino acid composition is superior to soy (94) and similar to milk. Assuming, as with isolated soy protein, that the anti-nutritional components of the quinoa plant can be removed (mainly fiber), then isolated quinoa may be a very beneficial protein source. To date, however, this protein has yet to be produced in supplemental form and certainly has yet to be systematically tested against animal proteins for the anabolic response after exercise.

Protein Quantity: How Much Protein Should an Athlete Consume After Resistance Training?

The optimal dose of protein to maximize the acute anabolic response after exercise is a classic debate on numerous levels (ie, from sport scientists to fitness enthusiasts). This notion is especially true for resistance-trained athletes, who often believe that the larger the dietary protein doses consumed per meal, the larger the increases in lean mass accretion. Recent data would suggest quite the contrary (72). It has been shown

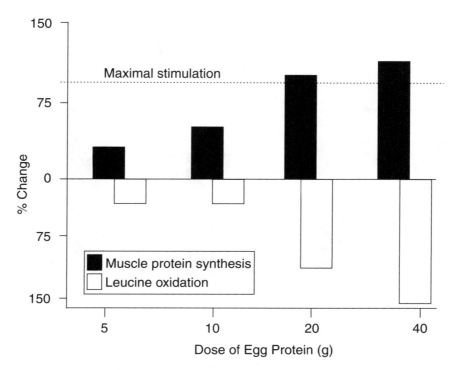

FIGURE 3.5   The relationship between protein dose and muscle protein synthesis. Twenty g of egg protein maximizes the anabolic response to resistance exercise. There is no additional benefit from consuming 40 g of egg protein. Protein consumed in excess is either used for energy or wasted.

that in experienced weight-trained men (~85 kg), the men who consumed varying doses of high-quality isolated egg protein experienced the greatest degree of stimulation of MPS at 20 g, and no further benefit was gained from consuming 20 g of protein compared to 40 g (Figure 3.5) after acute resistance exercise. Of interest, however, is that consuming excess amounts of protein actually increased leucine oxidation (ie, excess amino acids are being utilized for energy production or wasted). This finding of a graded response relationship with the dose of protein consumed and the extent of stimulation of muscle protein synthesis is in agreement with other data that illustrated that MPS is twice as great when 6 g of EAA is consumed compared to approximately 3 g of EAA (95), which is equivalent to approximately 15 g and 7.5 g of a high-quality protein, respectively.

A common and relevant question when attempting to advise athletes about the quantity of protein to consume is, "How does body mass or, more appropriately, lean body mass factor into this recommendation?" That is to say, do individuals with a greater degree of lean body mass (eg, ≥ 90 kg) require more protein than their smaller counterparts (≤ 50 kg)? This is an intriguing question that remains to be systematically investigated. However, considering that larger individuals have a greater absolute volume of blood (96) and, based on the notion that the blood amino acid concentrations after dietary protein consumption (specifically the leucine "trigger" hypothesis [Figure 3.4]) are a primary factor in determining the increase in MPS after acute exercise, it would not be completely inconceivable that larger individuals require more protein, and vice versa for their smaller counterparts (Figure 3.6). However, the maximal dose of protein, as noted in Figure 3.6, is most likely not too far off (ie, ± 5 g protein) from the maximal dose of 20 g that has been previously demonstrated (72).

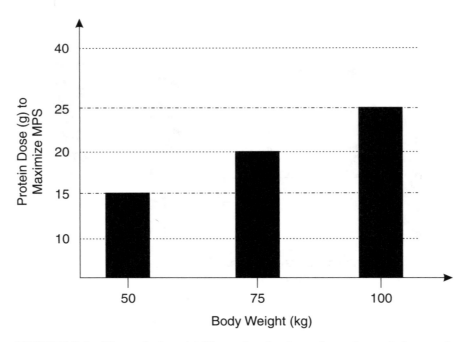

FIGURE 3.6 Theoretical model illustrating the dose of protein needed to maximally stimulate muscle protein synthesis (MPS) after an acute bout of resistance exercise. Note that this thesis has never been systematically tested and as such is purely speculative.

Recommendations for individuals who have been training for a period of time (≥ 8 weeks) may require special consideration. If a sports dietitian were to simply base recommendations on the fact that resistance exercise increases protein synthesis (9), then it would be quite possible that higher protein intakes are required to support this elevated response (97). However, recent data suggest this hypothesis is fallacious. Hartman et al have demonstrated that 12 weeks of resistance training decreases both whole-body protein synthesis and breakdown, with a resulting improved net protein balance when measured over the course of 24 hours (98), compared to the untrained state. These findings imply a greater retention of dietary nitrogen (ie, protein) after resistance training than before a person begins a training program, which is consistent with the anabolic nature of resistance exercise in stimulating muscle to "hang on" to more of its protein mass. It has been established that turnover of whole-body leucine (an essential amino acid that is largely oxidized in skeletal muscle) decreases in both the fasting and fed states after 12 weeks of resistance training, with a concomitant increase in fiber size (99). This suggests greater use of amino acids for protein accretion or simply a greater net retention, which further suggests that protein requirements are not elevated in strength-trained individuals (100–102). The underlying mechanisms for the decreased protein requirements with training may be 2-fold: (*a*) resistance exercise in the fasted state improves muscle net protein balance (9,14), suggesting a more efficient use of intracellular amino acids, and (*b*) aerobic exercise and resistance training preferentially stimulate specific muscle proteins (ie, aerobic exercise stimulates mitochondrial, and resistance exercise stimulates myofibrillar proteins) (13). This indicates skeletal muscle has the ability to direct signals to "turn on" specific proteins in response to a specific exercise stimulus. Thus, it would not be completely unlikely that repeated bouts of an anabolic stimulus on skeletal muscle may predispose muscle tissue to become a greater site of disposition of amino acids than in the untrained state.

BOX 3.1   Sources of High-Quality Protein

The following foods provide 20 g of high-quality protein when consumed in the portions indicated:

- 500 mL (about 2 cups) fat-free milk
- 3 oz beef
- 2.5 oz chicken or turkey
- ¾ cup cottage cheese

Finally, from a practical standpoint, combining differing research findings can illustrate how much and how often an individual could consume protein within a given day. If one assumes that intake of 20 g of a high-quality protein (see Box 3.1 for examples) maximizes the anabolic response for an individual weighing 85 kg (72); considers the data demonstrating that skeletal muscle becomes refractory to the stimulatory effect of amino acids after 2 hours of persistent exposure (103); and recognizes that resistance exercise increases MPS for at least 1 day after the exercise bout (9,104), then it can be hypothesized that an individual could consume 20 g of protein no more than five to six times a day to maximize muscle protein synthesis without excess loss to oxidation (72). However, an interesting thesis is that leucine oxidation may actually serve as a necessary signal to indicate a "leucine threshold" has been reached and sufficient substrate (ie, amino acids) is now available to build muscle proteins.

Protein Quantity: Is Protein Consumption Even Necessary After Endurance Exercise?

Carbohydrates and fats are the primary fuels utilized during endurance exercise (4,105,106), and protein consumption is often not of primary concern for endurance athletes. However, it is worth considering that if dietary protein is not consumed in adequate quantities, then MPB is the only other alternative to supply the amino acids to the intracellular free amino acid pool to ultimately support protein synthesis. Recommendations for nutrition practices in endurance athletes point to studies in nitrogen balance that report that these athletes require as much as 60% to 100% more protein than the Recommended Dietary Allowance (0.8 g/kg/d) to sustain nitrogen balance (107). Furthermore, it is has been established that mitochondrial protein synthesis is stimulated after endurance exercise (13) and this protein fraction is responsive to protein feeding (85). Therefore, consumption of dietary protein after endurance exercise is recommended to ensure an optimal adaptation and exploitation of the protein synthetic stimulus of the exercise itself. The quantity of protein to recommend to endurance athletes largely depends on the athlete's training status, training intensity, and duration of the workout. As highlighted by Tarnopolsky in a recent review (108), a recreational athlete training at a very moderate intensity (~40% VO_{2max}) for approximately 1 hour per day, 4 days per week, would expend approximately 2,000 kcal per week, whereas an elite athlete training at intensities of 60% to 80% VO_{2max} for 8 to 40 hours per week would expend approximately an additional 6,000 to 40,000 kcal per week more than resting energy requirements. The body size of the athlete should be considered because bigger athletes burn more energy than smaller athletes do (109). For these reasons, it is clear that any recommendation should be made on an individual basis and confirmation should be made by monitoring their body weight to ensure the athlete is obtaining adequate energy. Finally, if athletes who are expending large quantities of energy are matching this expenditure with intake, then it is unlikely, even at low percentage of total dietary energy derived from protein, that they are consuming insufficient protein. For example, a 70-kg athlete consuming 4,500 kcal/d and 15% energy from protein still would be consuming 170 g protein (2.4 g/kg) daily.

Current recommendations for endurance athletes' protein requirements are largely based on nitrogen balance studies (108) because studies using direct measures of muscle protein synthesis are lacking (110,111). If the dietary protein consumed contains amino acids and every amino acid contains nitrogen, then it seems quite reasonable that nitrogen balance would be a valid method to assess need. A positive nitrogen balance indicates that consumption of dietary protein was adequate or more than needed, and negative nitrogen balance indicates an inadequate protein intake. However, assessing dietary protein needs utilizing nitrogen balance methodology does have its shortcomings, and this topic has been reviewed elsewhere (2,108,112,113).

A study using stable isotope methodology demonstrated that active young men who performed two 90-minute cycling bouts (one in the morning and one in the afternoon) daily and consumed 1.0 g protein per kilogram per day achieved nitrogen balance during a 24-hour period (110). Another study compared subjects who were habitually fed a high-protein (1.8 g/kg/d) or low-protein (0.7 g/kg/d) diet for 7 days and then walked on a treadmill for 2 hours at a moderate intensity. In this study, leucine oxidation increased after the high-protein diet (114), which indicates the excess protein was utilized for energy. Interestingly, Bolster and colleagues recruited endurance athletes (running ≥ 56 km/wk) and had them consume a low-protein (0.8 g/kg/d), moderate-protein (1.8 g/kg/d), or high-protein (3.6 g/kg/d) diet for 4 weeks (115). Subsequently, the the athletes performed a 75-minute treadmill run at 70% VO_{2peak}. In this study, the fasted-state mixed muscle fractional synthetic rate (a direct measure of muscle protein synthesis) was attenuated during the recovery period following the high-protein dietary intervention as compared to low or moderate protein intakes (115). This result was in contrast to the authors' original hypothesis, which was that habitually consuming a high-protein diet would ultimately expand the free amino acid pool and therefore support greater rates of muscle protein synthesis (115). It was later highlighted in a review of a small subset of these subjects (n = 4) that fractional breakdown rate (a direct measure of muscle protein breakdown) was attenuated after high-protein intakes, such that NPB was improved to a greater extent compared to moderate or low protein intakes (62). These preliminary findings are not entirely surprising because muscle protein synthesis and breakdown have been shown to be tightly coordinated (9). Lastly, it has been demonstrated in highly trained cyclists who engaged in an exercise protocol similar to the Tour de France (ie, long exhausting cycling) that daily protein requirements of 1.5 to 1.8 g/kg are needed to maintain nitrogen balance under such vigorous exercise conditions (116,117).

It seems that diet manipulation can influence the anabolic response to endurance exercise; however, moderate endurance exercise does not increase dietary protein requirements above those of the general population. It seems that athletes engaged in vigorous training may need slightly more dietary protein; however, provided the athlete is consuming adequate energy and 10% to 15% of that is coming from dietary protein, then there is little need to consume excess amounts of protein.

Individual Amino Acids Supplementation: Fact or Fiction?

Glutamine and arginine are amino acids that are purported to have ergogenic effects if consumed in supplemental form. Glutamine, a highly abundant amino acid in the body, is largely synthesized in skeletal muscle and released in plasma during exercise (118,119). Muscle glutamine concentrations have been related to rates of MPS in skeletal muscle of rats, some of which were protein-deficient, endotoxemic, or starved (120), which begs the question of whether the findings can be extended to humans. Glutamine supplementation combined with 6 weeks of resistance training in young adults had no added effect on muscle strength and fat-free mass accretion as compared to a placebo group (121). Furthermore, data demonstrating glutamine ingestion in healthy adult men and women is associated with an approximately 4-fold increase (as compared to control subjects) in plasma growth hormone (122). It was suggested that an increase in plasma growth hormone concentrations following glutamine supplementation may be of significance for strength athletes to maximize training adaptations (80). However, it is not entirely clear whether elevated concentrations of growth hormone within normal physiological concentrations would benefit strength-training athletes. Specifically, West et al have established that exercise-induced "anabolic" hormones (ie, growth hormone, testosterone, insulin-like growth factor), within the physiological limits seen with protein and/or exercise-induced increments, have no influence on MPS (123), strength gains, or muscle hypertrophy (11). Furthermore, recombinant growth hormone has no effect on myofibrillar protein synthesis after resistance exercise in young men (124,125). Therefore, dietary supplementation with glutamine to maximize muscle hypertrophy or strength gains after resistance training is not recommended.

L-arginine is considered a conditionally essential amino acid that is in high demand after periods of rapid growth or physical or pathologic insult such that de novo synthesis cannot be met by normal dietary intake (126–128). However, in healthy adults, arginine can be synthesized in sufficient quantity to meet needs (128–130). Similar to glutamine, a purported benefit of arginine administered intravenously is its ability to stimulate growth hormone release (131). It was demonstrated that oral arginine can stimulate growth hormone (132); these results, however, could not be repeated in another study (133). Furthermore, oral arginine administration in doses of ≥ 10 g resulted in unwanted side effects (ie, abdominal cramps and diarrhea) (133). Regardless the method of administration, the relevance of stimulating growth hormone release in healthy nondeficient adults within physiological limits, insofar as muscle hypertrophy and strength are concerned, is questionable (11,123). It has been established that arginine is not required or stimulatory for muscle protein synthesis (134). Therefore, any ergogenic effect of L-arginine supplementation must be indirect and may be related to the stimulation of nitric oxide production (128). For example, L-arginine is the primary substrate for nitric oxide synthase, the enzyme responsible for nitric oxide production. This leads to the release of nitric oxide from the vascular endothelium, leading to vasodilation and subsequent increase in local blood flow. However, in a randomized and double-blind study, Lysecki et al found that after resistance exercise in young men that consumption of 10 g EAA in combination with 10 g L-arginine (ARG) or an isonitrogenous amount of glycine as a control had no influence on femoral artery blood flow despite an approximate 5-fold increase in blood L-arginine after ARG consumption (135). Furthermore, there was no effect on any markers of nitric oxide (nitrate, nitrite, endothelin-1) and no stimulatory effect on MPS at rest or after exercise (JE Tang and SM Phillips, unpublished observations). Therefore, L-arginine supplementation, provided that sufficient EAA are consumed, has no influence on the anabolic response after resistance exercise. As with glutamine supplementation, supplementation with free-form L-arginine cannot be recommended.

Summary

Recommendations for dietary protein intake should be individualized, but general recommendations are presented in Table 3.1 (27,28,33,45,46,80,85).

Resistance and endurance exercise both have the ability to stimulate MPS; however, the type of proteins that are accrued is related to the nature and stress of the stimulus as noted by diverse adaptations that occur after different modes of exercise. Specifically, resistance exercise preferentially stimulates myofibrillar proteins to aid in force production, and endurance training stimulates the accretion of mitochondria proteins

TABLE 3.1 Daily Protein Recommendations for Endurance- and Resistance-Training Athletes

Type of Training	Protein Recommendation, g/kg/d	Example of Total Daily Protein Intake
Endurance	1.2–1.4	84–98 g for 70-kg (154-1b) endurance athlete
Resistance	1.6–1.7	146–155 g for 91-kg (200-lb) strength athlete

Source: Data are from references 27, 28, 33, 45, 46, 80, and 85.

to assist in sustained energy production during exercise. Ingesting dietary protein after exercise, however, is paramount in supporting a high rate of MPS, which would elicit an optimal adaptation to the exercise stimulus. For example, many researchers have established that provision of protein soon after performance of resistance exercise results in a greater hypertrophic response than when no protein is consumed or when protein consumption is not close to the exercise stimulus (10,136,137). High-quality proteins such as milk, whey, casein, and soy can positively influence the MPS response, but differences in digestion rates and the subsequent rate of appearance of amino acids in the blood may also influence the MPS response such that milk and its isolated forms as whey may confer a further advantage to muscle anabolism. The leucine content of the protein may also be an important component to consider in regards to muscle anabolism. The quantity of protein to consume after exercise is less than what is commonly believed. However, consuming dietary protein within 1 hour after exercise may be of primary concern to elicit optimal training adaptations, provided the athlete is consuming adequate energy throughout the course of the day. Finally, supplementing dietary needs with individual amino acids, specifically glutamine and arginine, has no ergogenic effect in healthy adults.

References

1. Von Liebig J. *Animal Chemistry or Organic Chemistry in Its Application to Physiology*. London, UK: Taylor and Walton; 1842.
2. Phillips SM. Protein requirements and supplementation in strength sports. *Nutrition*. 2004;20:689–695.
3. Phillips SM, Atkinson SA, Tarnopolsky MA, MacDougall JD. Gender differences in leucine kinetics and nitrogen balance in endurance athletes. *J Appl Physiol*. 1993;75:2134–2141.
4. Tarnopolsky MA, Atkinson SA, Phillips SM, MacDougall JD. Carbohydrate loading and metabolism during exercise in men and women. *J Appl Physiol*. 1995;78:1360–1368.
5. Goldberg AL, Chang TW. Regulation and significance of amino acid metabolism in skeletal muscle. *Fed Proc*. 1978;37:2301–2307.
6. Burd NA, Tang JE, Moore DR, Phillips SM. Exercise training and protein metabolism: influences of contraction, protein intake, and sex-based differences. *J Appl Physiol*. 2009;106:1692–1701.
7. Rennie MJ, Edwards RH, Halliday D, Matthews DE, Wolman SL, Millward DJ. Muscle protein synthesis measured by stable isotope techniques in man: the effects of feeding and fasting. *Clin Sci*. 1982;63:519–523.
8. Martini WZ, Chinkes DL, Wolfe RR. The intracellular free amino acid pool represents tracer precursor enrichment for calculation of protein synthesis in cultured fibroblasts and myocytes. *J Nutr*. 2004;134:1546–1550.
9. Phillips SM, Tipton KD, Aarsland A, Wolf SE, Wolfe RR. Mixed muscle protein synthesis and breakdown after resistance exercise in humans. *Am J Physiol*. 1997;273:E99–E107.
10. Hartman JW, Tang JE, Wilkinson SB, Tarnopolsky MA, Lawrence RL, Fullerton AV, Phillips SM. Consumption of fat-free fluid milk after resistance exercise promotes greater lean mass accretion than does consumption of soy or carbohydrate in young, novice, male weightlifters. *Am J Clin Nutr*. 2007;86:373–381.

11. West DW, Burd NA, Tang JE, Moore DR, Staples AW, Holwerda AM, Baker SK, Phillips SM. Elevations in ostensibly anabolic hormones with resistance exercise enhance neither training-induced muscle hypertrophy nor strength of the elbow flexors. *J Appl Physiol.* 2010;108:60–67.

12. Kim PL, Staron RS, Phillips SM. Fasted-state skeletal muscle protein synthesis after resistance exercise is altered with training. *J Physiol.* 2005;568:283–290.

13. Wilkinson SB, Phillips SM, Atherton PJ, Patel R, Yarasheski KE, Tarnopolsky MA, Rennie MJ. Differential effects of resistance and endurance exercise in the fed state on signalling molecule phosphorylation and protein synthesis in human muscle. *J Physiol.* 2008;586:3701–3717.

14. Phillips SM, Parise G, Roy BD, Tipton KD, Wolfe RR, Tarnopolsky MA. Resistance training-induced adaptations in skeletal muscle protein turnover in the fed state. *Can J Physiol Pharmacol.* 2002;80:1045–1053.

15. Phillips SM, Tipton KD, Ferrando AA, Wolfe RR. Resistance training reduces the acute exercise-induced increase in muscle protein turnover. *Am J Physiol.* 1999;276:E118–E124.

16. Tang JE, Perco JG, Moore DR, Wilkinson SB, Phillips SM. Resistance training alters the response of fed state mixed muscle protein synthesis in young men. *Am J Physiol Regul Integr Comp Physiol.* 2008;294:R172–R178.

17. Carraro F, Stuart CA, Hartl WH, Rosenblatt J, Wolfe RR. Effect of exercise and recovery on muscle protein synthesis in human subjects. *Am J Physiol.* 1990;259:E470–E476.

18. Harber MP, Crane JD, Dickinson JM, Jemiolo B, Raue U, Trappe TA, Trappe SW. Protein synthesis and the expression of growth-related genes are altered by running in human vastus lateralis and soleus muscles. *Am J Physiol Regul Integr Comp Physiol.* 2009;296:R708–R714.

19. Miller BF, Olesen JL, Hansen M, Dossing S, Crameri RM, Welling RJ, Langberg H, Flyvbjerg A, Kjaer M, Babraj JA, Smith K, Rennie MJ. Coordinated collagen and muscle protein synthesis in human patella tendon and quadriceps muscle after exercise. *J Physiol.* 2005;567:1021–1033.

20. Dreyer HC, Fujita S, Cadenas JG, Chinkes DL, Volpi E, Rasmussen BB. Resistance exercise increases AMPK activity and reduces 4E-BP1 phosphorylation and protein synthesis in human skeletal muscle. *J Physiol.* 2006;576:613–624.

21. Kumar V, Selby A, Rankin D, Patel R, Atherton P, Hildebrandt W, Williams J, Smith K, Seynnes O, Hiscock N, Rennie MJ. Age-related differences in dose response of muscle protein synthesis to resistance exercise in young and old men. *J Physiol.* 2009;587:211–217.

22. Trappe S, Harber M, Creer A, Gallagher P, Slivka D, Minchev K, Whitsett D. Single muscle fiber adaptations with marathon training. *J Appl Physiol.* 2006;101:721–727.

23. Harber MP, Konopka AR, Douglass MD, Minchev K, Kaminsky LA, Trappe TA, Trappe S. Aerobic exercise training improves whole muscle and single myofiber size and function in older women. *Am J Physiol Regul Integr Comp Physiol.* 2009;297:R1452–R1459.

24. Trappe S, Godard M, Gallagher P, Carroll C, Rowden G, Porter D. Resistance training improves single muscle fiber contractile function in older women. *Am J Physiol Cell Physiol.* 2001;281:C398–C406.

25. Frontera WR, Meredith CN, O'Reilly KP, Knuttgen HG, Evans WJ. Strength conditioning in older men: skeletal muscle hypertrophy and improved function. *J Appl Physiol.* 1988;64:1038–1044.

26. Sheffield-Moore M, Yeckel CW, Volpi E, Wolf SE, Morio B, Chinkes DL, Paddon-Jones D, Wolfe RR. Postexercise protein metabolism in older and younger men following moderate-intensity aerobic exercise. *Am J Physiol Endocrinol Metab.* 2004;287:E513–E522.

27. Tipton KD, Rasmussen BB, Miller SL, Wolf SE, Owens-Stovall SK, Petrini BE, Wolfe RR. Timing of amino acid-carbohydrate ingestion alters anabolic response of muscle to resistance exercise. *Am J Physiol Endocrinol Metab.* 2001;281:E197–E206.

28. Tipton KD, Elliott TA, Cree MG, Aarsland AA, Sanford AP, Wolfe RR. Stimulation of net muscle protein synthesis by whey protein ingestion before and after exercise. *Am J Physiol.* 2007;292:E71–E76.

29. Durham WJ, Miller SL, Yeckel CW, Chinkes DL, Tipton KD, Rasmussen BB, Wolfe RR. Leg glucose and protein metabolism during an acute bout of resistance exercise in humans. *J Appl Physiol.* 2004;97:1379–1386.

30. Rasmussen BB, Tipton KD, Miller SL, Wolf SE, Wolfe RR. An oral essential amino acid-carbohydrate supplement enhances muscle protein anabolism after resistance exercise. *J Appl Physiol.* 2000;88:386–392.

31. Koopman R, Crombach N, Gijsen AP, Walrand S, Fauquant J, Kies AK, Lemosquet S, Saris WH, Boirie Y, van Loon LJ. Ingestion of a protein hydrolysate is accompanied by an accelerated in vivo digestion and absorption rate when compared with its intact protein. *Am J Clin Nutr.* 2009;90:106–115.

32. Beelen M, Tieland M, Gijsen AP, Vandereyt H, Kies AK, Kuipers H, Saris WH, Koopman R, van Loon LJ. Coingestion of carbohydrate and protein hydrolysate stimulates muscle protein synthesis during exercise in young men, with no further increase during subsequent overnight recovery. *J Nutr.* 2008;138:2198–2204.

33. Esmarck B, Andersen JL, Olsen S, Richter EA, Mizuno M, Kjaer M. Timing of postexercise protein intake is important for muscle hypertrophy with resistance training in elderly humans. *J Physiol.* 2001;535:301–311.

34. Trappe S, Williamson D, Godard M. Maintenance of whole muscle strength and size following resistance training in older men. *J Gerontol A Bio Sc Med Sci.* 2002;57:B138–B143.

35. Kosek DJ, Kim JS, Petrella JK, Cross JM, Bamman MM. Efficacy of 3 days/wk resistance training on myofiber hypertrophy and myogenic mechanisms in young vs. older adults. *J Appl Physiol.* 2006;101:531–544.

36. Fiatarone MA, Marks EC, Ryan ND, Meredith CN, Lipsitz LA, Evans WJ. High-intensity strength training in nonagenarians. Effects on skeletal muscle. *JAMA.* 1990;263:3029–3034.

37. Kalapotharakos VI, Michalopoulou M, Godolias G, Tokmakidis SP, Malliou PV, Gourgoulis V. The effects of high- and moderate-resistance training on muscle function in the elderly. *J Aging Phys Act.* 2004;12:131–143.

38. Slivka D, Raue U, Hollon C, Minchev K, Trappe S. Single muscle fiber adaptations to resistance training in old (>80 yr) men: evidence for limited skeletal muscle plasticity. *Am J Physiol Regul Integr Comp Physiol.* 2008;295: R273–R280.

39. Verdijk LB, Jonkers RA, Gleeson BG, Beelen M, Meijer K, Savelberg HH, Wodzig WK, Dendale P, van Loon LJ. Protein supplementation before and after exercise does not further augment skeletal muscle hypertrophy after resistance training in elderly men. *Am J Clin Nutr.* 2009;89:608–616.

40. Campbell WW, Crim MC, Young VR, Evans WJ. Increased energy requirements and changes in body composition with resistance training in older adults. *Am J Clin Nutr.* 1994;60:167–175.

41. Sallinen J, Pakarinen A, Fogelholm M, Sillanpaa E, Alen M, Volek JS, Kraemer WJ, Hakkinen K. Serum basal hormone concentrations and muscle mass in aging women: effects of strength training and diet. *Int J Sport Nutr Exerc Metab.* 2006;16:316–331.

42. Cribb PJ, Hayes A. Effects of supplement timing and resistance exercise on skeletal muscle hypertrophy. *Med Sci Sports Exerc.* 2006;38:1918–1925.

43. Hoffman JR, Ratamess NA, Tranchina CP, Rashti SL, Kang J, Faigenbaum AD. Effect of protein-supplement timing on strength, power, and body-composition changes in resistance-trained men. *Int J Sport Nutr Exerc Metab.* 2009;19:172–185.

44. Burk A, Timpmann S, Medijainen L, Vahi M, Oopik V. Time-divided ingestion pattern of casein-based protein supplement stimulates an increase in fat-free body mass during resistance training in young untrained men. *Nutr Res.* 2009;29:405–413.

45. Burd NA, Staples AW, West DWD, Moore DR, Holwerda AM, Baker SK, Phillips SM. Latent increases in fasting and fed-state muscle protein turnover with resistance exercise irrespective of intensity (abstract). *Appl Physiol Nutr Metab.* 2009;34:1122.

46. Drummond MJ, Glynn EL, Fry CS, Timmerman KL, Volpi E, Rasmussen BB. An increase in essential amino acid availability upregulates amino acid transporter expression in human skeletal muscle. *Am J Physiol.* 2010;298: E1011–E1018.

47. Ivy JL, Res PT, Sprague RC, Widzer MO. Effect of a carbohydrate-protein supplement on endurance performance during exercise of varying intensity. *Int J Sport Nutr Exerc Metab.* 2003;13:382–395.

48. Saunders MJ, Kane MD, Todd MK. Effects of a carbohydrate-protein beverage on cycling endurance and muscle damage. *Med Sci Sports Exerc.* 2004;36:1233–1238.

49. Saunders MJ, Luden ND, Herrick JE. Consumption of an oral carbohydrate-protein gel improves cycling endurance and prevents postexercise muscle damage. *J Strength Cond Res.* 2007;21:678–684.

50. van Essen M, Gibala MJ. Failure of protein to improve time trial performance when added to a sports drink. *Med Sci Sports Exerc.* 2006;38:1476–1483.

51. Cermak NM, Solheim AS, Gardner MS, Tarnopolsky MA, Gibala MJ. Muscle metabolism during exercise with carbohydrate or protein-carbohydrate ingestion. *Med Sci Sports Exerc.* 2009;41:2158–2164.

52. Breen L, Tipton KD, Jeukendrup AE. No Effect of carbohydrate-protein on cycling performance and indices of recovery. *Med Sci Sports Exerc.* 2010;42:1140–1148.

53. Jeukendrup AE, Tipton KD, Gibala MJ. Protein plus carbohydrate does not enhance 60-km time-trial performance. *Int J Sport Nutr Exerc Metab.* 2009;19:335–337; author reply 337–339.

54. Koopman R, Pannemans DL, Jeukendrup AE, Gijsen AP, Senden JM, Halliday D, Saris WH, van Loon LJ, Wagenmakers AJ. Combined ingestion of protein and carbohydrate improves protein balance during ultra-endurance exercise. *Am J Physiol Endocrinol Metab.* 2004;287:E712–E720.

55. Koopman R, Pannemans DL, Jeukendrup AE, Gijsen AP, Senden JM, Halliday D, Saris WH, van Loon LJ, Wagenmakers AJ. Combined ingestion of protein and carbohydrate improves protein balance during ultra-endurance exercise. *Am J Physiol.* 2004;287:E712–E720.

56. Holloszy JO, Booth FW. Biochemical adaptations to endurance exercise in muscle. *Ann Rev Physiol.* 1976;38:273–291.

57. Holloszy JO, Coyle EF. Adaptations of skeletal muscle to endurance exercise and their metabolic consequences. *J Appl Physiol.* 1984;56:831–838.

58. Hood DA. Invited Review: contractile activity-induced mitochondrial biogenesis in skeletal muscle. *J Appl Physiol.* 2001;90:1137–1157.

59. Hood DA, Takahashi M, Connor MK, Freyssenet D. Assembly of the cellular powerhouse: current issues in muscle mitochondrial biogenesis. *Exerc Sport Sci Rev.* 2000;28:68–73.

60. Howarth KR, Moreau NA, Phillips SM, Gibala MJ. Coingestion of protein with carbohydrate during recovery from endurance exercise stimulates skeletal muscle protein synthesis in humans. *J Appl Physiol.* 2009;106:1394–1402.

61. Fujita S, Rasmussen BB, Cadenas JG, Drummond MJ, Glynn EL, Sattler FR, Volpi E. Aerobic exercise overcomes the age-related insulin resistance of muscle protein metabolism by improving endothelial function and Akt/mammalian target of rapamycin signaling. *Diabetes.* 2007;56:1615–1622.

62. Rodriguez NR, Vislocky LM, Gaine PC. Dietary protein, endurance exercise, and human skeletal-muscle protein turnover. *Curr Opin Clin Nutr Metab Care.* 2007;10:40–45.

63. Dangin M, Boirie Y, Garcia-Rodenas C, Gachon P, Fauquant J, Callier P, Ballevre O, Beaufrere B. The digestion rate of protein is an independent regulating factor of postprandial protein retention. *Am J Physiol Endocrinol Metab.* 2001;280:E340–E348.

64. Dangin M, Boirie Y, Guillet C, Beaufrere B. Influence of the protein digestion rate on protein turnover in young and elderly subjects. *J Nutr.* 2002;132:3228S–3233S.

65. Dangin M, Guillet C, Garcia-Rodenas C, Gachon P, Bouteloup-Demange C, Reiffers-Magnani K, Fauquant J, Ballevre O, Beaufrere B. The rate of protein digestion affects protein gain differently during aging in humans. *J Physiol.* 2003;549:635–644.

66. Tang JE, Moore DR, Kujbida GW, Tarnopolsky MA, Phillips SM. Ingestion of whey hydrolysate, casein, or soy protein isolate: effects on mixed muscle protein synthesis at rest and following resistance exercise in young men. *J Appl Physiol.* 2009;107:987–992.

67. Phillips SM, Tang JE, Moore DR. The role of milk- and soy-based protein in support of muscle protein synthesis and muscle protein accretion in young and elderly persons. *J Am Coll Nutr.* 2009;28:343–354.

68. Tang JE, Phillips SM. Maximizing muscle protein anabolism: the role of protein quality. *Curr Opin Clin Nutr Metab Care.* 2009;12:66–71.

69. Tipton KD, Gurkin BE, Matin S, Wolfe RR. Nonessential amino acids are not necessary to stimulate net muscle protein synthesis in healthy volunteers. *J Nutr Biochem.* 1999;10:89–95.

70. Smith K, Barua JM, Watt PW, Scrimgeour CM, Rennie MJ. Flooding with L-[1-13C]leucine stimulates human muscle protein incorporation of continuously infused L-[1-13C]valine. *Am J Physiol.* 1992;262:E372–E376.

71. Cuthbertson D, Smith K, Babraj J, Leese G, Waddell T, Atherton P, Wackerhage H, Taylor PM, Rennie MJ. Anabolic signaling deficits underlie amino acid resistance of wasting, aging muscle. *FASEB J.* 2005;19:422–424.

72. Moore DR, Robinson MJ, Fry JL, Tang JE, Glover EI, Wilkinson SB, Prior T, Tarnopolsky MA, Phillips SM. Ingested protein dose response of muscle and albumin protein synthesis after resistance exercise in young men. *Am J Clin Nutr*. 2009;89:161–168.

73. Norton LE, Layman DK, Bunpo P, Anthony TG, Brana DV, Garlick PJ. The leucine content of a complete meal directs peak activation but not duration of skeletal muscle protein synthesis and mammalian target of rapamycin signaling in rats. *J Nutr*. 2009;13:1103–1109.

74. Greenhaff PL, Karagounis LG, Peirce N, Simpson EJ, Hazell M, Layfield R, Wackerhage H, Smith K, Atherton P, Selby A, Rennie MJ. Disassociation between the effects of amino acids and insulin on signaling, ubiquitin ligases, and protein turnover in human muscle. *Am J Physiol*. 2008;295:E595–E604.

75. Hagenfeldt L, Eriksson S, Wahren J. Influence of leucine on arterial concentrations and regional exchange of amino acids in healthy subjects. *Clin Sci (Lond)*. 1980;59:173–181.

76. Trappe TA, Burd NA, Louis ES, Lee GA, Trappe SW. Influence of concurrent exercise or nutrition countermeasures on thigh and calf muscle size and function during 60 days of bed rest in women. *Acta Physiol*. 2007;191:147–159.

77. Wolfe RR, Chinkes DL. *Isotope Tracers in Metabolic Research: Principles and Practice of Kinetic Analysis*. 2nd ed. Hoboken, NJ: Wiley; 2005.

78. Paddon-Jones D, Sheffield-Moore M, Katsanos CS, Zhang XJ, Wolfe RR. Differential stimulation of muscle protein synthesis in elderly humans following isocaloric ingestion of amino acids or whey protein. *Exp Gerontol*. 2006;41:215–219.

79. Ferrando AA, Tipton KD, Wolfe RR. Essential amino acids for muscle protein accretion. *Streng Cond J*. 2010;32: 87–92.

80. Paul GL. The rationale for consuming protein blends in sports nutrition. *J Am Coll Nutr*. 2009;28(suppl):464S–472S.

81. Boirie Y, Dangin M, Gachon P, Vasson MP, Maubois JL, Beaufrere B. Slow and fast dietary proteins differently modulate postprandial protein accretion. *Proc Natl Acad Sci USA*. 1997;94:14930–14935.

82. Bos C, Juillet B, Fouillet H, Turlan L, Dare S, Luengo C, N'Tounda R, Benamouzig R, Gausseres N, Tome D, Gaudichon C. Postprandial metabolic utilization of wheat protein in humans. *Am J Clin Nutr*. 2005;81;87–94.

83. Bohe J, Low A, Wolfe RR, Rennie MJ. Human muscle protein synthesis is modulated by extracellular, not intramuscular amino acid availability: a dose-response study. *J Physiol*. 2003;552:315–324.

84. Wilkinson SB, Tarnopolsky MA, MacDonald MJ, Macdonald JR, Armstrong D, Phillips SM. Consumption of fluid skim milk promotes greater muscle protein accretion following resistance exercise than an isonitrogenous and isoenergetic soy protein beverage. *Am J Clin Nutr*. 2007;85:1031–1040.

85. Josse AR, Tang JE, Tarnopolsky MA, Phillips SM. Body composition and strength changes in women with milk and resistance exercise. *Med Sci Sports Exerc*. 2010;42:1122–1130.

86. Gulliver P, Horwath C. Women's readiness to follow milk product consumption recommendations: design and evaluation of a "stage of change" algorithm. *J Hum Nutr Diet*. 2001;14:277–286.

87. Gulliver P, Horwath CC. Assessing women's perceived benefits, barriers, and stage of change for meeting milk product consumption recommendations. *J Am Diet Assoc*. 2001;101:1354–1357.

88. Rankin JW, Goldman LP, Puglisi MJ, Nickols-Richardson SM, Earthman CP, Gwazdauskas FC. Effect of post-exercise supplement consumption on adaptations to resistance training. *J Am Coll Nutr*. 2004;23:322–330.

89. Cribb PJ, Williams AD, Carey MF, Hayes A. The effect of whey isolate and resistance training on strength, body composition, and plasma glutamine. *Int J Sport Nutr Exerc Metab*. 2006;16:494–509.

90. Cribb PJ, Williams AD, Stathis CG, Carey MF, Hayes A. Effects of whey isolate, creatine, and resistance training on muscle hypertrophy. *Med Sci Sports Exerc*. 2007;39:298–307.

91. Teegarden D. The influence of dairy product consumption on body composition. *J Nutr*. 2005;135:2749–2752.

92. Zemel MB. Role of calcium and dairy products in energy partitioning and weight management. *Am J Clin Nutr*. 2004;79(suppl):907S–912S.

93. Candow DG, Burke NC, Smith-Plamer T, Burke DG. Effect of whey and soy protein supplementation combined with resistance training in young adults. *Int J Sport Nutr Exerc Metab*. 2006;16:233–244.

94. Ruales J, Nair BM. Nutritional quality of the protein in quinoa (Chenopodium quinoa Willd) seeds. *Plant Foods Hum Nutr*. 1992;42:1–11.

95. Borsheim E, Tipton KD, Wolf SE, Wolfe RR. Essential amino acids and muscle protein recovery from resistance exercise. *Am J Physiol Endocrinol Metab.* 2002;283:E648–E657.

96. Mier CM, Domenick MA, Turner NS, Wilmore JH. Changes in stroke volume and maximal aerobic capacity with increased blood volume in men and women. *J Appl Physiol.* 1996;80:1180–1186.

97. Lemon PW, Tarnopolsky MA, MacDougall JD, Atkinson SA. Protein requirements and muscle mass/strength changes during intensive training in novice bodybuilders. *J Appl Physiol.* 1992;73:767–775.

98. Hartman JW, Moore DR, Phillips SM. Resistance training reduces whole-body protein turnover and improves net protein retention in untrained young males. *Appl Physiol Nutr Metab.* 2006;31:557–564.

99. Moore DR, Del Bel NC, Nizi KI, Hartman JW, Tang JE, Armstrong D, Phillips SM. Resistance training reduces fasted- and fed-state leucine turnover and increases dietary nitrogen retention in previously untrained young men. *J Nutr.* 2007;137:985–991.

100. Campbell WW, Crim MC, Young VR, Joseph LJ, Evans WJ. Effects of resistance training and dietary protein intake on protein metabolism in older adults. *Am J Physiol.* 1995;268:E1143–E1153.

101. Campbell WW, Trappe TA, Jozsi AC, Kruskall LJ, Wolfe RR, Evans WJ. Dietary protein adequacy and lower body versus whole body resistive training in older humans. *J Physiol.* 2002;542:631–642.

102. Pikosky M, Faigenbaum A, Westcott W, Rodriguez N. Effects of resistance training on protein utilization in healthy children. *Med Sci Sports Exerc.* 2002;34:820–827.

103. Bohe J, Low JF, Wolfe RR, Rennie MJ. Latency and duration of stimulation of human muscle protein synthesis during continuous infusion of amino acids. *J Physiol.* 2001;532:575–579.

104. MacDougall JD, Gibala MJ, Tarnopolsky MA, MacDonald JR, Interisano SA, Yarasheski KE. The time course for elevated muscle protein synthesis following heavy resistance exercise. *Can J Appl Physiol.* 1995;20:480–486.

105. McKenzie S, Phillips SM, Carter SL, Lowther S, Gibala MJ, Tarnopolsky MA. Endurance exercise training attenuates leucine oxidation and BCOAD activation during exercise in humans. *Am J Physiol.* 2000;278:E580–E587.

106. Tarnopolsky LJ, MacDougall JD, Atkinson SA, Tarnopolsky MA, Sutton JR. Gender differences in substrate for endurance exercise. *J Appl Physiol.* 1990;68:302–308.

107. Joint Position Statement: nutrition and athletic performance. American College of Sports Medicine, American Dietetic Association, and Dietitians of Canada. *Med Sci Sports Exerc.* 2000;32:2130–2145.

108. Tarnopolsky M. Protein requirements for endurance athletes. *Nutrition.* 2004;20:662–668.

109. Loftin M, Sothern M, Koss C, Tuuri G, Vanvrancken C, Kontos A, Bonis M. Energy expenditure and influence of physiologic factors during marathon running. *J Strength Cond Res.* 2007;21:1188–1191.

110. el-Khoury AE, Forslund A, Olsson R, Branth S, Sjodin A, Andersson A, Atkinson A, Selvaraj A, Hambraeus L, Young VR. Moderate exercise at energy balance does not affect 24-h leucine oxidation or nitrogen retention in healthy men. *Am J Physiol.* 1997;273:E394–E407.

111. Forslund AH, El-Khoury AE, Olsson RM, Sjodin AM, Hambraeus L, Young VR. Effect of protein intake and physical activity on 24-h pattern and rate of macronutrient utilization. *Am J Physiol.* 1999;276:E964–E976.

112. Phillips SM, Moore DR, Tang JE. A critical examination of dietary protein requirements, benefits, and excesses in athletes. *Int J Sport Nutr Exerc Metab.* 2007;17(suppl):S58–S76.

113. Elango R, Humayun MA, Ball RO, Pencharz PB. Evidence that protein requirements have been significantly underestimated. *Curr Opin Clin Nutr Metab Care.* 2010;13:52–57.

114. Bowtell JL, Leese GP, Smith K, Watt PW, Nevill A, Rooyackers O, Wagenmakers AJ, Rennie MJ. Effect of oral glucose on leucine turnover in human subjects at rest and during exercise at two levels of dietary protein. *J Physiol.* 2000;525:271–281.

115. Bolster DR, Pikosky MA, Gaine PC, Martin W, Wolfe RR, Tipton KD, Maclean D, Maresh CM, Rodriguez NR. Dietary protein intake impacts human skeletal muscle protein fractional synthetic rates after endurance exercise. *Am J Physiol Endocrinol Metab.* 2005;289:E678–E683.

116. Brouns F, Saris WH, Stroecken J, Beckers E, Thijssen R, Rehrer NJ, ten Hoor F. Eating, drinking, and cycling. A controlled Tour de France simulation study, Part II. Effect of diet manipulation. *Int J Sports Med.* 1989;10 (suppl 1):S41–S48.

117. Brouns F, Saris WH, Stroecken J, Beckers E, Thijssen R, Rehrer NJ, ten Hoor F. Eating, drinking, and cycling. A controlled Tour de France simulation study, Part I. *Int J Sports Med.* 1989;10(suppl 1):S32–S40.

118. Bergstrom J, Furst P, Hultman E. Free amino acids in muscle tissue and plasma during exercise in man. *Clin Physiol.* 1985;5:155–160.

119. Henriksson J. Effect of exercise on amino acid concentrations in skeletal muscle and plasma. *J Exp Biol.* 1991; 160:149–165.

120. Jepson MM, Bates PC, Broadbent P, Pell JM, Millward DJ. Relationship between glutamine concentration and protein synthesis in rat skeletal muscle. *Am J Physiol.* 1988;255:E166–E172.

121. Candow DG, Chilibeck PD, Burke DG, Davison KS, Smith-Palmer T. Effect of glutamine supplementation combined with resistance training in young adults. *Eur J Appl Physiol.* 2001;86:142–149.

122. Welbourne TC. Increased plasma bicarbonate and growth hormone after an oral glutamine load. *Am J Clin Nutr.* 1995;61:1058–1061.

123. West DW, Kujbida GW, Moore DR, Atherton P, Burd NA, Padzik JP, De Lisio M, Tang JE, Parise G, Rennie MJ, Baker SK, Phillips SM. Resistance exercise-induced increases in putative anabolic hormones do not enhance muscle protein synthesis or intracellular signalling in young men. *J Physiol.* 2009;587:5239–5247.

124. Doessing S, Heinemeier KM, Holm L, Mackey AL, Schjerling P, Rennie M, Smith K, Reitelseder S, Kappel-gaard AM, Rasmussen MH, Flyvbjerg A, Kjaer M. Growth hormone stimulates the collagen synthesis in human tendon and skeletal muscle without affecting myofibrillar protein synthesis. *J Physiol.* 2010;588:341–351.

125. Burd NA, West DW, Churchward-Venne TA, Mitchell CJ. Growing collagen, not muscle, with weightlifting and growth hormone. *J Physiol.* 2010;588:395–396.

126. Saito H, Trocki O, Wang SL, Gonce SJ, Joffe SN, Alexander JW. Metabolic and immune effects of dietary argi-nine supplementation after burn. *Arch Surg.* 1987;122:784–789.

127. Witte MB, Barbul A. Arginine physiology and its implication for wound healing. *Wound Repair Regen.* 2003;11:419–423.

128. Paddon-Jones D, Borsheim E, Wolfe RR. Potential ergogenic effects of arginine and creatine supplementation. *J Nutr.* 2004;134(10 Suppl):2888S–2894S; discussion 2895S.

129. Castillo L, deRojas TC, Chapman TE, Vogt J, Burke JF, Tannenbaum SR, Young VR. Splanchnic metabo-lism of dietary arginine in relation to nitric oxide synthesis in normal adult man. *Proc Natl Acad Sci USA.* 1993;90:193–197.

130. Castillo L, Ajami A, Branch S, Chapman TE, Yu YM, Burke JF, Young VR. Plasma arginine kinetics in adult man: response to an arginine-free diet. *Metab Clin Exp.* 1994;43:114–122.

131. Kanaley JA. Growth hormone, arginine and exercise. *Curr Opin Clin Nutr Metab Care.* 2008;11:50–54.

132. Isidori A, Lo Monaco A, Cappa M. A study of growth hormone release in man after oral administration of amino acids. *Curr Med Res Opin.* 1981;7:475–481.

133. Gater DR, Gater DA, Uribe JM, Bunt JC. Effects of arginine/lysine supplementation and resistance training on glucose tolerance. *J Appl Physiol.* 1992;72:1279–1284.

134. Volpi E, Kobayashi H, Sheffield-Moore M, Mittendorfer B, Wolfe RR. Essential amino acids are primarily responsible for the amino acid stimulation of muscle protein anabolism in healthy elderly adults. *Am J Clin Nutr.* 2003;78:250–258.

135. Lysecki PJ, Manolakos JJ, Tang JE, Phillips SM. Bolus L-arginine supplementation in the fed state at rest and following resistance exercise does not affect bulk muscle blood flow [abstract]. *FASEB J.* 2007;21(Suppl):A123.

136. Holm L, Esmarck B, Suetta C, Matsumoto K, Doi T, Mizuno M, Miller BF, Kjaer M. Postexercise nutrient intake enhances leg protein balance in early postmenopausal women. *J Gerontol A Biol Sci Med Sci.* 2005;60:1212–1218.

137. Cribb PJ, Williams AD, Hayes A. A creatine-protein-carbohydrate supplement enhances responses to resistance training. *Med Sci Sports Exerc.* 2007;39:1960–1968.

Chapter 4

DIETARY FAT AND EXERCISE

MARK KERN, PHD, RD, CSSD

Introduction

Fats, also known as lipids, are molecules that have been characterized for their capacity to dissolve in non-polar solvents. Together with carbohydrate, fat serves as a major source of energy for athletes. Given their critical role in energy metabolism, dietary fats should be considered from performance-related perspectives as well as for implications in promoting or interfering with the wellness of active individuals. Endogenous fat stores, dietary fat, and other dietary components that influence fat metabolism work both separately and in concert. Research to date allows us to predict, at least to some degree, how various diet regimens and strategies that impact lipid metabolism influence fuel utilization, risk factors for chronic diseases, and athletic performance. This chapter provides practitioners with a review of lipids and their metabolism, particularly as they relate to exercise. The chapter will help the practitioner understand dietary practices that may benefit athletes.

Lipids are a diverse group of nutrients. Triglycerides are a class of lipids that makes up the majority (> 95%) of lipid in the human diet. There are several other varieties of lipids found in the diet and/or the human body, including fatty acids, monoglycerides, diglycerides, phospholipids, sterols (such as cholesterol and phytosterols), fat-soluble vitamins, eicosanoids, glycolipids, and other molecules. Lipids exhibit multiple functions in both foods and metabolism. Metabolic functions include energy production, imparting structure to cell membranes, emulsification, molecular signaling, and participation in many biochemical reactions and pathways.

Dietary Sources of Fat and Other Lipids

Lipids derived from diet play important roles in the health and the performance of athletes. The key lipids in the diet include triglycerides, phospholipids, and cholesterol. Other notable dietary lipids that may affect metabolism include diglycerides and phytosterols; however, relatively little research pertaining to athletes has been conducted on these dietary components.

Triglycerides and Fatty Acids

Triglycerides, also known as triacylglycerols, are composed of three acyl groups (fatty acids) attached by ester bonds to a glycerol backbone (see Figure 4.1). Generally referred to as "fat," these lipids account for the vast majority of lipids in the diet and are a substantial source of energy and the essential fatty acids (linoleic acid and alpha-linolenic acid). The Institute of Medicine (IOM) established an Acceptable Macronutrient Distribution Range (AMDR) for fat of 20% to 35% of total energy intake for adults (1). Intake of fat in this range will likely allow individuals to meet their needs for essential fatty acids without increasing the risk for coronary heart disease. The AMDR values for linoleic acid (often referred to as n-6 fatty acids) and alpha-linolenic acid (n-3 fatty acids) are 5% to 10% of energy and 0.6% to1.2% of energy, respectively (1).

Foods rich in triglycerides include oils, butter, margarine, spreads, salad dressings, fresh and processed meats, some fish, poultry (particularly when the skin is included), cheeses, milk products, avocados, most nuts and seeds, fried foods, some processed foods, cakes, cookies, chocolate, and some sport supplements (eg, medium-chain triglyceride [MCT] oil). However, lower fat food varieties are available for many of the foods that are traditionally rich in fat; therefore, not all versions of these foods are the best choices of foods for athletes. Furthermore, many other foods not listed can be rich in fat as well, so it is important to pay attention to food labels when determining the fat content of a food item. The types of fatty acids that comprise the triglycerides within a particular food are often as important as the total fat content.

Fatty acids differ in their physical structures as well as their metabolic effects. All fatty acid molecules are characterized by the presence of a hydrocarbon chain linked to a carboxylic acid group. One way of classifying fatty acids is based on the length of the hydrocarbon chain. Fatty acids with 2 to 4 carbons are considered short-chain fatty acids. Medium-chain fatty acids are those composed of 6 to10, or perhaps as many as 12 carbons. Long-chain fatty acids have 12 to 14 or more carbons in their chains. In general, longer fatty acid carbon chains have greater lipid solubility. By contrast, short- and medium-chain fatty acids tend to be quite soluble in water, which greatly affects their metabolism. The majority of dietary fatty acids are 16 to18 carbons in length. However, small amounts of short- and medium-chain fatty acids are obtained as naturally occurring components of foods such as dairy products and coconut oil. Commercially available supplements containing MCT oil are often marketed to athletes and can represent a substantial source of medium-chain fatty acids for those individuals who use them.

Another method of classifying fatty acids is based on their degree of saturation with hydrogen atoms. A fatty acid that is saturated (Figure 4.2), holds as many hydrogen atoms as possible, whereas unsaturated fatty acids have one or more double bonds, which displace hydrogen atoms. Fatty acids with a single double bond are referred to as monounsaturated fatty acids (MUFAs) and those with multiple double bonds are polyunsaturated fatty acids (PUFAs). The general structures of MUFAs and PUFAs are depicted in Figures

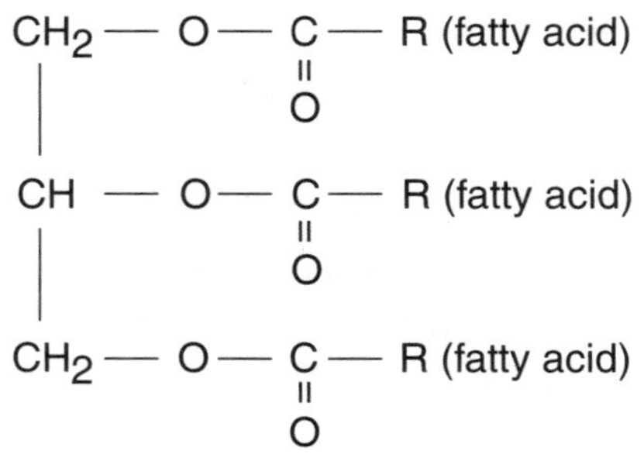

FIGURE 4.1   General structure of a triglyceride.

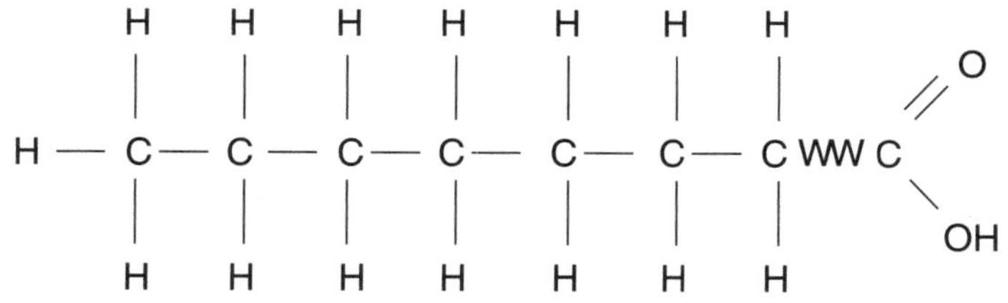

FIGURE 4.2   General structure of a saturated fatty acid.

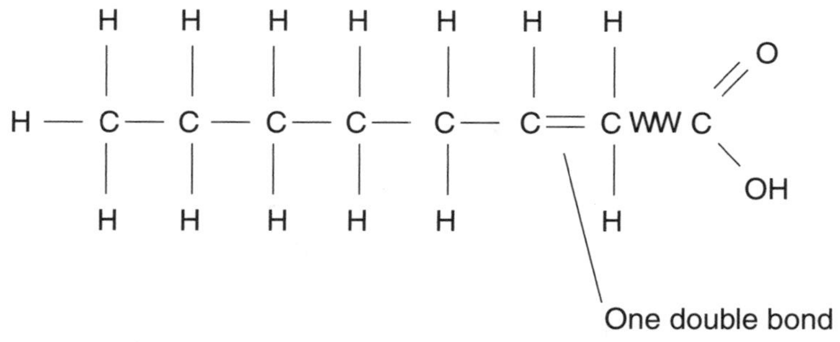

FIGURE 4.3   General structure of a monounsaturated fatty acid.

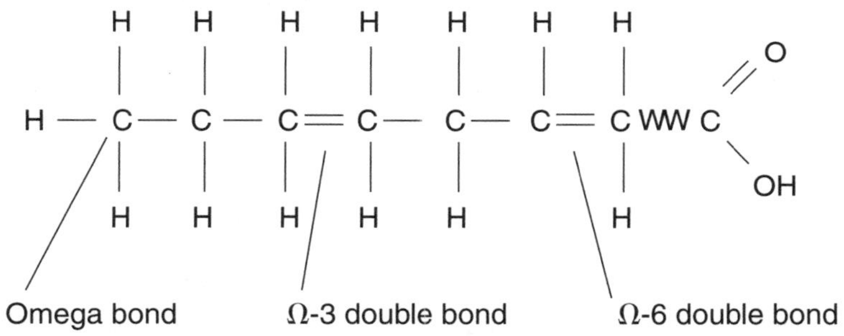

FIGURE 4.4   General structure of a polyunsaturated fatty acid with double bonds depicting omega classification highlighted.

4.3 and 4.4. Because saturated fatty acids are "saturated" with hydrogen ions, they possess no double bonds. Foods that are rich sources of saturated fatty acids include animal foods (eg, meat, fish, poultry, dairy, etc), cocoa butter, and tropical plant oils (ie, coconut oil, palm oil, and palm kernel oil). Plant foods such as canola oil, olives and olive oil, and avocados are good sources of MUFAs, whereas most other plant foods (eg, soy, corn, nuts, seeds, etc) and fish tend to be rich in PUFAs.

Unsaturated fatty acids are further classified by the position (eg, n-3, n-6, n-9, etc) of the double bond(s) within the hydrocarbon chain (Figure 4.4) as well as the configuration (ie, *cis* vs *trans* unsaturated fatty acids) of the molecules around the double bond (Figure 4.5). Although the amount of energy produced from the catabolism of fatty acids is similar regardless of the position or conformation of the double bond, these simple variations can produce profoundly different effects on both the metabolic and the health-related characteristics of fats. Dietary sources of n-3 PUFAs include fish, walnuts, and flaxseed, whereas n-6 fatty acids are found in relatively high levels in most, but not all, other plant foods. Most dietary sources of unsaturated fatty acids are found in *cis* conformation. Foods that are rich sources of *trans* unsaturated fatty acids include fats industrially produced through the process of hydrogenation (ie, shortening and other partially

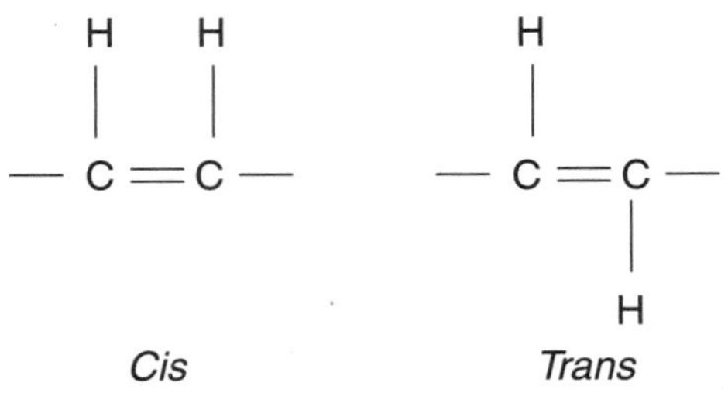

FIGURE 4.5   Depiction of the structures of *cis* vs *trans* double bonds.

hydrogenated oils), although some *trans* fatty acids occur naturally and are provided by meat and dairy products of ruminant animals. Hydrogenation involves the processing of fat sources, typically vegetable oils, by adding hydrogen at the site of the double bonds forming saturated fatty acids. When hydrogenation is incomplete, *trans* unsaturated fatty acids can form. Foods that are rich sources of various types of fatty acids are presented in Table 4.1

Essential fatty acids (EFA) must be obtained from the diet to avoid deficiency because they cannot be produced by the body. There are two EFAs: linoleic acid and alpha-linolenic acid. Clinical symptoms of EFA deficiency include dermatitis, decreased growth or weight loss, organ dysfunction, and abnormal reproductive status. Although these are the only fatty acids required in the diet, a portion of our needs can be met through consumption of longer, more unsaturated fatty acids. For example, eicosapentaenoic acid (EPA) and docosahexaenoic acid (DHA) can help meet n-3 fatty acid requirements.

Phospholipids and Cholesterol

The majority of the remaining dietary lipids are phospholipids and sterols such as cholesterol. Most dietary phospholipids are glycerophosphatides, which are composed of a glycerol molecule with fatty acids linked in the number 1 and number 2 carbon positions and a phosphate bound to choline, serine, ethanolamine, or inositol on the third carbon. A commonly consumed phospholipid is phosphatidyl choline, also known as lecithin. Phospholipids and cholesterol are key structural components of cell membranes and participate in many metabolic reactions.

Cholesterol (Figure 4.6) is a sterol that has several critical functions. It is required for the biosynthesis of vitamin D, bile acids, and sex hormones, and is critical to normal body processes. However, because the body can synthesize 100% of needed cholesterol, it is not necessary to consume cholesterol via dietary sources. Foods that provide cholesterol are animal products or plant products prepared with an animal product. Cholesterol-rich foods include organ meats, egg yolk, most seafood, meat, and some dairy products.

Athlete's Dietary Fat Intake

Researchers have assessed the dietary fat intake for various groups of athletes. The majority of the studies reported intakes that are within the range of the AMDR. In one study, fat intake of male collegiate cyclists in the United States during training was estimated to be approximately 27% of total energy (2). A study of Australian national-level triathletes and runners found that total fat consumption was approximately 27% and 32% of energy, respectively (3). In another study, female collegiate-level divers and swimmers consumed 22% to 23% of energy from fat at the end of the competitive season (4). Similar findings were

TABLE 4.1 Dietary Sources of Various Fatty Acids

Type of Fat	Food Sources
Polyunsaturated (n-6) fatty acids	Corn oil Corn oil margarine Cottonseed oil Pumpkin seeds Safflower oil Sesame seeds Soybean oil Walnuts
Polyunsaturated (n-3) fatty acids	Anchovies Catfish High–n-3 eggs Flax seed/flax oil Herring Mackerel Salmon Sardines Shrimp Tuna
Monounsaturated (n-9) fatty acids	Almonds Avocados Canola oil Cashews Peanut butter Peanut oil Peanuts Olive oil Olives
Saturated fatty acids	Bacon Butter Cheesecake Cheese Cream Cream cheese Coconut Coconut oil Half-and-half Highly marbled steaks Ice cream Palm kernel oil Ribs Sausage
Trans unsaturated fatty acid	Commercial baked goods (cookies, cakes, pies) Frozen, breaded foods (chicken nuggets, fish sticks) Frozen french fries Shortening Snack crackers and chips Stick margarines

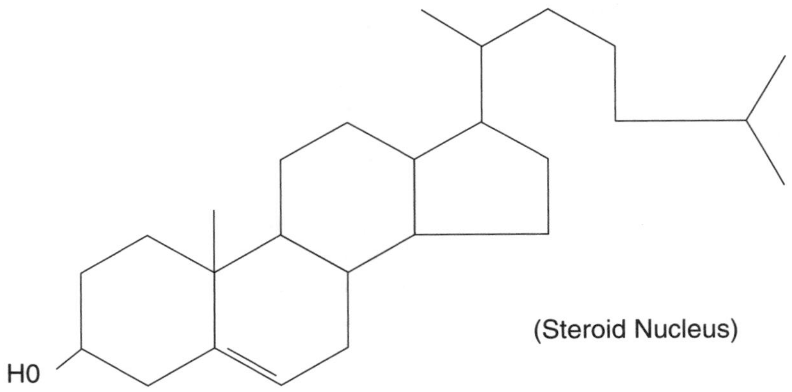

(Steroid Nucleus)

HO

FIGURE 4.6   Structure of cholesterol.

also reported during a taper from training in female swimmers (5). Researchers have reported higher fat consumption (30% to 43% of energy from fat) for swimmers in most other studies (6–10). Prepubescent girls from Croatia competing in gymnastics or ballet reportedly consume on average 29% to 36% of energy from fat, depending on their sport (11). During the 3 days before an ultra-endurance event, male cyclists averaged 30% to 31% of energy fat, and intake did not vary substantially within the 3 days leading up to the event (12). In an earlier study of ultra-endurance runners, fat intake decreased from approximately 35% to 30% of energy for women and 32% to 26% of energy for men during the 3 days before the event, in comparison to normal training diets (13). Some athletes (14) tend to consume an amount of fat less than the recommended range. For example, male Kenyan runners average approximately 13% of daily energy intake (46 ± 14 g) from fat (15). Given the variability in fat intake among athletes, it is not easy to recommend a single, universal level for fat consumption that will optimize performance. Professionals working with athletes should consider the athletes' sports and/or events, goals for body weight, risk factors for chronic diseases, and manipulations that may impact exercise performance before recommending total and specific dietary fat intake.

Metabolism

The vast majority (approximately 96%) of dietary fat that is consumed is digested and absorbed (16). Both of these processes occur primarily in the small intestine and require the emulsifying actions of bile acids secreted from the gallbladder in response to fat intake and the release of the gut hormone cholecystokinin. Digestion of triglycerides occurs by the actions of colipase and lipase (secreted by the pancreas), which hydrolyze two fatty acids from glycerol. Glycerophosphatides and cholesterol esters are also digested in the small intestine by the actions of the pancreatic enzymes phospholipase A-2 and cholesterol esterase, respectively. The ultimate products of digestion, primarily fatty acids, monoglycerides, lysophospholipids, and cholesterol, as well as other lipid-soluble dietary components, form small droplets (micelles) with the help of bile acids. This process readies them for uptake by the cells of the small intestine. Once absorbed, triglycerides, phospholipids, and cholesterol esters are reformed, transported to the endoplasmic reticulum along with other lipids, and packaged with protein (apoproteins) as lipoproteins (primarily chylomicrons) for secretion into lacteal (lymphatic) vessels lining the small intestine. The chylomicrons proceed through the lymphatic system via the left thoracic duct to the subclavian vein for ultimate dispersal into the systemic circulation via the heart. Short- and medium-chain fatty acids are much more water-soluble than long-chain fatty acids and most bypass this route of absorption and are taken up into the circulation from the small intestine for transport to the liver. There they are typically converted into ketones and exported to the peripheral circulation for catabolism by extrahepatic cells and tissues. These fatty acids represent a small fraction of total dietary lipids; therefore, most lipids are distributed into the circulation for uptake by tissues and subsequent metabolic processes as components of chylomicrons.

As chylomicrons pass through the capillaries, a portion of the triglyceride is hydrolyzed to free fatty acids (FFA) and glycerol by lipoprotein lipase (LPL) for uptake by target tissues. The remains of the chylomicrons (chylomicron remnants) are taken up by the liver for deposition and subsequent hepatic metabolism. The liver generally packages these lipids along with other lipids delivered to and produced within the hepatocytes as endogenous lipoproteins, principally very–low density lipoproteins (VLDL). After secretion from the liver, VLDL is metabolized by LPL in a manner that is similar to chylomicron metabolism; however, the resulting lipoprotein particle is a low-density lipoprotein (LDL).

Although lipids have a variety of important functions, a key function for the athlete is energy production. This occurs primarily from fatty acids that are made available from triglycerides along with some lipoprotein-bound triglyceride to provide a portion of the fatty acids available for energy production. Other substantial sources of fatty acids include triglycerides in adipose and muscle cells.

Fatty acids stored as a part of adipose tissue triglyceride are exported into the circulation by the action of the enzyme hormone sensitive lipase (HSL). Hormones that stimulate HSL activity include epinephrine, norepinephrine, glucagon, adrenocorticotropic hormone, thyroxine, thyroid stimulating hormone, and growth hormone. These fatty acids are transported through the circulation bound to protein, but are usually referred to as free fatty acids. After uptake by cells (such as muscle cells), the fatty acids can be subsequently catabolized for energy. Triglyceride stored within muscle cells (intramyocellular triglyceride) represents a small fraction of body triglyceride stores, but can provide critical energy to the muscle cells in which they are stored, particularly during long-term (ultra-endurance) exercise. Some triglyceride is also stored outside of muscles cells but still within the muscle tissue (intermyocellular triglyceride); however, these stores are very low in athletes.

Fatty acids that have been taken up by muscle cells are linked to coenzyme A (CoA) by fatty acyl CoA synthetase. These fatty acids must first be translocated to the mitochondria before they can be oxidized for energy. This occurs by the action of an elaborate transport mechanism that consists of carnitine and the enzymes carnitine-acylcarnitine translocase, carnitine palmitoyltransferase-I, and carnitine palmitoyltransferase-II. These molecules work in concert to transfer the fatty acids across the mitochondria membranes and to reesterify them to CoA. Once inside the mitochondria, these fatty acids can be catabolized through beta oxidation, resulting in multiple acetyl CoA molecules as well as one $FADH_2$ (reduced flavin adenine dinucleotide) and one NADH (reduced nicotinamide adenine dinucleotide) + H^+ for every 2 carbons cleaved, which can undergo further mitochondrial oxidation for energy (ATP) production via the electron transport system. The acetyl CoA molecules can also be used to provide energy by metabolism via the Krebs cycle and subsequent oxidative phosphorylation through the electron transport system. Fatty acid utilization increases in proportion to the plasma FFA concentrations, which has led to the development of many dietary strategies designed to increase plasma FFA concentrations and favor fat oxidation in preference to carbohydrate oxidation. These strategies are described in further detail later in the chapter.

Influences on Exercise and Lipid Metabolism

Most energy produced during exercise comes from fat and carbohydrate, with amino acids contributing a minor component under most circumstances. Sources of energy are determined by many variables; however, exercise intensity is the principal determinant of fuels utilized as well as total energy expended. Fatty acids found as a component of triglycerides represent the majority of lipids used for energy during exercise. As described earlier, these come principally from adipose tissue, intramuscular depots, and lipoproteins; the relative contributions of each vary depending on numerous factors, including exercise intensity. At lower intensities, intramuscular triglyceride contributes only a minor portion of energy expended in comparison to FFA obtained from the plasma. The relative contribution of intramuscular triglyceride utilization increases as exercise intensity increases (17). Likewise, the contribution of fat sources is influenced by the duration of the exercise bout, with plasma FFA contributing a higher percentage of fat utilized and a decrease in the relative utilization of intramuscular triglyceride as the duration progresses (17).

Because many strategies designed to enhance endurance exercise performance rely on increased fat utilization and "sparing" of carbohydrates, the relative contributions of fat and carbohydrate are often key concerns. These contributions are often measured by the nonprotein respiratory exchange ratio (RER). This physiological response is assessed by the collection of expired gasses at rest or during exercise and calculation of the volume of carbon dioxide produced divided by the volume of oxygen consumed. As RER approaches 1.00, carbohydrate is providing a greater percentage of fuel for metabolism, whereas an RER approaching 0.70 indicates greater fat utilization. The contribution of protein to energy expended is typically not determined, but can be assessed by determination of urinary urea excretion. At higher exercise intensities, the RER increases, indicating a greater reliance on carbohydrate as an energy source. This is largely due to enhanced carbohydrate utilization rather than a decrease in fat use; however, researchers have demonstrated a small decrease in absolute fat utilization as exercise intensity increased from 65% to 85% of maximal oxygen consumption (17).

Lipids and Exercise Performance

Many strategies related to intake of dietary lipids as well as alterations in metabolism by various dietary supplements have been assessed for potential influences on body composition of athletes and athletic performance. These include adaptations to a high total fat intake, consumption of specific dietary lipids (eg, MCT oil, conjugated linoleic acid, n-3 fatty acids, etc), and supplements such as carnitine and choline.

Fat Adaptation

Fat adaptation (fat loading) is a process in which high levels of dietary fat (typically 40% to 65% of energy) are consumed for up to several weeks, usually at the expense of carbohydrate. The goal of fat-loading is to enhance fat utilization for energy production by sparing carbohydrate during competition, thereby enhancing endurance capacity. Contrary to the relatively well-accepted concept of carbohydrate loading, relatively few research studies support the benefit of this type of diet regimen (18–20) and some studies have even suggested adverse effects on performance (21,22). Additionally, although many studies have detected increased fat utilization and reduced carbohydrate oxidation, no differences in performance have been detected in multiple studies assessing the effects of fat loading (23–27). At the present time, fat loading is an interesting hypothesis, but it is prudent to recommend a nutrient-dense diet that is high in carbohydrate and lower in fat (particularly saturated fat) until research conclusively demonstrates the benefits of fat adaptation and better elucidates an optimal range of fat intake.

Until then, athletes interested in testing the efficacy of fat adaptation might wish to do so outside of their competitive season and should closely monitor any adverse changes in body weight or performance. Fat intake should focus on incorporating fat-rich foods from plant sources rich in MUFAs and PUFAs. Athletes should monitor performance throughout a several-week regimen to determine the duration of fat adaptation that they require to observe any potential benefits. In that way, practitioners and athletes would be equipped to schedule a fat-loading regimen for peak performance at critical times during a competitive season. It should be noted that there is some concern about the potential adverse effects of fat adaptation on blood lipid profiles; however, exercise training typically improves blood lipid profiles (28) and adverse dietary effects of even saturated fat on blood lipids are often blunted in athletes (29,30).

A related regimen that has been studied combines a period of fat adaptation followed by a short-term carbohydrate restoration period. The goal of this method is to maximize fat utilization and carbohydrate stores at the time of the event to optimize performance. Early research using this strategy demonstrated improved cycling performance; Lambert et al (31) fed cyclists a high-fat diet providing at least 65% of energy from fat for 10 days followed by 3 days of a high-carbohydrate diet (> 70% of energy). They also fed subjects solutions containing MCTs before exercise and MCTs plus glucose during exercise.

Most other researchers using a similar protocol (but usually with a shorter fat-adaptation period and just a single day of high-carbohydrate intake) have not observed similar improvements (25,32,33). In fact, Havemann et al (33) demonstrated some negative effects: 1-km bursts during the endurance trial were performed poorly using this regimen. More research using longer diet alteration periods are warranted before conclusive recommendations on this strategy can be made.

Kiens and Burke propose that what was initially viewed as "glycogen sparing" following fat adaptation may actually represent a down-regulation of carbohydrate metabolism or "glycogen impairment" (34). Stellingwerff and colleagues (35) found that fat adaptation/carbohydrate restoration was associated with reduced activity of pyruvate dehydrogenase at rest and during exercise. This would impair rates of glycogenolysis at a time when muscle carbohydrate requirements are high. Endurance athletes that choose to evaluate the efficacy of such a regimen should consider doing so with a relatively long fat-adaptation period and a carbohydrate-loading phase longer than a single day.

MCT Oil

MCT oil is commonly marketed as a performance-enhancing lipid source. Because medium-chain fatty acids are absorbed into the portal circulation for transport to the liver and largely metabolized into ketones that are then exported to the peripheral circulation, they provide an alternative energy source to endogenous carbohydrate stores because they are quickly metabolized by peripheral tissues such as muscle cells (36–38). However, research demonstrating improved performance with MCT oil is limited. An animal study fed mice MCT oil at 17% of total energy intake for periods of 2 to 6 weeks and yielded improved swimming capacity and glycogen sparing, which seemed to be secondary to upregulation of enzymes of lipid metabolism (39). Human studies of longer-term feedings of MCT oil have not produced improvements in performance (40,41) and results from rodents do not necessarily translate to similar results in humans.

Most studies assessing the potential performance-enhancing effects of MCT oil have been acute research designs. One study demonstrated improvements when MCT oil was added to a carbohydrate feeding (42). However, that study has been criticized because the MCT oil increased the energy content of the feeding. Most other studies have failed to demonstrate improved performance with MCT oil consumption (43–48). One drawback to MCT oil feeding is increased risk for gastrointestinal discomfort (48), which is common during acute feeding and may limit its potential to improve performance; however, those symptoms seem to lessen over time (40,41). Given the potential for gastrointestinal distress along with the limited likelihood of performance enhancement, athletes should not experiment with MCT oil feeding on the day of an event, and any athlete interested in using MCT oil should do so over a period of a couple of weeks to eliminate the potential ergolytic effect of an upset stomach. Consumption of approximately 30 g twice per day seems to be sufficient to eliminate the gastrointestinal discomfort of a 30-g feeding before exercise (40).

Furthermore, registered dietitians (RDs) and athletes should be aware that chronic consumption of MCT oil has been shown to have a negative influence on blood lipids of athletes (ie, higher total cholesterol, LDL-cholesterol, and triglycerides after 2 weeks of feeding, in comparison to consumption of corn oil), which might be a concern for athletes with abnormal blood lipids or other risk factors for heart disease (49).

Conjugated Linoleic Acid

Conjugated linoleic acid (CLA) refers to a group of linoleic acid isomers in which the two double bonds are separated by only two carbons. Supplements available to athletes typically consist of equal amounts of the *cis*-9 and *trans*-11 and *trans*-10, *cis*-12 isomers. Dietary sources of CLA are primarily animal foods. The average intake from food is approximately 150 mg/d for women and 200 mg/d for men (50).

Most of the research on CLA that is applicable to athletes has focused on potential anabolic and fat-reducing effects of CLA supplementation during resistance training. Results of these studies are equivocal, with studies in which higher doses were examined providing slightly more promising results than lower-dose studies. Steck et al (51) demonstrated that 6.4 g of CLA per day (but not 3.2 g/d) for 12 weeks increased lean body mass in obese men and women, suggesting that a threshold of intake more than 3.2 g of CLA per day is needed to elicit positive responses. This notion has been supported by other research as well (52,53). One study demonstrated that 5 g of CLA per day increased lean body mass and reduced fat mass in men and women when supplemented during resistance training for 7 weeks (52). Researchers have also demonstrated that adding 6 g of CLA per day for 5 weeks to creatine and whey protein supplementation enhanced gains in lean mass and strength in weight-training men and women (53). Another study demonstrated improvements in body composition with supplementation of 3.6 g of CLA per day in women participating in an aerobic exercise program for 6 weeks (54). However, not all studies using high doses of CLA have obtained similar results. Researchers provided 6 g of CLA per day to resistance-training men for 28 days and failed to detect improved strength or lean body mass compared to a placebo (55). At a lower dosage, 3 g of CLA per day for 64 days failed to alter body composition of women (56).

Although not all studies are in agreement, athletes engaged in a strength-training regimen may benefit from higher-dose CLA supplementation. A dosage of at least 3.6 g/d for several weeks would be a good starting point to consider. Of note, one group of researchers did not detect ergogenic effects in exercisers consuming up to 6 g of CLA per day (55).

Very little research has evaluated potential endurance-enhancing effects of CLA. Supplementation of 3.6 g of CLA per day during 6 weeks of training in young women failed to enhance endurance (54). However, research in mice has demonstrated improvements in fat oxidation and swimming endurance after CLA consumption (57), which may have been due to norepinephrine-induced lipolysis (58) leading to enhanced mobilization of fatty acids from adipose tissue, thereby increasing plasma FFA concentrations. Before recommendations can be made for CLA supplementation for endurance performance, further research is needed to verify that a similar strategy is effective in trained athletes.

n-3 Fatty Acids

Supplements containing n-3 fatty acids, particularly fish oil supplements, have become very popular in recent years. Key dietary n-3 fatty acids include alpha-linolenic acid (ALA), EPA, and DHA. Fish oils are particularly rich sources of EPA and DHA, which are potent precursors for eicosanoids, hormone-like compounds synthesized by cyclooxgenase and lipoxygenase enzyme systems. Eicosanoids include thromboxanes, leukotrienes, and prostaglandins, and their functions (eg, blood vessel dilation, bronchiole dilation, platelet anti-aggregation, and anti-inflammatory properties) and potencies depend on their classes and the precursor fatty acids from which they are formed. Those produced from n-3 fatty acids have garnered attention for potential ergogenic effects as well as health benefits that they may provide to the athlete.

Because purified n-3 fatty acids are regulated as a drug by the Food and Drug Administration, these compounds are available in the United States only as a component of food and dietary supplements. In most studies, fish oil supplements are used as the source of n-3 fatty acids. Exercisers receiving fish oil containing 3 g EPA and 2 g DHA per day for 6 weeks exhibited improved brachial artery diameter and blood flow, suggesting that under the proper circumstances, n-3 supplementation may translate to improved performance (59). In earlier research, male soccer players took a daily supplement of 5.2 g of fish oil, providing 1.60 g of EPA and 1.04 g of DHA, for 10 weeks (60). This supplement regimen failed to improve maximal aerobic power, anaerobic power, or running performance in comparison to corn oil. Likewise, taking 6 g of fish oil supplement daily for 3 weeks failed to enhance endurance of trained cyclists (61). Although at high doses, fish oil, presumably due to its high concentration of n-3 fatty acids, produces metabolic effects that have the potential to improve athletic performance, clear evidence is not yet available to warrant that conclusion. Until solid evidence is available, it is not possible to establish recommended doses for fish oil or other n-3 fatty acid–rich foods. Furthermore, some research has indicated that fish oil supplementation may increase levels of markers of oxidative stress after exercise (62,63); therefore, some caution is recommended before beginning a fish oil supplementation regimen.

Athletes who have asthma or exercise-induced asthma are one group of athletes who may benefit from fish oil supplementation. Several studies have indicated that the anti-inflammatory properties seem to be responsible for the capacity of fish oil to improve pulmonary function indicators during exercise (64,65). Practitioners who work with these athletes should consult a physician to determine a dosing regimen; however, relatively large dosages of fish oil providing more than 5 g per day of EPA and DHA combined for 3 weeks have been demonstrated to be effective.

Carnitine and Choline

Several dietary supplements are marketed for their potential capacity to enhance lipid metabolism. These include caffeine, carnitine, choline, and other substances. Caffeine as an ergogenic aid is discussed in Chapter 7. Carnitine is required for the translocation of fatty acids from the cytosol to the mitochondria for ultimate energy production; therefore, enhanced carnitine status could theoretically enhance lipid oxidation and spare carbohydrates during exercise, promoting improved endurance capacity (66).

Carnitine is a nonessential nutrient provided in the average diet in amounts of 100 to 300 mg/d, primarily from foods such as red meats, chicken, fish, eggs, and milk (66). Those who consume a diet low in carnitine, such as vegetarians, compensate through increased biosynthesis and decreased renal carnitine clearance (67). Although carnitine is required for lipid oxidation, most research on carnitine supplementation fails to support its use for enhanced performance. A few studies, however, have demonstrated some positive effects on physiological variables, including increased fat utilization (68), a decrease in respiratory exchange ratio (69–71), and an increase in maximum oxygen consumption (VO_{2max}) (71,72). These data indicate that under some circumstances, metabolic changes may occur that could improve endurance performance. Notably, many studies have demonstrated no difference with carnitine supplementation in physiological variables such as heart rate, lactate, VO_{2max}, rate of perceived exertion, lipid metabolism, or exercise performance (73–79). However endurance was enhanced in one study in which carnitine was supplemented along with caffeine (80).

Although carnitine supplementation has been demonstrated increased plasma carnitine concentrations, increases in cellular carnitine levels are not typically observed (73,81–84). Simultaneous supplementation with choline (85) or carbohydrate (86) seems to enhance the incorporation of carnitine into muscle cells.

These combinations may enhance the efficacy of carnitine supplementation (87) and are worthy of continued investigation. Most notably, supplementation of 2 g of carnitine twice per day for 24 weeks along with 80 g of carbohydrate increased muscle carnitine, presumably by the action of insulin, spared muscle glycogen, and improved cycling performance (86).

Interestingly, endurance training seems to enhance the biosynthesis of carnitine (69), suggesting that athletes may be less likely to obtain benefits from supplementation than untrained individuals. However, some research indicates that carnitine status is diminished by exercise training (81), suggesting the opposite may be true, so the effect of carnitine supplementation remains unclear.

Supplementation with dosages ranging from 500 mg/d to 6 g/d for periods of 1 to 28 days seems to be safe (66); however, the dosage that is most likely to enhance lipid metabolism and therefore endurance is unknown, particularly because most studies report the absence of a positive effect. This suggests that if carnitine supplementation is effective, a different regimen than typically used in research studies is likely optimal. Most researchers have conducted studies with carnitine supplementation ranging between 1 to 12 weeks and providing 2 to 4 g/d. It is possible that a different dosage or a regimen that combines caffeine, choline, and/or carbohydrate for an extended period of time may be optimal. Practitioners should advise athletes interested in using carnitine to explore a regimen that combines carnitine at relatively high doses along with a substance that may enhance its efficacy, particularly carbohydrate, to maximize the potential for success.

In addition to enhancing cellular carnitine uptake, choline, as well as lecithin (phosphatidyl choline), has been studied for potential ergogenic effects due to choline's role with acetylcholine and muscular contraction. It is likely that choline deficiency would hamper optimal performance; however, there is no evidence to suggest that supplementation of choline in nondeficient individuals enhances exercise capacity (88,89). Interestingly, limited research suggests that an exercise-induced decrease in choline status may be prevented by choline supplementation (89). More research is needed to fully understand choline metabolism in athletes, but for now practitioners should consider including assessment of the intake of choline, now considered an essential nutrient, in the dietary assessments of athletes.

Summary

The potential roles of dietary fats for exercise performance are often overlooked, likely because most results to date for many strategies remain equivocal. RDs and athletes should consider lipid-based regimens or dietary supplements that could alter lipid metabolism in a manner that is potentially favorable for exercise performance and/or wellness. Likewise, dietary choices that might negatively impact lipid metabolism and therefore exercise performance, such as nicotinic acid supplementation, which can reduce fat utilization and enhance glycogen depletion at high doses (90), should be avoided. Researchers and practitioners should consider various dietary regimens and/or supplements or combinations of such strategies to optimize lipid metabolism, particularly under a variety of exercise conditions, possibly providing athletes with a winning edge.

References

1. Institute of Medicine. *Dietary Reference Intakes for Energy, Carbohydrate, Fiber, Fat, Fatty Acids, Cholesterol, Protein, and Amino Acids (Macronutrients)*. Washington, DC: National Academies Press; 2005.
2. Jensen CD, Zaltas ES, Whittam JH. Dietary intakes of male endurance cyclists during training and racing. *J Am Diet Assoc*. 1992;92:986–988.

3. Burke LM, Gollan RA, Read RSD. Dietary intakes and food use of groups of elite Australian male athletes. *Int J Sport Nutr*. 1991;1:378–394.

4. Petersen HL, Peterson CT, Reddy MB, Hanson KB, Swain JH, Sharp RL, Alekel DL. Body composition, dietary intake, and iron status of female collegiate swimmers and divers. *Int J Sport Nutr Exerc Metab*. 2006;16:281–295.

5. Ousley-Pahnke L, Black DR, Gretebeck RJ. Dietary intake and energy expenditure of female collegiate swimmers during decreased training prior to competition. *J Am Diet Assoc*. 2001;101:351–354.

6. Berning JR, Troup JP, VanHandel PJ, Daniels J, Daniels N. The nutritional habits of young adolescent swimmers. *Int J Sport Nutr*. 1991;1:240–248.

7. Barr SI. Relationship of eating attitudes to anthropometric variables and dietary intakes of female collegiate swimmers. *J Am Diet Assoc*. 1991;91:976–977.

8. Barr SI, Costill DL. Effect of increased training volume on nutrient intake of male collegiate swimmers. *Int J Sports Med*. 1992;13:47–51.

9. Smith MP, Mendez J, Druckenmiller M, Kris-Etherton PM. Exercise intensity, dietary intake and high-density lipoprotein cholesterol in young female competitive swimmers. *Am J Clin Nutr*. 1982;36:251–255.

10. Grandjean AC. Macronutrient intake of U.S. athletes compared with the general population and recommendations made for athletes. *Am J Clin Nutr*. 1989;49:1070–1076.

11. Soric M, Misigoj-Durakovic M, Pedisic Z. Dietary intake and body composition of prepubescent female aesthetic athletes. *Int J Sport Nutr Exerc Metab*. 2008;18:343–354.

12. Havemann L, Goedecke JH. Nutritional practices of male cyclists before and during an ultraendurance event. *Int J Sport Nutr Exerc Metab*. 2008;18:551–566.

13. Peters EM, Goetzsche JM. Dietary practices of South African ultradistance runners. *Int J Sport Nutr*. 1997;7:80–103.

14. Kopp-Woodroffe SA, Manore MM, Dueck CA, Skinner JS, Matt KS. Energy and nutrient status of amenorrheic athletes participating in a diet and exercise training intervention program. *Int J Sport Nutr*. 1999;9:70–88.

15. Onywera VO, Kiplamai FK, Tuitoek PJ, Boit MK, Pitsiladis YP. Food and macronutrient intake of elite Kenyan distance runners. *Int J Sport Nutr Exerc Metab*. 2004;14:709–719.

16. Carey MC, Small DM, Bliss CM. Lipid digestion and absorption. *Ann Rev Physiol*. 1983;45:651–677.

17. Romijn JA, Coyle EF, Sidossis LS, Gastaldelli A, Horowitz JF, Endert E, Wolfe RR. Regulation of endogenous fat and carbohydrate metabolism in relation to exercise intensity and duration. *Am J Physiol*. 1993:265;E380–E391.

18. Lambert EV, Speechly DP, Dennis SC, Noakes TD. Enhanced endurance in trained cyclists during moderate intensity exercise following 2 weeks adaptation to a high fat diet. *Eur J Appl Physiol*. 1994;69:287–293.

19. Muoio DM, Leddy JJ, Horvath PJ, Aw AB, Pendergast DR. Effects of dietary fat on metabolic adjustments to maximal VO_2 and endurance in runners. *Med Sci Sports Exerc*. 1994;26:81–88.

20. Horvath PJ, Eagen CK, Fisher NM, Leddy JJ, Pendergast DR. The effects of varying dietary fat on performance and metabolism in trained male and female runners. *J Am Coll Nutr*. 2000;19:52–60.

21. O'Keeffe KA, Keith RE, Wilson GD, Blessing DL. Dietary carbohydrate intake and endurance exercise performance of trained female cyclists. *Nutr Res*. 1989;9:819–830.

22. Helge JW, Richter EA, Kiens B. Interaction of training and diet on metabolism and endurance during exercise in man. *J Physiol*. 1996;492:293–306.

23. Phinney SD, Bistrian BR, Evans WJ, Gervino E, Blackburn GL. The human metabolic response to chronic ketosis without caloric restriction: preservation of submaximal exercise capability with reduced carbohydrate oxidation. *Metabolism*. 1973;32:769–776.

24. Burke LM, Hawley JA. Effects of short-term fat adaptation on metabolism and performance of prolonged exercise. *Med Sci Sports Exerc*. 2002;34:1492–1498.

25. Rowlands DS, Hopkins WG. Effects of high-fat and high-carbohydrate diets on metabolism and performance in cycling. *Metabolism*. 2002;51:678–690.

26. Goedecke JH, Christie C, Wilson G, Dennis SC, Noakes TD, Hopkins WG, Lambert EV. Metabolic adaptations to a high-fat diet in endurance cyclists. *Metabolism*. 1999;48:1509–1517.

27. Helge JW, Wulff B, Kiens B. Impact of a fat-rich diet on endurance in man: role of the dietary period. *Med Sci Sports Exerc*. 1998;30:456–461.

28. Durstine JL, Haskell WL. Effects of exercise training on plasma lipids and lipoproteins. *Exerc Sports Sci Rev.* 1994;22:477–521.

29. Brown RC, Cox CM. Effects of high fat versus high carbohydrate diets on plasma lipids and lipoproteins in endurance athletes. *Med Sci Sports Exerc.* 1998;30:1677–1683.

30. Leddy J, Horvath P, Rowland J, Pendergast D. Effect of a high or a low fat diet on cardiovascular risk factors in male and female runners. *Med Sci Sports Exerc.* 1997;29:17–25.

31. Lambert EV, Goedecke JH, Van Zyl C, Murphy K, Hawley JA, Dennis SC, Noakes TD. High-fat diet versus habitual diet prior to carbohydrate loading: effects of exercise metabolism and cycling performance. *Int J Sport Nutr Exerc Metab.* 2001;11:209–225.

32. Carey AL, Staudacher HM, Cummings NK, Stepto NK, Nikolopoulos V, Burke LM, Hawley JA. Effects of fat adaptation and carbohydrate restoration on prolonged endurance exercise. *J Appl Physiol.* 2001;91:115–122.

33. Havemann L, West SJ, Goedecke JH, McDonald IA, St Clair Gibson A, Noakes TD, Lambert EV. Fat adaptation followed by carbohydrate-loading compromises high-intensity sprint performance. *J Appl Physiol.* 2006;100: 194–202.

34. Kiens B, Burke LM. Fat adaptation for athletic performance: the nail in the coffin? *J Appl Physiol.* 2006;100:7–8.

35. Stellingwerff T, Spriet LL, Watt MJ, Kimber NF, Hargreaves M, Hawley JA, Burke LM. Decreased PDH activation and glycogenolysis during exercise following fat adaptation with carbohydrate restoration. *Am J Physiol Endocrinol Metab.* 2006;290:E380–E388.

36. Beckers EJ, Jeukendrup AE, Brouns F, Wagenmakers AJ, Saris WHM. Gastric emptying of carbohydrate-medium chain triglyceride suspensions at rest. *Int J Sports Med.* 1992;13:581–584.

37. Berning JR. The role of medium-chain triglycerides in exercise. *Int J Sports Nutr.* 1996;6:121–133.

38. Bach AC, Babayan VK. Medium-chain triglycerides: an update. *Am J Clin Nutr.* 1982;36:950–962.

39. Fushiki TK, Matsumoto K, Inoue K, Kawada T, Sugimoto E. Swimming capacity of mice is increased by chronic consumption of medium-chain triglycerides. *J Nutr.* 1995;125:531–539.

40. Misell LM, Lagomarcino ND, Schuster V, Kern M. Chronic medium-chain triacylglycerol consumption and endurance performance in trained runners. *J Sports Med Phys Fitness.* 2001;41:210–215.

41. Thorburn MS, Vistisen B, Thorp RM, Rockell MJ, Jeukendrup AE, Xu X, Rowlands DS. Attenuated gastric distress but no benefit to performance with adaptation to octanoate-rich esterified oils in well-trained male cyclists. *J Appl Physiol.* 2006;101:1733–1743.

42. Van Zyl CG, Lambert EV, Hawley JA, Noakes TD, Dennis SC. Effects of medium-chain triglyceride ingestion on fuel metabolism and cycling performance. *J Appl Physiol.* 1996;80:2217–2225.

43. Angus DJ, Hargreaves M, Dancey J, Febbraio MA. Effect of carbohydrate or carbohydrate plus medium-chain triglyceride ingestion on cycling time trial performance. *J Appl Physiol.* 2000;88:113–119.

44. Vistisen BL, Nybo L, Xuebing X, Hoy CE, Kiens B. Minor amounts of plasma medium-chain fatty acids and no improved time trial performance after consuming lipids. *J Appl Physiol.* 2003;94:2434–2443.

45. Goedecke JH, Elmer-English R, Dennis SC, Schloss I, Noakes TD, Lambert EV. Effects of medium-chain triacylglycerol ingested with carbohydrate on metabolism and exercise performance. *Int J Sport Nutr.* 1999;9:35–47.

46. Goedecke JH, Clark VR, Noakes TD, Lambert EV. The effects of medium-chain triacylglycerol and carbohydrate ingestion on ultra-endurance performance. *Int J Sport Nutr Exerc Metab.* 2005;15:15–28.

47. Satabin P, Portero P, Defer G, Bricout J, Guezennec CY. Metabolic and hormonal responses to lipid and carbohydrate diets during exercise in man. *Med Sci Sports Exerc.* 1987;19:218–223.

48. Jeukendrup AE, Thielen JJ, Wagenmakers AJ, Brouns F, Saris WHM. Effects of medium-chain triacylglycerol and carbohydrate ingestion during exercise on substrate utilization and subsequent cycling performance. *Am J Clin Nutr.* 1998;67:397–404.

49. Kern M, Lagomarcino ND, Misell LM, Schuster V. The effect of medium-chain triacylglycerols on the blood lipid profile of male endurance runners. *J Nutr Biochem.* 2000;11:288–293.

50. Ritzenthaler KL, McGuire MK, Falen R, Shultz TD, Dasgupta N, McGuire MA. Estimation of conjugated linoleic acid intake by written dietary assessment methodologies underestimates actual intake evaluated by food duplicate methodology. *J Nutr.* 2001;131:1548–1554.

51. Steck SE, Chalecki AM, Miller P, Conway J, Austin GL, Hardin JW, Albright CD, Thuillier P. Conjugated linoleic acid supplementation for twelve weeks increases lean body mass in obese humans. *J Nutr.* 2007;137:1188–1193.

52. Pinkoski C, Chilibeck PD, Candow DG, Esliger D, Ewaschuk JB, Facci M, Farthing JP, Zello GA. The effects of conjugated linoleic acid supplementation during resistance training. *Med Sci Sports Exerc.* 2006;38:339–348.

53. Cornish SM, Candow DG, Jantz NT, Chilibeck PD, Little JP, Forbes S, Abeysekara S, Zello GA. Conjugated linoleic acid combined with creatine monohydrate and whey protein supplementation during strength training. *Int J Sport Nutr Exerc Metab.* 2009;19:70–96.

54. Colakoglu S, Colakoglu M, Taneli F, Cetinoz F, Turkmen M. Cumulative effects of conjugated linoleic acid and exercise on endurance development, body composition, serum leptin and insulin levels. *J Sports Med Phys Fitness.* 2006;46:570–577.

55. Kreider RB, Ferreira MP, Greenwood M, Wilson M, Almada AL. Effects of conjugated linoleic acid supplementation during resistance training on body composition, bone density, strength, and selected hematological markers. *J Strength Cond Res.* 2002;16:325–334.

56. Zambell KL, Keim NL, Van Loan MD, Gale B, Benito P, Kelley DS, Nelson GJ. Conjugated linoleic acid supplementation in humans: effects on body composition and energy expenditure. *Lipids.* 2000;35:777–782.

57. Mizunoya W, Haramizu S, Shibakusa T, Okabe Y, Fushiki T. Dietary conjugated linoleic acid increases endurance capacity and fat oxidation in mice during exercise. *Lipids.* 2005;40:265–271.

58. Park Y, Albright KJ, Liu W, Storkson JM, Cook ME, Pariza MW. Effect of conjugated linoleic acid on body composition in mice. *Lipids.* 1997;32:853–858.

59. Raastad T, Hostmark AT, Stromme SB. Omega-3 fatty acid supplementation does not improve maximal aerobic power, anaerobic threshold and running performance in well-trained soccer players. *Scand J Med Sci Sports.* 1997;7:25–31.

60. Oostenbrug GS, Mensink RP, Hardeman MR, DeVries T, Brouns F, Hornstra G. Exercise performance, red blood cell deformability, and lipid peroxidation: effects of fish oil and vitamin E. *J Appl Physiol.* 1997;83:746–752.

61. Walser B, Giordano RM, Stebbins CL. Supplementation with omega-3 polyunsaturated fatty acids augments brachial artery dilation and blood flow during forearm contraction. *Eur J Appl Physiol.* 2006;97:347–354.

62. McAnulty SR, Nieman DC, Fox-Rabinovich M, Duran V, McAnulty LS, Henson DJ, Jin F, Landram MJ. Effects of n-3 fatty acids and antioxidants on oxidative stress after exercise. *Med Sci Sports Exerc.* 2010;42:1704–1711.

63. Filaire E, Massart A, Portier H, Rouveix M, Rosado F, Bage AS, Gobert M, Durand D. Effect of 6 weeks of n-3 fatty acid supplementation on oxidative stress in judo athletes. *Int J Sport Nutr Exerc Metab.* 2010;20:496–506.

64. Mickleborough TD, Murray RL, Ionescu AA, Lindley MR. Fish oil supplementation reduces severity of exercise-induced bronchoconstriction in elite athletes. *Am J Resp Crit Care Med.* 2003;168:1181–1189.

65. Mickleborough TD, Lindley MR, Ionescu AA, Fly AD. Protective effect of fish oil supplementation on exercise-induced bronchoconstriction in asthma. *Chest.* 2006;129:39–49.

66. Kanter MM, Williams MH. Antioxidants, carnitine, and choline as putative ergogenic aids. *Int J Sport Nutr.* 1995;5(Suppl):S120–S131.

67. Lombard KA, Olson AL, Nelson SE, Rebouche CJ. Carnitine status of lactoovovegetarians and strict vegetarian adults and children. *Am J Clin Nutr.* 1989;50:301–306.

68. Natali A, Santoro D, Brandi LS, Faraggiana D, Ciociaro D, Pecori N, Buzzigoli G, Ferrannini E. Effects of acute hypercarnitinemia during increased fatty substrate oxidation in man. *Metabolism.* 1993;45:594–600.

69. Gorostiaga EM, Maurer CA, Eclache JP. Decrease in respiratory quotient during exercise following L-carnitine supplementation. *Int J Sports Med.* 1989;10:169–174.

70. Vecchiet L, Di Lisa F, Pieralisi G, Ripari P, Menabo R, Giamberardino MA, Siliprandi N. Influence of L-carnitine administration on maximal physical exercise. *Eur J Appl Physiol.* 1990;61:486–490.

71. Wyss V, Ganzit GP, Rienzi A. Effects of L-carnitine administration on VO_{2max} and the aerobic-anaerobic threshold in normoxia and acute hypoxia. *Eur J Appl Physiol.* 1990;60:1–6.

72. Marconi C, Sassi G, Carpinelli A, Cerretelli P. Effects of L-carnitine loading on the aerobic and anaerobic performance of endurance athletes. *Eur J Appl Physiol.* 1985;54:131–135.

73. Wachter S, Vogt M, Kreis R, Boesch C, Bigler P, Hoppeler H, Krahenbuhl S. Long-term administration of L-carnitine to humans: effect on skeletal muscle carnitine content and physical performance. *Clin Chim Acta.* 2002;318:51–61.

74. Decombaz J, Olivier D, Acheson K, Gmuender B, Jequier E. Effect of L-carnitine on submaximal exercise metabolism after depletion of muscle glycogen. *Med Sci Sports Exerc.* 1993;25:733–740.

75. Oyono-Enguelle S, Freund H, Ott C, Gartner M, Heitz A, Marbach J, Maccari F, Frey A, Bigot H, Back AC. Prolonged submaximal exercise and L-carnitine in humans. *Eur J Appl Physiol.* 1988;58:53–61.

76. Greig C, Finch KM, Jones DA, Cooper M, Sargeant AJ, Forte CA. The effect of oral supplementation with L-carnitine on maximum and submaximum exercise capacity. *Eur J Appl Physiol.* 1985;56:457–460.

77. Colombani P, Wenk C, Kunz I, Krahenbuhl S, Kuhnt M, Arnold M, Frey-Rindova P, Frey W, Langhans W. Effects of L-carnitine supplementation on physical performance and energy metabolism of endurance-trained athletes: A double blind cross-over field study. *Eur J Appl Phys.* 1996;73:434–439.

78. Trappe SW, Costill DL, Goodpaster B, Vukovich MD, Fink WJ. The effects of L-carnitine supplementation on performance during interval swimming. *Int J Sports Med.* 1994;15:181–185.

79. Stuessi C, Hofer P, Meier C, Boutellier U. L-carnitine and the recovery from exhaustive endurance exercise: a randomised, double-blind, placebo-controlled trial. *Eur J Appl Physiol.* 2005;95:431–435.

80. Cha YS, Choi SK, Suh H, Lee SN, Cho D, Li K. Effects of carnitine coingested caffeine on carnitine metabolism and endurance capacity in athletes. *J Nutr Sci Vitaminol.* 2001;47:378–384.

81. Arenas J, Ricoy JR, Encinas AR, Pola P, D'Iddio S, Zeviani M, Didonato S, Corsi M. Carnitine in muscle, serum, and urine of nonprofessional athletes: effects of physical exercise, training, and L-carnitine administration. *Muscle Nerve.* 1991;14:598–604.

82. Barnett C, Costill DL, Vukovich MD, Cole KJ, Goodpaster BH, Trappe SW, Fink WJ. Effect of L-carnitine supplementation on muscle and blood carnitine content and lactate accumulation during high-intensity spring cycling. *Int J Sport Nutr.* 1994;4:280–288.

83. Soop M, Bjorkman O, Cederblad G, Hagenfeldt L, Wahren J. Influence of supplementation on muscle substrate and carnitine metabolism during exercise. *J Appl Physiol.* 1988;64:2394–2399.

84. Vukovich M, Costill D, Fink W. Carnitine supplementation: effect on muscle carnitine content and glycogen utilization during exercise. *Med Sci Sports Exerc.* 1994;26:1122–1129.

85. Daily JW, Sachan DS. Choline supplementation alters carnitine homeostasis in humans and guinea pigs. *J Nutr.* 1995;125:1938–1944.

86. Wall BT, Stephens FB, Constantin-Teodosiu D, Marimuthu K, Macdonald IA, Greenhaff PL. Chronic oral ingestion of L-carnitine and carbohydrate increases muscle carnitine content and alters muscle fuel metabolism during exercise in humans. *J Physiol.* 2011;589:963–973.

87. Hongu N, Sachan DS. Carnitine and choline supplementation with exercise alter carnitine profiles, biochemical markers of fat metabolism and serum leptin concentration in healthy women. *J Nutr.* 2003;133:84–89.

88. Spector SA, Jackman MR, Sabounjian LA, Sakkas C, Landers D, Willis WT. Effect of choline supplementation on fatigue in trained cyclists. *Med Sci Sports Exerc.* 1995;27:668–673.

89. Von Allworden HN, Horn S, Kahl J, Feldheim W. The influence of lecithin on plasma choline concentrations in triathletes and adolescent runners during exercise. *Eur J Appl Physiol.* 1993;67:87–91.

90. Pernow B, Saltin B. Availability of substrates and capacity for prolonged heavy exercise. *J Appl Physiol.* 1971;31:416–422.

Chapter 5

VITAMINS, MINERALS, AND EXERCISE

Stella Lucia Volpe, PhD, RD, FACSM, and Erica Bland, BSN, RN

Introduction

Micronutrients (vitamins and minerals) differ from macronutrients in that they are required in much smaller quantities than macronutrients. The use of macronutrients for all physiologic processes is enabled by micronutrients (1). Therefore, vitamins and minerals are necessary for many metabolic processes in the body, as well as to support growth and development (2). Vitamins and minerals are also key regulators in many reactions in exercise and physical activity, including energy metabolism, oxygen transfer and delivery, and tissue repair (2).

The vitamin and mineral needs of individuals who are physically active are a subject of debate. Some reports state that those who exercise require more vitamins and minerals than their sedentary counterparts, but other studies do not report greater micronutrient requirements. The intensity, duration, and frequency of activity, as well as the overall energy and nutrient intakes, affect micronutrient requirements (2–4). The purpose of this chapter is to review the vitamin and mineral needs of adults who are physically active.

Dietary Reference Intakes

Recommendations for all known vitamins and some essential minerals for healthy, moderately active people were updated beginning in 1997 (5–8). These recommendations are known as the Dietary Reference Intakes (DRIs). Adequate Intake (AI), Recommended Dietary Allowance (RDA), Estimated Average Requirement (EAR), and Tolerable Upper Intake Level (UL) are all types of DRIs. The RDA is the dietary intake level that is adequate for approximately 98% of healthy people. The AI is an estimated value that is used when an RDA cannot be determined. The EAR is a value used to approximate the nutrient needs of half of the healthy people in a group. The UL is the highest amount of a nutrient that most individuals can consume without adverse effects (9). DRI tables are published online by the Institute of Medicine (http://iom.edu/Activities/Nutrition/SummaryDRIs/DRI-Tables.aspx).

In general, if energy intakes are adequate, the vitamin and mineral needs of physically active individuals are similar to healthy, moderately active individuals. Thus, the use of the DRIs is appropriate. Some athletes may have increased requirements because of excessive losses of nutrients in sweat and urine, and supplementation may be needed. Because many individuals who are physically active choose to supplement with vitamins and minerals, the UL allows for practitioners to give guidelines to these individuals to prevent adverse reactions from excess consumption. Additional information about multivitamin and mineral and antioxidant supplements is provided in Chapter 7.

There are limitations to the research on micronutrients for athletes. Mixed results make it difficult for practitioners to give definitive advice to athletes. The research limitations include: (*a*) small numbers of subjects, most of whom are male; (*b*) differences in type of exercise performed and/or level of training and fitness; (*c*) lack of strong longitudinal data; (*d*) differences in assessment methodology or study design; and (*e*) various types and amounts of supplementation.

For micronutrients, an assessment of dietary intake is required because many athletes may not consume enough energy and therefore inadequate micronutrients, which could result in suboptimal exercise performance. Clark et al (10) assessed the pre- and postseason intakes of macro- and micronutrients in female soccer players and found that, despite meeting energy requirements (but not carbohydrate needs), intakes of the micronutrients vitamin E, folate, copper, and magnesium were marginal (< 75% of the RDA).

In an effort to assess if micronutrient supplementation affects performance, Telford et al (11) supplemented 82 male and female athletes from different sports with either a vitamin-mineral supplement or a placebo for 7 to 8 months. All subjects consumed diets that met the RDA for vitamins and minerals. Although vitamin-mineral supplementation did not improve performance in any of the sport-specific variables measured, an improved jumping ability in female basketball players was noted. Certainly, the area of supplementation and athletic performance needs to be further studied; however, it seems that individuals who consume adequate intakes of vitamins and minerals from food do not benefit from supplementation.

Water-Soluble Vitamins

Vitamins are classified by their solubility within the body. The water-soluble vitamins, which do not require fat for their absorption, include vitamin B-6, vitamin B-12, folate, thiamin, riboflavin, niacin, pantothenic acid, biotin, vitamin C, and choline. Table 5.1 lists the water-soluble vitamin needs for the athlete along with food sources.

Vitamin B-6

There are three major forms of vitamin B-6: pyridoxine (PN), pyridoxal (PL), and pyridoxamine (PM). The active coenzyme forms of vitamin B-6 are pyridoxal 5′-phosphate (PLP) and pyridoxamine 5′-phosphate (PMP) (12). Vitamin B-6 is involved in approximately 100 metabolic reactions, including those involving gluconeogenesis, niacin synthesis, and lipid metabolism (12).

Some researchers have reported that vitamin B-6 metabolism is affected by exercise and that poor vitamin B-6 status can impair exercise performance (13). Manore (14) reports that vitamin B-6 plays a key role in producing energy during exercise, and therefore individuals with an inadequate intake of vitamin B-6 have a reduced ability to optimally perform physical activity. It was once thought that exercise caused transient changes in vitamin B-6 status because exercise seems to increase the loss of vitamin B-6 through urinary excretion (14). However, this assumption may not be true (15,16). An animal study suggested that exercise itself causes retention of vitamin B-6 by decreasing excretion, even when intake of vitamin B-6 is restricted (17). This animal study demonstrates an adaptive mechanism that could occur as a result of exercise; however, over time this mechanism may not be sufficient for maintaining vitamin B-6 status if intake continues to be less than adequate.

TABLE 5.1   Water-Soluble Vitamin Needs for Athletes and Food Sources

Vitamin	Effect of Exercise on Requirements	Recommended Intake for Athletes	Food Sources	Comments
Vitamin B-6	Exercise does not cause transient changes in B-6 status.	RDA	Liver, chicken, bananas, potatoes, spinach	
Vitamin B-12	Exercise does not seem to increase needs.	RDA	Fish, milk and milk products, eggs, meat, poultry, fortified breakfast cereals	Vegan athletes may need to supplement to ensure adequate intake.
Folate	Exercise does not seem to increase needs.	RDA	Leafy greens (eg, spinach, turnip greens), dry beans, peas, fortified cereals, grain products, strawberries	
Thiamin	Exercise does not seem to increase needs.	RDA	Wheat germ, brewer's yeast, oysters, beef liver, peanuts, green peas, raisins, collard greens	Ergogenic effects are equivocal; positive effects are not strong.
Riboflavin	Exercise does not seem to increase needs.	RDA	Organ meats, milk, cheese, oily fish, eggs, dark leafy green vegetables	
Niacin	Exercise does not seem to increase needs.	RDA	Beef, pork, chicken, wheat flour, eggs, milk	Does not seem to have ergogenic effects; more research is needed.
Pantothenic acid	Not enough information.	AI	Eggs, whole grain cereals, meat	
Biotin	Not enough information.	AI	Kidney, liver, eggs, dried mixed fruit	
Vitamin C	Increased intakes may prevent upper respiratory tract infections.	At least the RDA; ultra-endurance athletes need more than the RDA, but less than the UL	Brussels sprouts, broccoli, chili and bell peppers, kiwi, oranges, papaya, guava	Strong antioxidant properties reported for endurance and ultra-endurance athletes.
Choline	Exercise does not seem to increase needs.	AI	Liver, egg yolks, peanuts, cauliflower, soybeans, grape juice, and cabbage	Does not seem to have an ergogenic effect; more research required.

Abbreviations: RDA, Recommended Dietary Allowance; AI, Adequate Intake; UL, Tolerable Upper Intake Level.

Considering the state of research, it seems that individuals who exercise do not have increased needs for vitamin B-6. However, Manore states that work capacity improves as vitamin B-6 status improves and deficiencies of vitamin B-6 negatively affect aerobic capacity (14). Therefore, if deficiencies exist, it may be necessary to supplement with vitamin B-6 at the level of the DRI. Dietary sources of vitamin B-6 can be found in Table 5.1.

Vitamin B-12 and Folate

Vitamin B-12 (cyanocobalamin) and folate (folic acid) are both necessary for DNA synthesis (18,19) and are interrelated in their synthesis and metabolism. Both vitamins are required for normal erythrocyte synthesis; it is this function by which these two vitamins may have an effect on exercise (20).

There is no evidence to suggest that exercise increases the need for either of these vitamins. Lukaski (1) states that while there is limited data assessing blood biochemical measures of folate status in physically active individuals, physical performance did not improve in folate-deficient athletes receiving folate supplementation. Inadequate intakes of either vitamin can lead to megaloblastic anemia. The adequate intake of vitamin B-12 is of special concern in vegan athletes because vitamin B-12 is almost exclusively found in animal foods (21,22). Vegetarians who consume dairy products and/or eggs are likely to have adequate intakes of vitamin B-12, but vegan athletes need to regularly consume vitamin B-12–fortified foods or may need to supplement (20,22). More information about vitamin B-12 and vegetarian athletes can be found in Chapter 16.

Although injections of vitamin B-12 are used clinically for individuals diagnosed with megaloblastic anemia, oral supplementation is sufficient if a frank anemia has not been diagnosed. A multivitamin and mineral supplement including 500 to 1,000 mg of vitamin C may decrease vitamin B-12 bioavailability from food but may also lead to vitamin B-12 deficiency (23,24). Because vitamin B-12 is secreted daily into the bile and then reabsorbed, it takes approximately 20 years for healthy people to show signs of deficiency (22). However, vitamin B-12 deficiency can be masked by high folate intake; thus, if a vitamin B-12 deficiency is suspected, an assessment of dietary intake will be necessary, especially if biochemical tests are negative for a B-12 deficiency.

Athletes who consume an adequate amount of vitamin B-12 and folate in their diets are probably not at risk for vitamin B-12 or folate deficiencies. Nonetheless, vitamin B-12 or folate deficiencies can lead to increased serum homocysteine levels, which is a risk factor for cardiovascular disease (25), pointing to the need for individuals who exercise to be concerned not only about nutrition and performance but also about overall health. Herrmann et al (16) assessed homocysteine, vitamin B-12, and folate serum concentrations in swimmers after high-volume and high-intensity swim training and during 5 days of recovery. Homocysteine levels were increased during both types of training as well as during recovery. Vitamin B-12 levels were unchanged during either type of training, but showed a decrease during the recovery phase, indicating a delayed response to the training. Folate levels, however, decreased during training, but blood levels returned to normal by the end of the recovery periods. Because vitamin B-12 and folate are metabolically interrelated, the changes in one and not the other at different times of exercise and recovery may indicate an adaptive response by each to "protect" the other. Konig et al (25) assessed the influence of training volume and acute physical exercise on homocysteine levels and the interactions with plasma folate and vitamin B-12. Contrary to what Herrmann et al found (16), Konig et al (25) found a decrease in homocysteine levels after training periods and an even lower level of homocysteine concentration after intense exercise. At the present time, it is difficult to determine if the increase in homocysteine levels are persistent with intense training or if they are transient; however, it is important for individuals who exercise to consume adequate levels of vitamin B-12 and folate. Dietary sources of folate and vitamin B-12 can be found in Table 5.1.

Thiamin

Thiamin participates in several energy-producing reactions as part of thiamin diphosphate (TDP) (also known as thiamin pyrophosphate [TPP]), including the citric acid cycle, branched-chain amino acid (BCAA) catabolism, and the pentose phosphate pathway (26). For example, thiamin is required for the conversion of pyruvate to acetyl-CoA during carbohydrate metabolism. This conversion is essential for the aerobic metabolism of glucose, and exercise performance and health will be impaired if this conversion does not occur (2). Thus, it is imperative that individuals who exercise consume adequate amounts of both thiamin and carbohydrates.

There seems to be a strong correlation between high carbohydrate intakes, physical activity, and thiamin requirements (26). This may be a concern for individuals who exercise because a high-carbohydrate diet is recommended for athletes; however, there has not been clear evidence indicating that individuals who exercise require more thiamin in their diets than sedentary individuals. Nonetheless, it is prudent to recommend that individuals who exercise obtain at least the DRI for thiamin to prevent depletion.

To date, the studies that have been published have had equivocal outcomes of the effects of thiamin supplementation on exercise performance. In three studies, including two with cycle ergometry (27–29), supplementation with thiamin derivatives did not enhance exercise performance. However, Suzuki and Itokawa (30) reported that daily supplementation with 100 mg of thiamin significantly decreased fatigue during cycle ergometry. In a study conducted on the effects of thiamin, riboflavin, and vitamin B-6 depletion on exercise performance, van der Beek and colleagues (31) found no adverse effects on exercise performance.

Although there is limited research about the effects of exercise on thiamine, a few cross-sectional studies report that a small percentage of active individuals may have a thiamin deficiency (14). However, more research is required to determine if thiamin requirements are greater in individuals who exercise. Thiamin requirements may parallel the intensity, duration, and frequency of exercise. Because so little research has been done, practitioners should not recommend thiamin intakes more than the DRI for physically active individuals unless a thiamin deficiency has been determined. Dietary sources of thiamin are listed in Table 5.1.

Riboflavin

Riboflavin is involved in several key metabolic reactions that are important during exercise: glycolysis, the citric acid cycle, and the electron transport chain (32). Riboflavin is the precursor in the synthesis of the flavin coenzymes, flavin mononucleotide (FMN), and flavin-adenine dinucleotide (FAD), which assist in oxidation reduction reactions by acting as 1- and 2-electron transfers (32). Riboflavin status may be altered in individuals who are initiating an exercise program (32); however, it is unclear if it is a transient or long-term effect of exercise. Human studies of longer duration are necessary to evaluate the long-term effects of exercise on riboflavin status (32).

It seems that individuals who are physically active and consume adequate amounts of dietary riboflavin are not at risk for depletion of riboflavin and do not require levels more than the RDA (32). Riboflavin deficiency is uncommon in Western countries because it is found in a wide variety of foods. However, athletes who restrict their food intake for weight loss may be at greater risk for riboflavin deficiency (1). Dietary sources of riboflavin are listed in Table 5.1.

Niacin

Niacin is a family of molecules that include both nicotinic acid and nicotinamide (32). The coenzyme forms of niacin are nicotinamide adenine dinucleotide (NAD) and NAD phosphate (NADP). Both are involved in glycolysis, the pentose pathway, the citric acid cycle, lipid synthesis, and the electron transport chain (32). Nicotinic acid is often prescribed and used in pharmacologic doses to reduce serum cholesterol and C-reactive protein levels (32,33). It seems that pharmacological doses of nicotinic acid may augment the use of carbohydrate as a substrate during exercise by decreasing the availability of free fatty acids (32).

Despite this strong connection to exercise metabolism, no solid data presently support increased niacin supplementation for individuals who exercise (32).

Furthermore, pharmacologic doses of niacin can result in a "niacin rush," whereby individuals have blood vessel dilation resulting in flushing, notably reddening in the face, and extreme itching. Athletes may take high doses of niacin with the thought that "more is better." However, taking too much niacin, as with taking too much of any vitamin or mineral, can be detrimental to health and exercise performance because vitamins and minerals can compete with one another and affect metabolism of other nutrients. Because of niacin's role in vasodilation, several researchers have studied the effect of niacin supplementation on thermoregulation and reported mixed results, likely due to differences in methodology (34,35).

It is important that individuals who exercise obtain the DRI for niacin to ensure adequate intake and prevent alterations in fuel utilization that could possibly impair performance. More research needs to be conducted to evaluate the role of niacin on exercise performance. It is important to evaluate this relationship because an adverse effect of niacin may accelerate the depletion of glycogen stores and therefore indirectly affect performance (1). Dietary sources of niacin are listed in Table 5.1.

Pantothenic Acid

Pantothenic acid, whose biologically active forms are coenzyme A (CoA) and acyl carrier protein, is involved in acyl group transfers such as the acylation of amino acids (36,37). Pantothenic acid coenzymes are also involved in lipid synthesis and metabolism and oxidation of pyruvate and alpha ketoglutarate (37). Acetyl CoA is an important intermediate in fat, carbohydrate, and protein metabolism (37). To date, only a few studies have examined the effects of pantothenic acid supplementation on exercise performance (37,38) and there have been no recent human studies (39). Definite conclusions cannot be made; however, it would be prudent to suggest that athletes consume the AI for pantothenic acid. Dietary sources include sunflower seeds, mushrooms, peanuts, brewer's yeast, yogurt, and broccoli (2).

Biotin

Biotin is an essential cofactor in four mitochondrial carboxylases (one carboxylase is in both the mitochondria and cytosol) (40). These carboxylase-dependent reactions are involved in energy metabolism; thus, biotin deficiency could potentially result in impaired exercise performance. To date, no studies have been done on the role of biotin on exercise performance or biotin requirements for individuals who are physically active. Controlled, well-designed studies are needed to establish whether biotin is needed in larger amounts by individuals who exercise.

Good dietary sources of biotin include peanut butter, boiled eggs, toasted wheat germ, egg noodles, Swiss cheese, and cauliflower (2). It is hypothesized that biotin is synthesized by bacteria in the gastrointestinal tract of mammals; however, there are no published reports proving that this actually occurs (40).

Vitamin C

Vitamin C, also referred to as ascorbic acid, ascorbate, or ascorbate monoanion (41), is involved in the maintenance of collagen synthesis, oxidation of fatty acids, and formation of neurotransmitters. It is also an antioxidant (41,42). It has been fairly well-documented that vitamin C protects against oxidative stress in endurance and ultra-endurance athletes, especially preventing upper respiratory tract infections (43). It should also be mentioned here that although aerobic exercise increases oxidative stress, it also results in an increase in the enzymatic and nonenzymatic antioxidants as an adaptation to training. Vitamin C levels in the blood can be increased up to 24 hours after exercise but decreased to less than pre-exercise levels in the days after prolonged exercise; thus, one must be cautious when blood measurements of vitamin C are used as assessment parameters in research studies (43–46) because they may not be truly reflective of status.

Tauler et al (47) reported that high vitamin C intake positively influenced the response of neutrophils and lymphocytes to oxidative stress induced by exercise (duathlon competition), increasing the neutrophil activation. Robson et al (48) also reported a significantly greater neutrophil oxidative burst following exercise after only 7 days of supplementing athletes with an antioxidant combination of 18 mg beta carotene, 900 mg vitamin C, and 90 mg vitamin E. The positive response could not be solely attributed to vitamin C. However, it could be speculated that vitamin C had the greatest impact of the three antioxidant vitamins because it was given at such a high dose. It has been reported that higher plasma vitamin C levels were associated with greater skeletal muscle strength in individuals older than 65 years (49).

Vitamin C is often supplemented in very high doses in the hope that it may prevent colds. Although it had been believed that supplementation with vitamin C in high doses (≥ 1 g/d) reduced the severity and duration of colds, more recent research has not shown this to be true (50,51).

Most of the existing data from supplementation and dietary studies do not support the concept that athletes require an increased amount of vitamin C for a variety of reasons (43). First, the dietary intake of vitamin C is similar in athletes and sedentary control subjects, as is the response to supplementation (43). Second, a strong association is lacking between the concentration of ascorbic acid in the blood and dietary intake of vitamin C (43). Lastly, no difference has been found between athletes and nonathletes in the excretion of ascorbic acid in urine, which is an assessment of the utilization of vitamin C within the body (43).

However, individuals who consistently exercise (at any level) may require at least 100 mg vitamin C per day, which can easily be consumed in food, to maintain normal vitamin C status and protect the body from oxidative damage caused by exercise (42). Individuals who are competing in ultra-endurance events may require up to 500 mg or more of vitamin C per day (42) consumed as supplements. Nonetheless, athletes should not exceed the UL for vitamin C. Dietary sources of vitamin C can be found in Table 5.1.

Choline

Choline is a vitamin-like compound required for the synthesis of all cell membranes (52). It can be synthesized from the amino acid methionine (53). Choline is also involved in carnitine and very low–density lipoprotein cholesterol (VLDL-C) synthesis (52,54). It has been suggested that choline may affect nerve transmission by serving as a structural and signaling component for cells and may expedite the loss of body fat due to its role in fat metabolism (53).

Overt choline deficiencies have not been reported in humans (55). However, inadequate choline stores have been associated with increased levels of homocysteine and thus an increased risk for cardiovascular disease (56). Although there have been reports that plasma choline concentrations are significantly decreased after long-distance swimming, running, and triathlons (57,58), not all researchers observe this phenomena (59). Deuster et al (60) found that although choline supplementation significantly increased plasma choline concentrations, supplementation did not affect physical or cognitive performance after exhaustive physical activity.

There is insufficient research to suggest that athletes need more than the AI for choline. Beef liver, peanuts, peanut butter, iceberg lettuce, cauliflower, and whole-wheat bread are some of the highest sources of choline. Potatoes, grape juice, tomatoes, bananas, and cucumbers are also good sources (52) (see Table 5.1). Consuming a wide variety of foods will likely provide sufficient amounts and there is no evidence to support choline supplementation.

Fat-Soluble Vitamins

The fat-soluble vitamins include vitamins A, D, E, and K. Aside from vitamin E, data about the relationship of the fat-soluble vitamins and exercise are not as abundant as for other micronutrients. Table 5.2 shows the fat-soluble vitamin needs for the athlete along with food sources.

Vitamin A

Vitamin A, which is considered a subset of the retinoids, is a fat-soluble vitamin best known for the role it plays in the visual cycle (61). Other important functions of vitamin A include its role in cell differentiation, reproduction, fetal development, and bone formation (61,62), and as an antioxidant. Plants can synthesize carotenoids that are precursors of vitamin A; however, humans and other animals convert carotenoids to retinol or acquire preformed vitamin A from animal foods or supplements (61). Assessment of vitamin A intake in individuals who are physically active has shown varied results; however, some of these assessments are faulty in that they did not necessarily specify the source of vitamin A (plant vs animal) (62). Individuals with low fruit and vegetable intake typically have lower beta carotene intakes than those with high fruit and vegetable consumption. Lukaski (1) attributes food restriction to inadequate consumption of vitamin A.

Although preformed vitamin A is a well-known antioxidant, beta carotene is a weak antioxidant and may be a pro-oxidant. Beta carotene quenches singlet oxygen, but there are limited data to suggest in vivo antioxidant activity in humans (63). It seems that derivatives of beta carotene may manifest in the lungs and arterial blood, possibly encouraging tumor growth, especially in smokers and individuals exposed to second-hand smoke and automobile fumes (63). Thus, individuals who exercise, and especially those who

TABLE 5.2 Fat-Soluble Vitamin Needs for Athletes and Food Sources

Vitamin	Effect of Exercise on Requirements	Recommended Intake for Athletes	Food Sources	Comments
Vitamin A	Exercise may increase needs; results equivocal, and beta carotene may be better, but not definitive.	RDA	Carrots, broccoli, tomatoes	Although vitamin A can be an antioxidant, intakes more than the DRI may result in adverse effects in athletes.
Vitamin D	Exercise does not seem to increase needs.	RDA, although higher levels may be needed in the winter if living in northern states (to prevent bone loss)	Oily fish, liver, eggs, fortified foods such as margarine, breakfast cereals, bread, milk, and powdered milk	
Vitamin E	Exercise may increase needs.	RDA, but not more than the UL	Plant oils (eg, soybean, corn, olive oils), nuts, seeds, wheat germ	Strong antioxidant effects in endurance athletes and older athletes.
Vitamin K	Exercise does not seem to increase needs.	AI, but not more than the UL	Leafy green vegetables (eg, spinach, turnip greens), cabbage, green tea, alfalfa, oats, cauliflower	Increased needs may be needed for bone formation.

Abbreviations: RDA, Recommended Dietary Allowance; AI, Adequate Intake; UL, Tolerable Upper Intake Level.

exercise in cities where there are greater numbers of automobiles, would be wise not to supplement with beta carotene.

Aguilo and colleagues found decreased blood levels of beta carotene in well-trained professional cyclists after a cycling stage, but this was not found in amateur cyclists (64). Perhaps this is a preventative response for trained endurance athletes. Nonetheless, vitamin A supplementation for 60 days (in combination with vitamin C and E supplementation) was shown to be effective in decreasing the oxidative response after a 45-minute bout of cycling at 70% of maximum oxygen consumption (VO_{2max}) in untrained, healthy individuals (65). As with other studies that combined antioxidant vitamins, it is difficult to determine if any one vitamin had a greater effect than another.

Athletes are encouraged to consume fruits and vegetables containing beta carotene, but supplementation is not recommended. Because vitamin A is a fat-soluble vitamin and stored in body tissues, athletes should not exceed the UL. There are limited studies about excessive intake of vitamin A by humans; however, Barker and Blumsohn (66) reviewed animal data and found that consumption of large amounts of vitamin A can increase bone resorption and blood calcium levels, ossify cartilage, and suppress parathyroid hormone levels. It has also been reported that excessive intakes of vitamin A may lead to reduced bone mineral density and increased risk for hip fractures (67). Although more research is needed in this area, it underscores the fact that levels more than the UL can have detrimental effects on the body. Table 5.2 lists some dietary sources of vitamin A.

Vitamin D

Vitamin D is considered both a hormone and a vitamin (68). Its roles in maintaining calcium homeostasis and in bone remodeling are well established. Vitamin D can be obtained from foods as well as from sunlight because 7-dehydrocholesterol is converted to pre–vitamin D_3 in the skin (68). Conversion of vitamin D to its more active forms begin in the liver, then in the kidney where the 1-alpha-hydroxylase adds another hydroxyl group to the first position on 25-hydroxyvitamin D. This results in 1,25-dihydroxyvitamin D_3 [$1,25-(OH)_2 D_3$], also known as calcitriol, the most active form of vitamin D (68). The effects of calcitriol on calcium metabolism are discussed in more detail later in this chapter in the section on calcium.

To date, little research has been conducted on the effects of physical activity on vitamin D requirements and the effects of vitamin D on exercise performance (69). However, it is well recognized that vitamin D is a necessity for optimal bone growth, and emerging research suggests that a vitamin D deficiency increases the risk of autoimmune diseases, nonskeletal chronic diseases, and can affect human immunity, muscle function, and inflammation (70).

There have been reports that weightlifting may increase serum calcitriol and serum Gla-protein (an indicator of bone formation) levels that may result in enhanced bone accretion (71). Bell et al (71) reported changes in serum calcitriol levels without observing changes in serum calcium, phosphate, or magnesium levels. Furthermore, there is evidence that $1,25-(OH)_2D_3$ may affect muscle function because receptors for $1,25-(OH)_2 D_3$ have been found in cultured human muscle cells (72,73). However, 6 months of daily supplementation with 0.50 mcg 1–25 dihydroxyvitamin D_3 did not improve muscle strength in ambulatory men and women older than 69 years (74). Vitamin D supplementation by itself does not improve performance in older adults. More research is needed to determine if vitamin D combined with calcium supplements is beneficial for athletic performance (75).

Vitamin D deficiency is prevalent in the older population and may be due to low sunlight exposure, decreased ability of older skin to synthesize vitamin D, or low intake of dietary vitamin D (76). There is no generally accepted criterion for vitamin D deficiency. However, in a study of vitamin D in the older Dutch population, Wicherts et al (76) considered serum levels of 25-hydroxy vitamin D (25-OHD) less than 10 ng/mL to be vitamin D deficient and serum levels of 25-OHD less than 20 ng/mL to be vitamin D insufficient. These conservative categorizations were based on proposed classifications for bone health. In this study, almost 50% of the participants were vitamin D insufficient and nearly 12% of them were vitamin D deficient. This study confirms the high prevalence of low serum 25-OHD concentrations in older people in the general population and concludes that vitamin D status is associated with a decrease in physical performance over time (76).

The effect of vitamin D on muscle was explored by Cannell et al (77) in an animal model. Vitamin D–deficient rats that were administered vitamin D showed an improved muscle protein anabolism, an increase in weight gain and muscle mass, and a decrease in myofibrillar protein degradation (77). These animal findings were confirmed by human muscle biopsy studies. The biopsies on vitamin D–deficient patients found atrophy of muscle fibers before treatment and substantial improvement after treatment (77).

Athletes who may be consuming inadequate energy should be evaluated for vitamin D status because of the risk of long-term negative effects on calcium homeostasis and bone mineral density. Furthermore, individuals who live at or north of 42 degrees latitude (eg, the northern states and Canada) may require more vitamin D during the winter months to prevent increases in parathyroid hormone secretion and decreased bone mineral density (78,79).

The best dietary sources of vitamin D include fatty fish and fortified foods such as milk, breakfast cereals, and orange juice (also see Table 5.2). Exposure to 15 minutes of sunlight per day in light-skinned individuals, and 30 minutes per day in dark-skinned individuals, will also result in sufficient amounts of vitamin D, but not all individuals obtain this amount of sunlight per day because of geographic location and/or use of sun block lotion. Older individuals may be less able to convert vitamin D (80).

Vitamin E

Vitamin E refers to a family of eight related compounds known as the tocopherols and the tocotrienols (81). Like vitamin A, vitamin E is well known for its antioxidant function in the prevention of free radical damage to cell membranes (81). Vitamin E also plays a role in immune function (81).

Cesari et al (49) reported that plasma alpha tocopherol was significantly correlated with knee extension strength, whereas plasma gamma tocopherol was associated only with knee extension strength in individuals older than 65 years. Bryant et al (82) assessed different levels and combinations of antioxidant supplements in seven trained male cyclists (approximately 22 years of age), who participated in four separate supplementation phases. They ingested two capsules per day containing the following treatments: placebo (placebo plus placebo); vitamin C (1 g/d plus placebo); vitamins C and E (1 g/d vitamin C plus 200 IU/kg vitamin E); and vitamin E (400 IU/kg vitamin E plus placebo). Researchers found that the vitamin E treatment was more effective than vitamin C alone or vitamins C and E together. Plasma malondialdehyde (MDA) concentrations, a general measure of oxidative damage, were lowest with vitamin E supplementation. Others have reported decreased serum creatine kinase levels, a measure of muscle damage, in marathoners supplemented with vitamins E and C (83).

Although vitamin E may be protective during endurance exercise, a persistent question has been whether vitamin E supplementation has any effect on resistance performance. Avery and colleagues (84) assessed the effects of 1,200 IU vitamin E per day vs a placebo on the recovery responses to repeated bouts of resistance training. There were no significant differences between the vitamin E–supplemented group and the placebo group in muscle soreness, exercise performance, or plasma MDA concentrations. In an earlier study, McBride et al (85) assessed whether resistance training would increase free radical production and whether supplemental vitamin E would affect free radical production. Twelve men who were recreational weight trainers were supplemented with 1,200 IU vitamin E (RRR-d-alpha-tocopherol succinate) or a placebo daily for 2 weeks. In both the placebo- and vitamin E–supplemented groups, plasma creatine kinase and MDA levels increased pre- to postexercise; however, vitamin E diminished the increase in these variables postexercise, thus decreasing muscle membrane disruption (85).

To date, data on the vitamin E status of athletes have been sparse. However, those who have assessed dietary intakes have reported that in female figure skaters and female heptathletes, dietary intake of vitamin E tended to be less than other nutrients, and less than what the athletes may need (86,87). Vitamin E supplementation does not seem to be effective as an ergogenic aid (88). Although vitamin E has been shown to sequester free radicals in exercising individuals by decreasing membrane disruption (85), there have not been reports indicating that supplemental vitamin E improves exercise performance. Takanami and colleagues (89) proposed that exercise may cause a mobilization of vitamin E from store tissues and redistribution in the body, which may prevent oxidative damage. Therefore, vitamin E contributes to the prevention of exercise-induced lipid peroxidation. Nonetheless, vitamin E's role in prevention of oxidative damage due to exercise may be significant, and more long-term research is needed to assess its effects. Dietary sources of vitamin E are listed in Table 5.2.

Vitamin K

Vitamin K, a group of three related substances, is a fat-soluble vitamin. Phylloquinone or phytonadione (vitamin K-1) is found in plants (90). Menaquinone (MK) once referred to as vitamin K-2 is produced by bacteria in the intestines, supplying an undetermined amount of the daily requirement of vitamin K (91). Menadione (K-3) is the synthetic form of vitamin K (90).

All vitamin K variants are fat-soluble and stable to heat. Alkalis, strong acids, radiation, and oxidizing agents can destroy vitamin K. It is absorbed from the upper small intestine with the help of bile or bile salts and pancreatic juices, and then carried to the liver for the synthesis of prothrombin, a key blood-clotting factor (92).

Vitamin K is necessary for normal blood clotting. It is required for the posttranslational modification of prothrombin and other proteins (eg, factors IX, VII, and X) involved in blood coagulation by carboxylating glutamate residues (93). Vitamin K is necessary for conversion of prothrombin to thrombin with the aid of potassium and calcium. Thrombin is the important factor needed for the conversion of fibrinogen to the active fibrin clot (92). Coumarin acts as an anticoagulant by preventing conversion of vitamin K to its active form, thus preventing carboxylation of the glutamate residues. Coumarin, or synthetic dicumarol, is used medically primarily as an oral anticoagulant to decrease functional prothrombin (93). The salicylates, such as aspirin, often taken by patients who have had a myocardial infarction, increase the need for vitamin K (94).

Vitamin K is known to influence bone metabolism by facilitating the synthesis of osteocalcin, also known as bone gla protein (BGP) (95). Bone contains proteins with vitamin K–dependent gamma carboxyglutamate residues (94). Impaired vitamin K metabolism is associated with undercarboxylation of the noncollagenous bone-matrix protein osteocalcin (which contains gamma carboxyglutamate residues) (96). If osteocalcin is not in its fully carboxylated state, normal bone formation will be impaired (96).

Because strenuous exercise can lead to decreased bone mineral density, Craciun et al (97) assessed 1 month of vitamin K supplementation (10 mg/d) on various bone markers before and after supplementation. At baseline, athletes not using oral contraceptives were biochemically vitamin K–deficient. In all subjects, vitamin K supplementation was associated with an increased calcium-binding capacity of osteocalcin. In the low-estrogen group, vitamin K supplementation increased bone formation by 15% to 20%, with a concomitant decrease of 20% to 25% in bone resorption markers. Because vitamin K may not be absorbed as efficiently as once thought, its role in the prevention of bone loss has become more apparent. Further research may establish a need for increased intake of vitamin K in athletes, especially female athletes.

Braam et al (98) studied the effects of estrogen and vitamin K supplementation on bone loss in female endurance athletes. The subjects were divided into three groups based on their menstrual cycle status and then were randomly assigned to treatment with either vitamin K or placebo. The rate of bone loss in all three subgroups was significantly high and neither estrogen nor vitamin K supplementation prevented bone loss (98).

An average diet will usually provide at least 75 to 150 mcg/d of total vitamin K, which is the suggested minimum, although 300 to 750 mcg/d may be optimal (99). Absorption of vitamin K may vary from person to person, but is estimated to be 20% to 60% of total intake (99). Vitamin K toxicity rarely occurs from natural sources (vitamin K-1 or MK), but toxic side effects from the synthetic vitamin K used in medical treatment are possible (100). Vitamin K deficiency is more common than previously thought. Western diets high in sugar and processed foods, intakes of vitamins A and E more than the ULs, and antibiotics may contribute to a decrease in intestinal bacterial function, resulting in a decrease in the production and/or metabolism of vitamin K (101). The best dietary sources of vitamin K include green leafy vegetables, liver, broccoli, peas, and green beans (Table 5.2).

Major Minerals

Minerals are equally as important as vitamins in exercise metabolism. They play a variety of roles, with some having a greater impact on performance than others. Minerals are classified as either major or trace minerals. The major minerals include calcium, phosphorus, magnesium, sulfur, potassium, sodium, and chloride (2). Table 5.3 lists the major mineral requirements and food sources.

Calcium

Calcium, a well-studied mineral, is the fifth most common element in the human body (102,103). Ninety-nine percent of calcium exists in the bones and teeth, with the remaining 1% distributed in extracellular fluids, intracellular structures, cell membranes, and various soft tissues (102,104,105). The major functions of calcium include bone metabolism, blood coagulation, neuromuscular excitability, cellular adhesiveness, transmission of nerve impulses, maintenance and functionality of cell membranes, and activation of enzymatic reactions and hormonal secretions.

Calcium Homeostasis

The level of calcium in the serum is tightly managed within a range of 2.2 to 2.5 mmol/L (8.5 to 10.2 mg/dL) by parathyroid hormone (PTH), vitamin D, and calcitonin (102,104–106). When serum calcium levels decrease to less than the normal range, PTH responds by increasing the synthesis of calcitriol in the kidney (104,105). Calcitriol increases calcium reabsorption in the kidneys, calcium absorption in the intestines, and osteoclastic activity in the bone (releasing calcium into circulation) (102,104,105). When serum calcium levels are higher than normal values, the hormone calcitonin increases renal excretion of calcium, decreases calcium absorption in the intestines, and increases osteoblastic activity (102,104,105).

Average Calcium Intakes

Calcium intakes are typically lower in females than in males. Teenage girls and women tend to consume less calcium than teenage boys and men. Master women athletes (older than 50 years) consume approximately 79% of the recommended intake (107).

Individuals who are physically active should strive to consume at least the RDA for calcium. If an individual has a high sweat rate or exercises in hot conditions, more calcium than the RDA may be needed. Bergeron et al (108) reported a mean loss of 0.9 mmol/L in female athletes who exercised in the heat for 90

TABLE 5.3 Major Mineral Needs for Athletes and Food Sources

Mineral	Effect of Exercise on Requirements	Recommended Intake for Athletes	Food Sources	Comments
Calcium	Individuals who consistently exercise in the heat may have greater requirements.	RDA, but not more than the UL (those who exercise in the heat should take more than the RDA, but should not exceed the UL)	Milk, cheese, yogurt, tofu processed with calcium, kale, almonds, collard greens, spinach, canned salmon with bones, bok choy, soy milk fortified with calcium	Higher calcium intakes may also be related to fat loss—important for athletes in sports that require a low body weight (eg, gymnastics, distance running) or have weight requirements for competition (eg, rowing/crew).
Phosphorus	Exercise does not seem to increase needs.	RDA	Milk, cheese, yogurt, nuts, oatmeal, sardines, asparagus	Phosphate loading has not been researched enough; may be more harmful than helpful.
Magnesium	Exercise does not seem to increase needs; however, those exercising in hot environments may require more.	RDA	Peanuts, tofu, broccoli, spinach, Swiss chard, tomato paste, nuts, seeds	No ergogenic effects established.
Sulfur	Exercise does not seem to increase needs.	No RDA or AI; needs are generally met by consuming foods with the sulfur-containing amino acids	Garlic, legumes, nuts, seeds, red meat, eggs, asparagus	
Potassium	Exercise does not seem to increase needs; however, individuals with a high sweat rate may need more.	AI	Oranges, bananas, tomatoes, sardines, flounder, salmon, potatoes, beans, blackstrap molasses, milk	No ergogenic effects observed at this time.
Sodium	Exercise typically results in increased needs, especially for those who exercise in the heat.	AI	Luncheon and cured meats, processed cheese, most prepared foods	
Chloride	Exercise typically results in increased needs, especially for those who exercise in the heat.	AI	Foods with high sodium levels; also found in salt substitutes with potassium chloride	

Abbreviations: RDA, Recommended Dietary Allowance; AI, Adequate Intake; UL, Tolerable Upper Intake Level.

minutes. Currently, it is difficult to determine how much more calcium athletes should consume; however, consuming more than the RDA but less than the UL for calcium should be safe for most athletes, especially those who consistently exercise in the heat or sweat heavily.

Calcium has been studied for its possible effects on decreasing body weight (109). Any such effects could be consequential, especially for athletes in sports in which body weight is a concern (eg, wrestlers, jockeys, gymnasts, figure skaters, or lightweight rowers). It has been reported that a higher calcium intake is inversely related to body weight. Skinner et al (110) reported that calcium intake was negatively related to body fat in growing children. Lorenzen and colleagues (111) examined whether a calcium supplement (500 mg/d) had an effect on change in body fat and weight during a 1-year period in young girls. This study reported that habitual dietary calcium intake was inversely associated with body fat. However, supplementation with low-dose calcium had no effect on body weight, fat, or height during the study. Lorenzen et al (111) suggest that the effect of calcium on body weight may only be exerted if it is ingested as part of a meal and not as a supplement.

Some of the early studies on calcium and weight loss were done in animals. Lower fat pad mass and body weight gains were also reported in transgenic mice fed either a diet with calcium carbonate (1.2% calcium), or a diet with nonfat dry milk (1.2% or 2.4% calcium) than in mice fed a control diet (112). The mice on all three calcium diets had significantly less weight gain and fat pad mass than the control group; however, the effect was greater in the 2.4% calcium group (derived from nonfat dry milk). In addition, Melanson et al (113) reported that higher acute calcium intake is associated with higher rates of whole-body fat oxidation in humans. They also found that total calcium intake was a more important predictor of fat oxidation than calcium intake from dairy sources alone. Nonetheless, increased calcium intake was not correlated with decreased body weight in 100 pre- and postmenopausal women who were given 1,000 mg supplemental calcium per day (114).

Despite the mixed results of studies on calcium and body weight and the fact that other variables in the diet affect body weight, it would be prudent to encourage increased calcium consumption because increased calcium intakes have been shown to increase bone mineral density. Calcium from low-fat dairy sources will also provide an individual with vitamin D, riboflavin, potassium, and protein. (For a review on calcium and body weight, see reference 115).

Sources of calcium are listed in Table 5.3. Dairy sources have the highest bioavailability. For individuals not consuming adequate dietary calcium, supplementation with calcium citrate or calcium carbonate is recommended. Individuals should avoid calcium supplements containing bone meal, oyster shell, and shark cartilage due to the increased lead content in these supplements, which can be toxic (2). Calcium supplements are best absorbed if taken in doses of 500 mg or less and when taken between meals. Because calcium citrate does not require gastric acid for optimal absorption, it is considered the best calcium supplement for older women (116).

Factors Affecting Calcium Absorption

Certain factors can inhibit or enhance calcium absorption. High-protein and high-sodium diets have been shown to result in increased urinary calcium excretion in postmenopausal women (117). Although high-sodium diets have been well documented to increase urinary calcium excretion, lower-protein diets may actually reduce intestinal calcium absorption. Kerstetter et al (118) reported that dietary protein intakes of 0.8 g/kg or less per day have been associated with a reduction in intestinal calcium absorption, which can cause secondary hyperparathyroidism. Fiber and caffeine have small effects on calcium loss; a cup of brewed coffee results in a 3.5 mg loss of calcium (103). Phytates, however, greatly decrease calcium absorption, and oxalates greatly reduce calcium bioavailability (2,103). Conversely, vitamin D, lactose, glucose, a healthy digestive system, and higher dietary requirements (eg, pregnancy) all enhance calcium absorption (2). Thus, it is important to convey the need for a well-balanced, varied diet for optimal absorption of calcium.

Phosphorus

Phosphorous is the second most abundant mineral in the body, with approximately 85% of total body phosphorous in bone, mainly as hydroxyapatite crystals (102,119). Phosphate is important in bone mineralization in both animals and humans (119). Even in the presence of a high amount of calcitriol, rickets can result from a phosphate deficiency in humans (119). Although phosphorous is required for bone growth, excessive amounts of phosphorous may harm the skeleton, especially when accompanied by a low calcium intake (119). Excessive phosphorus intakes have been negatively correlated with radial bone mineral density (120).

High phosphorous intakes reduce serum calcium levels, especially when calcium intake is low, because phosphorous carries calcium with it into soft tissues (105,119). The resulting hypocalcemia activates PTH secretion, which results in increased bone loss (resorption) to maintain serum calcium homeostasis (119). High phosphorous intakes can also decrease active vitamin D production, further reducing calcium absorption and producing secondary hyperparathyroidism (119). Because of its ubiquitous nature, phosphorus intakes are usually more than the recommended intakes (5).

Because most individuals consume enough phosphorus in their diets, overconsumption is usually the concern. A special concern is the amount of soft drinks that individuals consume because many contain high amounts of phosphate and often replace milk. Several studies reported that the greater the consumption of carbonated beverages, especially cola beverages, the greater the risk of fracture (121–123). This association was stronger in women and girls. These results may have important health implications due to the 300% increase in carbonated beverage consumption combined with a decrease in milk consumption over the past several decades (121).

Another way that individuals who exercise, especially competitive athletes, may consume excessive phosphorus is via "phosphate loading." Phosphate loading is thought to decrease the buildup of hydrogen ions that increase during exercise and negatively affect energy production (124). Research on phosphate loading as an ergogenic aid has shown equivocal results (124). Bremner et al (125) reported a 30% increase in plasma inorganic phosphate levels with a 25% increase in erythrocyte 2,3-bisphosphoglycerate (2,3-BPG) levels after 7 days of phosphate loading in healthy subjects. They concluded that phosphate loading increased both plasma and erythrocyte phosphate pools, but that the increase in erythrocyte 2,3-BPG was probably a result of the increase in cell inorganic phosphate. These researchers did not assess phosphate loading on exercise performance. The long-term negative consequences of phosphate loading on bone mineral density have not been documented and should be considered before an athlete tries this practice. Furthermore, there has been limited research in this area, and thus the risk-benefit ratio of loading with phosphate has not been established.

Phosphorus content is highest in protein foods. Table 5.3 lists some food sources of phosphorus.

Magnesium

Approximately 60% to 65% of the body's magnesium is present in bone, 27% is in muscle, 6% to 7% is in other cells, and 1% is in extracellular fluid (126). Magnesium plays an important role in several metabolic processes required for exercise, such as mitochondrial function; protein, lipid, and carbohydrate synthesis; energy-delivering processes; electrolyte balance; and neuromuscular coordination (127–129).

Urinary and sweat magnesium excretion may be exacerbated in individuals who exercise, especially in hot, humid conditions (130). A female tennis player who suffered from hypomagnesemia was supplemented daily with 500 mg of magnesium gluconate, which dissipated her muscle spasms (131). It has been shown that a marginal magnesium deficiency actually impairs performance as well as amplifies the negative effects of strenuous exercise (129). If individuals are consuming inadequate energy and are exercising intensely on a daily basis, especially in the heat, they may lose a large amount of magnesium through sweat (2,10). Mineral sweat loss is typically assessed by using sweat patches, which are placed on different parts of the body (because different parts of the body sweat at different rates). Once collected, magnesium can be assessed through specific instruments that measure mineral status, such as atomic absorption spectrophotometry, inductively coupled mass spectrometry, and thermal ionization spectrophotometry. Clinical signs of magnesium deficiency, such as muscle spasms, should be monitored. Nevertheless, hypomagnesemia during exercise is the exception rather than the norm. For example, Kuru et al (132) reported unchanged tissue magnesium levels in older rats that underwent a 1-year swimming program. Table 5.3 lists some food sources of magnesium.

Sulfur

Sulfur is present in the body in a nonionic form and is a constituent of some vitamins (eg, thiamin and biotin), amino acids (eg, methionine and cysteine), and proteins. Sulfur also assists with acid-base balance. If protein needs are met, sulfur is not required in the diet because it is provided by protein foods (2).

Because sulfur is part of several proteins, the small body of research on its effects on exercise performance is limited to sulfur-containing amino acids. It has been established that dietary sulfur-containing amino acids affect glutathione synthesis; however, their acute effect under conditions of oxidative stress, such as exercise, is not understood. Mariotti et al (133) fed rats different types of protein or glucose 1 hour before a 2-hour run on a treadmill. They found that cysteine from dietary proteins displayed a dose-dependent and short-term stimulatory effect on liver glutathione during exercise, but did not immediately benefit whole-body glutathione homeostasis. At this point, increased sulfur intake does not seem warranted. Individuals consuming adequate high-quality protein in their diets will be consuming adequate sulfur.

Potassium

One of the three major electrolytes, potassium is the major intracellular cation (134,135). The two major roles of potassium in the body are maintaining intracellular ionic strength and maintaining transmembrane ionic potential (134).

An increase in extracellular potassium concentrations in human skeletal muscle may play a substantial role in development of fatigue during intense exercise (136). Nielsen and colleagues (136) found that intense intermittent training reduced the accretion of potassium in human skeletal muscle interstitium during exercise. This may occur through a reuptake of potassium because of greater activity of the sodium potassium–adenosine triphosphatase (ATPase) pumps in muscle. This decreased potassium accretion in muscle was associated with delayed fatigue during intense exercise. Thus, another response to intense training is the reduction of potassium accumulation in the skeletal muscle. Millard-Stafford et al (137) found that female runners had a greater increase in serum potassium concentrations than did male runners after a simulated 40-km road race in a hot, humid environment. It seems that serum potassium shifts into the extracellular space during and immediately after exercise; this shift may occur to a greater extent in highly trained individuals. However, this shift seems to be transient because most researchers report a return to baseline in extracellular serum potassium concentrations at 1 hour or more after exercise (136,137).

If an individual becomes hyperkalemic or hypokalemic, cells may become nonfunctional (135). If the observed shift in potassium after exercise is not transient, serious consequences may occur. However, because potassium is ubiquitous in foods, individuals who exercise may not require more potassium in their diets. Individuals who exercise at lower levels (eg, walking, gardening, recreational jogging) probably do not experience significant shifts in serum potassium concentrations. Table 5.3 lists some food sources of potassium.

Sodium and Chloride

Sodium and chloride are the most abundant cation and anion, respectively, in extracellular fluid (138) and assist in nerve transmission. In these respects they are important in exercise.

The need for proper hydration and electrolyte replacement before, during, and after exercise has been well established (139,140). Sweat sodium is often measured to assess sodium changes. In a study of 14 women, sweat sodium was increased after 60 minutes of cycling in dry heat, and the amount of sodium in the sweat was greater in the winter than in the summer (141). Millard-Stafford et al (137) reported that females had higher serum sodium concentrations than males after a 40-km run. Stachenfeld et al (142) reported similar results in sodium concentrations in their female subjects 120 minutes after cycling. As with potassium, this increase in serum sodium concentration seems to be transient. Nonetheless, it seems that increased dietary sodium is warranted in individuals who exercise, especially if they are exercising in hot, humid conditions. Increased sodium is required to maintain fluid balance and prevent cramping. The increase in dietary sodium may be met by either consuming higher sodium foods or by adding salt to foods. Because sodium also increases urinary calcium excretion, a balance between sodium and calcium intake is required. See Chapter 6 for a detailed discussion on fluids, electrolytes, and exercise.

Physically active individuals typically consume more dietary sodium than nonactive individuals do, and some researchers have wondered if sodium could be ergogenic. Jain et al (143) assessed whether 0.5 g of sodium citrate per kg of body weight has an ergogenic effect on oxygen debt and exercise endurance in untrained, healthy men. They reported a decrease in oxygen debt postexercise and an increase in high-intensity exercise performance (on a bicycle ergometer). It is not known what effect sodium citrate supplementation would have on trained athletes.

Physically active individuals should consume varied, balanced diets that include the proper amount of sodium for maintenance of hydration and performance. Specific sodium recommendations for athletes, including those who are salty sweaters, can be found in Chapter 6. Table 5.3 lists some food sources of sodium and chloride. Foods high in sodium are typically high in salt (sodium chloride), and therefore are also high in chloride.

Trace Minerals

The trace minerals include iron, zinc, copper, selenium, iodide, fluoride, chromium, manganese, molybdenum, boron, and vanadium (2). Table 5.4 lists trace mineral requirements and food sources.

Iron

Total body iron constitutes approximately 5 mg per kg of body weight in men and 3.8 mg/kg in women (144). Iron is utilized for many functions related to exercise, such as hemoglobin and myoglobin synthesis (145), as well as incorporation into mitochondrial cytochromes and nonheme iron compounds (146). Some iron-dependent enzymes (ie, nicotinamide adenine dinucleotide and succinate dehydrogenase) are involved in oxidative metabolism (146,147).

The incidence of iron-deficiency anemia among athletes and nonathletes alike is only approximately 5% to 6% (148,149). However, some have reported that as many as 60% of female athletes may have some degree of iron depletion (150), with ranges of 30% and 50%, especially among female athletes and those athletes who participate in endurance sports (148,151–154). Researchers have reported decreased hemoglobin levels, but not other iron indexes, in college-age males and females who participated in 12 weeks of weight training (155). According to some estimates, a 1% drop in hemoglobin results in 1.5% to 2% decrease in work capacity and output (156).

Because female athletes do not typically consume adequate amounts of dietary iron (as a result of lower energy consumption and/or reduction in meat content of the diet), coupled with iron losses in sweat,

TABLE 5.4 Trace Mineral Needs for Athletes and Food Sources

Mineral	Effect of Exercise on Requirements	Recommended Intake for Athletes	Food Sources	Comments
Iron	Exercise may increase requirements if a person becomes iron-depleted or iron-deficient anemic.	RDA, but may need more if iron-depleted or iron deficient-anemic	Clams, red meat, oysters, egg yolks, salmon, tofu, raisins, whole grains	May have an ergogenic effect if the athlete is iron-depleted or iron-deficient anemic.
Zinc	Exercise does not seem to increase needs; however, transient losses are often observed.	RDA, but not more than the UL	Oysters, red meat, poultry, fish, wheat germ, fortified cereals	May have ergogenic effects, but not definitive and mostly animal studies; may impact thyroid hormone function if zinc-deficient.
Copper	Exercise does not seem to increase needs.	RDA	Red meat, fish, soy products, mushrooms, sweet potatoes	
Selenium	Despite antioxidant properties, exercise does not seem to increase needs.	RDA, not more than the UL	Fish, meat, poultry, cereal, grains, mushrooms, asparagus	More research is needed.
Iodine	Exercise does not seem to increase needs.	RDA	Eggs, milk, strawberries, mozzarella cheese, cantaloupe	
Fluoride	Exercise does not seem to increase needs.	AI	Fluoridated water, fish, tea	
Chromium	Exercise does not seem to increase needs, although more research is required due to transient losses seen.	AI	Broccoli, potatoes, grape juice, turkey ham, waffles, orange juice, beef	Was thought to increase muscle mass, but research has consistently shown that it does not; may improve glucose tolerance in individuals with type 2 diabetes.
Manganese	Exercise does not seem to increase needs.	AI	Liver, kidneys, wheat germ, legumes, nuts, black tea	
Molybdenum	Exercise does not seem to increase needs.	RDA	Peas, leafy green vegetables (eg, spinach, broccoli), cauliflower	
Boron	Exercise does not seem to increase needs.	No RDA or AI; UL = 20 mg/d	Apples, pears, grapes, leafy green vegetables, nuts	Despite research on its possible effects on bone and muscle, boron does not seem to have ergogenic effects.
Vanadium	Exercise does not seem to increase needs.	No RDA or AI; UL = 1.8 mg/d	Mushrooms, shellfish, black pepper, parsley, dill weed, grains, grain products	May have an insulin-like effect on glucose metabolism, but data are limited to animal studies.

Abbreviations: RDA, Recommended Dietary Allowance; AI, Adequate Intake; UL, Tolerable Upper Intake Level.

gastrointestinal bleeding, myoglobinuria from myofibrillar stress, hemoglobinuria due to intravascular hemolysis, and menstruation (157), health and optimal exercise performance may be compromised. Decreased exercise performance is related not only to anemia and a decreased aerobic capacity, but also to tissue iron depletion and diminished exercise endurance (158–160) Dietary iron-deficiency anemia negatively impacts the oxidative production of adenosine triphosphate (ATP) in skeletal muscle, as well as the capacity for prolonged exercise (161,162). There have been reports that iron-depleted women have decreased VO_{2max} as a result of decreased iron storage (163).

Other studies have reported alterations in metabolic rate, thyroid hormone status, and thermoregulation with iron depletion and iron-deficiency anemia (164–167), although some researchers have not observed these alterations (168). Mild iron-deficiency anemia has also been shown to negatively affect psychomotor development and intellectual performance (169) as well as immune function (170).

Iron Supplementation

For individuals who are diagnosed with iron-deficiency anemia, iron supplementation is the most prudent way to increase iron stores and prevent adverse physiological effects (171). Ferrous sulfate is the least expensive and most widely used form of iron supplementation (171,172). For adults diagnosed with iron-deficiency anemia, a daily dose of at least 60 mg elemental iron taken between meals is recommended (171).

Supplementation may also be warranted for athletes with iron depletion (low serum ferritin levels) without iron-deficiency anemia (173). Hinton and colleagues (174) assessed time to complete a 15-km cycle ergometry test in 42 women with iron depletion. Half received a daily supplement of 100 mg of ferrous sulfate, and the other half received a placebo for 6 weeks. At baseline, there were no differences between the groups in serum ferritin status or in their 15-km time. The iron supplementation increased serum ferritin concentrations in the supplemented group, while subsequently decreasing their 15-km cycle ergometry time. These results suggest that iron depletion may impair aerobic exercise performance, and thus practitioners should consider assessing iron depletion in athletes.

Factors Affecting Iron Absorption

Several factors inhibit or enhance iron absorption. Factors that inhibit iron absorption include phytates and oxalates; tannins in tea and coffee; adequate iron stores; excessive intake of other minerals such as zinc, calcium, and manganese; reduced gastric acid production; and certain antacids.

Factors that enhance iron absorption include heme iron, meat protein factor, ascorbic acid, low iron stores, normal gastric acid secretion, and a high demand for red blood cells, such as occurs with blood loss, exercise training (especially at altitude), and during pregnancy (2).

Consuming vitamin C–containing foods or beverages with meals and consuming tea or coffee at least an hour before or after a meal rather than with a meal will enhance dietary iron absorption. Table 5.4 lists some dietary sources of iron.

Zinc

Zinc exists in all organs, tissues, fluids, and secretions. Approximately 60% of total body zinc is present in muscle, 29% in bone, and 1% in the gastrointestinal tract, skin, kidney, brain, lung, and prostate (175). Zinc plays a role in more than 300 metabolic reactions in the body (2). Alkaline phosphatase, carbonic anhydrase, and zinc-copper superoxide dismutase are just a few of the zinc metalloenzymes (2). Low zinc status can also impair immune function (170), which can be detrimental to exercise as well as to overall health.

Many individuals in the United States, including athletes, do not consume the recommended amount of zinc (176,177). It has been reported that approximately 50% of female distance runners consume less than the recommended amount of zinc (178), but some researchers have reported zinc intakes in female and male collegiate swimmers greater than 70% of recommended intakes (179). It seems that when dietary zinc intake is sufficient, zinc status is not negatively affected by exercise training (180).

The studies conducted on zinc and exercise also show a transient effect of exercise on zinc status. Lukaski (181) reports that it is well known that exercise acutely changes circulating zinc concentrations. Plasma and serum zinc concentrations are thought to be increased immediately after brief, intense, and prolonged endurance exercise. This can be explained by the effect of muscle breakdown on the movement of zinc (181). Muscle breakdown causes zinc to move from contracting skeletal muscle into extracellular fluid, thus increasing zinc concentration (181). The increase in zinc concentrations usually decreases within a brief period of time postexercise because of increased urinary excretion (181). Zinc status has been shown to directly affect basal metabolic rate, thyroid hormone levels, and protein utilization (182), which can have a negative effect on exercise performance and health.

Baltaci et al (183) assessed the effects of zinc supplementation and zinc deficiency on rats performing an acute swimming exercise. They reported that zinc-deficient rats had lower glycogen stores than the rats supplemented with zinc. This same group of researchers also reported greater MDA concentrations in zinc-deficient rats compared with rats supplemented with zinc, which were all placed on a swimming program of 30 min/d for 4 weeks (184). These animal findings demonstrate zinc's important role in exercise performance and overall health.

Consumption of a varied diet with adequate amounts of zinc should be emphasized. Table 5.4 includes some dietary sources of zinc.

Copper

Approximately 50 to 120 mg of copper is found in the human body (185). Some of the functions of copper include enhancing iron absorption (via metalloenzyme ceruloplasmin), forming collagen and elastin, participating in the electron transport chain (cytochrome C oxidase), and acting as an antioxidant (zinc-copper superoxide dismutase) (185).

Deficiencies of copper are unlikely, but because copper plays a role in red blood cell maturation, anemia can develop with copper deficiency (185). Gropper et al (186) surveyed 70 female collegiate athletes and found that intakes (including supplementation) ranged from 41% to 118% of the recommended intakes for copper, but athletes across all sports had normal copper status (as measured by serum copper and ceruloplasmin levels).

Because the copper content of food is greatly affected by soil conditions, it is rarely listed in nutrient analysis computer databases. Some good dietary sources of copper are organ meats (eg, liver), seafood (eg, oysters), cocoa, mushrooms, various nuts, seeds (eg, sunflower seeds), and whole-grain breads and cereals (Table 5.4).

Selenium

Selenium is well known for its role as an antioxidant in the body (metalloenzyme glutathione peroxidase) and also functions in normal thyroid hormone metabolism (2). Limited data are available about whether individuals who exercise require more selenium than sedentary individuals. Because of the increased oxidation with exercise, it seems that more selenium in the diet would be necessary for individuals who are physically active. In a double-blind study, Tessier et al (187) assigned 12 men to 180 mcg selenomethionine and 12 men to a placebo for 10 weeks and reported that endurance training enhanced the antioxidant potential of glutathione peroxidase, but the selenium supplementation had no effect on performance.

It has also been reported that a combination of 150 mcg selenium, combined with 2,000 IU retinol, 120 mg ascorbic acid, and 30 IU alpha tocopherol increased total plasma antioxidant status after exercise (188). However, because little data are available and excess selenium is toxic, individuals who exercise should consume no more than the RDA for selenium and never exceed the UL.

Like copper, the selenium content of food can vary greatly with the soil content. Good sources of selenium include brazil nuts, sunflower seeds, mushrooms, fish, shellfish, meat, eggs, and milk (see Table 5.4).

Iodide/Iodine

The thyroid hormones are synthesized from iodide and tyrosine (2); thus, iodide is required for normal metabolic rate.

No data on iodide requirements for individuals who are physically active have been reported; however, Smyth and Duntas (189) reviewed data about exercise-induced iodine deficiency. It is well known that profuse sweating, during vigorous exercise or in hot and humid temperatures, leads to substantial losses of electrolytes and minerals (189). Although electrolyte replacement after sweat has been well established, little attention has been given to iodine losses in sweat. Smyth and Duntas (189) reviewed various studies about urinary and sweat iodine loss. They concluded that subjects who partake in occasional physical exercise do not have considerable loss of iodine through sweat (189); however, elite and competitive athletes who partake in frequent vigorous exercise may experience a greater loss of iodine, resulting in an iodine deficiency. In such a situation, thyroid hypofunction may result if iodine is not replaced (189). Iodide is mainly found in saltwater fish, molasses, iodized salt, and seafood (see Table 5.4).

Fluoride

Fluoride's main function is to maintain teeth and bone health (2). It has long been known that fluoride in adequate amounts in the water can prevent tooth decay (190). Fluoride is important to bone health because it stimulates bone growth (osteoblasts), increases trabecular bone formation, and increases vertebral bone mineral density (191).

To date, studies are lacking on the fluoride requirements for individuals who exercise. Most research on fluoride has been done to assess its effect on bone mineral density and prevention of osteoporosis. Because of fluoride's important role in bone metabolism, more studies with fluoride and female athletes are warranted.

Dietary sources of fluoride are limited to tea, seaweed, seafood, and, in some communities, naturally fluoridated water or fluoridated public water systems (see Table 5.4).

Chromium

Chromium potentiates the action of insulin and thus influences carbohydrate, lipid, and protein metabolism (192). Chromium may also have antiatherogenic effects by reducing serum cholesterol levels (193), but these reports have not been well documented. Supplement manufacturers have marketed chromium to increase lean body mass and decrease body weight. However, a number of researchers have shown that chromium does not increase lean body mass or decrease body weight (194–196).

Urinary chromium excretion has been reported to be greater on the days that individuals exercise compared with days they do not exercise (197,198). Increased chromium excretion coupled with inadequate dietary intake suggests that individuals who exercise need more chromium in their diets; however, it has not been established that individuals who exercise require more than the AI for chromium. Whether chromium may enhance muscle mass has not been established (196,199,200), despite what is written in the popular press. More information about chromium picolinate supplements can be found in Chapter 7. Dietary sources of chromium include whole grains, organ meats, beer, egg yolks, mushrooms, and nuts (see Table 5.4).

Manganese

Manganese plays a role in antioxidant activity in the body because it is part of superoxide dismutase. Manganese also plays a role in carbohydrate metabolism and bone metabolism (2).

There are no data about whether individuals who exercise require more manganese in their diets or if it is an ergogenic aid. Dietary sources of manganese include whole grains, leafy vegetables, nuts, beans, and tea (see Table 5.4).

Molybdenum

Molybdenum interacts with copper and iron, and excessive intakes of molybdenum may inhibit absorption of these two minerals (2). Molybdenum also plays a role in glucocorticoid metabolism (142).

There are no data about molybdenum requirements for individuals who are physically active. Beans, nuts, whole grains, milk, and milk products are all good dietary sources of molybdenum (see Table 5.4).

Boron

Presently, boron has not been found to be essential for humans, but it may play a role in bone metabolism through its interactions with calcitriol, estradiol, testosterone, magnesium, and calcium (201–204). Many athletes believe that boron will increase lean body mass and increase bone mineral density, but research studies have not shown boron to have these effects (203–205).

Most of the research on boron has been limited to its effect on bone mineral density and lean body mass (202,203). Whether individuals who exercise require more boron in their diets has not been established. Dietary sources of boron include fruits and vegetables as well as nuts and beans (see Table 5.4).

Vanadium

Like chromium, vanadium has been shown to potentiate the effects of insulin (206). In addition, supplements of vanadium, as vanadyl sulfate, have been theorized to increase lean body mass, but these anabolic effects have not been demonstrated in research studies (206).

Vanadyl sulfate supplements are discussed in Chapter 7. Dietary sources of vanadium include grains, mushrooms, and shellfish (see Table 5.4).

Summary

Overall, the vitamin and mineral needs of physically active individuals are similar to the requirements for all healthy individuals. If dietary intakes are adequate (ie, the individual is meeting 70% or more of the RDA/ AI for nutrients), supplementation is unnecessary. However, sweat and urinary losses may require some individuals to consume higher amounts of some micronutrients, quantities that can be obtained with a varied diet of properly selected foods. Supplementation may be necessary when intake is inadequate. Care must be taken so that individuals do not exceed the UL, which could impair both exercise performance and health.

BOX 5.1   Online Resources of Vitamins and Minerals

Food and Nutrition Board of the Institute of Medicine
http://www.iom.edu/About-IOM/Leadership-Staff/Boards/Food-and-Nutrition-Board.aspx
Established in 1940, the Food and Nutrition Board (FNB) studies issues of national and global importance on the safety and adequacy of the US food supply; establishes principles and guidelines for good nutrition; and provides authoritative judgment on the relationships among food intake, nutrition, and health maintenance and disease prevention.

Institute of Medicine Dietary Reference Intakes (DRIs)
http://iom.edu/Activities/Nutrition/SummaryDRIs/DRI-Tables.aspx
Tables of DRIs as well as summaries and full reports can be found at the IOM Web site.

Vitamin D Health
http://www.vitamindhealth.org
Dr. Michael Holick's Web site on vitamin D contains research articles, presentations, and information on emerging science on vitamin D.

Food and Nutrition Information Center
http://fnic.nal.usda.gov
The Food and Nutrition Information Center provides credible, accurate, and practical resources for nutrition and health professionals, educators, government personnel, and consumers.

Special attention must be given to individuals who are physically active to assess their micronutrient needs. In assessing these individuals, consider the following: frequency, intensity, duration, and type(s) of physical activity; environment (hot or cold) in which exercise is done; sex; and dietary intakes and food preferences. It is particularly important to assess usual dietary intakes of calcium and iron in female athletes.

Proper assessment by the professional can help individuals who are physically active consume adequate amounts of micronutrients for optimal health and performance. In particular, athletes should be encouraged to consume adequate energy intake, and by doing so, they will typically consume adequate vitamins and minerals. Encouraging all of those who exercise to consume sufficient fruit and vegetables will also help to ensure they too will obtain the adequate amounts of vitamins and minerals needed for overall health and optimal performance.

A general summary of all the vitamins and minerals discussed in this chapter, including the effect of exercise on their requirements, recommended intakes for athletes, general food sources, and possible ergogenic effects, can be found in Tables 5.1 through 5.4. These tables can act as a quick reference guide for registered dietitians. Box 5.1 provides a list of online resources.

References

1. Lukaski HC. Vitamin and mineral status: effects on physical performance. *Nutrition.* 2004;20:632–644.
2. Byrd-Bredbenner C, Berning J, Beshgetoor D. *Perspectives in Nutrition.* 8th ed. Boston, MA: McGraw-Hill Science/Engineering/Math; 2008.
3. Burke L, Desbrow B, Minehan M. Dietary supplements and nutritional ergogenic aids in sport. In: Burke L, Deakin V, eds. *Clinical Sports Nutrition.* 3rd ed. Sydney, Australia: McGraw-Hill; 2006:455–513.

4. Kimura N, Fukuwatari T, Sasaki R, Hayakawa F, Shibata K. Vitamin intake in Japanese women college students. *J Nutr Sci Vitaminol.* 2003;49:149–155.

5. Institute of Medicine. *Dietary Reference Intakes for Calcium and Vitamin D.* Washington, DC: National Academies Press; 2010. http://books.nap.edu/openbook.php?record_id=13050. Accessed November 5, 2011.

6. Institute of Medicine. *Dietary Reference Intakes for Thiamin, Riboflavin, Niacin, Vitamin B6, Folate, Vitamin B12, Pantothenic Acid, Biotin, and Choline.* Washington, DC: National Academies Press; 1998.

7. Institute of Medicine. *Dietary Reference Intakes for Vitamin C, Vitamin E, Selenium, and Carotenoids.* Washington, DC: National Academies Press; 2000.

8. Institute of Medicine. *Dietary Reference Intakes for Vitamin A, Vitamin K, Arsenic, Boron, Chromium, Copper, Iodine, Iron, Manganese, Molybdenum, Nickel, Silicon, Vanadium, and Zinc.* Washington, DC: National Academies Press; 2000.

9. Barr S. Introduction to Dietary Reference Intakes. *Appl Physiol Nutr Metab.* 2006;31:61–65.

10. Clark M, Reed DB, Crouse SF, Armstrong RB. Pre- and post-season dietary intake, body composition, and performance indices of NCAA division I female soccer players. *Int J Sport Nutr Exerc Metab.* 2003;13:303–319.

11. Telford RD, Catchpole EA, Deakin V, Hahn AG, Plank AW. The effect of 7 to 8 months of vitamin/mineral supplementation on athletic performance. *Int J Sport Nutr.* 1992;2:135–153.

12. McCormick DB. Vitamin B6. In: Bowman BA, Russell RM, eds. *Present Knowledge in Nutrition.* 9th ed. Washington, DC: ILSI Press; 2006:269–277.

13. Kim Y-N, Driskell JA. Vitamins. In: Driskell JA, Wolinsky I, eds. *Nutritional Concerns in Recreation, Exercise, and Sport.* Boca Raton, FL: CRC Press; 2009:91–121.

14. Manore M. Effect of physical activity on thiamine, riboflavin, and vitamin B-6 requirements. *Am J Clin Nutr.* 2000;72(suppl):598S–606S.

15. Crozier PG, Cordain L, Sampson DA. Exercise-induced changes in plasma vitamin B-6 concentrations do not vary with exercise intensity. *Am J Clin Nutr.* 1994;60:552–558.

16. Herrmann M, Wilkinson J, Schorr H, Obeid R, Georg T, Urhausen A, Scharhag J, Kindermann W, Herrmann W. Comparison of the influence of volume-oriented training and high-intensity interval training on serum homocysteine and its cofactors in young, healthy swimmers. *Clin Chem Lab Med.* 2003;41:1525–1531.

17. Okada M, Goda H, Kondo Y, Murakami Y, Shibuya M. Effect of exercise on the metabolism of vitamin B6 and some PLP-dependent enzymes in young rats fed a restricted vitamin B6 diet. *J Nutr Sci Vitaminol.* 2001;47:116–121.

18. Stabler SP. Vitamin B12. In: Bowman BA, Russell RM, eds. *Present Knowledge in Nutrition.* 9th ed. Washington, DC: ILSI Press; 2006:302–313.

19. Bailey LB, Gergory JF. Folate. In: Bowman BA, Russell RM, eds. *Present Knowledge in Nutrition.* 9th ed. Washington, DC: ILSI Press; 2006:278–301.

20. McMartin K. Folate and vitamin B-12. In: Wolinsky I, Driskell JA, eds. *Sports Nutrition.* Boca Raton, FL: CRC Press; 1997:75–84.

21. American Dietetic Association, Dietitians of Canada. Position of the American Dietetic Association and Dietitians of Canada: Vegetarian diets. *J Am Diet Assoc.* 2003;103:748–765.

22. Cox G. Special needs: the vegetarian athlete. In: Burke L, Deakin V, eds. *Clinical Sports Nutrition.* 3rd ed. Sydney, Australia: McGraw-Hill; 2006:656–671.

23. Herbert V. Vitamin C supplements and disease: counterpoint (editorial). *J Am Coll Nutr.* 1995;14:112–113.

24. Herbert V. Folic acid and vitamin B12. In: Rothfield B, ed. *Nuclear Medicine in vitro.* Philadelphia, PA: JB Lippincott; 1983:337–354.

25. Konig D, Bisse E, Deibert P, Muller H-M, Wieland H, Berg A. Influence of training volume and acute physical exercise on the homocysteine levels in endurance-trained men: interactions with plasma folate and vitamin B-12. *Ann Nutr Metab.* 2003;47:114–118.

26. Peifer JJ. Thiamin. In: Wolinsky I, Driskell JA, eds. *Sports Nutrition.* Boca Raton, FL: CRC Press; 1997:47–55.

27. Webster MJ, Scheett TP, Doyle MR, Branz M. The effect of a thiamin derivative on exercise performance. *Eur J Appl Physiol Occup Physiol.* 1997;75:520–524.

28. Doyle MR, Webster MJ, Erdmann LD. Allithiamine ingestion does not enhance isokinetic parameters of muscle performance. *Int J Sport Nutr.* 1997;7:39–47.

29. Webster MJ. Physiological and performance responses to supplementation with thiamin and pantothenic acid derivatives. *Eur J Appl Physiol Occup Physiol.* 1998;77:486–491.

30. Suzuki M, Itokawa Y. Effects of thiamine supplementation on exercise-induced fatigue. *Metab Brain Dis.* 1996; 11:95–106.

31. van der Beek EJ, van Dokkum W, Wedel M, Schrijver J, van den Berg H. Thiamin, riboflavin and vitamin B6: impact of restricted intake on physical performance in man. *J Am Coll Nutr.* 1994;13:629–640.

32. Lewis RD. Riboflavin and niacin. In: Wolinsky I, Driskell JA, eds. *Sports Nutrition.* Boca Raton, FL: CRC Press; 1997:57–73.

33. Backes JM, Howard PA, Moriarty PM. Role of C-reactive protein in cardiovascular disease. *Ann Pharmacother.* 2004;38:110–118.

34. Murray R, Bartoli WP, Eddy DE, Horn MK. Physiological and performance responses to nicotinic-acid ingestion during exercise. *Med Sci Sports Exerc.* 1995;27:1057–1062.

35. Stephenson LA, Kolka MA. Increased skin blood flow and enhanced sensible heat loss in humans after nicotinic acid ingestion. *J Therm Biol.* 1995;20:409.

36. Miller JW, Rogers LM, Rucker RB. Pantothenic acid. In: Bowman BA, Russell RM, eds. *Present Knowledge in Nutrition.* 9th ed. Washington, DC: ILSI Press; 2006:327–339.

37. Thomas EA. Pantothenic acid and biotin. In: Wolinsky I, Driskell JA, eds. *Sports Nutrition.* Boca Raton, FL: CRC Press; 1997:97–100.

38. Smith CM, Narrow CM, Kendrick ZV, Steffen C. The effect of pantothenate deficiency in mice on their metabolic response to fast and exercise. *Metabolism.* 1987;36:115–121.

39. Nice C, Reeves AG, Brinck-Johnsen T, Noll W. The effects of pantothenic acid supplementation on human exercise capacity. *J Sports Med Phys Fitness.* 1984;24:26–29.

40. Camporeale G, Zempleni J. Biotin. In: Bowman BA, Russell RM, eds. *Present Knowledge in Nutrition.* 9th ed. Washington, DC: ILSI Press; 2006:314–326.

41. Johnston C. Vitamin C. In: Bowman BA, Russell RM, eds. *Present Knowledge in Nutrition.* 9th ed. Washington, DC: ILSI Press; 2006:233–241.

42. Keith RE. Ascorbic acid. In: Wolinsky I, Driskell JA, eds. *Sports Nutrition.* Boca Raton, FL: CRC Press; 1997: 29–45.

43. Peake JM. Vitamin C: effects of exercise and requirements with training. *Int J Sport Nutr Exerc Metab.* 2003;13: 125–151.

44. Duthie GG, Robertson JD, Maughan RJ, Morrice PC. Blood antioxidant status and erythrocyte lipid peroxidation following distance running. *Arch Biochem Biophys.* 1990;282:78–83.

45. Fishbaine B, Butterfield G. Ascorbic acid status of running and sedentary men. *Int J Vitam Nutr Res.* 1984;54:273.

46. Gleeson M, Robertson JD, Maughan RJ. Influence of exercise on ascorbic acid status in man. *Clin Sci.* 1987;73:501–505.

47. Tauler P, Aguilo A, Gimeno I, Noguera A, Agusti A, Tur JA, Pons A. Differential response of lymphocytes and neutrophils to high intensity physical activity and to vitamin C diet supplementation. *Free Radic Res.* 2003;37: 931–938.

48. Robson PJ, Bouic PJ, Myburgh KH. Antioxidant supplementation enhances neutrophil oxidative burst in trained runners following prolonged exercise. *Int J Sport Nutr Exerc Metab.* 2003;13:369–381.

49. Cesari M, Pahor M, Bartali B, Cherubini A, Penninx BW, Williams GR, Atkinson H, Martin A, Guralnik JM, Ferrucci L. Antioxidants and physical performance in elderly persons: the Invecchiare in Chianti (InChianti) study. *Am J Clin Nutr.* 2004;79:289–294.

50. Audera C, Patulny RV, Sander BH, Douglas RM. Mega-dose vitamin C in treatment of the common cold: a randomized controlled trial. *Med J Aust.* 2001;175:359–362.

51. Douglas RM, Chalker EB, Treacy B. Vitamin C for preventing and treating the common cold. *Cochrane Database Syst Rev.* 2000;2:CD000980.

52. Zeisel SH, Niculescu MD. Choline and Phosphatidylcholine. In: Shils ME, Shike M, Ross CA, Caballero B, Cousins RJ, eds. *Modern Nutrition in Health and Disease.* 10th ed. Philadelphia, PA: Lippincott Williams & Wilkins; 2006:525–536.

53. Burke ER. Nutritional ergogenic aids. In: Berning JR, Steen SN, eds. *Nutrition for Sport & Exercise.* 2nd ed. Gaithersburg, MD: Aspen Publishers; 1998:119–142.

54. McChrisley B. Other substances in foods. In: Wolinsky I, Driskell JA, eds. *Sports Nutrition.* Boca Raton, FL: CRC Press; 1997:205–219.

55. Kanter MM, Williams MH. Antioxidants, carnitine, and choline as putative ergogenic aids. *Int J Sport Nutr.* 1995;5(suppl):S120–S131.

56. Zeisel S, da Costa KA. Choline: an essential nutrient for public health. *Nutr Rev.* 2009;67:615–623.

57. Sandage BW, Sabounjian LA, White R, et al. Choline citrate may enhance athletic performance. *Physiologist.* 1992;35:236a.

58. Von Allworden HN, Horn S, Kahl J, Feldheim W. The influence of lecithin on plasma choline concentrations in triathletes and adolescent runners during exercise. *Eur J Appl Physiol.* 1993;67:87–91.

59. Spector SA, Jackman MR, Sabounjian LA, Sakkas C, Landers DM, Willis WT. Effect of choline supplementation on fatigue in trained cyclists. *Med Sci Sports Exerc.* 1995;27:668–673.

60. Deuster PA, Singh A, Coll R, Hyde DE, Becker WJ. Choline ingestion does not modify physical or cognitive performance. *Mil Med.* 2002;167:1020–1025.

61. Ross CA. Vitamin A and carotenoids. In: Shils ME, Shike M, Ross CA, Caballero B, Cousins RJ, eds. *Modern Nutrition in Health and Disease.* 10th ed. Philadelphia, PA: Lippincott Williams & Wilkins; 2006.

62. Stacewicz-Sapuntzakis M. Vitamin A and carotenoids. In: Wolinsky I, Driskell JA, eds. *Sports Nutrition.* Boca Raton, FL: CRC Press; 1997:101–109.

63. Omenn GS. An assessment of the scientific basis for attempting to define the Dietary Reference Intake for beta carotene. *J Am Diet Assoc.* 1998;98:1406–1409.

64. Aguilo A, Tauler P, Pilar Guix M, Villa G, Cordova A, Tur JA, Pons A. Effect of exercise intensity and training on antioxidants and cholesterol profile in cyclists. *J Nutr Biochem.* 2003;14:319–325.

65. Vassilakopoulos T, Karatza MH, Katsaounou P, Kollintza A, Zakynthinos S, Roussos C. Antioxidants attenuate the plasma cytokine response to exercise in humans. *J Appl Physiol.* 2003;94:1025–1032.

66. Barker M. and Blumsohn A. Is vitamin A consumption a risk factor for osteoporotic fracture? *Proc Nutr Soc.* 2003;62:845–850.

67. Melhus H, Michaelsson K, Kindmark A, Bergstrom R, Holmberg L, Mallmin H, Wolk A, Ljunghall S. Excessive dietary intake of vitamin A is associated with reduced bone mineral density and increased risk for hip fracture. *Ann Intern Med.* 1998;129:770–778.

68. Holick MF. Vitamin D. In: Shils ME, Shike M, Ross CA, Caballero B, Cousins RJ, eds. *Modern Nutrition in Health and Disease.* 10th ed. Philadelphia, PA: Lippincott Williams & Wilkins; 2006:376–395.

69. Lewis NM, Frederick AM. Vitamins D and K. In: Wolinsky I, Driskell JA, eds. *Sports Nutrition.* Boca Raton, FL: CRC Press; 1997:111–117.

70. Willis KS, Peterson NJ, Larson-Meyer DE. Should we be concerned about the vitamin D status of athletes? *Int J Sport Nutr Exerc Metab.* 2008;18:204–224.

71. Bell NH, Godsen RN, Henry DP, Shary J, Epstein S. The effects of muscle-building exercise on vitamin D and mineral metabolism. *J Bone Miner Res.* 1988;3:369–373.

72. Simpson R, Thomas G, Arnold A. 1,25 dihydroxyvitamin D receptors in skeletal and heart muscle. *J Biol Chem.* 1985;260:8882–8884.

73. Costa E, Blau H, Feldman D. 1,25(OH)$_2$-D$_3$ receptors and humoral responses in cloned human skeletal muscle cells. *Endocrinology.* 1986;119:2214–2217.

74. Grady D, Halloran B, Cummings S, Leveille S, Wells L, Black D, Byl N. 1,25-dihydroxyvitamin D$_3$ and muscle strength in the elderly: a randomized controlled trial. *J Clin Endocrinol Metab.* 1991;73:1111–1117.

75. Latham NK, Anderson CS, Reid IR. Effects of vitamin D supplementation on strength, physical performance, and falls in older persons: a systematic review. *J Am Geriatr Soc.* 2003;51:1219–1226.

76. Wicherts IS, van Schoo NM, Boeke JP, Visser M, Deeg D, Smit J, Knol DL, Lips P. Vitamin D status predicts physical performance and its decline in older persons. *J Endocrinol Metab.* 2007;92:2058–2065.

77. Cannell JJ, Hollis BW, Sorneson MB, Taft TN, Anderson JB. Athletic performance and vitamin D. *Med Sci Sports Exerc.* 2009;41:1102–1110.

78. Krall EA, Sahyoun N, Tannenbaum S, Dallal GE, Dawson-Hughes B. Effect of vitamin D intake on seasonal variations in parathyroid hormone secretion in postmenopausal women. *N Engl J Med.* 1989;321:1777–1783.

79. Dawson-Hughes B, Dallal GE, Krall EA, Harris S, Sokoll LJ, Falconer G. Effects of vitamin D supplementation on wintertime and overall bone loss in healthy postmenopausal women. *Ann Intern Med.* 1991;115:505–512.

80. Simon J, Leboff M, Wright J, Glowacki J. Fractures in the elderly and vitamin D. *J Nutr Health Aging.* 2002;6: 406–412.

81. Traber MG. Vitamin E. In: Shils ME, Shike M, Ross CA, Caballero B, Cousins RJ, eds. *Modern Nutrition in Health and Disease.* 10th ed. Philadelphia, PA: Lippincott Williams & Wilkins; 2006:396–411.

82. Bryant RJ, Ryder J, Martino P, Kim J, Craig BW. Effects of vitamin E and C supplementation either alone or in combination on exercise-induced lipid peroxidation in trained cyclists. *J Strength Cond Res.* 2003;17:792–800.

83. Rokitzi L, Logemann E, Sagredos AN, Murphy M, Wetzel-Roth W, Keul J. Lipid peroxidation and antioxidant vitamins under extreme endurance stress. *Acta Physiol Scand.* 1994;154:149–154.

84. Avery NG, Kaiser JL, Sharman MJ, Scheett TP, Barnes DM, Gomez AL, Kraemer WJ, Volek JS. Effects of vitamin E supplementation on recovery from repeated bouts of resistance exercise. *J Strength Cond Res.* 2003;17:801–809.

85. McBride JM, Kraemer WJ, Triplett-McBride T, Sebastianelli W. Effect of resistance exercise on free radical production. *Med Sci Sports Exerc.* 1998;30:67–72.

86. Mullins VA, Houtkooper LB, Howell WH, Going SB, Brown CH. Nutritional status of U.S. elite female heptathletes during training. *Int J Sport Nutr Exerc Metab.* 2001;11:299–314.

87. Ziegler PJ, Nelson JA, Jonnalagadda SS. Nutritional and physiological status of U.S. national figure skaters. *Int J Sport Nutr.* 1999;9:345–360.

88. Meydani M, Fielding RA, Fotouhi N. Vitamin E. In: Wolinsky I, Driskell JA, eds. *Sports Nutrition.* Boca Raton, FL: CRC Press; 1997:119–135.

89. Takanami Y, Iwane H, Kawai Y, Shimomitsu T. Vitamin E supplementation and endurance exercise. *Sports Med.* 2000;2:73–83.

90. Suttie JW. Vitamin K. In: DeLuca HF, ed. *The Fat Soluble Vitamins.* London, England: Plenum Press; 1978.

91. Binkley NC, Suttie JW. Vitamin K nutrition and osteoporosis. *J Nutr.* 1995;125:1812–1821.

92. Tortora GJ, Derrickson BH. *Principles of Anatomy and Physiology.* Hoboken, NJ: Wiley; 2009.

93. Brown WH, Foote CS. Vitamin K, blood clotting, and basicity. In: Brown WH, Foote CS, eds. *Organic Chemistry.* 2nd ed. Orlando, FL: Saunders College Publishing; 1998:635,1026.

94. Mayers PA. Structure and function of the lipid-soluble vitamins. In: Murray RK, Granner DK, Mayers PA, Rodwell VW, eds. *Biochemistry.* Sydney, Australia: Prentice-Hall International; 1990.

95. Kanai T, Takagi T, Masuhiro K, Nakamura M, Iwata M, Saji F. Serum vitamin K level and bone mineral density in post-menopausal women. *Int J Gynecol Obstetr.* 1997;56:25–30.

96. Philip WJ, Martin JC, Richardson JM, Reid DM, Webster J, Douglas AS. Decreased axial and peripheral bone density in patients taking long-term warfarin. *QJM.* 1995;88:635–640.

97. Craciun AM, Wolf J, Knapen MH, Brouns F, Vermeer C. Improved bone metabolism in female elite athletes after vitamin K supplementation. *Int J Sports Med.* 1998;19:479–484.

98. Braam L, Knapen M, Geusena P, Brouns F, Vermeer C. Factors affecting bone loss in female endurance athletes. A two-year follow-up study. *Am J Sports Med.* 2003;31:889–895.

99. Booth SL, Suttie JW. Dietary intake and adequacy of vitamin K. *J Nutr.* 1998;128:785–788.

100. Shearer MJ, Bach A, Kohlmeier M. Chemical, nutritional sources, tissue distribution, and metabolism of vitamin K with specific reference to bone health. *J Nutr.* 1996;126(4 Suppl):1181S–1186S.

101. Suttie JW. Vitamin K. In: Shils ME, Shike M, Ross CA, Caballero B, Cousins RJ, eds. *Modern Nutrition in Health and Disease.* 10th ed. Philadelphia, PA: Lippincott Williams & Wilkins; 2006:412–425.

102. Weaver CM. Calcium. In: Bowman BA, Russell RM, eds. *Present Knowledge in Nutrition.* 9th ed. Washington, DC: ILSI Press; 2006:373–382.

103. Heaney RP. Osteoporosis. In: Krummel DA, Kris-Etherton PM, eds. *Nutrition in Women's Health.* Gaithersburg, MD: Aspen Publishers; 1996:418–439.

104. Allen LH, Wood RJ. Calcium and phosphorous. In: Shils ME, Olson JA, Shike M, eds. *Modern Nutrition in Health and Disease.* 8th ed. Philadelphia, PA: Lea & Febiger; 1994:144–163.

105. Clarkson PM, Haymes EM. Exercise and mineral status of athletes: calcium, magnesium, phosphorus, and iron. *Med Sci Sports Exerc*. 1995;27:831–843.

106. Zeman FJ, Ney DM. *Applications in Medical Nutrition Therapy*. 2nd ed. Upper Saddle River, NJ: Prentice Hall; 1996.

107. Beshgetoor D, Nichols JF. Dietary intake and supplement use in female master cyclists and runners. *Int J Sport Nutr Exerc Metab*. 2003;13:166–172.

108. Bergeron MF, Volpe SL, Gelinas Y. Cutaneous calcium losses during exercise in the heat: a regional sweat patch estimation technique [abstract]. *Clin Chem*. 1998;44(suppl):A167.

109. Moyad MA. The potential benefits of dietary and/or supplemental calcium and vitamin D. *Urol Oncol*. 2003;21: 384–391.

110. Skinner JD, Bounds W, Carruth BR, Zeigler P. Longitudinal calcium intake is negatively related to children's body fat indexes. *J Am Diet Assoc*. 2003;103:1626–1631.

111. Lorenzen JK, Molgaard C, Michaelsen KF, Astrup A. Calcium supplementation for 1 y does not reduce body weight or fat mass in young girls. *Am J Clin Nutr*. 2006;83:18–23.

112. Zemel MB, Shi H, Greer B, Dirienzo D, Zemel PC. Regulation of adiposity by dietary calcium. *FASEB J*. 2000;14:1132–1138.

113. Melanson EL, Sharp TA, Schneider J, Donahoo WT, Grunwald GK, Hill JO. Relation between calcium intake and fat oxidation in adult humans. *Int J Obes Relat Metab Disord*. 2003;27:196–203.

114. Shapses SA, Heshka S, Heymsfield SB. Effect of calcium supplementation on weight and fat loss in women. *J Clin Endocrinol Metab*. 2004;89:632–637.

115. Christensen R, Lorenzen JK, Svith CR, Batels EM, Melanson EL, Saris WH, Tremblay A, Astrup A. Effect of calcium from dairy and dietary supplements on faecal fat excretion: a meta-analysis of randomized controlled trials. *Obes Rev*. 2009;10:475–486.

116. Dawson-Hughes B, Dallal GE, Krall EA, Sadowski L, Sahyoun N, Tennenbaum S. A controlled trial of the effect of calcium supplementation on bone density in postmenopausal women. *N Engl J Med*. 1990;323:878–883.

117. Harrington M, Bennett T, Jakobsen J, Ovesen L, Brot C, Flynn A, Cashman KD. The effect of a high-protein, high-sodium diet on calcium and bone metabolism in postmenopausal women and its interaction with vitamin D receptor genotype. *Br J Nutr*. 2004;91:41–51.

118. Kerstetter JE, O'Brien KO, Insogna KL. Dietary protein, calcium metabolism, and skeletal homeostasis revisited. *Am J Clin Nutr*. 2003;78(3 Suppl):584S–592S.

119. US Department of Health and Human Services. *The Surgeon General's Report on Nutrition and Health*. Rocklin, CA: Prima Publishing and Communications; 1988.

120. Metz JA, Anderson JJ, Gallagher PN. Intakes of calcium, phosphorus, and protein, and physical activity level are related to radial bone mass in young adult women. *Am J Clin Nutr*. 1993;58:537–542.

121. Wyshak G, Frisch RE, Albright TE, Albright NL, Schiff I, Witschi J. Nonalcoholic carbonated beverage consumption and bone fractures among former college athletes. *J Orthopaedic Res*. 1989;7:91–99.

122. Wyshak G. Teenaged girls, carbonated beverage consumption, and bone fractures. *Arch Pediatr Adolesc Med*. 2000;154:610–613.

123. Wyshak G, Frisch RE. Carbonated beverages, dietary calcium, the dietary calcium/phosphorus ratio, and bone fractures in girls and boys. *J Adolesc Health*. 1994;15:210–215.

124. Horswill CA. Effects of bicarbonate, citrate, and phosphate loading on performance. *Int J Sport Nutr*. 1995;5 (suppl):S111–S119.

125. Bremner K, Bubb WA, Kemp GJ, Trenell MI, Thompson CH. The effect of phosphate loading on erythrocyte 2,3-bisphosphoglycerate levels. *Clin Chim Acta*. 2002;323:111–114.

126. Volpe SL. Magnesium. In: Bowman BA, Russell RM, eds. *Present Knowledge in Nutrition*. 9th ed. Washington, DC: ILSI Press; 2006:400–408.

127. Haymes EM, Clarkson PC. Minerals and trace minerals. In: Berning JR, Steen SN, eds. *Nutrition for Sport & Exercise*. 2nd ed. Gaithersburg, MD: Aspen Publishers; 1998:77–107.

128. Konig D, Weinstock C, Keul J, Northoff H, Berg A. Zinc, iron, and magnesium status in athletes: influence on the regulation of exercise-induced stress and immune function. *Exerc Immunol Rev*. 1998;4:2–21.

129. Nielsen FH, Lukaski HC. Update on the relationship between magnesium and exercise. *Magnesium Res.* 2006; 19:180–189.

130. McDonald R, Keen CL. Iron, zinc and magnesium nutrition and athletic performance. *Sports Med.* 1988;5:171–184.

131. Liu L, Borowski G, Rose LI. Hypomagnesemia in a tennis player. *Phys Sportsmed.* 1983;11:79–80.

132. Kuru O, Senturk MK, Gunduz F, Aktekin B, Aktekin MR. Effect of long-term swimming exercise on zinc, magnesium, and copper distribution in aged rats. *Biol Trace Elem Res.* 2003;93:105–112.

133. Mariotti F, Simbelie KL, Makarios-Lahham L, Huneau JF, Laplaize B, Tome D, Even PC. Acute ingestion of dietary proteins improves post-exercise liver glutathione in rats in a dose-dependent relationship with their cysteine content. *J Nutr.* 2004;134:128–131.

134. Oh MS, Uribarri J. Electrolytes, water, and acid-base balance. In: Shils ME, Shike M, Ross CA, Caballero B, Cousins RJ, eds. *Modern Nutrition in Health and Disease.* 10th ed. Philadelphia, PA: Lippincott Williams & Wilkins; 2006:149–193.

135. Electrolytes: sodium, chloride, and potassium. In: Bowman BA, Russell RM, eds. *Present Knowledge in Nutrition.* 9th ed. Washington, DC: ILSI Press; 2006:409–421.

136. Nielsen JJ, Mohr M, Klarskov C, Kristensen M, Krustrup P, Juel C, Bangsbo J. Effects of high-intensity intermittent training on potassium kinetics and performance in human skeletal muscle. *J Physiol.* 2004;554:857–870.

137. Millard-Stafford M, Sparling PB, Rosskopf LB, Snow TK, DiCarlo LJ, Hinson BT. Fluid intake in male and female runners during a 4-km field run in the heat. *J Sports Sci.* 1995;13:257–263.

138. Luft FC. Salt, water, and extracellular volume regulation. In: Ziegler EE, Filer LJ Jr, eds. *Present Knowledge in Nutrition.* 7th ed. Washington, DC: ILSI Press; 1996:265–271.

139. Shirreffs SM, Armstrong LE, Cheuvront SN. Fluid and electrolyte needs for preparation and recovery from training and competition. *J Sports Sci.* 2004;22:57–63.

140. Coyle EF. Fluid and fuel intake during exercise. *J Sports Sci.* 2004;22:39–55.

141. Keatisuwan W, Ohnaka T, Tochihara Y. Physiological responses of women during exercise under dry-heat condition in winter and summer. *Appl Human Sci.* 1996;15:169–176.

142. Stachenfeld NS, Gleim GW, Zabetakis PM, Nicholas JA. Fluid balance and renal response following dehydrating exercise in well-trained men and women. *Eur J Appl Physiol.* 1996;72:469–477.

143. Jain P, Jain P, Tandon HC, Babbar R. Effect of sodium citrate ingestion on oxygen debt and exercise endurance during supramaximal exercise. *Indian J Med Res.* 2003;118:42–46.

144. Huebers H, Finch CA. Transferrin: physiologic behavior and clinical implications. *Blood.* 1984;64:763–767.

145. Finch CA, Lenfant L. Oxygen transport in men. *N Engl J Med.* 1972;286:407–410.

146. Dallman PR. Tissue effects of iron deficiency. In: Jacobs A, Worwood M, eds. *Iron in Biochemistry and Medicine.* London, England: Academic Press; 1974:437–476.

147. Dallman PR. Biochemical basis for the manifestations of iron deficiency. *Annu Rev Nutr.* 1986;6:13–40.

148. Balaban EP, Cox JV, Snell P, Vaughan RH, Frenkel EP. The frequency of anemia and iron deficiency in the runner. *Med Sci Sports Exerc.* 1989;21:643–648.

149. Fogelholm GM, Himberg JJ, Alopaeus K, Gref CG, Laakso JT, Lehto JJ, Mussalo-Rauhamaa H. Dietary and biochemical indices of nutritional status in male athletes and controls. *J Am Coll Nutr.* 1992;11:181–191.

150. Cowell BS, Rosenbloom CA, Skinner R, Summers SH. Policies on screening female athletes for iron deficiency in NCAA division I-A institutions. *Int J Sport Nutr Exerc Metab.* 2003;13:277–285.

151. Brown RT, McIntosh SM, Seabolt VR, Daniel WA. Iron status of adolescent female athletes. *J Adolesc Health Care.* 1985;6:349–352.

152. Parr RB, Bachman LA, Moss RA. Iron deficiency in female athletes. *Phys Sportsmed.* 1984;12:81–86.

153. Plowman SA, McSwegin PC. The effects of iron supplementation on female cross-country runners. *J Sports Med.* 1981;21:407–416.

154. Schena F, Pattini A, Mantovanelli S. Iron status in athletes involved in endurance and in prevalently anaerobic sports. In: Kies C, Driskell JA, eds. *Sports Nutrition: Minerals and Electrolytes.* Philadelphia, PA: CRC Press; 1995:65–79.

155. Deruisseau KC, Roberts LM, Kushnick MR, Evans AM, Austin K, Haymes EM. Iron status of young males and females performing weight-training exercise. *Med Sci Sports Exerc.* 2004;36:241–248.

156. Gera T, Sachdev HPS, Nestel P. Effect of iron supplementation on physical performance in children and adolescents: systematic review of randomized controlled trials. *Indian Pediatr.* 2007;44:15–23.

157. Bank WJ. Myoglobinuria in marathon runners: possible relationship to carbohydrate and lipid metabolism. *Ann N Y Acad Sci.* 1977;301:942–950.

158. Woolf K, St Thomas M, Hahn N, Vaughan L, Carlson A, Hinton P. Iron status in highly active and sedentary young women. *Int J Sport Nutr Exerc Metab.* 2009;19:519–535.

159. Viteri FE, Torun B. Anemia and physical work capacity. *Clin Hematol.* 1974;3:609–626.

160. Santolo MD, Stel G, Banfi G, Gonano F, Cauci S. Anemia and iron status in young fertile non-professional female athletes. *Eur J Appl Physiol.* 2008;102:703–709.

161. Finch CA, Miller LR, Inamdar A, Person R, Seiler K, Mackler B. Iron deficiency in the rat: physiological and biochemical studies of muscle dysfunction. *J Clin Invest.* 1976;58:447–453.

162. McLane JA, Fell RD, McKay RH, Winder WW, Brown EB, Holloszy JO. Physiological and biochemical effects of iron deficiency on rat skeletal muscle function. *Am J Physiol.* 1981;241:C47–C54.

163. Zhu YI, Haas JD. Iron depletion without anemia and physical performance in young women. *Am J Clin Nutr.* 1997;66:334–341.

164. Martinez-Torres C, Cubeddu L, Dillmann E, Brengelmann GL, Leets I, Layrisse M, Johnson DG, Finch C. Effect of exposure to low temperature on normal and iron-deficient subjects. *J Physiol.* 1984;246:R380–R383.

165. Beard JL, Borel MJ, Derr J. Impaired thermoregulation and thyroid function in iron-deficiency anemia. *Am J Clin Nutr.* 1990;52:13–19.

166. Beard J, Tobin B, Green W. Evidence for thyroid hormone deficiency in iron-deficient anemic rats. *J Nutr.* 1989;119:772–778.

167. Rosenzweig PH, Volpe SL. Iron, thermoregulation, and metabolic rate. *Crit Rev Food Sci Nutr.* 1999;39:131–148.

168. Harris Rosenzweig P, Volpe SL. Effect of iron supplementation on thyroid hormone levels and resting metabolic rate in two college female athletes: a case study. *Int J Sport Nutr Exerc Metab.* 2000;10:434–443.

169. Lozoff B. Behavioral alterations in iron deficiency. *Adv Pediatr.* 1988;35:331–359.

170. Gleeson M, Nieman DC, Pedersen BK. Exercise, nutrition and immune function. *J Sports Sci.* 2004;22:115–125.

171. Beard J. Iron. In: Bowman BA, Russell RM, eds. *Present Knowledge in Nutrition.* 9th ed. Washington, DC: ILSI Press; 2006:430–444.

172. Solvell L. Oral iron therapy: side effects. In: Hallberg L, ed. *Iron Deficiency: Pathogenesis, Clinical Aspects, Therapy.* London, England: Academic Press; 1970:573–583.

173. Nielsen P, Nachtigall D. Iron supplementation in athletes. *Sports Med.* 1998;26:207–216.

174. Hinton PS, Giordano C, Brownlie T, Haas JD. Iron supplementation improves endurance after training in iron-depleted, nonanemic women. *J Appl Physiol.* 2000;88:1103–1111.

175. Cunnane SC. *Zinc: Clinical and Biochemical Significance.* Boca Raton, FL: CRC Press; 1988.

176. Ganapathy S, Volpe SL. Zinc, exercise, and thyroid hormone function. *Crit Rev Food Sci Nutr.* 1999;39:369–390.

177. Micheletti A, Rossi R, Rufini S. Zinc status in athletes: relation to diet and exercise. *Sports Med.* 2001;31:577–582.

178. Deuster PA, Day BA, Singh A, Douglass L, Moser-Veillon PB. Zinc status of highly trained women runners and untrained women. *Am J Clin Nutr.* 1989;49:1295–1301.

179. Lukaski HC, Siders WA, Hoverson BS, Gallagher SK. Iron, copper, magnesium and zinc status as predictors of swimming performance. *Int J Sports Med.* 1996;17:534–540.

180. Lukaski HC, Hoverson BS, Gallagher SK, Bolonchuk WW. Physical training and copper, iron, and zinc status of swimmers. *Am J Clin Nutr.* 1990;51:1093–1099.

181. Lukaski HC. Magnesium, zinc, and chromium nutriture and physical activity. *Am J Clin Nutr.* 2000;72(suppl):585S–593S.

182. Wada L, King J. Effect of low zinc intakes on basal metabolic rate, thyroid hormones and protein utilization in adult men. *J Nutr.* 1986;48:1045–1053.

183. Baltaci AK, Ozyurek K, Mogulkoc R, Kurtoglu E, Ozkan Y, Celik I. Effects of zinc deficiency and supplementation on the glycogen contents of liver and plasma lactate and leptin levels of rats performing acute exercise. *Biol Trace Elem Res.* 2003;96:227–236.

184. Ozturk A, Baltaci AK, Mogulkoc R, Oztekin E, Sivrikaya A, Kurtoglu E, Kul A. Effects of zinc deficiency and supplementation on malondialdehyde and glutathione levels in blood and tissues of rats performing swimming exercise. *Biol Trace Elem Res.* 2003;94:157–166.

185. O'Dell BL. Copper. In: Brown ML, ed. *Sports Nutrition.* 6th ed. Washington, DC: International Life Sciences Institute-Nutrition Foundation; 1990:261–273.

186. Gropper SS, Sorrels LM, Blessing D. Copper status of collegiate female athletes involved in different sports. *Int J Sport Nutr Exerc Metab.* 2003;13:343–357.

187. Tessier F, Margaritis I, Richard M-J, Moynot C, Marconnet P. Selenium and training effects on the glutathione system and aerobic performance. *Med Sci Sports Exerc.* 1995;27:390–396.

188. Margaritis I, Palazzetti S, Rousseau AS, Richard MJ, Favier A. Antioxidant supplementation and tapering exercise improve exercise-induced antioxidant response. *J Am Coll Nutr.* 2003;22:147–156.

189. Smyth PPA, Duntas LH. Iodine uptake and loss—can frequent strenuous exercise induce iodine deficiency? *Horm Metab Res.* 2005;37:555–558.

190. Phipps KR. Fluoride. In: Ziegler EE, Filer LJ Jr, eds. *Present Knowledge in Nutrition.* 7th ed. Washington, DC: ILSI Press; 1996:329–333.

191. Phipps KP. Fluoride and bone health. *J Public Health Dent.* 1995;55:53–56.

192. Stoecker BJ. Chromium. In: Shils ME, Shike M, Ross CA, Caballero B, Cousins RJ, eds. *Modern Nutrition in Health and Disease.* 10th ed. Philadelphia, PA: Lippincott Williams & Wilkins; 2006:332–337.

193. McCarty MF. Up-regulation of intracellular signalling pathways may play a central pathogenic role in hypertension, atherogenesis, insulin resistance, and cancer promotion—the "PKC syndrome." *Med Hypotheses.* 1996;46: 191–221.

194. Hallmark MA, Reynolds TH, Desouza CA, Dotson CO, Anderson AA, Rogers MA. Effect of chromium and resistive training on muscle strength and body composition. *Med Sci Sports Exerc.* 1996;28:139–144.

195. Lukaski HC, Bolonchuk WW, Siders WA, Miline DB. Chromium supplementation and resistance training: effects on body composition, strength, and trace element status of men. *Am J Clin Nutr.* 1996;63:954–965.

196. Volpe SL, Huang HW, Larpadisorn K, Lesser II. Effect of chromium supplementation and exercise on body composition, resting metabolic rate and selected biochemical parameters in moderately obese women following an exercise program. *J Am Coll Nutr.* 2001;20:293–306.

197. Anderson RA, Polansky MM, Bryden NA. Strenuous running: acute effects on chromium, copper, zinc, and selected clinical variables in urine and serum of male runners. *Biol Trace Elem Res.* 1984;6:327–336.

198. Anderson RA, Bryden NA, Polansky MM, Deuster PA. Exercise effects on chromium excretion of trained and untrained men consuming a constant diet. *J Appl Physiol.* 1988;64:249–252.

199. Campbell WW, Joseph LJ, Anderson RA, Davey SL, Hinton J, Evans WJ. Effects of resistive training and chromium picolinate on body composition and skeletal muscle size in older women. *Int J Sport Nutr Exerc Metab.* 2002;12:125–135.

200. Kobla HV, Volpe SL. Chromium, exercise, and body composition. *Crit Rev Food Sci Nutr.* 2000;40:291–308.

201. Nielsen FH. Boron, manganese, molybdenum, and other trace elements. In: Bowman BA, Russell RM, eds. *Present Knowledge in Nutrition.* 9th ed. Washington, DC: ILSI Press; 2006:506–526.

202. Meacham SL, Taper LJ, Volpe SL. The effect of boron supplementation on blood and urinary calcium, magnesium, phosphorus, and urinary boron in female athletes. *Am J Clin Nutr.* 1995;61:341–345.

203. Volpe SL, Taper LJ, Meacham SL. The effect of boron supplementation on bone mineral density and hormonal status in college female athletes. *Med Exerc Nutr Health.* 1993;2:323–330.

204. Volpe SL, Taper LJ, Meacham SL. The relationship between boron and magnesium status, and bone mineral density: a review. *Magnes Res.* 1993;6:291–296.

205. Ferrando AA, Green NR. The effect of boron supplementation on lean body mass, plasma testosterone levels, and strength in male bodybuilders. *Int J Sport Nutr.* 1993;3:140–149.

206. Bucci L. Dietary supplements as ergogenic aids. In: Wolinsky I, ed. *Nutrition in Exercise and Sport.* 3rd ed. Boca Raton, FL: CRC Press; 1998:315–368.

Chapter 6

FLUID, ELECTROLYTES, AND EXERCISE

Bob Murray, PhD, FACSM

Introduction

Maintaining adequate hydration during physical activity is one of the most important nutrition practices for optimizing performance and protecting health and well-being. Even a slight amount of dehydration (eg, 1% loss of body weight, which is 1.5 lb [0.7 kg] in a 150-lb [68-kg] athlete) can adversely affect the body's ability to cope with physical activity, particularly when that activity occurs in a warm environment (1,2). Greater dehydration (eg, > 1% loss of body weight) is known to impair performance when the exercise occurs in warm environments. The physiological consequences of dehydration are comprehensively reviewed in the scientific literature (for selected reviews, see references 3–6), but when educating coaches and athletes, the emphasis is better placed on the physiological and performance benefits of staying well-hydrated (7–9).

This chapter focuses on the practical relevance of ingesting adequate amounts of fluid and electrolytes before, during, and after physical activity to replace sweat losses, with the goals of maintaining physiological function, safeguarding health, and improving performance. The information in this chapter is gleaned from decades of research on the physiological and performance-related responses to changes in hydration status. In addition, numerous position stands on the topic of hydration and exercise have been published by a variety of professional organizations (10–20), and the key points from those documents are also included in this chapter.

For individuals who engage in vigorous physical activity or who spend considerable time in warm environments, water and electrolyte losses can be prodigious and can have a large impact on daily fluid and electrolyte needs (21,22). For that reason, it is important for sports health professionals to have a fundamental understanding of the science that underpins daily water and electrolyte balance, starting with an appreciation of the incredible uniqueness of the water molecule.

The Uniqueness of Water

To understand why the hydration status of the human body has such a great impact on every physiological function, it is essential to understand that water is the most biological active molecule in the body. No other nutrient is as essential or is needed in as great an amount on a daily basis, and for good reason. Water's central role in life is not just because it is a solvent, but because it is also solute, reactant, product, carrier, lubricant, shock absorber, coolant, catalyst, ionizing agent, messenger, controller, and primary volumetric constituent of most cells. It is this compendium of unique characteristics that makes water the most important molecule in biology.

Yet, until recent decades water has been a somewhat neglected molecule in biology. After all, water molecules are rarely portrayed in structural drawings of other biological molecules, yet without water, those molecules could not function (23). Water is a small molecule; 1 liter of water at room temperature contains a septillion molecules, in other words, a million, million, million, million molecules. In fact, water (H_2O) is smaller and lighter than even gases such as oxygen (O_2) and carbon dioxide (CO_2), yet most water is found as liquid or solid (ice). Picture an individual water molecule as a plumpish sphere in which one portion bears a negative charge, while the other portion is positively charged. That bipolar charge characteristic is what attracts one water molecule to the next, allowing water to exist mostly in liquid and solid form rather than as a gas. The bipolar charge also governs water's interaction with all other elements and compounds.

In cells, water molecules not only allow proteins to form three-dimensional shapes, they are also indispensable for allowing proteins to perform their various functions (eg, enzymes and contractile proteins). For example, some proteins use bound water molecules as extension units that allow the proteins to perform their functions; water molecules can also cause some protein structures to stiffen while causing others to become more flexible (23). It is now thought that proteins, water, and ions are organized within cells into various clusters associated with membranes and the cytoskeleton; metabolites are channeled through these clusters (referred to as *metabolons*) rather than existing as free solutes in an aqueous solution, which has been the classic vision of how the cytoplasm was organized (24).

Among water's unique properties are a high heat capacity, a high thermal conductivity, and a high latent heat of evaporation, all of which help keep the body and its various parts (most of which have a high water content) from overheating during exercise. For example, the unique thermal characteristics of water prevent a runner's leg muscles from being destroyed by local overheating, allowing the heat produced by muscles to be quickly transferred, with the help of circulating blood, away from active muscle and distributed throughout the body.

Considering the central importance of water to every aspect of life, it should be no surprise that the human body has developed intricate physiological systems responsible for maintaining water balance.

Daily Fluid and Electrolyte Balance

Control of Fluid Balance

At rest in thermoneutral conditions (thermoneutral refers to environmental temperatures and activity levels that do not provoke sweating or shivering), body fluid balance is maintained at ± 0.2% of total body weight (25), a very narrow tolerance befitting the critical importance of hydration status on physiological function, even in nonexercise conditions. Under thermoneutral sedentary conditions, the daily intake of fluid usually matches or exceeds the volume of fluid that is lost through urine, feces, and sweat; through respiration; and via transcutaneous water loss. In other words, over 24 hours most people drink enough fluid to replace fluid losses. Maintaining fluid balance requires the constant integration of input from hypothalamic osmoreceptors (to gauge the osmolality of the blood) and vascular baroreceptors (to gauge the pressure within major vessels) so that fluid intake matches or modestly exceeds fluid loss. In this regard, the combination of thirst-driven and spontaneous drinking is such that fluid balance is normally maintained in most people over the course of a day. Interestingly, thirst-driven fluid intake accounts for only a small percentage of daily fluid intake; most fluid is spontaneously consumed with meals or snacks during the day and not directly in response to being thirsty (22).

When sweating occurs, body fluid balance is regulated by mechanisms that reduce urinary water and sodium excretion and stimulate thirst. Sweat loss is accompanied by a decrease in plasma volume and an increase in plasma osmolality (because more water than salt is lost in sweat, the sodium and chloride concentrations in blood plasma increase). These changes are sensed by vascular pressure receptors (these baroreceptors respond to a decrease in blood volume) and hypothalamic osmoreceptors, which respond to an increase in plasma sodium concentration (ie, increased plasma osmolality). In response to dehydration, integrated input from baroreceptors and osmoreceptors results in an increase in vasopressin (antidiuretic hormone; also identified as ADH or AVP) release from the pituitary gland and in renin release from the kidneys. These hormones, including angiotensin II and aldosterone, which result from an increase in plasma renin activity, increase water and sodium retention by the kidneys and provoke an increase in thirst (25,26).

During the course of a day, ingesting adequate water and electrolytes in foods and beverages eventually restores plasma volume and osmolality to normal levels and, whenever excess fluid is ingested, water balance is restored by the kidneys (ie, excess fluid is excreted). However, for physically active people, body fluid balance is often compromised because the human thirst mechanism is an imprecise gauge of immediate fluid needs and because it is sometimes difficult to ingest enough fluid to offset the large volume of sweat that can be lost during physical activity.

Daily Fluid Needs

Some people are confused by well-intended, but errant hydration recommendations, such as advice that everyone should consume eight 8-oz glasses of water per day to maintain proper hydration (27). Although the genesis of this advice is a matter of debate, it is interesting that eight 8-oz servings amounts to 2 quarts (approximately 2 liters), the volume that had been often cited as the daily fluid requirement for sedentary adults (27). In point of fact, no one fluid-intake recommendation will suffice for everyone because of the wide disparity in daily fluid needs due to differences in body size, physical activity, and environmental conditions (22). For a small, elderly individual living in an assisted-care facility, 2 L/d might be too much fluid, but for a physically active person, 2 liters might represent the fluid needs of just 1 hour of activity. The 2004 Dietary Reference Intake recommendations for water and electrolytes (22) identify the Adequate Intake (AI) for water to be 3.7 L/d in males (130 oz/d; the equivalent of 16 cups/day of fluid) and 2.7 L/d for females (95 oz/d; about 12 cups/d) (22). The AI is an estimate of the daily nutrient intake that is assumed to be adequate for most people. In other words, there is a low probability of inadequacy if sedentary females and males ingest 2.7 to 3.7 liters of fluid per day.

The 12 cups of fluid per day that represent the AI for water intake in adult females does not mean that women should literally drink at least 12 cups of water each day. Rather, it means that a total of 12 cups of fluid from all sources will meet the hydration needs of most adult females. This important distinction should be stressed when educating and counseling people about their hydration needs. Regardless of the extent of daily water needs, water can be supplied by a variety of foods and fluids such as fruit and vegetables, milk, soft drinks, fruit juices, sport drinks, water, coffee, tea, and soups. Approximately 20% of daily water needs is consumed from water found in food, and the remaining 80% is provided by fluids ingested throughout the day (22). In brief, the prevailing scientific consensus is that sedentary individuals living in temperate environments can rely on the combination of thirst and spontaneous drinking to successfully maintain daily fluid balance, whereas physically active people and those living in warm environments often find it difficult to keep pace with their daily fluid needs.

Between 45% and 75% of body weight is water, a value that varies inversely with fat mass (22). Regardless of the volume of total body water, maintenance of fluid balance in physically active people can be an ongoing challenge. Fluid is constantly lost from the body by way of the kidneys (urine), gastrointestinal tract (feces), respiratory tract, and skin (the latter two routes represent insensible water loss), and periodically lost from the eccrine sweat glands during exercise and heat exposure (4,25). (Eccrine sweat glands are responsible for secreting sweat onto the skin in response to physical activity and heat stress. Apocrine glands are found in the armpits and groin and are not part of the thermoregulatory response.)

The total volume of fluid lost from the body on a daily basis is determined by the environmental conditions, the size (and surface area) of the individual, the individual's metabolic rate, physical activity, sweat loss, the composition of the diet, and the volume of excreted fluids. Insensible water loss via the skin is relatively constant (see Table 6.1) (25), but water loss via the respiratory tract is affected by the ambient temperature, relative humidity, and ventilatory volume. Inhaled air is humidified during its passage through the respiratory tract, and, as a result, exhaled air has a relative humidity of 100%. Inhaling warm, humid air reduces insensible water loss because the inhaled air already contains substantial water vapor. As indicated in Table 6.1, athletes and workers experience more insensible water losses via the respiratory tract merely because of the overall increase in breathing that accompanies exercise. The air inhaled during cold-weather activity contains relatively little water vapor, so as it is warmed and humidified during its transit through the respiratory tract, additional water loss occurs. For this reason, during cold-weather activity, especially when conducted at altitude, transcutaneous and respiratory water loss can be quite high, at times exceeding 1 L/d (28).

What is the absolute minimum water need for a sedentary individual? That value is difficult to accurately discern, but it is likely to be no less than 1 L/d. The reasoning for this is that minimum urine flow is approximately 500 mL/d, transcutaneous water loss is approximately 400 mL/day, and respiratory loss is a minimum of 200 mL/d. Keep in mind that this minimum value would apply only to someone who was completely sedentary for the entire day in a temperate environment. Current thinking is that the water requirement in most minimally active adults ranges between 3 and 4 L/d due to the transcutaneous, respiratory, and urinary water loss that accompanies normal daily living (22).

When individuals work, train, and compete in warm environments, their daily water needs can be considerably larger and might increase to more than 10 L/d (29). For example, an athlete who trains 2 hours each day can easily lose an additional 4 liters of body fluid, resulting in a daily fluid requirement in excess of 7 to 8 liters. Some people are active more than 2 hours each day, further increasing their fluid needs. Such losses can strain the capacity of the fluid regulatory system such that thirst becomes an inadequate stimulus

TABLE 6.1 Typical Daily Fluid Losses (mL) for a 70-kg (154-lb) Athlete

	Normal Weather (68°F/20°C)	Warm Weather (85°F/29°C)	Exercise in Warm Weather (85°F/29°C)
Insensible losses:			
Skin	350	350	350
Respiratory tract	350	250	650
Urine	1,400	1,200	500
Feces	100	100	100
Sweat	100	1,400	5,000
TOTAL	**2,300**	**3,300**	**6,600**

Note: Daily fluid loss varies widely among athletes and can exceed 10 L/d under some circumstances.
Source: Adapted from Guyton AC, Hall JE. *Textbook of Medical Physiology.* 10th ed. Philadelphia, PA: WB Saunders Co; 2000, with permission from Elsevier. Copyright © 2000, Elsevier, Inc.

for fluid intake and, coupled with limited opportunities for spontaneous drinking, persistent dehydration (hypohydration) can occur.

To put these volumes of fluid loss in perspective, consider that the body of a 60-kg (132-lb) individual contains approximately 36 kg water (60% of body weight). If that person remains sedentary in a moderate environment, daily fluid requirements will be approximately 3 liters or 8.3% of total body water ($3 \div 36 \times 100$). In other words, every 12 days that person's body water will completely turn over. Now consider an 80-kg (176-lb) American football player who sweats profusely during two-a-day practices in the summer heat. That individual's water needs might be 10 L/d, representing approximately 20% of his total body water. If such large volumes seem unreasonably high, consider that most athletes will lose between 1 and 2 L of sweat per hour of exercise, and some people are capable of sweating more than 3 L/h (5). For example, Palmer and Spriet (30) reported an average sweat loss of 1.8 L/h in competitive ice hockey players during a training session. Three of the 44 players tested lost less than 1 L/h, while 12 players lost in excess of 2 L/h.

During physical activity, urine production is reduced as the kidneys attempt to conserve water and sodium to offset losses due to sweating. When fluid intake is limited and dehydration occurs, the kidneys are capable of concentrating the urine to four to five times the concentration of blood. However, some renal fluid loss (approximately 500 mL/d) is obligatory for waste removal. Daily urine losses in some athletes and workers tend to be less than in sedentary individuals, a trend that is exacerbated by warm weather as the body strives to conserve fluid. However, most athletes consume large volumes of fluid during the day and as a result produce more urine than their sedentary counterparts. Reduced urine volume in physically active individuals usually indicates inadequate fluid intake. In general, urine volumes tend to be 800 to 1,500 mL/d in sedentary individuals, but can exceed 4 L/d in physically active individuals who ingest large volumes of fluid (26).

What impact does the composition of the diet have on daily water needs? The simple answer to this question is that in sedentary individuals, the water required to excrete urea from protein (amino acid) degradation and to excrete excess electrolyte intake can represent a meaningful increase in daily water needs. However, for physically active people who already have an increased water requirement, the effect of diet on overall water need is usually quite small. For example, to excrete the urea produced from the degradation of 100 g protein would require approximately 700 mL water to be excreted from the body.

How much water is contributed by the oxidation of macronutrients? This volume is also relatively small, approximately 130 mL per 1,000 kcal in a mixed diet (31), and is relatively inconsequential for those individuals consuming more than 2 liters of fluid per day. To be more specific, the oxidation of carbohydrate, fat, and protein produces 15, 13, and 9 mL of water per 100 kcal of oxidized substrate, respectively (31).

Control of Electrolyte Balance

The concentrations of electrolytes across cell membranes must be tightly regulated to assure proper function of cells throughout the body. In the case of cardiac muscle, for example, an electrolyte imbalance such as hyperkalemia can have fatal consequences if plasma potassium concentration increases just a few mmol per liter. For this and other reasons, the kidneys are well equipped to maintain electrolyte balance by conserving or excreting minerals such as sodium, chloride, potassium, calcium, and magnesium. Although an "appetite" for sodium chloride does exist in humans (32), there is little evidence to suggest that the intake of other minerals is governed in a similar way. In most individuals, when dietary energy intake is adequate, mineral intake is usually in excess of mineral needs, assuring positive mineral balance. However, repeated days of profuse sweating can result in substantial electrolyte loss, especially sodium and chloride, the two minerals found in greatest concentrations in sweat. When dietary mineral intake (especially sodium intake) is not sufficient to compensate for such large losses, severe muscle cramping (33) and hyponatremia (34) might result.

Daily Electrolyte Needs

Electrolytes are lost in urine and sweat. Some athletes, soldiers, and workers lose large volumes of sweat on a daily basis (eg, 4 to 10 liters or more), and that loss is accompanied by a similarly large electrolyte loss. As shown in Table 6.2, the concentrations of potassium, magnesium, and calcium in sweat are low and relatively constant compared with the higher, more variable concentrations of sodium and chloride. The fact that sodium concentration in sweat varies widely among individuals means that some people will be prone to large sodium deficits whereas others will not. Increased risk of heat-related problems, hyponatremia, and muscle cramps has been linked to large sodium chloride losses in sweat (29,33–35). Increased salt intake mitigates severe whole-body muscle cramping that seems to result from chronic sodium deficits caused by large sweat losses. However, increased salt intake is not helpful in cramps of other origin (eg, from neuro-muscular imbalance).

Some people mistakenly believe that potassium loss is what causes muscle cramps and suggest eating oranges and bananas to replace the potassium lost in sweat. However, potassium loss is not the culprit. Potassium is lost in sweat (22,34,35), but the concentration of potassium in sweat (usually less than 10 mmol/L) is far less than that of sodium (20 to more than 100 mmol/L). In addition, the amount of potassium lost in even a large volume of sweat represents a small fraction of total body potassium content, whereas sweat sodium losses in a single 2-hour training session can approximate 20% of total body sodium content.

For some individuals, the amount of sodium chloride lost in sweat is not trivial. Consider, for example, a football player who practices for 5 hours per day, during which time he loses 8 liters of sweat (average sweat loss of 1.6 L/h). If his sweat contains 50 mmol Na^+/L, his total sodium loss will be 9,200 mg sodium (ie, 23 g NaCl). This sodium loss, which does not include the 50 to 200 mmol (1,150 to 4,600 mg) of sodium that is typically lost in urine, illustrates that physically active people often require a large salt intake to replace losses in sweat. The 2004 Dietary Reference Intakes recommend (22) restricting daily sodium intake to only 1.5 g/d (3.8 g salt per day), with a Tolerable Upper Intake Level for salt of 5.8 g/d (2.3 g sodium per day). The basis of this recommendation is that a reduction in dietary sodium intake can blunt the age-related increase in blood pressure. Clearly, these stringent dietary recommendations are inadequate for athletes, fitness enthusiasts, and workers who lose considerably more salt in their sweat. However, this discrepancy is recognized in the DRI report: "This [recommendation] does not apply to highly active individuals . . . who lose large amounts of sweat on a daily basis" (22).

Human sweat contains small amounts of dozens of organic and inorganic substances (eg, amino acids, urea, lactic acid, calcium, magnesium, iron), some of which are minerals. Even when sweat losses are large, it is unlikely that minerals such as magnesium, iron, and calcium will be lost in sufficient quantities in sweat to provoke a mineral imbalance in most people. However, there may be some individuals for whom such

TABLE 6.2 Mineral (Electrolyte) Losses in Sweat

Mineral	Concentration in Sweat, mmol/L (mg/L)	AI Values, mg/d	Possible AI Lost in Sweat, % AI/L
Sodium	20–80 (460–1,840)	1,300	35–140
Chloride	20–80 (710–2,840)	1,300	35–140
Potassium	4–10 (160–390)	4,700	3–8
Magnesium	0–1.5 (0–36)	240–420	0–15
Calcium	0–3 (0–120)	1,000–1,300	0–12

Abbreviation: AI, Adequate Intake.

losses could constitute an additional dietary challenge, as might be the case with sweat calcium losses in physically active females (see Table 6.2). For example, a female athlete who loses 3 liters of sweat in a day could lose up to 120 to 360 mg calcium. Although this amount of calcium can be easily replaced by consuming a cup of milk, sweat calcium loss does increase the dietary calcium needs of active males and females.

Position Stands on Fluid and Electrolyte Replacement

There are numerous position stands published by a variety of professional organizations that address fluid and electrolyte replacement before, during, and after physical activity (10–20). Table 6.3 provides a summary of the key recommendations from those documents. The recommendations vary and have evolved over time, although the differences among the recommendations are relatively small and the central intent of each is to assure that physically active individuals remain well hydrated. The common message is that proper hydration practices reduce the risk of dehydration and heat illness, maintain cardiovascular and thermoregulatory function, and improve performance during vigorous physical activity.

Fluid and Electrolyte Replacement Before Exercise

Adequate hydration before physical activity helps assure optimal physiologic and performance responses. For example, laboratory subjects who ingest fluid in the hour before exercise exhibit lower core temperatures and heart rates during exercise than when no fluid is ingested (36–38). Unfortunately, many athletes enter training sessions and competitive events already dehydrated. For example, Volpe et al (39) reported that more than 60% of the college athletes (n = 174) in their study had prepractice urine specific gravity measures indicative of hypohydration. Palmer and Spriet (30) noted similar findings in half of the ice-hockey players they studied (n = 44).

Clearly, athletes who enter competition in a dehydrated state are often at a competitive disadvantage (6). For example, in a study by Armstrong et al (40), subjects ran 5,000 meters (approximately 19 minutes) and 10,000 meters (approximately 40 minutes) in either a normally hydrated or dehydrated condition. When dehydrated by approximately 2% of body weight (by a diuretic given prior to exercise), their running speeds decreased significantly (by 6% to 7%) in both events. To make matters worse, exercise in the heat exacerbates the performance-impairing effects of dehydration (41).

When people live and are physically active in warm environments, voluntary fluid intake is often insufficient to meet fluid needs, as verified by a study conducted with soccer players in Puerto Rico (42). The athletes were studied during 2 weeks of training. When the players were allowed to drink fluids throughout the day as they wished (average intake = 2.7 L/d), their total body water at the end of 1 week was approximately 1.1 liters less than when they were mandated to drink 4.6 liters of fluid per day. In other words, their voluntary fluid consumption did not match their fluid losses, causing them to enter training and competition already dehydrated.

How do individuals know when they are adequately hydrated? This simple question continues to perplex scientists and clinicians because there is no one method that can accurately and reliably determine adequate hydration status. Measuring plasma osmolality is often used in laboratory settings to assess hydration status, but a blood draw and expensive equipment are required. The specific gravity of urine from the first void after awaking in the morning can provide useful information about hydration status, but some equipment is needed (eg, a refractometer or hydrometer), although the cost of such equipment is reasonable (eg, less than $200).

TABLE 6.3 Recommendations for Fluid and Electrolyte Replacement When Exercising

Position Stand (Reference)	Before Exercise	During Exercise	After Exercise	Electrolyte Replacement
American College of Sports Medicine Position Stand: Exercise and Fluid Replacement, 2007 (11)	Drink 5–7 mL per kg body weight at least 4 h prior to exercise. If needed, drink 3–5 mL per kg body weight 2 h prior.	Follow a customized fluid replacement program to prevent excessive dehydration (ie, > 2% weight loss).	Fully replace fluid and electrolyte deficits. For rapid rehydration, drink 1.5 L fluid (with electrolytes) per kg weight loss.	Consuming snacks and beverages with sodium will help stimulate thirst and retain fluids.
American College of Sports Medicine Roundtable on Hydration and Physical Activity: Consensus Statements, 2005 (20)	No recommendation.	Replace, but do not exceed, sweat losses. Limit fluid deficits to < 2% loss of body weight.	Rehydration within 6 h of exercise requires drinking 125%–150% of weight loss. Fluids should contain sodium. If 24 h before next exercise, rely on normal food and fluid intake.	Rely on salty foods, fluids, and sport drinks.
National Athletic Trainers Association, 2000 (13)	Consume approximately 500–600 mL (17–20 oz) of water or sport drink 2–3 h before exercise and 200–300 mL (7–10 oz) 10–20 min before exercise.	Fluid replacement should approximate sweat and urine losses, with the goal of keeping weight loss < 2% body mass. Example: 200–300 mL (7–10 oz) every 10–20 min, but individualized recommendations should be followed.	To ensure hydration within 4–6 h after exercise, drink about 25%–50% more than existing weight loss.	Adding a modest amount of salt (0.3–0.7 g/L) is acceptable to stimulate thirst, increase voluntary fluid intake, and decrease the risk of hyponatremia.
American Academy of Pediatrics, 2000 (14)	Before prolonged physical activity, the child should be well hydrated.	Periodic drinking should be enforced, even if a child is not thirsty. Example: a child weighing 40 kg (88 lb) should drink 150 mL water or a flavored, salted beverage every 20 min.	No recommendation.	Make water or a flavored, salted beverage available for active children.
American Dietetic Association,[a] Dietitians of Canada, and the American College of Sports Medicine, 2009 (15)	At least 4 h before exercise, drink 5–7 mL water or sport drink per kg body weight (2–3 mL/lb).	Follow individualized hydration plan to limit dehydration to < 2% loss of body weight.	Drink at least 16–24 oz (450–675 mL) for every pound (0.45 kg) of body weight loss.	Consume rehydration beverages and salty foods to help replace electrolyte losses.

continues

TABLE 6.3 Recommendations for Fluid and Electrolyte Replacement When Exercising (continued)

Position Stand (Reference)	Before Exercise	During Exercise	After Exercise	Electrolyte Replacement
International Marathon Medical Directors Association–Association of International Marathons, 2006 (17)	No recommendation.	Drink to thirst but have an idea of individual fluid needs.	No recommendation.	Foods and beverages containing sodium should be available at marathon aid stations.
Inter-Association Task Force on Exertional Heat Illnesses, 2003 (18)	Athletes should begin exercise properly hydrated.	Fluid intake should nearly approximate fluid losses. Individualized recommendations must be followed.	No recommendation.	Hydrating with a sport drink containing carbohydrates and electrolytes before and during exercise is optimal to replace losses and provide energy. Replacing lost sodium after exercise is best achieved by consuming food, in combination with a rehydration beverage.
USA Track and Field Advisory, 2003 (19)	Consume approximately 500–600 mL (17–20 oz) of water or sport drink 2–3 h before exercise and 300–360 mL (10–12 oz) 0–10 min before exercise.	During the race drink no more than 1 cup (8–10 oz) every 15–20 min.	Drink about 25% more than sweat losses to ensure optimal hydration 4–6 h after the event.	Addition of modest amounts of sodium (0.5–0.7 g/L) can offset sodium lost in sweat and may minimize medical events associated with electrolyte imbalances (eg, muscle cramps, hyponatremia).

[a]In January 2012, American Dietetic Association changed its name to Academy of Nutrition and Dietetics.

Noting the color and volume of urine is practical way to help physically active people subjectively assess their hydration status. Darkly colored urine of relatively small volume is an indication of dehydration, a signal to ingest more fluid prior to activity. Monitoring urine output is a common recommendation in occupational settings such as the mining industry, in which the workers are constantly exposed to conditions of high heat and humidity. In addition to measuring body weight after awakening, the use of some measure of urine concentration (eg, specific gravity, osmolality, or color) will often allow for the detection of dehydration (11,43). It should be noted that the intake of B-vitamin supplements, specifically riboflavin, can cause brightly colored urine even when an individual is well hydrated.

It has been suggested that ingesting a glycerol solution before physical activity in the heat might confer cardiovascular and thermoregulatory advantages resulting from hyperhydration. In fact, ingesting glycerol solutions prior to exercise does result in a reduction in urine production and in the temporary retention of fluid (37,38). Glycerol-induced hyperhydration is accompanied by weight gain that is proportional to the amount of water retained (usually approximately 0.5 to 1 kg). Fluid retention occurs because after glycerol molecules are absorbed and distributed throughout the body water (with the exception of the aqueous-humor and the cerebral-spinal fluid compartments), their presence provokes a transient increase in plasma osmolality, prompting a temporary decrease in urine production. As glycerol molecules are removed from the body water in subsequent hours, plasma osmolality decreases, urine production increases, and the excess water is excreted.

There are several reasons why it is unwise to recommend glycerol-induced hydration to athletes:

- Athletes pay a metabolic cost for carrying extra body weight.
- There is no compelling evidence that glycerol-induced hyperhydration results in a physiological benefit (38).
- The side effects of ingesting glycerol can range from mild sensations of bloating and lightheadedness to more severe symptoms of headaches, dizziness, and nausea (44).
- Glycerol-induced hyperhydration can cause blood sodium levels to decrease (45), possibly predisposing to hyponatremia.
- In 2010, glycerol was added to the World Anti-Doping Agency (WADA) list of prohibited substances (for use as a plasma-volume expander in masking the presence of banned substances) (46).

As noted in Table 6.3, there are several similar recommendations for fluid intake before exercise (when heavy sweating is anticipated), but a general recommendation is this: drink approximately 5 to 7 mL of water or sport drink per kilogram body weight (about 1 oz per each 10 lb of body weight) 4 hours before exercise (11). This will allow ample time for excess fluid to be excreted or for additional fluid to be consumed. If profuse sweating is expected, as would be the case with a vigorous workout in a warm environment, drink an additional 3 to5 mL/kg weight (0.6 oz per each 10 lb of body weight) approximately 2 hours before exercise (11). For example, a 70-kg (154-lb) individual would ingest 500 mL (approximately 16 oz) of fluid 4 hours before exercise and an additional 200 to 350 mL (7 to 12 oz) 2 hours before exercise. There is no need to drink large volumes of fluid immediately before exercise. In fact, doing so can lead to gastrointestinal discomfort and an increased risk of hyponatremia, a dangerously low blood sodium level that can be prompted by excessive fluid intake.

There is currently no specific recommendation regarding electrolyte intake before physical activity, although some football players, tennis players, endurance athletes, and workers have learned to stave off muscle cramps and reduce the risk of hyponatremia by consuming salty food or drink prior to exercise. Individuals who excrete large volumes of salty sweat (skin and clothing caked in the white residue of salt after exercise) are advised to take steps to assure adequate salt intake throughout the day (11,33). Some endurance athletes rely on salt tablets to help assure adequate sodium replacement during long training sessions and competition. If used judiciously and taken with ample fluid, salt tablets can be an acceptable way to replace sodium. However, the risk is that insufficient fluid is ingested with the tablets. Doing so would cause a concentrated saline solution to be introduced into the small intestine, prompting the movement of water from the bloodstream into the intestinal lumen to dilute the saline solution as it empties from the stomach. To prevent such an occurrence, a tablet that contains 180 mg sodium should be consumed with at least 8 oz (240 mL) of water or sport drink. Salty foods such as pretzels, tomato juice, and various soups can also serve as additional sources of dietary sodium.

Fluid and Electrolyte Replacement During Exercise

Research has shown that cardiovascular, thermoregulatory, and performance responses are optimized by replacing sweat loss during exercise (see Table 6.4) (2,7–9,47–49). These and similar research findings are reflected in the various recommendations for fluid and electrolyte intake during exercise.

TABLE 6.4 Beneficial Responses to Adequate Fluid Intake During Exercise

Characteristic	Response
Heart rate	Lower
Stroke volume	Higher
Cardiac output	Higher
Skin blood flow	Higher
Core temperature	Lower
Perceived exertion	Lower
Performance	Better

Source: Data are from references 4–6.

The American College of Sports Medicine position stand recognizes the physiological and performance benefits of minimizing dehydration by simply recommending that "individuals should develop customized fluid replacement programs that prevent excessive (> 2% body weight reductions from baseline body weight) dehydration" (10). In some cases, minimizing dehydration during exercise may require little more than athletes drinking whenever they are thirsty (50); in most cases, however, athletes are best advised to create a personal hydration plan to guide the frequency and volume of their fluid intake during exercise. Developing a personal hydration plan requires that the athletes periodically record body weights before and after activity. Using the simplest approach, weight loss indicates inadequate drinking, while weight gain indicates excessive drinking (see Figure 6.1) (51). That basic feedback is often all athletes need to fine tune their hydration practices. For a hydration continuum with recommendations for fluid and sodium intake for a variety of activities, see Table 6.5 (52). For athletes who continue to struggle with dehydration, calculations based on pre- and postexercise body weights, fluid intake, and urine output can be used to prescribe the volume and frequency of fluid intake required to minimize dehydration. Such measurements should be made periodically throughout the season to adjust for changes in environment, training intensity, fitness, and acclimation. Beginning activity with a comfortable volume of fluid already in the stomach, followed by additional fluid intake at 10- to 30-minute intervals (depending on sweat rate), will help assure a rapid gastric emptying rate by maintaining gastric volume, an important driver of gastric emptying during exercise (53).

Why is thirst often an imprecise regulator of fluid needs during exercise? There are at least three reasons. The first is behavioral—there are often many distractions during physical activity, so thirst signals can easily be missed or disregarded. The second reason is that fluid is often not readily available, so even if thirst is perceived, it might not be convenient to act on it. The third reason is rooted in the physiology of the thirst mechanism (54,55). Consider that the plasma osmolality of a well-hydrated (euhydrated) person is 285 mOsm/kg (some would argue that 280 mOsm/kg is the correct value, but for this example, we will use 285). The thirst threshold is the plasma osmolality above which thirst is triggered and this is thought to be 293 mOsm/kg (this varies among people, but usually is within 290 to 295 mOsm/kg). A simple calculation relying on total body water (TBW) shows the amount of fluid that has to be lost from the body before thirst is stimulated: TBW − [(TBW × 285)/293]. For example, if TBW is 36 liters (as it would be for a 60-kg [132-lb] person), then 1 liter of water must first be lost from the body for thirst to be initiated: 36 − [(36 × 285)/293] = 1 liter. This is the scientific rationale for the admonition that by the time thirst is perceived, some dehydration has already occurred.

An example of the inadequacy of the human thirst mechanism during exercise can be found in the study by Passe et al (56). Experienced runners participated in a 10-mile race conducted on a 400-meter track. The

FIGURE 6.1 Calculating sweat rates. Reproduced with permission from Murray R. Fluid replacement: the American College of Sports Medicine position stand. *Sports Sci Exch.* 1996;9(63):6.

Drinking fluid during exercise to keep pace with sweat loss goes a long way toward helping fitness enthusiasts, athletes, and workers feel good and work hard. Because sweat rates can vary widely, it is important to be aware of how much sweat is lost during physical activity. Knowing how much fluid is typically lost through an hour of activity becomes a goal for fluid replacement. Here are some simple steps to take to determine hourly sweat rate. In the example given below, Kelly K. should drink about 1 liter (32 oz) of fluid during each hour of activity to remain well hydrated.

A	B	C	D	E	F	G	H	I	J
		Body Weight							
Name	**Date**	**Before Exercise**	**After Exercise**	**Δ BW (C − D)**	**Drink Volume**	**Urine Volume***	**Sweat Loss (E + F − G)**	**Exercise Time**	**Sweat Rate (H/I)**
Kelly K.	9/15	61.7 kg	60.3 kg	1400 g	420 mL	90 mL	1730 mL	90 min	19 mL/min
		(lb/2.2)	(lb/2.2)	(kg × 1000)	(oz × 30)	(oz × 30)	(oz × 30)	1.5 h	1153 mL/h
		kg	kg	g	mL	mL	mL	min	mL/min
		(lb/2.2)	(lb/2.2)	(kg × 1000)	(oz × 30)	(oz × 30)	(oz × 30)	h	mL/h
		kg	kg	g	mL	mL	mL	min	mL/min
		(lb/2.2)	(lb/2.2)	(kg × 1000)	(oz × 30)	(oz × 30)	(oz × 30)	h	mL/h
		kg	kg	g	mL	mL	mL	min	mL/min
		(lb/2.2)	(lb/2.2)	(kg × 1000)	(oz × 30)	(oz × 30)	(oz × 30)	h	mL/h

Abbreviation: ΔBW, change in body weight.

*Weight of urine should be subtracted *if urine was excreted prior to postexercise body weight.*

TABLE 6.5 Hydration Continuum with Recommendations for Fluid and Sodium Intake During Various Activities

	Sedentary (24 h)	Low-Intensity, Short-Duration (30 min)	Moderate-Intensity, Moderate-Duration (60 min)	High-Intensity, Moderate-Duration (60–120 min)	Moderate-Intensity, Long-Duration (2–8+ h)	Low-Intensity, Long-Duration (8+ h)
Typical sweat loss[a]	0 mL	0–0.5 L	0.5–1.5 L	1–3 L	1–16+ L	2–12+L
Typical sodium loss[b]	1.5–3 g	0–0.5 g	0.5–1.5 g	1–3 g	1–16 g	2–12 g
Drink schedule	2–4 L/d	0–0.5 L	0.5–1.5 L	1–3 L	1–14 L	2–12 L
Beverage options	Water, coffee, tea, milk, fruit juice, soft drinks, soup	Nothing, water, fitness waters, sport drinks	Nothing, water, fitness waters, sport drinks	Sport drinks, water	Sport drinks, water, extra sodium	Sport drinks, water, coffee, tea, milk, fruit juice, soft drinks, soup

[a]Typical sweat rates for most people under most conditions; some people may sweat more.
[b]Assumes a loss of 1 g sodium per liter of sweat (43 mmol Na+ per liter).
Adapted with permission from Murray R. SSI Hydration Continuum. http://sportsscienceinsights.com/2009/10/ssi-hydration-continuum. Accessed July 11, 2011.

environmental conditions were moderate (69°F, 77% relative humidity), but sufficient for ample sweating to occur. Every 2 miles, the runners had the opportunity to grab a 24-oz sports bottle containing a commercial sport drink. They could drink from the bottle ad libitum; when they desired no more, the runners tossed the bottles onto the infield where the bottles were collected, part of a measurement system whereby drink volumes for each runner were calculated. As in a road race, if the runners chose not to drink, they had to wait until the next 2-mile opportunity. After the race, each runner completed a questionnaire so that their impressions of the adequacy of their fluid intake could be recorded. On average, the runners replaced only 30% of sweat loss (range = 5% to 67%), even though the conditions for fluid intake were purposefully optimized. Had thirst been an adequate stimulus for fluid intake, the runners would have done a better job hydrating. The fact they did not is evidence that other factors often conspire to produce the voluntary dehydration that is so often reported in the literature (54). The postrun questionnaires revealed that the runners grossly underestimated the extent of their sweat loss while accurately estimating their fluid intake. These results led the investigators to conclude that the inability to accurately estimate sweat loss contributed to the runners' inadequate fluid intake.

Are there circumstances in which thirst might be an adequate gauge of fluid needs during physical activity? Undoubtedly there are. For example, it is relatively easy to drink during long-duration, low-intensity activity such as slow marathon runs (eg, > 4 hours), ultra-endurance biking and running, hiking and backpacking, military marches, and similar activities. Under those circumstances, thirst may be an adequate stimulus for fluid intake in many people because there is ample opportunity to sense the presence of thirst and to drink accordingly. However, perceptions of thirst can also be inadequate in these circumstances, leading to dehydration and volume depletion in some participants and hyperhydration and hyponatremia in others.

Not surprisingly, most humans prefer—and drink more of—beverages that are flavored and sweetened (57–59). This is an important consideration in preventing dehydration because any step that can be taken to increase voluntary fluid intake will help reduce the risk of health issues associated with dehydration and heat stress. In addition to having palatable beverages available for athletes to drink (60), it is also important for athletes to periodically record body weights before and after vigorous physical activity as a way to assess the effectiveness of fluid intake and as a reminder of the importance of drinking adequate volumes of fluid during exercise (61). For tips for encouraging drinking and for education on hydration, see Boxes 6.1 and 6.2.

When performance is a key consideration in a workout or competition, a sport drink has well-documented advantages over plain water. Carbohydrate is an important component of a fluid-replacement beverage because it improves palatability by conferring sweetness, provides a source of fuel for active muscles, and stimulates fluid absorption from the intestine (47,48). The performance benefits of carbohydrate feeding during physical activity are covered in more detail in other chapters. Although it is clear that carbohydrate feeding benefits performance (4,11,13,15,29,49), more carbohydrate in a beverage is not necessarily better.

BOX 6.1   Tips for Encouraging Drinking Before, During, and After Sweaty Physical Activity

Preparation
- Know the warning signs of dehydration (thirst, unusual fatigue, lightheadedness, headache, dark urine, dry mouth, infrequent urination, unusually rapid heartbeat).
- Know where to find fluid (water fountains, stores, etc).
- Freeze fluid bottles overnight to allow the drink to stay cold longer during workouts.
- Ideally, have a variety of beverage flavors to choose from.
- Pre-hydrate to produce a light-colored urine.

Training
- When sweating is anticipated, start activity with a stomach comfortably full of fluid.
- Practice drinking during training.
- Take fluid with you. Wear a bottle belt or fluid pack; take along a cooler full of drinks.
- Keep a comfortably full stomach during activity.
- Train yourself to drink more during exercise.
- One medium mouthful of fluid = about 1 oz.
- Always carry money to buy drinks.
- Periodically record your body weight before and after activity.
- Complete rehydration requires full replacement of fluid *and* sodium losses.
- After activity, drink 24 oz for every pound of weight lost during activity.

Competition
- Better hydration means better performance—plan to drink during competition.
- When sweating, drink early and often, but don't overdrink.
- In distance running, stop to drink if that's what it takes to assure adequate intake. You will more than make up the time by staying well hydrated.
- During a road race, pinch the top of the drink cup to form a spout that will make drinking easier.
- You can carry fluid with you during a road race by folding the top of the cup to prevent the fluid from spilling out.
- Put more in your stomach than on your head. Pouring water over your head does *nothing* to reduce body temperature.
- If prone to dehydration, drink by schedule—not by thirst.

BOX 6.2   Tips for Hydration Education

- Educate coaches, trainers, supervisors, parents, and athletes about the benefits of proper hydration.
- Create educational posters, flyers, brochures, or presentations.
- Have palatable fluids readily available.
- Help athletes compare weights before and after exercise.
- Establish individualized fluid replacement regimens.

Research has demonstrated that ingesting drinks containing more than 6% to 7% carbohydrate (ie, more than 14 to 17 g per 8-oz serving) will decrease the rate of gastric emptying (51,53) and fluid absorption (62).

Table 6.3 (pages 113–114) includes recommendations about sodium intake during exercise as a way to improve beverage palatability, promote rehydration, and reduce the risk of hyponatremia and severe muscle cramps. Electrolyte intake becomes important whenever sweat loss is high (eg, more than 4 L/d), as commonly occurs during two-a-day practices and prolonged training and competition. Sweat contains more sodium and chloride than other minerals, and although sodium content of sweat is normally substantially less than the plasma value (plasma = 138 to 142 mmol/L; sweat = 20 to 80 mmol/L), large sweat losses can result in considerable salt loss (refer to Table 6.2). Normally, sodium deficits are uncommon among athletes and military personnel (63), in large part because a normal diet often provides more than enough salt to replace that lost in sweat.

However, persistent sodium losses can present problems, as illustrated by Bergeron (64) in a case study of a nationally ranked tennis player who suffered from frequent muscle cramps. A high sweat rate (2.5 L/h) coupled with a higher-than-normal sweat sodium concentration (90 mmol/L) predisposed the player to severe cramping. The cramps were eliminated when the player increased his daily dietary intake of sodium chloride from less than 10 g/d to 15 to 20 g/d, relied on a sport drink during practices and games, and increased his daily fluid intake to assure adequate hydration. A link between sweat sodium loss and cramping has also been reported in American football players (65).

It is also important to understand that ingesting sodium chloride in a beverage consumed during physical activity not only helps ensure adequate fluid intake (66) but also stimulates more complete rehydration after activity (67). Both of these responses reflect the critical role that sodium plays in maintaining the osmotic drive to drink and in providing an osmotic stimulus to retain fluid in the extracellular space (ie, in the plasma and interstitial fluid compartments).

The sodium content of a sport drink does not directly affect the rate of fluid absorption (68). This is because the amount of sodium that can be included in a beverage is small compared with the amount of sodium that can be provided from the bloodstream. Whenever fluid is ingested, sodium diffuses from plasma into the gut, driven by an osmotic gradient that strongly favors sodium influx. In brief, sodium chloride is an important constituent of a properly formulated sport drink because it improves beverage palatability, helps maintain the osmotic drive for drinking, reduces the amount of sodium that the blood has to supply to the intestine prior to fluid absorption, helps maintain plasma volume during exercise, and serves as the primary osmotic impetus for restoring extracellular fluid volume after exercise (66,67,69).

A good example of the effect that beverage composition has on voluntary fluid intake is demonstrated by the work of Wilk and Bar-Or (58). Preadolescent boys (ages 9 to 12 years) completed 3 hours of intermittent exercise in the heat, during which time they could drink one of three beverages ad libitum. The boys completed this protocol on three occasions. The beverages tested included water, a sport drink, and a placebo (a flavored, artificially sweetened replica of the sport drink). The boys drank almost twice as much sport drink as they did water, whereas consumption of the placebo decreased in between. Flavoring and sweetness increased voluntary fluid intake (more intake with placebo vs water), and the presence of sodium chloride in the sport drink further increased consumption (ie, the subjects drank more sport drink than placebo).

These results are consistent with the physiology of the thirst mechanism. In humans, the sensation of thirst is a function of changes in plasma sodium concentration (plasma osmolality) and of changes in blood volume (54,55,66,69). Drinking plain water removes the osmotic drive to drink (by quickly diluting the sodium concentration of the blood) and reduces the volume-dependent drive (by partially restoring blood volume), causing the premature satiation of thirst. Unfortunately, the resulting decrease in fluid intake occurs before adequate fluid has been ingested. As the Wilk and Bar-Or research (58) demonstrated, the osmotic drive for drinking can be maintained by the presence of low levels of sodium chloride in a beverage, resulting in greater fluid intake. This application of basic physiology is nothing new. For centuries, bartenders have known that salty foods and snacks help sustain fluid intake among their patrons.

Some individuals mistakenly interpret the current recommendations for fluid intake to mean that dehydration is to be avoided at all costs and that there is no such thing as drinking too much fluid. Unfortunately, this is not true. Excessive water intake, even at rest, can result in life-threatening hyponatremia. Ingesting too much water, beer, or other low-sodium fluid can quickly dilute the plasma sodium concentration. When this occurs, the osmotic balance across the blood-brain barrier is disrupted and water quickly enters the brain, causing swelling that can lead to seizures, coma, and even death (34,70–72). In similar fashion, excessive drinking during prolonged exercise can also result in hyponatremia (72). For that reason, physically active individuals should be counseled to limit their fluid intake to no more than is needed to minimize dehydration and to ingest sodium in food or drink during prolonged exercise (eg, > 2 hours) (see Box 6.3) (11,15,34,71,72).

Fluid and Electrolyte Replacement After Exercise

On those occasions when a fluid deficit (ie, dehydration) exists after physical activity, it is often important to rehydrate quickly. An afternoon of working in the yard, two-a-day football practices, a daylong sports tournament, and 8 hours of manual labor are all examples of activities in which dehydration (more precisely referred to in these instances as *hypohydration*) is likely. Fluid and electrolyte intake after physical activity is a critical factor in helping people recover quickly—both physically and mentally. Maughan et al (67) concluded that ingesting plain water is ineffective at restoring euhydration because water absorption causes plasma osmolality to decrease, suppressing thirst and increasing urine output. When sodium is provided in fluids or foods, the osmotic drive to drink is maintained (67,69,73), and urine production is decreased.

Plain water is a good thirst quencher, but not an effective rehydrator. Only when water is ingested in combination with foods that contain sodium, chloride, and other minerals will sufficient water be retained to promote complete rehydration. For example, low-fat, high-sodium foods and beverages such as tomato juice, baked potato chips, pretzels, pickles, and crackers can be consumed as snacks on days when large sweat sodium losses are expected.

Maughan et al (67) also emphasized the importance of ingesting fluid in excess of the deficit in body weight to account for obligatory urine losses. In other words, the advice normally given athletes—"drink a pint [454 mL] of fluid for every pound [454 g] of body weight deficit"—must be amended to "drink *at least* a pint of fluid for every pound of body weight deficit." More precise recommendations for how much fluid athletes should ingest to assure rapid and complete rehydration will evolve from future research; existing data indicate that ingestion of 150% of weight loss is required to achieve normal hydration within 6 hours after exercise (69).

BOX 6.3   Drinking Dos and Don'ts

Dehydration is the most common performance-sapping mistake, but it is also the most preventable. Here are some guidelines to help physically active people stay well hydrated.

DO	DON'T
Do start exercise well hydrated. When heavy sweating is expected, drink 2–3 cups (475–700 mL; ~7 mL/kg body weight or ~1 oz/10 lb body weight) of fluid 4 hours before exercise to allow excess fluid to be lost as urine. If urine output is still low 2 hours before exercise, drink 5–12 oz (150–300 mL; ~3–5 mL/kg body weight or ~0.6 oz/10 lb body weight). There is no benefit to hyperhydration, so don't drink excessively.	*Don't* rely solely on water. If sweating lightly, water is an acceptable fluid replacement beverage. For heavier sweating (eg, > 0.5 L/h), sport drinks help replace the electrolytes lost in sweat and supply performance-boosting carbohydrates to aid exercise performance. Excessive water drinking can lead to dangerous electrolyte disturbances (hyponatremia).
Do weigh yourself. The best way to determine if you'd had enough to drink during a workout is to check to see how much weight you've lost. Minimal weight loss (eg, < 1 lb; ~0.5 kg) means that you've done a good job staying hydrated. Remember that weight loss during an exercise session is water loss, not fat loss, and must be replaced.	*Don't* overdrink. Water is definitely a good thing, but you *can* get too much of a good thing. Drinking large amounts of fluid is not only unnecessary, but can be downright dangerous. A bloated stomach, puffy fingers and ankles, a bad headache, and confusion are warning signs of hyponatremia.
Do drink during exercise. When sweating, drink every 10 to 20 minutes during a workout. Those who sweat heavily can benefit from drinking more often (eg, every 10 minutes) whereas individuals who sweat lightly should drink less often (every 20+ minutes).	*Don't* gain weight during exercise. If you weigh more after exercise than you did before, that means that you drank more than you needed. Be sure to cut back the next time so that no weight is gained.
Do ingest sodium during exercise. The best time to begin replacing the sodium lost in sweat is during exercise. That's one reason why a good sport drink is better than plain water. Sodium intake of 1 g per hour is recommended during prolonged exercise where heavy sweat loss is expected.	*Don't* restrict salt in your diet. Ample salt (sodium chloride) in the diet is essential to replace the salt lost in sweat. Because athletes sweat a lot, their need for salt is often much more than for non-athletes.
Do follow your own plan. Everyone sweats differently, so every athlete should have a drinking plan tailored to his or her individual needs.	*Don't* use dehydration to lose weight. Restricting fluid intake during exercise impairs performance and increases the risk of heat-related problems. Dehydration should be kept to a minimum by following an individualized fluid-replacement plan.

continues

BOX 6.3   Drinking Dos and Don'ts (continued)

DO	DON'T
Do drink plenty during meals. If you weren't able to drink enough during practice to keep from losing weight, be sure to drink enough before the next practice. Mealtime makes it easy to drink and to consume the sodium that comes along with food. When rapid rehydration is required, drink 50% more than the existing fluid deficit (eg, if a 2-lb [~ 1-kg] fluid deficit exists, drink 48 oz [1,500 mL] of fluid to get caught up).	*Don't* delay drinking during exercise. Stick to a drinking schedule so that you avoid dehydration early in exercise. Once dehydrated, it's next to impossible to catch up to what your body needs because dehydration actually slows the speed at which fluid exits the stomach.

Source: Adapted with permission from Murray R, Stofan J, Eichner ER. Hyponatremia in athletes. *Sports Sci Exch.* 2003;16:1–6.

Finally, when rapid rehydration is the goal, consumption of alcoholic beverages is contraindicated because of alcohol's diuretic properties. Caffeine is, by comparison, a much milder diuretic and, in those who regularly ingest caffeine, might not be much of a diuretic at all (21). The 2004 DRI recommendations conclude that, "While consumption of beverages containing caffeine and alcohol have been shown in some studies to have diuretic effects, available information indicates that this may be transient in nature, and that such beverages can contribute to total water intake and thus can be used in meeting recommendations for dietary intake of total water" (22). However, when rapid rehydration is required, athletes should rely on noncaffeinated and nonalcoholic beverages. Education efforts with athletes should reflect the fact that many individuals will choose to consume alcoholic and caffeinated beverages. For those who do drink coffee, colas, beer, and similar beverages, the best advice is to do so in moderation, avoiding such drinks before and in the first few hours after physical activity.

Fluid and Electrolyte Balance at Environmental Extremes

The environment has a major impact on fluid and electrolyte balance (74). Exposure to extreme heat, high humidity, prolonged cold, water immersion, altitude, and reduced gravity increases the need for water and electrolytes to match the increased losses that occur in those circumstances (4–6,28,74). In extreme dry heat, combined water loss from sweating, respiration, and transcutaneous routes can increase water and salt needs to high levels, often exceeding 10 liters and 20 g, respectively. Not surprisingly, a high proportion of children who reside in hot and arid environments were found to be in a state of moderate to severe dehydration (75). Although respiratory water loss is minimal during exposure to wet heat, sweating is profuse as the body struggles to lose heat through the evaporation of sweat from the skin. This can be particularly troublesome for unacclimatized individuals exposed to high humidity; the inability of the sweat glands to respond maximally to environmental heat and humidity imposes a limit on both thermal comfort and the physiological capacity to sustain even mild exercise. During physical activity in cold environments, respiratory water loss increases because of the low humidity and increased ventilatory rate, and it is also possible for sweat rates to exceed 1 L/h due to the warm, humid microenvironment created underneath the clothing. Being immersed in water increases urine production because the increase in plasma volume that accompanies immersion triggers high-pressure baroreceptors. It should also be noted that competitive swimmers can sweat during tough workouts whenever internal body temperature exceeds the sweat threshold. Physical activity at altitude provokes the same responses as activity in the cold, with additional challenges to hydration posed by an altitude-induced reduction in food and fluid intake and increased urinary water and salt loss. Astronauts who spend days in zero-gravity conditions lose considerable water and salt as a result of the inevitable diuresis that occurs. All of these conditions promote fluid loss and increase the risk of dehydration.

Diarrheal disease also promotes rapid dehydration and claims the lives of millions of people around the world each year. Each year in the United States, diarrheal illnesses in children result in roughly 3 million physician visits, 220,000 hospitalizations, and roughly 400 deaths (76). The World Health Organization and various medical bodies recommend the use of oral rehydration solutions—simple concoctions of carbohydrates and electrolytes—to combat diarrheal fluid loss and save lives (77). As is the case with sport drinks, a small amount of carbohydrate stimulates rapid water absorption in the small intestine, with sodium, chloride, and potassium replacing electrolytes lost in diarrhea and thereby helping sustain fluid balance. Oral rehydration has been shown to be as effective as intravenous rehydration, and is a home remedy that can be administered at a much lower cost and risk (76). Interestingly, fluid replacement during diarrheal disease does not reduce stool volume or disease duration; fluid replacement saves lives by maintaining body fluid balance until the disease runs its course (78).

Summary

Water is constantly lost from the body with each water-saturated breath, with the seeping of water through the skin, with the obligatory production of urine and feces, in substantial volumes in sweat, and, when ill, through emesis and diarrhea. Fortunately, the combination of thirst and spontaneous drinking usually does a good job of matching fluid intake to losses so that progressive, chronic dehydration is typically not an issue, even for the elderly. However, for any individual who sweats profusely day after day, adequate water and salt replacement can pose a considerable challenge that can only be met by following practical yet scientifically founded recommendations for fluid and electrolyte intake.

The human body relies on an adequate volume of body water for all physiological and biochemical processes, so it should be no surprise that dehydration can adversely affect the health and performance of athletes and nonathletes. For that reason, it is essential that physically active people ingest ample fluids throughout the day to replace what is lost in sweat and urine. Two hours before a physical activity during which heavy sweating is expected, approximately 7 mL per kilogram body weight (~1 oz per each 10 lb of body weight) of water or sport drink should be consumed. During exercise, the goal is to drink enough to minimize weight loss (ie, minimize dehydration). Light sweaters require only modest volumes of fluid intake (eg, < 500 mL/h [16 oz/h]), whereas heavy sweaters may have to ingest in excess of 1.5 L/h (~50 oz/h) to minimize dehydration. To fully restore hydration status after exercise, it is necessary to ingest 150% of the existing fluid deficit. For example, if the fluid deficit is 2 lb (0.9 kg), 48 oz (1.4 liters) of fluid should be consumed. For those who exercise only once per day, fluid deficits are usually corrected during the course of normal eating and drinking. Those who train more than once each day or who sweat throughout the day (eg, workers and soldiers) have to adopt a more aggressive fluid replacement plan, along with adequate salt intake, to avoid chronic dehydration.

References

1. Cheuvront S, Carter R, Castellani JW, Sawka MN. Hypohydration impairs endurance exercise performance in temperate but not cold air. *J Appl Physiol.* 2005;99:1972–1976.

2. Murray R. Hydration and physical performance. *J Am Coll Nutr.* 2007;26(suppl):542S–548S.

3. Murray R. Nutrition for the marathon and other endurance sports: environmental stress and dehydration. *Med Sci Sports Exerc.* 1992;24(suppl):S319–S323.

4. Sawka MN. Body fluid responses and dehydration during exercise and heat stress. In: Pandolf KB, Sawka MN, Gonzalez RR, eds. *Human Performance Physiology and Environmental Medicine at Terrestrial Extremes.* Indianapolis, IN: Benchmark Press; 1988:227–266.

5. Sawka MN, Pandolf KB. Effects of body water loss on physiological function and exercise performance. In: Gisolfi CV, Lamb DR, eds. *Perspectives in Exercise Science and Sports Medicine: Fluid Homeostasis During Exercise.* Indianapolis, IN: Benchmark Press; 1990:1–38.

6. Sawka MN. Physiological consequences of dehydration: exercise performance and thermoregulation. *Med Sci Sports Exerc.* 1992;24:657–670.

7. Below PR, Coyle EF. Fluid and carbohydrate ingestion individually benefit intense exercise lasting one hour. *Med Sci Sports Exerc.* 1995;27:200–210.

8. Coyle EF, Montain SJ. Benefits of fluid replacement with carbohydrate during exercise. *Med Sci Sports Exerc.* 1992;24(suppl):S324–S330.

9. Montain SJ, Coyle EF. The influence of graded dehydration on hyperthermia and cardiovascular drift during exercise. *J Appl Physiol.* 1992;73:1340–1350.

10. American College of Sports Medicine. Position stand on the prevention of thermal injuries during distance running. *Med Sci Sports Exerc.* 1985;17:ix–xiv.

11. American College of Sports Medicine. Exercise and fluid replacement. *Med Sci Sports Exerc.* 2007;39:377–390.

12. American College of Sports Medicine. Position stand on heat and cold illnesses during distance running. *Med Sci Sports Exerc.* 1996;38:i–x.

13. National Athletic Trainers' Association. Position statement: fluid replacement for athletes. *J Athl Train.* 2000;35:212–224.

14. American Academy of Pediatrics. Climatic heat stress and the exercising child and adolescent. *Pediatrics.* 2000;106:158–159.

15. American Dietetic Association. Position of the American Dietetic Association, Dietitians of Canada, and the American College of Sports Medicine: nutrition and athletic performance. *J Am Diet Assoc.* 2009;100:709–731.

16. Noakes T. IMMDA advisory statement on guidelines for fluid replacement during marathon running. *Clin J Sports Med.* 2003;13:309–318. http://www.usatf.org/groups/coaches/library/2007/hydration/IMMDAAdvisory Statement.pdf. Accessed February 24, 2010.

17. Hew-Butler T, Verbalis JG, Noakes TD. Updated fluid recommendation: position statement from the International Marathon Medical Directors Association (IMMDA). *Clin J Sport Med.* 2006;16:283–292.

18. Inter-Association Task Force. Exertional heat illness consensus statement. *NATA News.* 2003;6:24–29.

19. Casa D. Proper hydration for distance running: identifying individual fluid needs. A USA Track and Field advisory. April 2003. http://www.usatf.org/groups/coaches/library/2007/hydration/ProperHydrationForDistanceRunning.pdf. Accessed February 24, 2010.

20. Casa DJ, Clarkson PM, Roberts WO. American College of Sports Medicine Roundtable on Hydration and Physical Activity: Consensus Statements. *Curr Sports Med Reports.* 2005;4:115–127.

21. Grandjean AC, Reimers KJ, Buyckx ME. Hydration: issues for the 21st century. *Nutr Rev.* 2003;61:261–271.

22. Institute of Medicine. *Dietary Reference Intakes for Water, Potassium, Sodium, Chloride, and Sulfate.* Washington, DC: National Academies Press; 2004. http://www.nap.edu. Accessed February 18, 2005.

23. Ball P. Water as an active constituent in cell biology. *Chem Rev.* 2008;108:74–108.

24. Shepherd VA. The cytomatrix as a cooperative system of macromolecular and water networks. *Curr Topics Develop Biol.* 2006;75:171–223.

25. Guyton AC, Hall JE. *Textbook of Medical Physiology.* 10th ed. Philadelphia, PA: WB Saunders Co; 2000.

26. Zambraski EJ. Renal regulation of fluid homeostasis during exercise. In: Gisolfi CV, Lamb DR, eds. *Perspectives in Exercise Science and Sports Medicine: Fluid Homeostasis During Exercise.* Indianapolis, IN: Benchmark Press; 1990:3:247–280.

27. Valtin H. "Drink at least eight glasses of water a day?" Really? Is there scientific evidence for "8 x 8"? *Am J Physiol Regul Integr Comp Physiol.* 2002;283:R993–R1004.

28. Hoyt RW, Honig A. Environmental influences on body fluid balance during exercise: altitude. In: Buskirk ER, Puhl SM. *Body Fluid Balance.* Boca Raton, FL: CRC Press; 1996;186–193.

29. Maughan RJ, Shirreffs SM, Galloway DR, Leiper JB. Dehydration and fluid replacement in sport and exercise. *Sports Exerc Inj.* 1995;1:148–153.

30. Palmer MS, Spriet LL. Sweat rate, salt loss, and fluid intake during an intense on-ice practice in elite Canadian male junior hockey players. *App Physiol Nutr Metab.* 2008;33:263–271.

31. Jéquier E, Constant F. Water as an essential nutrient: the physiological basis of hydration. *Eur J Clin Nutr.* 2010; 64:116–123.

32. Ladell WS. Water and salt (sodium chloride) intakes. In: Edholm O, Bacharach A, eds. *The Physiology of Human Survival.* New York, NY: Academic Press. 1965:235–299.

33. Bergeron MF. Heat cramps: fluid and electrolyte challenges during tennis in the heat. *J Sci Med Sport.* 2003;6: 19–27.

34. Montain SJ, Sawka MN, Wenger CB. Hyponatremia associated with exercise: risk factors and pathogenesis. *Exerc Sports Sci Rev.* 2001;3:113–117.

35. Shirreffs SM, Maughan RJ. Whole body sweat collection in humans: an improved method with preliminary data on electrolyte content. *J Appl Physiol.* 1997;82:336–341.

36. Bauman A. The epidemiology of heat stroke and associated thermoregulatory disorders. In: Sutton JR, Thompson MW, Torode ME, eds. *Exercise and Thermoregulation.* Sydney, Australia: University of Sydney; 1995:203–208.

37. Riedesel ML, Allen DY, Peake GT, Al-Qattan K. Hyperhydration with glycerol solutions. *J Appl Physiol.* 1987;63: 2262–2268.

38. Latzka WA, Sawka MN, Montain SJ, Skrinar GS, Fielding RA, Matott RP, Pandolf KB. Hyperhydration: tolerance and cardiovascular effects during uncompensable exercise-heat stress. *J Appl Physiol.* 1998;84:1858–1864.

39. Volpe SL, Poule KA, Bland EG. Estimation of prepractice hydration status of National Collegiate Athletic Association Division I athletes. *J Athl Train.* 2009;44:624–629.

40. Armstrong LE, Costill DL, Fink WJ. Influence of diuretic-induced dehydration on competitive running performance. *Med Sci Sports Exerc.* 1985;17:456–461.

41. Sawka MN, Francesconi RP, Young AJ, Pandolf KB. Influence of hydration level and body fluids on exercise performance in the heat. *JAMA.* 1984;252:1165–1169.

42. Rico-Sanz J, Frontera WA, Rivera MA, Rivera-Brown A, Mole PA, Meredith CN. Effects of hyperhydration on total body water, temperature regulation and performance of elite young soccer players in a warm climate. *Int J Sports Med.* 1995;17:85–91.

43. Cheuvront SN, Sawka MN. Hydration assessment of athletes. *Sports Sci Exch.* 2005;18:1–12. http://gssiweb.org/Article_Detail.aspx?articleid=706. Accessed February 24, 2010.

44. Murray R, Eddy DE, Paul GL, Seifert JG, Halaby GA. Physiological responses to glycerol ingestion during exercise. *J Appl Physiol.* 1991;71:144–149.

45. Freund BJ, Montain SJ, Young AJ, Sawka MN, DeLuca JP, Pandolf KB, Valeri CR. Glycerol hyperhydration: hormonal, renal, and vascular fluid responses. *J Appl Physiol.* 1995;79:2069–2077.

46. World Anti Doping Agency. The 2010 Prohibited List—International Standard. http://www.wada-ama.org/rtecontent/document/2010_Prohibited_List_FINAL_EN_Web.pdf. Accessed November 15, 2010.

47. Coyle EF, Montain SJ. Carbohydrate and fluid ingestion during exercise: are there trade-offs? *Med Sci Sports Exerc.* 1992;24:671–678.

48. Gisolfi CV, Duchman SD. Guidelines for optimal replacement beverages for different athletic events. *Med Sci Sports Exerc.* 1992;24:679–687.

49. Walsh RM, Noakes TD, Hawley JA, Dennis SC. Impaired high-intensity cycling performance time at low levels of dehydration. *Int J Sports Med.* 1994;15:392–398.

50. Noakes TD. Hydration in the marathon: using thirst to gauge safe fluid replacement. *Sports Med.* 2007:37:463–466.

51. Murray R. Fluid replacement: the American College of Sports Medicine position stand. *Sports Sci Exch.* 1996;9:1–6.

52. Murray, Robert. SSI Hydration Continuum at http://sportsscienceinsights.com/2009/10/ssi-hydration-continuum. Accessed July 11, 2011.

53. Maughan RJ. Gastric emptying during exercise. *Sports Sci Exch.* 1993;6:1–6.

54. Greenleaf JE. Problem: thirst, drinking behavior, and involuntary dehydration. *Med Sci Sports Exerc.* 1992;24: 645–656.

55. Phillips PA, Rolls BJ, Ledingham ML, Morton JJ. Body fluid changes, thirst and drinking in man during free access to water. *Physiol Behav.* 1984;33:357–363.

56. Passe D, Horn M, Stofan J, Horswill C, Murray R. Voluntary dehydration in runners despite favorable conditions for fluid intake. *Int J Sports Nutr Exerc Metab.* 2007:17:284–295.

57. Hubbard RW, Szlyk PC, Armstrong LE. Influence of thirst and fluid palatability on fluid ingestion during exercise. In: Gisolfi CV, Lamb DR, eds. *Perspectives in Exercise Science and Sports Medicine: Fluid Homeostasis During Exercise.* Vol 3. Indianapolis, IN: Benchmark Press; 1990:39–96.

58. Wilk B, Bar-Or O. Effect of drink flavor and NaCl on voluntary drinking and hydration in boys exercising in the heat. *J Appl Physiol.* 1996;80:1112–1117.

59. Greenleaf JE. Environmental issues that influence intake of replacement beverages. In: Marriott BM, ed. *Fluid Replacement and Heat Stress.* Vol 15. Washington, DC: National Academies Press; 1991:1–30.

60. Broad E. Fluid requirements of team sport players. *Sports Coach.* 1996(Summer):20–23.

61. Horswill CA. Effective fluid replacement. *Int J Sport Nutr.* 1998;8:175–195.

62. Ryan AJ, Lambert GP, Shi X, Chang RT, Summers RW, Gisolfi CV. Effect of hypohydration on gastric emptying and intestinal absorption during exercise. *J Appl Physiol.* 1998;84:1581–1588.

63. Armstrong LE, Costill DL, Fink WJ. Changes in body water and electrolytes during heat acclimation: effects of dietary sodium. *Aviat Space Environ Med.* 1987;58:143–148.

64. Bergeron MF. Heat cramps during tennis: a case report. *Int J Sport Nutr.* 1996;6:62–68.

65. Stofan JR, Zachwieja JJ, Horswill CA, Murray R, Anderson SA, Eichner ER. Sweat and sodium losses in NCAA football players: a precursor to heat cramps? *Int J Sports Nutr Exerc Metab.* 2005;15:641–652.

66. Nose H, Mack GW, Shi X, Nadel ER. Role of osmolality and plasma volume during rehydration in humans. *J Appl Physiol.* 1988;65:325–331.

67. Maughan RJ, Shirreffs SM, Leiper JB. Rehydration and recovery after exercise. *Sport Sci Exch.* 1996;9:1–5.

68. Gisolfi CV, Summers RW, Schedl HP, Bleiler TL. Effect of sodium concentration in a carbohydrate-electrolyte solution on intestinal absorption. *Med Sci Sports Exerc.* 1995;27:1414–1420.

69. Shirreffs SM, Taylor AJ, Leiper JB, Maughan RJ. Post-exercise rehydration in man: effects of volume consumed and drink sodium content. *Med Sci Sports Exerc.* 1996;28:1260–1271.

70. Booth DA. Influences on human fluid consumption. In: Ramsay DJ, Booth DA, eds. *Thirst: Physiological and Psychological Aspects.* London, England: Springer-Verlag; 1991:56–72.

71. Murray R, Stofan J, Eichner ER. Hyponatremia in athletes. *Sports Sci Exch.* 2003;16:1–6.

72. Eichner ER. Six paths to hyponatremia. *Curr Sports Med Rep.* 2009;8:280–281.

73. Gonzalez-Alonso J, Heaps CL, Coyle EF. Rehydration after exercise with common beverages and water. *Int J Sports Med.* 1992;13:399–406.

74. Piantodosi CA. *The Biology of Human Survival.* New York, NY: Oxford University Press; 2003.

75. Bar-David Y, Urkin J, Landau D, Bar-David Z, Pilpel D. Voluntary dehydration among elementary school children residing in a hot arid environment. *J Hum Nutr Diet.* 2009;22:455–460.

76. Diggins KC. Treatment of mild to moderate dehydration in children with oral rehydration therapy. *J Am Acad Nurse Pract.* 2008;20:402–406.

77. World Health Organization. WHO position paper on oral rehydration salts to reduce mortality from cholera. http://www.who.int/cholera/technical/en/index.html. Accessed March 5, 2010.

78. Atia AN, Buchman AL. Oral rehydration solutions in non-cholera diarrhea: a review. *Am J Gastroenterol.* 2009;104:2596–2604.

Chapter 7

ERGOGENIC AIDS, DIETARY SUPPLEMENTS, AND EXERCISE

MARIE DUNFORD, PhD, RD, AND ELLEN J. COLEMAN, MA, MPH, RD, CSSD

Introduction

Athletes spend billions of dollars on dietary supplements each year for the purpose of improving performance, changing weight or body composition, or enhancing health. Athletes are particularly interested in those substances known as ergogenic aids. An ergogenic aid is any substance or strategy that improves athletic performance by improving the production of energy. Although some ergogenic aids and dietary supplements may be beneficial, others may actually impair performance and health.

Supplement use among athletes of all ages and abilities is high. It is estimated that approximately 85% of elite track and field athletes and 60% of all elite athletes use one or more dietary supplement (1,2). Similarly, collegiate athletes are frequent users of dietary supplements, particularly energy drinks and calorie-replacement beverages. The most popular supplements among college males are protein powders and drinks, creatine, multivitamins, and vitamin C. Among college females, the most-used supplements are multivitamins and vitamin C (3). Clearly, athletes are regular users of dietary supplements and they need up-to-date, reliable information.

Adolescent athletes report similar usage patterns, with approximately70% consuming at least one supplement. Energy drinks, protein supplements, and creatine are popular, especially in sports such as football and baseball (4). Use of supplements has been reported as early as middle school. Adolescents may try to emulate top athletes in their sport, who sometimes acknowledge supplement use in media interviews. Some adolescents have reported that they feel pressure to obtain an athletic scholarship as a means of attending college and look to performance-enhancing drugs and dietary supplements as a way to help them achieve their goal. They may also feel peer pressure from teammates who use supplements (5). Although adolescents use supplements, there is little scientific information about safety and effectiveness of supplement use in adolescents or children.

Regulation of Dietary Supplements

In the United States, dietary supplements are regulated under the 1994 Dietary Supplement Health and Education Act (DSHEA), which establishes legal definitions and label guidelines. The legal definition for the term *dietary supplement* is as follows: "A dietary supplement is a vitamin, mineral, herb, botanical, amino acid, metabolite, constituent, extract, or a combination of any of these ingredients" (6). Such a broad definition puts supplements with different structures, functions, or safety profiles in the same category. Prior to 1994, botanicals and herbals were considered neither food nor drugs, but DSHEA currently classifies them as dietary supplements (6). This is in contrast to most European countries, which regulate herbals and botanicals as medicines (7).

DSHEA establishes supplement label guidelines. The Supplements Facts label uses a format similar to the Nutrition Facts label found on food. The label is an important source of information about suggested serving size, type, and quantity of ingredients and percent Daily Values (if established). However, the term *proprietary blend* may be used. The ingredients in a proprietary blend are listed, but the amounts of the substances are not. This term is used to prevent competitors from knowing the exact formulation of a company's product, but it also prohibits consumers and professionals from knowing the amount of each ingredient contained in the supplement.

Health claims, but not therapeutic claims, may also be found on the labels. Therapeutic claims involve the diagnosis, treatment, or prevention of disease. The Food and Drug Administration (FDA) requires the following statement to appear on the label: "This product is not intended to diagnose, treat, cure, or prevent any disease." However, it is often difficult for consumers to understand the difference between health claims (eg, calcium builds strong bones) and therapeutic claims (eg, calcium restores lost bone). More information about structure/function claims on supplement labels can be found on the FDA Web site (www.fda.gov).

There are three critical questions regarding any supplement:

- Is it safe?
- Is it effective?
- Is it contaminated?

Consumers may mistakenly believe that the safety, efficacy, and purity of dietary supplements are tightly regulated. It is imperative that athletes and those who advise them understand that safety, effectiveness, and purity of dietary supplements are *not* comparable to over-the-counter medications or prescription drugs, which are subject to stricter regulation.

Under DSHEA, the FDA does not have the authority to require that supplements be approved for safety before they are marketed. In other words, any dietary supplement that appears on the market is *presumed* to be safe. The FDA must prove that a supplement is unsafe or that it is adulterated before it can be removed from the market. Likewise, the FDA does not conduct premarket reviews to determine if a supplement is effective. There is no law that requires the manufacturer to show evidence of effectiveness before or after a supplement is marketed (6).

The purity of dietary supplements has become a critical issue for athletes as more supplements have been identified as tainted (8–13). Some supplements may contain ingredients that could cause athletes to test positive for substances banned by the governing body of their sport. Some of these substances may be due to poor manufacturing practices and use of tainted ingredients, but there is also evidence that some ingredients, such as precursors to anabolic steroids, are added intentionally (8). An athlete who tests positive for a banned substance will likely be penalized even if the substance was unknowingly ingested via a dietary supplement.

Athletes should be aware that some weight loss supplements and muscle-building supplements might be contaminated. As of March 2009, more than 70 weight loss supplements have been found to contain prescription drugs (6). Analysis of muscle-building supplements has revealed that some contain anabolic steroids or their precursors, substances that are banned by most sports governing bodies. For example, a 2002 study by the International Olympic Committee found that approximately 15% of the 634 samples tested contained substances not listed on the label that would have led to the athlete testing positive for banned substances (10). A 2007 study of 52 supplements found that 25% contained a small amount of steroids (11). Athletes should be especially cautious of supplements described as "testosterone boosters."

The active ingredient(s) in herbal dietary supplements can vary tremendously. In 2000, before ephedrine-containing dietary supplements were banned by the FDA, Gurley et al (9) found that the ephedrine alkaloid content of half of the 20 dietary supplements studied varied by more than 20% when compared with the amount listed on the label. Of the products studied, one product had no active ingredient, one contained more than 150%, and five contained norpseudoephedrine, a controlled substance (drug).

In the past, there have also been reports of toxicity in some herbal preparations. In the case of acute toxicity, the usual cause is the use of a toxic herb as a substitute for a nontoxic species or contamination with a pharmaceutical agent. In the case of chronic toxicity, the cause is typically contamination with a heavy metal or other agent. Most toxicity problems associated with herbal supplements can be avoided if good agricultural and manufacturing practices are followed (7).

In 2007 the FDA finalized regulations requiring current good manufacturing practices (CGMP) for dietary supplements. The goal of these rules is to ensure to consumers that dietary supplements meet quality standards, are free from contamination, and are accurately labeled (14). However, reports continue to surface about contaminated dietary supplements, which would suggest that not all supplements are manufactured using CGMP. The following organizations test and certify dietary supplements for purity:

- ConsumerLab (www.consumerlab.com)
- NSF (www.nsf.org/consumer/dietary_supplements)
- United States Pharmacopeia (www.usp.org/USPVerified)

Evaluation of Ergogenic Aids and Dietary Supplements

Practitioners who simply dismiss the use of dietary supplements may lose credibility with athletes. When working with athletes, it is important to understand their goals and motivations. For elite athletes, competitions are won by slim margins, and some dietary supplements could make a performance difference. Practitioners and athletes must seriously discuss if, and how much of, a supplement would be safe and effective. Athletes need to be aware that dietary supplements sometimes contain banned substances, and that they are subject to disqualification even if they were unaware that the supplement was contaminated. In other words, the athlete must weigh the relative risks with the known benefits.

Recommendations should be evidence based. Beneficial effects may have been found under certain conditions, such as those who are well trained or who performed a certain intensity or duration of activity. It is important to communicate this information. For example, creatine supplements would not be recommended to a marathon runner because evidence has been shown of effectiveness in those performing repeated high-intensity, short-duration (< 30 seconds) exercise bouts, not those engaged in endurance exercise. Advertisements often quote research studies, sometimes out of context, and the practitioner should explain to the athlete the physiological mechanisms, the effects of training, the potential side effects, and the conditions of use.

It is the professional's role to provide as much unbiased information as possible to the athlete considering supplementation and it is appropriate to express concerns about safety. It is unethical to suggest that the information is unbiased if the athlete's supplement purchase would mean monetary gain for the person giving the information. In other words, anyone selling a supplement is not an unbiased source of information.

Practitioners should also consider talking with athletes about the use of multiple dietary supplements at the same time. In many cases, supplements are studied individually and information about safety and effectiveness is for that supplement only at the doses used in the study. Supplement-to-supplement interactions are possible and the safety of an individual supplement taken with other supplements is not typically known. It is also not possible for an athlete to know if a particular supplement is effective if multiple supplements are consumed.

The use of dietary supplements is an ever-changing and ever-challenging aspect of sports nutrition. Sports dietitians should be open-minded skeptics. If a supplement is safe, working with the athlete to determine effectiveness may be a better approach than dismissing supplement use out of hand. Box 7.1 lists questions and resources for evaluating dietary supplements and ergogenic aids.

Commonly Used Supplements

The number of new products introduced to the market is dizzying. Sports dietitians must constantly update their knowledge base. Coverage of all of the available supplements would be impossible, but this chapter does review those that athletes commonly use and ask about. They are listed here in alphabetical order.

AAKG (Arginine Alpha-ketoglutarate)

See Nitric Oxide.

BOX 7.1   Guidelines for Evaluating Dietary Supplements and Ergogenic Aids

Is the supplement safe?
- Check the Food and Drug Administration (FDA) Web site (www.fda.gov) for recalls, withdrawals, and safety alerts (can follow via Twitter: @FDArecalls).

Is the supplement effective?
- Determine whether the claims being made are physiologically plausible.
- Review the scientific literature:
  - Search reputable free databases such as PubMed (www.ncbi.nlm.nih.gov/PubMed).
  - Search member-only databases such as ADA Evidence Analysis Library (www.ada evidencelibrary.com); Natural Medicine Comprehensive Database (www.naturaldatabase .com); or EBSCO (ebscohost.com).
  - Read review articles about the specific supplement.
  - Search Web sites with evidence-based supplement information such as Lewis Gale Hospital Alleghany Natural Pharmacist-Consumer (www.alleghanyregional.com/healthcontent .asp?page=/choice/demonstration/TheNaturalPharmacist-Consumer) or SupplementWatch (www.supplementwatch.com).

Is the supplement likely to be free from contamination?
- Check Web sites such as ConsumerLab.com (Athletic Banned Substances Screened Products) (www.consumerlab.com); NSF (Certified for Sport) (www.nsf.org); United States Pharmacopeia (www.usp.org/USPVerified); and Informed-Choice (www.informed-choice.org).

Amino Acids

See Protein Supplements.

Androstenedione

Androstenedione is an anabolic steroid used to increase blood testosterone. It received widespread media attention when professional baseball player Mark McGwire admitted use during his home run record-setting season in 1998. This admission influenced use in others, including adolescents, and drove up the sale of androstenedione (15).

Androstenedione, androstenediol, and, to a lesser extent, dehydroepiandrosterone (DHEA) are often referred to as *prohormones*. The human body potentially converts oral androstenedione into testosterone so such supplements have been marketed as ways to increase skeletal muscle mass and strength. However, numerous studies have shown that androstenedione or other prohormone supplements are not effective for increasing muscle mass (16,17).

There are also major concerns about safety. The FDA, in a white paper released in March 2004, listed more than 25 potential androgenic and estrogenic effects (18). Side effects may include a decrease in high-density lipoprotein (HDL) cholesterol and an increase in serum estrogen concentration. Safety concerns prompted the US Congress to pass the Anabolic Steroid Control Act of 2004, which lists androstenedione as a controlled substance that cannot be sold without a prescription. Most sports governing bodies list andro-stenedione as a banned substance.

Bottom line: Androstenedione is not safe and not effective; a banned substance.

Antioxidants

See Vitamin C and Vitamin E Supplements (Antioxidants).

Arginine

See Growth Hormone Releasers.

Arginine Alpha-ketoglutarate (AAKG)

See Nitric Oxide.

Beet Juice

Beet juice, which is also called beetroot juice, is naturally high in nitrate. Preliminary research suggests that consumption of a large dose of nitrate may have an effect on skeletal muscle efficiency. The possible mechanisms include reducing the adenosine triphosphate (ATP) cost of muscle force production and the ability to tolerate high-intensity exercise for a longer period of time (19). Larsen et al (20) found that the consumption of sodium nitrate at a dose of 0.1 mmol/kg/d for 3 days resulted in a lower oxygen demand when well-trained males performed submaximal exercise on a cycle ergometer. A study by Bailey et al (21) used 500 mL of beet juice per day as a source of the sodium nitrate. Eight recreational athletes consumed the beet juice over 6 days and performed both moderate- and high-intensity cycling. The study found a lower oxygen demand during moderate-intensity exercise in those who consumed beet juice. Additionally, those subjects had an increased time to exhaustion associated with the high-intensity cycling when compared to those who received the placebo. Positive results have also been reported in studies of walking, running, and cycling (22,23). The results of these studies have influenced some endurance athletes to consume beet juice in an effort to increase skeletal muscle efficiency. Although the results of these studies are promising, more research needs to be done.

In response to these studies, questions about the safety of a concentrated dose of nitrate were raised. Nitrate is not carcinogenic; however, nitrite that is formed from dietary nitrate may combine with dietary amines and result in nitrosamines, which may be carcinogenic. The acceptable daily intake (ADI) of nitrate recommended by the World Health Organization is 3.65 mg/kg/d. For perspective, the dose used in the Larsen et al study (20) was 6.2 mg/kg/d of sodium nitrate and the dose in the Bailey et al study (19) was 4.16 mg/kg/d. The amount used in both studies exceeded the ADI. The ADI has a large margin of safety and the amounts used in these research studies represent a very small risk (24). However, more research is needed to better understand both the risks and benefits of beet juice for endurance athletes.

Bottom line: Studies indicate that beet juice has promise as a way to increase skeletal muscle efficiency due to a lower oxygen demand in endurance athletes; there are safety concerns; further research is needed.

Beta-alanine

Beta-alanine is a nonessential amino acid and the only naturally occurring beta amino acid. It is the rate-limiting precursor for carnosine, which buffers lactic acid. Carnosine is found in high concentrations in skeletal muscles under normal conditions, and studies suggest that beta-alanine supplementation can substantially increase muscle carnosine levels (25–27). In theory, both aerobic and anaerobic performance could be improved due to increased buffering capacity as a result of increased muscle carnosine levels. Beta-alanine supplementation may also delay neuromuscular fatigue.

Enhanced buffering of muscle pH is particularly important during high-intensity exercise. Studies have shown improved performance with beta-alanine supplementation during multiple bouts of high-intensity exercise as well as a single bout of exercise lasting greater than 60 seconds (25,26,28). However, not all studies of beta-alanine supplementation in those performing repeated sprints have shown an effect (29).

Although most of the research has been done with athletes performing high-intensity exercise, a few researchers are studying the effect of beta-alanine supplementation in endurance athletes. Endurance events often require a sprint to the finish line. Van Thienen et al (30) found that beta-alanine supplementation improved sprint performance in endurance cyclists.

Study dosages are approximately 3.2 to 6.4 g/d, with a higher initial dose followed by a lower maintenance dose. Such doses seem to be safe. Beta-alanine shows promise as an ergogenic aid. Further studies on safety and effectiveness are warranted.

Bottom line: Beta-alanine is safe and shows promise as a way to effectively buffer muscle pH in athletes performing high-intensity (sprint) exercise. More research is needed.

Beta-Hydroxy-Beta-Methylbutyrate (HMB)

See HMB.

Bitter Orange

See Citrus aurantium (Bitter Orange).

Branched-Chain Amino Acids (BCAA)

The branched-chain amino acids (BCAA), named for their chemical structure, are leucine, isoleucine, and valine. During prolonged endurance exercise when glycogen stores are low, skeletal muscle can metabolize these amino acids for energy. BCAA also competes with tryptophan, an amino acid associated with mental fatigue, and is involved in the immune system (31–34).

In theory, greater availability of BCAA late in prolonged exercise could provide a much needed fuel source. Higher blood levels of BCAA in the presence of tryptophan could help to delay fatigue. However, supplemental BCAA has not been shown to delay fatigue or improve endurance performance in elite athletes (31).

Although the trials are small, some positive effects have been reported in studies that examined immune response (31). Immunosuppression in endurance-trained athletes, such as triathletes, may be a result of decreased glutamine levels. BCAA supplementation reverses the decline in glutamine because BCAA is metabolized to glutamine in skeletal muscle. BCAA supplements may play a role in supporting immune function, but more research is needed (31).

Another area of research is the use of BCAA supplements to reduce exercise-induced muscle damage. Preliminary studies with a small number of untrained subjects found that 5 g of BCAA before doing squat exercises reduced delayed-onset muscle soreness (DOMS) and muscle fatigue for several days after exercise (32–34). The mechanism is not known, but a possibility is that BCAA could reduce protein breakdown and stimulate protein synthesis in the exercised muscle. This has become a more active area of research.

Supplemental BCAA, often consumed 5 to 20 g/d in divided doses, seems to be safe. (*See also* Glutamine section of this chapter.)

Bottom line: BCAA is safe at recommended doses; it is not effective for improving performance; positive effects on immune response and reduction of postexercise muscle fatigue are under investigation.

Caffeine

Athletes use caffeine as an ergogenic aid to improve endurance performance as well as to delay fatigue and enhance fat loss. There have been a considerable number of studies and review articles (35–38), and the consensus opinion is that caffeine is an effective ergogenic aid for some athletes. The strongest evidence is that caffeine can enhance endurance performance. Most of these studies have been conducted in runners, cyclists, and cross-country skiers. There is also evidence that caffeine can improve performance for those engaged in high-intensity activities lasting 1 to 20 minutes. Those studies have been conducted in runners, cyclists, swimmers, and rowers. At the present time, there are not enough scientific studies with sufficient rigor to draw conclusions about athletes in other sports (35).

In the past, caffeine was thought to improve endurance performance by enhancing free fatty acid release, which in turn would spare muscle glycogen. Although caffeine may enhance free fatty acid mobilization during endurance exercise, fat oxidation is not significantly increased, nor is muscle glycogen spared. The ergogenic benefit of caffeine is likely due to its role as a central nervous system stimulant resulting in a heightened sense of awareness and a decreased perception of effort (35–37).

Many athletes who strength train use caffeine to delay fatigue while training. In theory, the caffeine would have an indirect performance effect by allowing athletes to train harder or longer (35). Caffeine may enhance contractile force in skeletal muscle during submaximal contractions. It may also increase the athlete's threshold for pain or perceived exertion, which could result in longer training sessions (38). Although caffeine is touted as a "fat burner," there is no evidence to support that caffeine alone has a substantial effect on fat or weight loss, although there may be a slight increase in resting metabolic rate for a few hours after consumption. Caffeine does potentiate the effect of ephedrine, which is used for weight loss. More information about caffeine and ephedrine together is found under the Ephedra section.

To achieve the desired ergogenic effect, users must have a significant amount of caffeine in their blood. In the past, the recommended dose for endurance athletes was 5 to 6 mg per kilogram body weight. Newer studies in endurance athletes suggest that a more moderate dose, 2 to 3 mg per kilogram body weight, is effective (35). High doses are not beneficial because as caffeine dose increases, performance does not increase and because caffeine does cause side effects, such as increased heart rate. The athlete will likely need to establish the optimal dose by trial and error. A reasonable starting point is 2 mg per kilogram body weight. For the 110-lb (50-kg) person, this recommended dose would be 100 mg caffeine. At the highest dose, 6 mg/kg body weight, a 50-kg person would need to consume 300 mg caffeine. The optimal timing of caffeine intake (eg, 1 hour before performance, during performance, etc) is being studied, but the results are not conclusive (38).

Caffeine could be consumed in a variety of ways, including the consumption of strongly brewed coffee (8 oz = ~85 mg), caffeine-containing soft drinks (12 oz = ~36 mg), energy bars with caffeine (1 bar = 50 or 100 mg), caffeinated gels, (1 oz = ~50 mg), or caffeine-containing pills (1 tablet = 100 mg). The latter are used because they contain a standardized concentrated dose; the caffeine content of brewed coffee can vary considerably. Coffee may also contain chemicals that may impair exercise performance (35).

Caffeine is legally and socially acceptable throughout the world, but at certain levels is considered a controlled/restricted substance. For a National Collegiate Athletic Association (NCAA) athlete, urinary caffeine levels exceeding 15mcg/mL would subject the athlete to disqualification. Such levels would be very difficult to reach via food intake (ie, the equivalent of approximately 17 caffeine-containing soft drinks) and the equivalent amount of caffeine-containing tablets would likely impair performance in other ways (ie, shaking, rapid heartbeat, etc). However, some athletes have achieved this level and were disqualified. The International Olympic Committee (IOC) moved caffeine from its Prohibited List to its Monitoring Program in 2004. This allows athletes to take common cold remedies containing caffeine and drink caffeinated drinks without risk of disqualification. The IOC continues to monitor urinary caffeine levels, but there is no evidence of caffeine abuse by Olympic athletes (35).

Caffeine is considered safe to use by most adults, but it is has several known adverse effects. Blood pressure is increased both at rest and during exercise, heart rate is increased, gastrointestinal distress can occur, and insomnia may result. The adverse effects are more likely to occur in those people who are caffeine-naïve or at higher doses (6 to 9 mg/kg body weight). For routine users, caffeine is addictive and sudden withdrawal results in severe headaches. In the past, athletes were cautioned not to consume caffeinated beverages because they were thought to contribute to dehydration. There is no evidence that consuming caffeine at the levels recommended to improve performance causes dehydration or electrolyte imbalance (35,39).

Caffeine recommendations are intended for adults and there is concern about caffeine use by adolescents and children (35,40). Many energy drinks are marketed to youth and there is growing concern about the "ratcheting up" of caffeine levels in these products. For example, some energy drinks have 200 mg of caffeine as well as herbal sources of caffeine in 75 mL (2.5 oz). At the extreme end are products that contain approximately 500 mg of caffeine in 20 oz. These are concentrated sources of caffeine, particularly for small-bodied individuals, and there is potential for caffeine intoxication (40).

Bottom line: Caffeine is safe at recommended doses, effective for endurance performance and high-intensity activities lasting up to 20 minutes, and effective as a central nervous system stimulant, which can mask mental and physical fatigue. Caffeine is listed as a banned substance by the NCAA, but it is unlikely that the testing threshold would be exceeded due to intolerable adverse effects.

Carnitine

Carnitine is essential in the human body to transport fatty acids into the mitochondria to be used for energy. It is found in the diet and can be synthesized in the body from the amino acid lysine. Deficiencies have occurred, but typically not in healthy adults. Carnitine supplementation is known to normalize long-chain fatty acid metabolism in carnitine-deficient individuals (41), but the benefits to healthy people are questionable. Because carnitine is used in fat oxidation, claims for supplemental carnitine include increased fat metabolism and, as a result of enhanced fat utilization, loss of body fat.

Despite decades of study, there is no compelling evidence that carnitine supplements improve performance (42–45). Several studies have shown that supplementation does not change fat metabolism during exercise (43–45). Research has turned to use of carnitine supplements for recovery (43,46). More research is needed in this area.

Most study protocols use an oral dose of 2 to 4 g/d, which is the dose typically recommended by manufacturers. Carnitine supplementation seems to be safe at recommended doses (42,43,47).

Bottom line: Carnitine is safe at recommended doses; it is not effective for improving performance.

Chondroitin Sulfate

See Glucosamine/Chondroitin Sulfate.

Chromium (Chromium Picolinate)

Chromium is an essential mineral that augments the action of insulin. It enhances insulin sensitivity by increasing the number of insulin receptors, thus improving glucose utilization (48,49). Enhanced insulin sensitivity could also promote the uptake of amino acids into muscle cells, stimulate protein synthesis, and enhance glycogen stores. These biological functions make chromium supplements attractive to athletes who want to increase muscle mass, decrease body fat, and improve performance.

Chromium is found in a variety of foods, such as beef, poultry, eggs, nuts, whole grains, and wheat germ. The Dietary Reference Intake (DRI) for adults ranges from 20 to 35 mcg/d, depending on age and sex. Mean daily dietary intake by adults is approximately 25 mcg for females and 33 mcg for males. Athletes who consume sufficient energy and a variety of foods would not likely be deficient. No Tolerable Upper Intake Level (UL) has been established (50).

Chromium is a popular supplement and is usually found as chromium picolinate. The picolinate makes the compound extremely stable and this stability results in much greater gastrointestinal absorption of supplemental chromium than food-based chromium (51). There is concern that chromium picolinate supplements can result in an increase in free radical production, and other forms are available. These forms vary in their ability to be absorbed (52). Chromium supplementation of 50 to 200 mcg/d seems to be safe. However, some supplement manufacturers recommend that a 200 mcg dose be taken several times per day and such high doses pose some safety concerns. Higher intakes may decrease iron absorption. Accumulated chromium in the body can damage DNA (53).

Supplemental chromium's initial popularity was based on animal and early human studies that reported an increase in muscle mass and a decrease in body fat. Later studies, with stricter methodology including better measurements of body composition, did not replicate the initial results (54). The consensus opinion is that chromium supplementation is not effective for changing body composition in athletes either by increasing muscle mass or decreasing body fat (49,55). Supplemental chromium is also not effective as a weight loss aid for obese individuals (49,56). There is no evidence that it promotes faster resynthesis of glycogen stores after high-intensity exercise (57). Although chromium supplementation can help to improve blood glucose levels in those with diabetes, there is no evidence that such an effect occurs in individuals who do not have diabetes (58).

Bottom line: Chromium is safe at recommended doses; there are some safety concerns with doses more than 200 mcg or forms that have high bioavailability. It is not effective for increasing muscle mass, decreasing body fat, or improving performance.

Citrus aurantium *(Bitter Orange)*

Citrus aurantium, also known as bitter orange, contains synephrine, octopamine, and other stimulatory compounds. Synephrine is chemically similar to epinephrine; octopamine to norepinephrine (59–61). Supplements containing bitter orange have become more popular as ephedrine-containing supplements have been removed from the US market. Supplements advertised as ephedra-free may contain a combination of *citrus aurantium* and caffeine, both of which can be derived from herbal sources.

In small studies, exercise tolerance is modestly improved with caffeine-containing bitter orange supplements, probably due to the stimulatory effects of the ingredients, which may mask physical and mental fatigue. Under both resting and exercise conditions, these compounds increase blood pressure and plasma glucose (59,60). Some adverse events, both minor (temporary elevation in heart rate) and serious (stroke) have been reported (59).

Citrus aurantium is marketed as a weight-loss aid that enhances fat metabolism. Although bitter orange and similar stimulants can slightly increase resting metabolic rate (RMR), the temporary and small increase in RMR is unlikely to result in clinically significant weight loss (61). There is some promise for bitter orange's effect on enhancing fat metabolism, but there are many questions about safety and efficacy that need to be better answered (62).

Bottom line: There are concerns about the safety of bitter orange; it is effective as a central nervous stimulant; more research needed to establish efficacy as a weight-loss aid.

Conjugated Linoleic Acid

Conjugated linoleic acid (CLA) is an isomer of the essential fatty acid linoleic acid and part of a group of polyunsaturated fatty acids found in lamb, beef, and dairy products. The major isomer found naturally is *cis*-9, *trans*-11, but most supplements have a mixture of the natural isomer and a *trans*-10, *cis*-12 isomer. In animal studies it is the *trans*-10, *cis*-12 isomer that can reduce the deposition of fat in adipose tissue; however, this isomer is also associated with deposition of fat in the liver and spleen and insulin resistance in the test animals (63). CLA supplements are often marketed to athletes as a way to reduce body fat, change body composition, and improve performance.

Studies in animals who received CLA supplements for the purpose of weight loss were promising, but results of human studies are mixed (63–65). At the present time the results in humans are too inconsistent to warrant recommendation of CLA supplements as a weight-loss aid. As for a performance effect, there are no studies that suggest the CLA supplements directly impact performance, although changes in body composition can contribute to a positive effect on performance.

The safety of CLA supplements has not been established. The two isomers may have opposite effects and there is concern because some animal studies detected insulin resistance and fatty liver. More research is needed to determine a safe dose in humans, including types of isomers used, duration of use, and dose/response (63).

Bottom line: Safety in humans not established for CLA; evidence of effectiveness as a weight-loss aid is mixed in humans.

Creatine

Creatine is a nitrogen-containing compound found in meat and fish in small amounts. It is used in the body as a source of muscle energy in the form of creatine phosphate (also known as phosphocreatine). Supplemental creatine increases total creatine by approximately 10% to 30% and phosphocreatine stores by approximately 10% to 40% (66). Creatine supplementation also increases muscle cell volume and muscle fiber hypertrophy (67).

Numerous studies have documented that creatine supplements result in a small but significant increase in lean body mass with repeated high-intensity, short-duration (< 30 seconds) exercise bouts (66–72). Volek and Rawson (67) report that most studies of creatine show an ergogenic effect for a variety of athletes and a performance effect for weightlifters. Creatine supplementation may help the athlete maintain or sustain force output for a longer period of time, thus completing more repetitions. For example, creatine supplements may allow an athlete to train harder by completing more weightlifting repetitions. This increase in training stimulus over time may result in the athlete becoming stronger, faster, or more powerful.

In the past, the safety of creatine supplementation was debated, but current scientific research suggests that creatine supplementation is safe. There is no evidence that creatine supplements negatively affect hydration status or heat tolerance (67–72), although athletes are always advised to be properly hydrated. Supplemental creatine is consumed as creatine monohydrate. The usual dose is 3 to 5 g/d. Some athletes use a short-term loading period—up to 20 to 25 g/d for 5 to 7 days—but the initial "loading" dose has not been shown to be more beneficial. The typical dose in research studies is about 20 g/d for the first 5 days, and 5 to 10 g/d thereafter. Some complaints of minor side effects such as gastrointestinal disturbances and cramps have been reported (67).

Some athletes respond to creatine supplements with significant increases in muscle creatine levels, but others are nonresponders. This is likely explained by the amount of creatine in the muscle prior to supplementation and may depend on the usual diet. In one study, vegetarians showed larger increases in muscle creatine after supplementation than nonvegetarians because the vegetarians had lower muscle creatine levels prior to supplementation (73).

Bottom line: Creatine is safe at recommended doses; it is effective for a small but significant increase in lean body mass with repeated high-intensity, short-duration (< 30 seconds) exercise bouts; it is also effective for increasing performance in weightlifters.

Dehydroepiandrosterone (DHEA)

Dehydroepiandrosterone (DHEA) is a precursor to testosterone and estrogen but it is considered a weak androgen. The biochemical link to testosterone has made it a popular prohormone among athletes. Such athletes hope that the prohormones—androstenedione, androstenediol, and DHEA—will increase blood testosterone levels, which in turn will increase muscle mass (74). Masters' athletes have expressed an interest in DHEA because natural DHEA in the body diminishes substantially with age; in fact, it is one of the steepest hormonal decreases in humans (74,75). DHEA supplements are often advertised as being "a fountain of youth."

Studies do not suggest that DHEA, the weakest of the three androgens, has an anabolic effect or can enhance athletic performance (74). There is also no evidence that DHEA supplementation improves cognitive function (eg, awareness, perception) or enhances quality of life in older people (75). There are also concerns about the safety of supplemental DHEA. Before the passage of the Dietary Health and Supplement Education Act in 1994, DHEA was a prescription drug. In the United States, it is now available over-the-counter and in dietary supplements; in other countries it remains a controlled substance due to abuse potential. Although other prohormones, such as androstenedione, are banned for sale under the Anabolic Steroid Control Act of 2004, DHEA is not. The effects of high doses or long-term use are not known. Because of its unknown safety profile and lack of proven effectiveness, DHEA supplementation for athletes and older individuals is not recommended at this time (74,75).

Bottom line: DHEA is neither safe nor effective.

Dihydroxyacetone (DHA)

See Pyruvate and Dihydroxyacetone.

Ephedra (Ephedrine-Containing Supplements)

No dietary supplement has been as controversial as ephedra. In December 2003, the FDA issued a consumer alert that advised consumers to stop buying and using products containing ephedra. Sales were banned in April 2004, based on the FDA ruling that dietary supplements containing ephedrine alkaloids presented an unreasonable risk of illness or injury (76). A federal court later struck down parts of the ban. At present, low-dose (≤ 10 mg) ephedrine-containing supplements are legal to sell and purchase in the United States, unless a state enacts its own ban, as California and New York have. Ephedrine is also found in over-the-counter medications.

Even the terminology has caused confusion. *Ephedra, ephedrine alkaloids,* and *ephedrine* are different terms, although they are frequently used interchangeably. Scientifically, *ephedra* refers to a genus of plants. Some species in this genus contain *ephedrine alkaloids* in the stems and branches. One of the ephedrine alkaloids is *ephedrine.* Although there is a scientific distinction, in common usage ephedra refers to any dietary supplement that contains ephedrine alkaloids.

Ma huang, a traditional Chinese herbal medicine, is extracted from the species *Ephedra sinica* Stapf and contains six different ephedrine alkaloids. Of the six, the main active ingredient is ephedrine. Ephedrine can also be synthesized in the laboratory. Ma huang has been used for centuries to treat asthma and nasal congestion. In the United States, ephedrine is added to over-the-counter medications for the same purposes. But ephedrine use in athletes has more often been related to weight loss, increased energy, and enhanced performance. So the critical questions are whether ephedrine-containing supplements are safe and effective for these purposes.

In some respects, ephedra is the poster child for the DSHEA of 1994. At the time that the act was passed, many health professionals thought that herbal medicines, which prior to this act were considered neither a food nor drug, were inappropriately categorized as dietary supplements. Their concern was that some herbal products were being used as medications, and as such, dose was an important issue. The FDA shared these concerns.

What made the ephedra issue more contentious was that experts did not agree on what dosage was safe. The FDA proposed that not more than 8 mg of ephedrine alkaloids be used in a 6-hour period *and* not more than 24 mg in a 24-hour period. Usage should not exceed 7 days (77). However, another group of scientists suggested that a single dose should not exceed 30 mg ephedrine alkaloids and that up to 90 mg in a 24-hour period is safe, and that usage should not exceed 6 months (78). Such differing dosage recommendations make it confusing for both consumers and health professionals.

Within a few years after the passage of the DSHEA, the FDA became increasingly concerned about the safety of ephedrine. By 1997, half of the adverse event reports (AERs) that consumers telephoned to a hotline involved ephedrine. The adverse events reported included known side effects such as headache, increased heart rate, increased blood pressure, and insomnia. The AERs also included deaths to otherwise healthy middle-aged and young adults, which alarmed the FDA.

The adverse events reports are hard to interpret. Data collected from self-reports lack scientific rigor. Many of the AERs do not contain information about dose, even though dose is a critical factor. Some consumers may have used these supplements despite the manufacturers' warnings. Most warn against use by those with a history of heart disease, diabetes, or high blood pressure, or by pregnant or lactating women.

The safety of ephedrine-containing dietary supplements has been hotly debated. Shekelle et al (79) reviewed 16,000 AERs and found that 21 were serious events: two deaths, nine strokes, four heart attacks, one seizure, and five psychiatric problems. In these cases, ephedrine was believed to be the sole contributor, but there was not enough evidence to establish a cause-and-effect relationship. In addition to the 21 serious adverse effects, 10 other cases involved ephedrine as a contributing (but not sole) factor. Based on this and other evidence, the FDA concluded that ephedrine-containing dietary supplements presented an unreasonable safety risk.

"Significant or unreasonable risk of illness or injury" (76) is the basis for the ban on ephedrine-containing dietary supplements. Proponents of the ban point to documented deaths and serious cardiovascular and psychiatric events. They believe that the risk-benefit ratio meets the "unreasonable risk" portion of the FDA criterion (80). Opponents of the ban counter that the risk is very small. In 1999, approximately 3 million people purchased ephedrine-containing dietary supplements and consumed an estimated 3 billion "servings." The risk of a serious adverse event is estimated to be less than 1 in 1,000 and opponents point out that a cause-and-effect relationship has not been established. They argue that the deaths, although tragic, do not represent a significant risk (78).

Of particular importance to athletes is the risk associated with using ephedrine before strenuous workouts in the heat. In 2001 the National Football League (NFL) banned ephedra after the death of lineman Korey Stringer, who collapsed and died from heatstroke. Practice was held in hot and humid conditions (approximating 110°F on the heat index) and his body temperature upon hospital admission was reported to have been 108.8°F. Toxicology tests were not conducted on autopsy, but an ephedrine-containing dietary supplement was found in his locker.

In 2003 Major League pitching prospect Steve Bechler, age 23, also suffered heatstroke while training in hot and humid conditions. His body temperature rose to 108°F. In this case, the coroner cited the use of ephedrine as a cause of death. In Bechler's case, there seems to have been several contributing circumstances, including a history of borderline hypertension and liver abnormalities and a restriction of both food and fluid in the previous 24 hours in an effort to lose weight.

Another safety issue is quality control. In 2000 Gurley et al (9) published a study of the ephedrine alkaloid content of 20 dietary supplements. The content of 10 of the products varied by more than 20% when compared with the amount listed on the label. One product contained more than 150% of the amount listed on the label and one had no active ingredient. Five contained norpseudoephedrine, a controlled substance (drug). "Spiked" products are especially problematic because most athletes are subject to testing for banned substances (81).

In addition to safety, effectiveness must be considered. Regarding weight loss, most study protocols use ephedrine and caffeine in combination because caffeine is known to enhance the effect of ephedrine. Studies report that the use of ephedrine and caffeine by obese people can produce a short-term weight loss of 8 to 9 lb. Studies to date have not been conducted for longer than 6 months, so it is unknown what the long-term effect might be or the effect of discontinuing the ephedrine and caffeine. It is also not known if an ephedrine-induced short-term weight loss has long-term health benefits (79).

Most athletes are not obese, but they may use ephedrine-containing dietary supplements before and during training camp to lose weight that was gained in the off-season. There have been no studies to date in athletes who use this combination for short-term weight loss.

Results of studies using ephedrine and caffeine as a performance enhancer have been mixed (79,82–86). In two trials using bicycle ergometers (82,83), ephedrine and caffeine significantly increased time to exhaustion.

Military subjects ran 3.2 km with 11 kg of gear, and individuals in the ephedrine-caffeine trial recorded faster times than those in the control group (84). No effect of ephedrine and caffeine was reported in a trial of treadmill walking (85). A 2008 study of resistance-trained males reported no effect on muscle strength or anaerobic performance (86). Some athletes claim that ephedrine- and caffeine-containing dietary supplements give them "more energy." This is likely due to the stimulant effect of these compounds, which can mask fatigue. It is known that some brands are "spiked" with norpseudoephedrine and such drugs are stimulatory. With the current ban on ephedrine supplements containing more than 10 mg, there is concern that bitter orange *(citrus aurantium)* or similar compounds will become a substitute herbal stimulant source in some dietary supplements. Bitter orange contains synephrine, which is considered a drug (see *citrus aurantium*).

The NCAA and many professional sports organizations ban ephedrine-containing supplements. The IOC allows ephedrine at urinary concentrations less than 10 mcg/mL. This level could be exceeded with multiple doses of over-the-counter ephedrine-containing medications (eg, decongestants) or dietary supplements (87).

Bottom line: Safety is a concern for ephedra at doses more than 10 mg; it has a narrower safety profile than most dietary supplements. Ephedra is effective in combination with caffeine for a short-term weight loss of 8 to 9 lb in obese individuals and may be effective for masking physical and mental fatigue due to central nervous system stimulation. It is not effective for improving muscle strength or anaerobic performance. Multiple doses may result in a positive banned substances test.

Glucosamine/Chondroitin Sulfate

Glucosamine and chondroitin are sold as dietary supplements to reduce joint pain and improve function and range of motion. They are used as an alternative therapy for osteoarthritis (OA). Glucosamine is an amino sugar that may help form and repair cartilage. Chondroitin is part of a protein that aids in elasticity of cartilage. The mechanism of action is unknown, but glucosamine and chondroitin may stimulate cartilage protein synthesis or inhibit breakdown. The body manufactures glucosamine and chondroitin and the amount produced is not associated with dietary intake (88).

Early studies were promising, but they were also controversial because they lacked scientific rigor. The National Institutes of Health funded a well-designed study, GAIT, to determine the effect of glucosamine and chondroitin on osteoarthritis of the knee (89). The researchers found that 1,500 mg/d of glucosamine and 1,200 mg/d chondroitin sulfate, either alone or in combination, for 24 weeks did not reduce pain effectively in the overall group of patients with osteoarthritis of the knee. Further data analysis suggested that the combination of glucosamine and chondroitin sulfate may be effective in the small subgroup of patients with moderate-to-severe knee pain. A continuation of the GAIT study found that glucosamine did not slow the narrowing of the knee joint space (90). A 2010 meta analysis found that neither glucosamine nor chondroitin, alone or in combination, reduced joint pain or affected the narrowing of the joint space in those with osteoarthritis of the hip or knee (91).

The typical recommended dosage of glucosamine and chondroitin is 1,500 mg/d and 1,200 mg/d, respectively. Improvement of symptoms would not be expected for 6 to 8 weeks. However, if improvement does not occur after 8 weeks of continuous use, it is not likely that supplementation will help. Minimal adverse effects have been reported, especially compared with frequent use of nonsteroidal anti-inflammatory drugs (NSAIDs), such as ibuprofen. Those considering taking glucosamine and chondroitin should discuss this decision with their physician as part of their osteoarthritis treatment plan.

Bottom line: Glucosamine and chondroitin are safe. They are generally not effective for reducing joint pain or increasing functionality in those with osteoarthritis of the knee; however, they may be beneficial for some individuals with moderate-to-severe knee pain.

Glutamine

Glutamine is a nonessential amino acid under normal conditions, but a conditionally essential amino acid under physiological stress in which glutamine is a fuel source for immune system cells. Plasma glutamine in endurance athletes can be decreased after strenuous exercise. Supplemental glutamine is theorized to be beneficial for decreasing exercise-induced stress and susceptibility to infections (92). Some athletes use glutamine to increase cell volume to stimulate protein synthesis in an effort to increase muscle mass.

A 2008 review by Gleeson (92) concluded that glutamine supplementation is not an effective countermeasure for immunologic stress and does not decrease exercise-induced immunosuppression. Claims related to glutamine supplementation in weight training, such as improved recovery, decreased muscle catabolism, and muscle gain has not been substantiated by research studies. Research also suggests that glutamine is not effective for increasing muscle mass (93).

Recommendations made by manufacturers range from 5 to 10 g/d to more than 20 g/d. Because glutamine is found in the amino acid profile of dietary proteins, no specific DRI or Recommended Dietary Allowance has been established. The estimated daily intake of glutamine is approximately 3 to 6 g (based on a dietary protein intake of 0.8 to 1.6 g per kg body weight). Athletes who consume protein supplements may consume more. It is known that some endurance athletes consume diets low or marginal in protein, and increasing protein intake, and therefore glutamine intake, would likely be beneficial. Glutamine supplements are considered safe (92).

Bottom line: Glutamine is safe but not effective.

Green Tea Extract

A popular supplement to aid weight loss is green tea extract. The extract contains several antioxidant compounds known as catechins. In the presence of caffeine, some of these catechins influence energy metabolism and fat oxidation (94,95).

A 2010 meta-analysis (94) compared the effects of green tea catechins with and without caffeine in randomized controlled trials. Studies showed that green tea extract in the presence of caffeine resulted in statistically significant decreases in body mass index (BMI), body weight, and waist circumference. The actual losses were small—a decrease of approximately 1.38 kg (3 lb) of body weight. In the absence of caffeine, green tea catechins do not produce these changes.

Although green tea is widely consumed as a beverage and generally regarded as safe, green tea extract may not be safe. There have been case reports of acute liver toxicity and thrombotic thrombocytopenic purpura (low platelet count and bruising) associated with the use of green tea extract (96–98). Consumers must be aware that green tea and green tea extract are not the same.

Bottom line: Green tea extract is not the same as green tea and should be used with caution due to some reports of liver toxicity and thrombotic thrombocytopenic purpura; It is effective for small loss of body weight.

Growth Hormone Releasers

Exercise is a very potent stimulator of growth hormone. Certain amino acids, such as arginine, ornithine, and lysine, can also stimulate growth hormone release when infused intravenously or administered orally (99–101). Some individuals consume these amino acids before strength training to accentuate the exercise-induced release of growth hormone and to promote greater gains in muscle mass and strength.

These amino acids may be consumed individually or together and are often advertised as growth hormone releasers.

More research has been conducted with arginine than with ornithine or lysine. Oral ingestion of 5 to 9 g of arginine at rest results in a dose-dependent increase in growth hormone. A higher dose of 13 g causes considerable gastrointestinal distress without further increasing growth hormone concentration (100). Ingesting arginine alone increases resting growth hormone level at least 100%. By comparison, exercise increases growth hormone level by 300% to 500% (101). Ingesting arginine before exercise, however, *decreases* the growth hormone response to exercise to approximately 200% (99,101).

Because consuming arginine attenuates the effect of exercise on growth hormone concentration, athletes should not take arginine supplements before exercise. Although studies have found that arginine is capable of stimulating growth hormone release, there is no evidence that such supplements independently increase muscle mass or strength.

Bottom line: Growth hormone releasers are safe at recommended doses and effective for stimulating growth hormone release. If taken before exercise, these supplements decrease the effectiveness of exercise as a stimulator of growth hormone release; they are not effective for increasing muscle mass or strength.

HMB

Beta-hydroxy-beta-methylbutyrate (HMB) is a metabolite of the amino acid leucine. This branched-chain amino acid has some anticatabolic properties. Therefore, HMB is promoted to enhance lean body mass and to increase strength gains. Taken as a supplement, HMB theoretically minimizes the protein breakdown caused by intense exercise, but the mechanism by which it works is unknown (102).

Over the years, the results of individual research studies have been mixed. A 2009 meta-analysis (103) analyzed the effects of HMB supplements on muscle strength, muscle damage, and body composition in trained and untrained lifters. In untrained lifters, HMB supplementation was effective for small increases in lower body and average strength and very small increases in upper-body strength. In trained lifters, any gains were very small. There were no substantial effects on body composition in either trained or untrained subjects. HMB supplementation holds the most promise for untrained individuals who begin resistance training.

More research is needed to determine the ability of HMB supplements to reduce muscle damage in response to resistance training. Although there are reports of reduced muscle damage (104), a 2009 meta-analysis was not able to draw conclusions based on the studies to date (103).

HMB supplements seem to be safe (105,106). Subjects who consumed 3 g HMB per day for 6 to 8 weeks showed no adverse effects on lipid profiles or hepatic, renal, or immune function. The recommended dosage is 3 g/d in three 1-g doses. There is no evidence that larger doses will be beneficial (106). Further research is needed to determine the long-term safety profile of HMB.

Bottom line: HMB is safe. It is not effective in resistance-trained athletes. It may contribute to a small to very small increase in overall, upper-body, and lower-body strength in untrained individuals.

L-Carnitine

See Carnitine.

Lysine

See Growth Hormone Releasers.

Medium-Chain Triglycerides

Medium-chain triglycerides (MCT) contain fatty acids with 6 to 10 carbon atoms. MCT are quickly emptied from the stomach, rapidly absorbed via the portal vein and easily transported into the mitochondria. These features give MCT distinct advantages over long-chain triglycerides as a readily available energy source (107).

As the intensity of exercise increases, the body shifts its fuel usage from fat to carbohydrate. One of the adaptations that the body makes to endurance training is the increased ability to oxidize fat during moderate- to high-intensity exercise (107). Athletes have considered many methods to increase fat availability and oxidation in an effort to spare glycogen and prolong performance, especially in ultra-endurance events. The ingestion of supplemental MCT oil is one such method (108).

Several studies of well-trained endurance cyclists have reported that the ingestion of MCT oil does not enhance endurance performance (109–112). The MCT oil did not significantly alter fat oxidation during exercise and did not spare muscle glycogen. There seems to be no ergogenic benefit for endurance athletes. MCT is cleverly advertised to bodybuilders as "the oil for the well-tuned human machine." However, there have been no research studies of MCT use in strength athletes and no plausible theory for how such a supplement would enhance performance.

Kern et al (113) posed questions about the safety of MCT supplementation. In a 2-week study of male endurance runners, the ingestion of 30 g MCT oil twice per day resulted in altered blood lipids. Total cholesterol, low-density lipoprotein cholesterol, and triacylglycerol were increased, although none exceeded established desirable ranges. Because there seems to be no performance benefit, these increases in blood lipids further support the case for not recommending MCT supplements for athletes. When exercise intensity is increased, such as during a sprint portion of an endurance event, MCT supplementation can result in mild to severe gastrointestinal stress and diarrhea (112).

Bottom line: MCT's effect on blood lipids is unknown. It may cause some GI symptoms. It is not effective for enhancing endurance performance.

Multivitamin and Mineral Supplements

Multivitamin and mineral supplements (MVM) are among the most popular dietary supplements consumed by athletes, particularly female athletes (3). They represent an easy, convenient, and fairly inexpensive way to obtain nutrients that are lacking in the diet. Because athletes have busy schedules, they often perceive a one-a-day type multivitamin and mineral supplement to be an "insurance policy." However, a multivitamin and mineral supplement may not fill as many "gaps" as the athlete believes it will. Studies suggest that MVM tend to substantially increase the intakes of zinc and vitamins A, E, and B-6. MVM are less likely to substantially increase calcium, magnesium, and potassium intakes (114) and have relatively low amounts of vitamin D.

A comprehensive review of vitamins and minerals is found in Chapter 5. There is no scientific evidence at this time that all athletes should consume a daily multivitamin and mineral supplement. With the inclusion of energy bars, cereal, and other highly fortified products in the diet, many athletes may already be consuming the equivalent of a multivitamin and mineral supplement. However, athletes who chronically restrict energy or who are recovering from eating disorders are generally deficient in one or more nutrients. They would benefit from supplementation, as would those who are pregnant or lactating.

Fortunately, there are good tools to help determine if dietary deficiencies may be present. Computerized nutrient analysis compares self-reported intake with the current recommendations. The UL is helpful in determining if total intake from food and supplements is potentially harmful. Thorough nutrition assessment is necessary before multivitamin and mineral supplements are recommended to individual athletes. In some cases, it may be more beneficial to take a single supplement, such as iron, calcium, or vitamin D, which would provide a more appropriate dose than that found in a multivitamin and mineral supplement (114).

The routine use of multivitamin supplements by the general population for the prevention of cancer or cardiovascular disease has been controversial. There is a growing body of literature that vitamin supplementation in those who are not vitamin deficient is unlikely to prevent cancer or chronic diseases. There is also some evidence to suggest that disease risk may be increased in some people who use MVM supplements (115–117).

Bottom line: Multivitamin/mineral supplements are considered safe, although there is potential to consume high doses. They are effective to increase nutrient intake to some degree but are not likely to improve performance (unless nutrient deficiencies were present) or to prevent chronic disease.

Nitric Oxide (NO)/Arginine Alpha-ketoglutarate (AAKG)

Nitric oxide (NO) supplements contain arginine alpha-ketoglutarate (AAKG). Arginine is a nonessential amino acid that is the substrate for the nitric oxide synthase enzyme. This enzyme catalyzes the oxidation of arginine to produce nitric oxide (a gas) and citrulline. NO is a key signaling molecule in the cardiovascular system and promotes vasodilation (118).

In theory, the nitric oxide-induced vasodilation increases blood flow and oxygen transport to the muscles and promotes an extended "muscle pump" during resistance training. The increased blood flow also enhances delivery of nutrients and removal of wastes. NO supplements are marketed as a way to produce dramatic increases in muscle size and strength.

Few studies have evaluated the safety and efficacy of supplements containing arginine alpha-ketoglutarate in resistance-trained adult men (119,120). Campbell and colleagues (121) found that AAKG supplementation (12 g/d for 8 weeks) significantly increased one-repetition max bench press, Wingate peak power performance, and plasma arginine levels, but had no effect on body composition, total body water, isokinetic quadriceps muscle endurance, or aerobic capacity.

Little and associates (122) compared the effect of 10 days of supplementation with creatine (0.1 g/kg/d or 8 g/d) alone or creatine plus AAKG (0.075 g/kg/d or 6 g/d) on exercise performance and body composition. Bench-press repetitions over three sets significantly increased with creatine plus AAKG and creatine alone compared to placebo. Peak power significantly increased with creatine plus AAKG compared with no changes in creatine alone or placebo. Thus, creatine alone and in combination with AAKG improved upper-body muscle endurance and creatine plus AAKG improved peak power output on repeated Wingate tests.

In patients with atherosclerosis, the blood vessel endothelium has a reduced capacity to produce nitric oxide and dilate effectively. However, healthy people do not have reduced nitric oxide production or impaired endothelial vasodilation. There is no evidence that AAKG supplements increase nitric oxide levels or blood flow to the muscles of healthy people (118).

Arginine alpha-ketoglutarate appears to be safe in doses up to 12 g/d for short-term use (1 to 8 weeks). High doses can cause gastrointestinal distress and diarrhea (123). There are case reports of palpitations, dizziness, syncope, vomiting, and headache associated with the use of AAKG supplements (124).

On the basis of two studies, AAKG (eg, nitric oxide supplements) *may* increase muscle strength but not muscle size. Further research on AAKG is warranted before AAKG can be considered a safe and effective sports supplement for increasing muscle strength.

Bottom line: The safety and effectiveness of NO/AAKG are questionable due to limited research; preliminary results suggest AAKG *may* increase muscle strength but not muscle size.

Omega-3 (n-3) Fatty Acid Supplements

n-3 fatty acid (fish oil) supplements are marketed to athletes as a way to reduce inflammation, reduce the effects of oxidative stress, and counteract the negative effects of strenuous exercise on the immune system. Typically, n-3 fatty acid supplements contain eicosapentaenoic acid (EPA) and docosahexaenoic acid (DHA), with the greatest proportion being EPA. The amounts used in research studies are generally more than 2.4 g of n-3 fatty acids per day, with various mixtures of EPA, DHA, and, sometimes, alpha-linolenic acid (ALA).

In studies of trained athletes, n-3 fatty acid supplements do not seem to positively affect inflammation or immune responses or improve performance (125–128). There is emerging evidence that n-3 fatty acid supplements containing EPA and DHA may have a protective effect for athletes who have exercise-induced bronchoconstriction due to asthma (129). Malaguti et al (130) found damage to red blood cell membranes in the study group that received 3 g of fish oil supplements daily, suggesting that excessive amounts may negatively affect some of the mechanisms the body has to counteract oxidative stress.

A common recommendation for athletes is 1 to 2 g of n-3 fatty acids daily. Recommendations for higher dosages for trained athletes, particularly endurance athletes, have been made (131); however, there is a lack of evidence to support such recommendations and there are concerns about high-dose supplementation with n-3 fatty acids. The FDA recommends that consumers not exceed a daily total of 3 g EPA and DHA from all sources, with no more than 2 g/d from a dietary supplement (http://www.fda.gov). No DRI has been established.

Bottom line: n-3 fatty acid supplements are promising for use in athletes with exercise-induced bronchoconstriction due to asthma. They are not effective to reduce inflammation, enhance the immune system, or improve performance. The FDA recommends that intake of EPA and DHA not exceed 3 g/d with no more than 2 g/d from supplement sources.

Ornithine

See Growth Hormone Releasers.

Protein Supplements

To promote muscle growth athletes must consume adequate calories, adequate protein, and engage in resistance training. In general, athletes in training need between 1.2 and 1.7 g protein/kg body weight/d, assuming that caloric intake is adequate (132). Many athletes report intakes more than the top end of the range (133,134). Surveys suggest that bodybuilders and other muscle strength/size-focused athletes consume more than 2 g protein per kg daily. Bodybuilders sometimes report intakes as high as 2.5 to 3.5 g/kg/d.

Many factors contribute to protein needs, including overall energy intake, carbohydrate availability, protein quality, exercise intensity, duration, and time, training status, sex, age, and timing of intake (133,134). Once protein needs are met, the overall energy content of the diet affects body composition more than any other variable (135). Each athlete should be individually assessed to determine estimated protein need. Most male strength athletes, with the exception of those who have weight class restrictions (eg, wrestlers) consume adequate protein from food. Thus, the protein needs of athletes can be achieved without supplementation (133). However, some athletes believe protein supplements are necessary, particularly when they are adolescents or college freshman (136). Athletes may find that protein supplements are more convenient and portable than eating food proteins. Goals and motivations should be considered when translating daily protein intake into actual foods and/or supplements.

Protein supplements are often advertised as an effective way to increase muscle mass and strength. A meta-analysis that evaluated all trials between 1967 and 2001 relating to protein supplementation with resistance training for 2 or more days per week for 3 weeks showed no change in lean weight gain or strength (69). However, since that time some studies have shown that protein supplementation in combination with resistance training significantly increased lean tissue mass over placebo (135,137). Such results have led to more research about the type and timing of protein from both food and supplements. Protein foods and supplements contain a variety of proteins, including whey, casein, and soy. Whey has always been a popular source because of its high biological value (equivalent to egg protein). Whey and casein are milk proteins. Whey is the liquid portion of coagulated milk, whereas casein is found in the curds (semisolid portion). During processing of protein supplements, the whey proteins are concentrated and the fat and lactose are removed. Whey protein isolate is lactose-free whereas whey powder and whey protein concentrate can contain substantial amounts of lactose (138). These differences also affect the cost of the supplement.

Because whey has greater solubility than casein, the amino acids found in whey enter the bloodstream faster. Studies have shown that whey protein supplements, with or without creatine, promote skeletal muscle gains (139–141). Cribb and colleagues (139) evaluated the effect of supplementation with whey or casein (1.5 g/kg/d) during 10 weeks of resistance training. Whey supplementation promoted greater gains in lean mass, greater decreases in fat mass, and greater improvements in strength (even when expressed relative to body weight). Candow and associates (140) found that whey and soy protein (1.2 g/kg/d) equally increased muscle mass and strength compared to an isocaloric placebo during 6 weeks of resistance training. Although not all subjects experienced the same gains, such research suggests that whey protein may be superior to other proteins for increasing muscle size and strength (142). Evidence suggests consumption of whey protein or dairy-based protein to promote muscle protein synthesis, net muscle protein accretion, and ultimately hypertrophy. There is also evidence that whey is better than casein and soy protein (143).

Timing is another protein issue that is being investigated. Consuming some protein after resistance exercise promotes muscle growth (141,144–146). Tipton and colleagues (141) found that despite different patterns of blood amino acid responses, acute ingestion of both whey and casein after exercise resulted in similar increases in muscle protein synthesis. This has led to recommendations about protein timing with protein supplements or foods with a similar amino acid profile such as milk or low-fat chocolate milk. From a physiological perspective, there is an advantage during the recovery period to having elevated blood levels of glucose (hyperglycemia), amino acids (hyperaminoacidemia), and insulin (hyperinsulinemia) (146,147).

Protein supplements seem to be safe for athletes without latent or known kidney or liver disease. It does not seem that excessive protein intake by athletes harm healthy kidneys (134,145). Those who consume high levels of protein should monitor their health and follow up with a physician if problems occur. From a practical perspective, daily protein intakes exceeding 2.5 g per kg body weight put athletes at risk for dehydration, low carbohydrate intake, excessive energy intake, and increased excretion of urinary calcium. Athletes should consider protein intake, both from food and supplementation, in the context of their total energy, macronutrient, and fluid needs. For healthy athletes, protein supplements are generally considered safe and can be part of their overall plan for an appropriately timed, adequate daily consumption of protein (145).

Bottom line: Protein supplements are safe and can be an effective source of protein (as are food proteins) for increasing muscle size and strength when part of proper caloric and protein intake in the presence of resistance training. Whey protein may be more effective than casein for increasing muscle size and strength.

Pyruvate and Dihydroxyacetone

Pyruvate is the end product of glycolysis, a cellular energy process that takes place outside of the mitochondria. Once transported into the mitochondria, pyruvate can be converted to acetyl-CoA. Dihydroxyacetone

(DHA) is also produced during glycolysis. Both are 3-carbon compounds; thus, they are referred to as trioses, but pyruvate is the more popular and better-known supplement. Pyruvate supplements are probably safe for adults, although minor side effects, such as gas or diarrhea, have been reported (148).

It has been suggested that pyruvate supplements can increase aerobic endurance and decrease body fat. Bodybuilders in particular have been interested in the fat-reducing effects. Pyruvate is often advertised as a weight-loss aid to both athletes and sedentary individuals. Although studies in the early 1990s were promising, those promises have not been realized with more recent studies.

In 1990 Stanko et al (149,150) published two studies suggesting that endurance capacity could be enhanced with pyruvate and DHA supplementation. The studies were conducted in untrained males, so their application to athletes was immediately questioned. High levels of pyruvate (> 20 g/d) were used and there were adverse gastrointestinal effects, such as gas and nausea, from the high doses. This raised further questions about the feasibility of pyruvate supplementation.

A 2000 study (151) cast doubt on previous research results, which had not been replicated by the original researchers or others. This study found that aerobic performance was not improved in trained, recreational athletes. In fact, blood pyruvate concentrations were not increased even with 7 g supplemental pyruvate. All subjects complained of increased gastrointestinal effects as the dose was increased, and some subjects could not complete the study because of these adverse effects. There is no evidence that pyruvate supplements are an effective ergogenic aid.

Pyruvate supplementation is also linked to weight-loss claims. Animal studies suggested a possible mechanism. The results of two studies by Stanko et al (152,153) are widely cited as evidence that pyruvate supplements reduce body weight and body fat in humans. These studies were conducted in morbidly obese inactive women in a metabolic ward, and energy intake was restricted to 500 or 1,000 kcal/d. Additionally, study doses of pyruvate were more than 20 g/d. Although there were small but statistically significant weight and fat losses in these subjects when living in a metabolic ward, the conditions under which the studies were conducted limit any application of the results to active, free-living people.

Pyruvate is expensive to produce and most supplements contain approximately 1 g per tablet. The usual dose sold is unlikely to increase blood pyruvate levels. Even at the more than 20-g levels used in research studies, there is no evidence to suggest that pyruvate supplements will improve performance or result in weight or fat loss in athletes or other active people.

Bottom line: Pyruvate and DHA are safe, but may have some unacceptable side effects. They are not effective to improve performance or weight loss.

Quercetin

Phytochemicals are compounds that have biological activity. There are thousands of phytochemicals in foods, including a group known as flavonoids. Some flavonoids are associated with the prevention of cardiovascular disease or cancer because of their antioxidant and anti-inflammatory properties. Quercetin is a flavonoid that has received attention and study because it is a powerful antioxidant, five times more potent than vitamin C (154,155).

Quercetin supplementation has become popular with athletes for its potential antioxidant and anti-inflammatory effects and the promise of improved performance. A 2011 meta-analysis of 11 studies found quercetin supplementation of 1,000 mg/d had a significant positive effect on endurance capacity (VO_{2max}) and endurance performance. The effect was approximately a 3% improvement, which the authors described as between trivial and small (156). Quercetin, like caffeine, may have a stimulant effect due to its ability to block adenosine receptors in the brain. It may also reduce skeletal muscle fatigue by decreasing free radical (reactive oxygen species) production (157).

There is some evidence that supplementation can help to counter inflammation in well-trained athletes. In a study of trained cyclists, 1,000 mg/d of quercetin for 2 weeks was an effective anti-inflammatory agent after 3 days of heavy training (158). Other studies of cyclists have not found a similar effect (159). In ultra-endurance runners, quercetin supplementation (3 weeks of 1,000 mg/d) did not reduce perceived exertion during a 160-km (100-mile) run or prevent oxidative damage (160,161).

At the present time, it seems that Quercetin supplementation may improve endurance performance to a small degree or reduce oxidative damage in trained athletes. It may have an anti-inflammatory effect, although more study is needed. The usual study dose, 1,000 mg/d, seems to be safe.

Bottom line: Quercetin is safe. It is effective for improving endurance performance to a small degree or preventing oxidative damage in trained athletes. It may have some anti-inflammatory effects.

Ribose

Ribose is a 5-carbon sugar formed from glucose via the pentose phosphate pathway. Most sugars found in food, such as glucose and fructose, are 6-carbon sugars. Thus, little ribose is obtained from dietary sources, but cells can easily synthesize ribose, which is needed for ATP synthesis. The theoretical question posed is whether ribose supplementation could increase ATP production or enhance ATP recovery and improve high-intensity exercise performance.

Studies have not been able to demonstrate that ribose supplementation (5 g/d for 5 days) positively affects anaerobic capacity, enhances ATP restoration, or alters the body's metabolic response to exercise. Such supplements, although they seem to be safe, are not effective in improving high-intensity exercise performance (162,163).

Bottom line: Ribose is safe but not effective.

Vanadium (Vanadyl Sulfate)

Vanadium is a trace element that is essential for animals and may be essential for humans, although the latter has not yet been established. Daily dietary intake is approximately 10 to 30 mcg, with a total body pool of approximately 100 to 200 mcg. Supplemental vanadium is usually sold as vanadyl sulfate or a similar compound because of enhanced bioavailability (164). The UL has been established at 1.8 mg for adults (50).

Early studies in rats and in humans with type 2 diabetes have shown that supplemental vanadyl sulfate has insulin-mimetic properties. Effects include increased hepatic and muscle insulin sensitivity, augmented glucose uptake, and a stimulation of glycogen synthesis (165). These properties, all of which could be beneficial to athletes, have resulted in increased popularity of this supplement among active people. However, the effects demonstrated in studies with subjects with type 2 diabetes have not been replicated in humans without diabetes (164). At this time, vanadium supplements are not recommended to athletes without type 2 diabetes because there is no evidence of a beneficial insulin-mimicking effect.

The evidence for the use of vanadyl sulfate with those with type 2 diabetes is weak (165,166). Studies that have reported improved insulin sensitivity and increased glucose uptake were nonrandomized trials, and randomized clinical trials are needed. It should be noted that the doses used in research studies, typically 30 to 150 mg, exceed levels that would be possible through food intake alone. Therefore, it seems that any effect of vanadium supplements is pharmacological. Athletes with diabetes should be counseled to regard the use of vanadyl supplements as a medication even though they are legally sold as dietary supplements in the United States. Use of vanadyl supplements for glycemic control in those with type 2 diabetes is not recommended at this time (165).

Bottom line: Vanadium supplements are safe at intakes below the UL; higher doses are pharmacological and should be treated as such. The supplements are not effective as performance enhancers.

Vitamin C and Vitamin E Supplements (Antioxidants)

Vitamins C and E are powerful antioxidants that work in conjunction with each other and glutathione to guard against oxidative stress. Endurance athletes are subject to great oxidative stress, which can lead to damaged cells, tissues, and organs. All humans experience cellular damage by reactive oxygen species (free radicals), substances that are generated as a result of normal metabolic processes, but these free radicals can be neutralized by antioxidants. The goal is to have the proper balance between free radical production and antioxidant protection. When free radicals, known as oxidants, outnumber antioxidants, cellular damage can occur (138,167).

Aerobic exercise increases the production of free radicals. However, a positive result of aerobic training is a buildup of the body's natural defenses against free radicals, the enzymatic and nonenzymatic antioxidants. A critical issue for athletes is whether enough antioxidants are present to interact with the increased amount of free radicals being produced. There needs to be a balance between rate of production of free radicals and rate of clearance by antioxidants. At high concentrations, antioxidant vitamins can act as pro-oxidants, so athletes need sufficient but not excessive amounts of the antioxidant vitamins (138,167,168).

Vitamin C is found in both fruits (eg, oranges, grapefruits, strawberries) and vegetables (eg, tomatoes, peppers, broccoli, cabbage). Peake (169) reports that except for those who chronically restrict energy, athletes tend to consume more dietary vitamin C than the general population and meet the DRI. All athletes are highly encouraged to consume a variety of fruits and vegetables daily and those who are restricting energy especially benefit because fruits and vegetables are nutrient-dense foods. The DRI for vitamin E can be obtained through diet alone if excellent food sources are chosen, such as vegetable oils, nuts, and seeds (170). One concern is that endurance athletes tend to follow a low-fat diet and have low vitamin E intake (171).

To address the question of whether supplemental vitamin C and E may reduce oxidative stress in athletes, Williams et al (171) reviewed the results of studies of vitamin E, C and/or beta carotene supplements in endurance athletes prior to 2005. Of the 47 trials, 20 reported that oxidative stress was decreased, 23 reported no effect, and four reported an increase in oxidative stress. These mixed results suggest that that more research is needed and that there may be a threshold above which intake is counterproductive.

Endurance athletes sometimes choose to supplement with vitamin C and E as an "insurance policy" to guard against oxidative stress. However, some recent study results raise questions about such an approach for several reasons. Studies suggest that antioxidant supplements may delay muscle recovery (119,168,172) and interfere with some of the benefits of exercise, such as less insulin resistance (120). To guard against excessive intakes, it is highly recommended that athletes consume the DRI for vitamins C and E through the consumption of food. Those who choose to supplement should consider low-dose supplements.

Vitamin C is an antioxidant, but athletes may use it as a supplement for other reasons. Recurring upper respiratory tract infections and colds are the bane of endurance athletes (strenuous endurance exercise may be immunosuppressive). The effectiveness of such supplements on the incidence and prevalence of the common cold has been well studied in the general population over the past 20 years. Vitamin C does not seem to prevent colds, but it does seem to modestly reduce the duration of a cold (173). Once the cold begins and until symptoms disappear, recommendations for supplemental vitamin C range from 250 to 1,000 mg/d, with some evidence to support the higher doses (173). Supplemental vitamin C is likely effective because of its mild antihistamine effect. This constitutes the use of vitamin C as a disease treatment and in this respect should be evaluated like an over-the-counter cold medication.

Both vitamin C and E have an established UL. The UL for vitamin C is 2,000 mg; higher doses may result in diarrhea. Vitamin E has a very low toxicity and the UL is 1,000 mg (170).

Bottom line: Vitamins C and E are safe; the effectiveness of these supplements as an antioxidant is mixed, with their effectiveness likely related to the balance of oxidants and antioxidants; excessive amounts are not beneficial and may upset the balance. Vitamin C is not effective for preventing colds, but it does decrease the duration of a cold.

Vitamin D Supplements

The vitamin D status of athletes has received more attention as the prevalence of low vitamin D intake and the use of sunscreen to block ultraviolet (UV) light exposure (a precursor to vitamin D production) has increased among people of all ages. Vitamin D plays a very important role in bone health, and evidence of its importance in exercise-related inflammation and prevention of chronic disease is accumulating. Very limited data in athletes would suggest that some athletes have a vitamin D deficiency and that more have an insufficiency. Data collection is hampered by vitamin D databases with missing values and the difficulty in assessing UV exposure (174).

Vitamin D status can be determined by measuring 25-OH D_3 (also known as 25-hydroxy vitamin D or 25-hydroxycholecalciferol) in the blood. A concentration of less than 10 to 11 ng/mL (25–27.5 nmol/L) is considered a clinical deficiency because this range is associated with rickets in children and the equivalent disease in adults, osteomalacia. A blood level of less than 10 to 15 ng/mL (25–37.5 nmol/L) is reflective of a subclinical deficiency due to its association with inadequate bone health and overall health. However, there is a controversy about the concentration that defines insufficiency. A concentration more than 15 ng/mL (37.5 nmol/L) is generally considered adequate, but some vitamin D researchers feel that an insufficiency is present unless the 25-OH D_3 concentration is more than 30 ng/mL (75 nmol/L) (http://ods.od.nih.gov/factsheets/vitamind.asp). As would be expected, adequate vitamin D may improve the performance of vitamin D–deficient athletes (175).

The DRI for vitamin D was updated in 2010 (176). The current DRI is 15 mcg (600 IU) for individuals ages 1 to 70 years, and 20 mcg (800 IU) for those older than 70 years. The UL is 100 mcg (4,000 IU). Although vitamin D toxicities can occur, they are rare.

Recommendations for athletes are speculative at this time. One recommendation is 20 to 50 mcg (800 to 2,000 IU) daily, an amount unlikely to be obtained from food alone (174). Safe UV sun exposure, which is defined as 5 to 30 minutes between 10 AM and 3 PM twice a week based on latitude, season of the year, and skin pigment, or vitamin D supplementation is recommended (174).

Bottom line: Vitamin D supplements are safe, but high doses can be toxic when taken for long periods of time. Vitamin D supplements are effective for improving vitamin D status in those with low or marginal intake or UV exposure.

Weight Loss Supplements

See Citrus aurantium (Bitter Orange); Ephedra (Ephedrine-Containing Supplements); Green Tea Extract.

Summary

Table 7.1 summarizes the safety and effectiveness of the dietary supplements discussed in this chapter. Because the body of scientific literature is always changing, practitioners must continually update their

TABLE 7.1   Safety and Effectiveness of Selected Dietary Supplements and Ergogenic Aids

Supplement	Safety (at Recommended Doses)	Effectiveness
Androstenedione [Banned substance]	Not safe.	Not effective.
Beet juice	Concerns about the safety of excess nitrate consumption.	Early studies show promise as a way to increase skeletal muscle efficiency due to lower oxygen demand.
Beta-alanine	Seems to be safe.	Shows promise as an effective buffer of muscle pH.
Branched-chain amino acid (BCAA)	Seems to be safe.	Not effective for improving performance; some promising studies related to immune system support and reduction of postexercise fatigue.
Caffeine [Banned substance at a certain threshold but not likely to be reached by athletes due to side effects that are detrimental to performance.]	Seems to be safe.	Effective as a central nervous system stimulant; effective for improving endurance performance and high-intensity activities lasting up to 20 minutes.
Carnitine	Seems to be safe.	Not effective.
Chromium (chromium picolinate)	Low doses seem to be safe; doses > 200 mcg or forms with high availability raise safety concerns.	Not effective for increasing muscle mass, decreasing body fat, or improving performance.
Citrus aurantium (bitter orange)	Concerns about safety.	Effective as a central nervous system stimulant.
Conjugated linoleic acid (CLA)	Safety in humans not established.	Effectiveness is unknown because study results are mixed.
Creatine	Seems to be safe.	Effective for increasing lean body mass in athletes performing repeated high-intensity, short-duration (< 30 seconds) exercise bouts. Performance benefit in weightlifters.
Dehydroepiandrosterone (DHEA)	Not safe.	Not effective.
Ephedrine [Banned substance in many sports; banned by the International Olympic Committee at a certain threshold, which can be reached with multiple doses.]	Safety concerns hotly debated. Doses > 10 mg banned by the FDA due to significant safety risks. Narrower safety profile than most dietary supplements.	Effective as a central nervous system stimulant. With caffeine, effective for short-term, 8- to 9-lb weight loss in obese people. Not effective for improving muscle strength or anaerobic performance.
Glucosamine/Chondroitin sulfate	Seems to be safe.	Generally not effective for reducing joint pain or increasing functionality in those with osteoarthritis, although individual responses vary.
Glutamine	Seems to be safe.	Not effective.
Green tea extract	Use with caution (some reports of liver toxicity).	Effective for small loss of body weight.

continues

TABLE 7.1   Safety and Effectiveness of Selected Dietary Supplements and Ergogenic Aids (continued)

Supplement	Safety (at Recommended Doses)	Effectiveness
Growth hormone releasers (arginine)	Seems to be safe.	Effective for stimulating growth hormone release. If taken before exercise, decreases the effectiveness of exercise as a stimulator of growth hormone. Not effective for increasing muscle mass or strength.
Beta-hydroxy-beta-methylbutyrate (HMB)	Seems to be safe.	Not effective in resistance-trained athletes. Small to very small increases in overall, upper-body, and lower-body strength in untrained individuals.
Medium-chain triglycerides (MCT)	Seems to be safe but unknown effect on blood lipids.	Not effective.
Multivitamin and mineral supplements	Seems to be safe, although there is potential to consume high doses.	Effective to increase nutrient intake to a degree, which can help to reverse nutrient deficiencies. Not likely to improve performance or prevent chronic disease in those without nutrient deficiencies.
Nitric oxide (NO)/Arginine alpha-ketoglutarate (AAKG)	Safety in humans not established.	Effectiveness unknown due to lack of research. Preliminary results suggest it may increase muscle strength but not muscle size.
n-3 fatty acid supplements	FDA recommends intake of EPA and DHA not exceed 3 g/d with no more than 2 g/d from supplement sources.	Promising for use in athletes with exercise-induced bronchoconstriction due to asthma; not effective to reduce inflammation, enhance the immune system, or improve performance.
Protein	Seems safe for those without latent or known kidney or liver disease.	Effective source of protein (as are food proteins). Whey protein may be more effective than casein for increasing muscle size and strength.
Pyruvate	Seems to be safe.	Not effective.
Quercetin	Seems to be safe.	In trained athletes, effective for improving endurance performance to a small degree or preventing oxidative damage; may have some anti-inflammatory effects.
Ribose	Seems to be safe.	Not effective.
Vanadium (vanadyl sulfate)	Seems to be safe.	Not effective.
Vitamin C and/or E supplements	Seems to be safe.	Effectiveness as an antioxidant likely depends on the balance of oxidants and antioxidants. Excessive amounts are not beneficial and may upset the balance. Vitamin C not effective for preventing colds, but effective for decreasing the duration of a cold.
Vitamin D	Seems to be safe, although can be toxic when consumed in high doses.	Effective for improving vitamin D status in those with low or marginal intake or ultraviolet exposure.

knowledge. Supplements that show promise based on early human studies or those with mixed results require that practitioners pay attention to new developments. For some of the supplements that show promise, more studies may mean that effectiveness in trained athletes is confirmed. For other promising supplements, the opposite will be true.

Even with the large number of questionable supplements flooding the market, it is important to consider the possibility of an athlete benefiting from a particular supplement. The placebo effect cannot be overlooked. Athletes will always be looking for a competitive edge and it is likely that use of ergogenic aids and dietary supplements will remain high. There are some supplements that are safe but not effective. There also may be some supplements that are effective but not safe, and these pose serious risk-benefit questions that ultimately can only be answered by the athlete. For those select few dietary supplements determined to be safe and effective, it still remains crucial that the practitioner assesses the individual athlete's needs and goals, and educate accordingly.

References

1. Tscholl P, Alonso JM, Dollé G, Junge A, Dvorak J. The use of drugs and nutritional supplements in top-level track and field athletes. *Am J Sports Med.* 2010;38:133–140.
2. Schroder H, Navarro E, Mora J, Seco J, Torregrosa JM, Tramullas A. The type, amount, frequency and timing of dietary supplement use by elite players in the first Spanish basketball league. *J Sports Sci.* 2002;20:353–358.
3. Froiland K, Koszewski W, Hingst J, Kopecky L. Nutritional supplement use among college athletes and their sources of information. *Int J Sport Nutr Exerc Metab.* 2004;14:104–120. Erratum in: *Int J Sport Nutr Exerc Metab.* 2004;14:606.
4. Hoffman JR, Faigenbaum AD, Ratamess NA, Ross R, Kang J, Tenenbaum G. Nutritional supplementation and anabolic steroid use in adolescents. *Med Sci Sports Exerc.* 2008;40:15–24.
5. Calfee R, Fadale P. Popular ergogenic drugs and supplements in young athletes. *Pediatrics.* 2006;117:e577–e589.
6. Food and Drug Administration. 1994 Dietary Supplement Health and Education Act (DSHEA). http://www.fda.gov/Food/DietarySupplements/default.html. Accessed January 4, 2009.
7. van Breemen RB, Fong HH, Farnsworth NR. Ensuring the safety of botanical dietary supplements. *Am J Clin Nutr.* 2008;87(suppl):509S–513S.
8. Maughan R. Contamination of dietary supplements and positive drug tests in sport. *J Sports Sci.* 2005;23:883–889.
9. Gurley BJ, Gardner SF, Hubbard MA. Content versus label claims in ephedra-containing dietary supplements. *Am J Health Syst Pharm.* 2000;57:963–969.
10. Geyer H, Parr MK, Mareck U, Reinhart U, Schrader Y, Schänzer W. Analysis of non-hormonal nutritional supplements for anabolic-androgenic steroids: results of an international study. *Int J Sports Med.* 2004;25:124–129.
11. Judkins C, Hall D, Hoffman K. Investigation into supplement contamination levels in the US market. HFL. 2007. http://www.usatoday.com/sports/hfl-supplement-research-report.pdf. Accessed March 9, 2010.
12. Baume N, Mahler N, Kamber M, Mangin P, Saugy M. Research of stimulants and anabolic steroids in dietary supplements. *Scand J Med Sci Sports.* 2006;16:41–48.
13. Martello S, Felli M, Chiarotti M. Survey of nutritional supplements for selected illegal anabolic steroids and ephedrine using LC-MS/MS and GC-MS methods, respectively. *Food Addit Contam.* 2007;24:258–265.
14. Food and Drug Administration. FDA issues dietary supplements final rule. June 22, 2007. www.fda.gov/NewsEvents/Newsroom/PressAnnouncements/2007/ucm108938.htm. Accessed March 9, 2010.
15. Brown WJ, Basil MD, Bocarnea MC. The influence of famous athletes on health beliefs and practices: Mark McGwire, child abuse prevention, and androstenedione. *J Health Commun.* 2003;8:41–57.
16. Tipton KD, Ferrando AA. Improving muscle mass: response of muscle metabolism to exercise, nutrition and anabolic agents. *Essays Biochem.* 2008;44:85–98.

17. Brown GA, Vukovich M, King DS. Testosterone prohormone supplements. *Med Sci Sports Exerc*. 2006;38: 1451–1461.

18. Food and Drug Administration. FDA White Paper: health effects of androstenedione. Released March 11, 2004. http://www.fda.gov/oc/whitepapers/andro.html. Accessed March 9, 2010.

19. Bailey SJ, Fulford J, Vanhatalo A, Winyard PG, Blackwell JR, DiMenna FJ, Wilkerson DP, Benjamin N, Jones AM. Dietary nitrate supplementation enhances muscle contractile efficiency during knee-extensor exercise in humans. *J Appl Physiol*. 2010;109:135–148.

20. Larsen FJ, Weitzberg E, Lundberg JO, Ekblom B. Effects of dietary nitrate on oxygen cost during exercise. *Acta Physiol (Oxf)*. 2007;191:59–66.

21. Bailey SJ, Winyard P, Vanhatalo A, Blackwell JR, Dimenna FJ, Wilkerson DP, Tarr J, Benjamin N, Jones AM. Dietary nitrate supplementation reduces the O2 cost of low-intensity exercise and enhances tolerance to high-intensity exercise in humans. *J Appl Physiol*. 2009;107:1144–1155.

22. Lansley KE, Winyard PG, Fulford J, Vanhatalo A, Bailey SJ, Blackwell JR, DiMenna FJ, Gilchrist M, Benjamin N, Jones AM. Dietary nitrate supplementation reduces the O2 cost of walking and running: a placebo-controlled study. *J Appl Physiol*. 2011;110:591–600.

23. Lansley KE, Winyard PG, Bailey SJ, Vanhatalo A, Wilkerson DP, Blackwell JR, Gilchrist M, Benjamin N, Jones AM. Acute dietary nitrate supplementation improves cycling time trial performance. *Med Sci Sports Exerc*. 2011; 43:1125–1131.

24. Derave W, Taes Y. Beware of the pickle: health effects of nitrate intake. *J Appl Physiol*. 2009;107:1677; author reply 1678.

25. Artioli GG, Gualano B, Smith A, Stout J, Lancha HA Jr. The role of beta-alanine supplementation on muscle carnosine and exercise performance. *Med Sci Sports Exerc*. 2010;42:1162–1173.

26. Stout JR, Cramer JT, Zoeller RF, Torok D, Costa P, Hoffman JR, Harris RC, O'Kroy J. Effects of beta-alanine supplementation on the onset of neuromuscular fatigue and ventilatory threshold in women. *Amino Acids*. 2007; 32:381–386.

27. Harris RC, Tallon MJ, Dunnett M, Boobis L, Coakley J, Kim HJ, Fallowfield JL, Hill CA, Sale C, Wise JA. The absorption of orally supplied beta-alanine and its effect on muscle carnosine synthesis in human vastus lateralis. *Amino Acids*. 2006;30:279–289.

28. Hill CA, Harris RC, Kim HJ, Harris BD, Sale C, Boobis LH, Kim CK, Wise JA. Influence of beta-alanine supplementation on skeletal muscle carnosine concentrations and high intensity cycling capacity. *Amino Acids*. 2007;32:225–233.

29. Sweeney KM, Wright GA, Brice GA, Doberstein ST. The effect of beta-alanine supplementation on power performance during repeated sprint activity. *J Strength Cond Res*. 2010;24:79–87.

30. Van Thienen R, Van Proeyen K, Vanden Eynde B, Puype J, Lefere T, Hespel P. Beta-alanine improves sprint performance in endurance cycling. *Med Sci Sports Exerc*. 2009;41:898–903.

31. Negro M, Giardina S, Marzani B, Marzatico F. Branched-chain amino acid supplementation does not enhance athletic performance but affects muscle recovery and the immune system. *J Sports Med Phys Fitness*. 2008;48: 347–351.

32. Shimomura Y, Yamamoto Y, Bajotto G, Sato J, Murakami T, Shimomura N, Kobayashi H, Mawatari K. Nutraceutical effects of branched-chain amino acids on skeletal muscle. *J Nutr*. 2006;136(suppl):529S–532S.

33. Jackman SR, Witard OC, Jeukendrup AE, Tipton KD. Branched-chain amino acid ingestion can ameliorate soreness from eccentric exercise. *Med Sci Sports Exerc*. 2010;42:962–970.

34. Greer BK, Woodard JL, White JP, Arguello EM, Haymes EM. Branched-chain amino acid supplementation and indicators of muscle damage after endurance exercise. *Int J Sport Nutr Exerc Metab*. 2007;17:595–607.

35. Burke LM. Caffeine and sports performance. *Appl Physiol Nutr Metab*. 2008;33:1319–1334.

36. Davis JK, Green JM. Caffeine and anaerobic performance: ergogenic value and mechanisms of action. *Sports Med*. 2009;39:813–832.

37. Ganio MS, Klau JF, Casa DJ, Armstrong LE, Maresh CM. Effect of caffeine on sport-specific endurance performance: a systematic review. *J Strength Cond Res*. 2009;23:315–324.

38. Tarnopolsky MA. Effect of caffeine on the neuromuscular system—potential as an ergogenic aid. *Appl Physiol Nutr Metab.* 2008;33:1284–1289.

39. Armstrong LE. Caffeine, body fluid-electrolyte balance, and exercise performance. *Int J Sport Nutr Exerc Metab.* 2002;12:189–206.

40. Reissig CJ, Strain EC, Griffiths RR. Caffeinated energy drinks—a growing problem. *Drug Alcohol Depend.* 2009; 99:1–10.

41. Muller DM, Seim H, Kiess W, Loster H, Richter T. Effects of oral L-carnitine supplementation on in vivo long-chain fatty acid oxidation in healthy adults. *Metabolism.* 2002;51:1389–1391.

42. Brass EP. Carnitine and sports medicine: use or abuse? *Ann N Y Acad Sci.* 2004;1033:67–78.

43. Kraemer WJ, Volek JS, Dunn-Lewis C. L-carnitine supplementation: influence upon physiological function. *Curr Sports Med Rep.* 2008;7:218–223.

44. Broad EM, Maughan RJ, Galloway SD. Carbohydrate, protein, and fat metabolism during exercise after oral carnitine supplementation in humans. *Int J Sport Nutr Exerc Metab.* 2008;18:567–584.

45. Broad EM, Maughan RJ, Galloway SD. Effects of four weeks L-carnitine L-tartrate ingestion on substrate utilization during prolonged exercise. *Int J Sport Nutr Exerc Metab.* 2005;15:665–679.

46. Kraemer WJ, Spiering BA, Volek JS, Ratamess NA, Sharman MJ, Rubin MR, French DN, Silvestre R, Hatfield DL, Van Heest JL, Vingren JL, Judelson DA, Deschenes MR, Maresh CM. Androgenic responses to resistance exercise: effects of feeding and L-carnitine. *Med Sci Sports Exerc.* 2006;38:1288–1296. Erratum in: *Med Sci Sports Exerc.* 2006;38:1861.

47. Rubin MR, Volek JS, Gomez AL, Ratamess NA, French DN, Sharman MJ, Kraemer WJ. Safety measures of L-carnitine L-tartrate supplementation in healthy men. *J Strength Cond Res.* 2001;15:486–490.

48. Speich M, Pineau A, Ballereau F. Minerals, trace elements and related biological variables in athletes and during physical activity. *Clin Chim Acta.* 2001;312:1–11.

49. Volpe SL. Minerals as ergogenic aids. *Curr Sports Med Rep.* 2008;7:224–229.

50. Institute of Medicine. *Dietary Reference Intakes for Vitamin A, Vitamin K, Arsenic, Boron, Chromium, Copper, Iodine, Iron, Manganese, Molybdenum, Nickel, Silicon, Vanadium, and Zinc.* Washington, DC: National Academies Press; 2001.

51. Vincent J. The biochemistry of chromium. *J Nutr.* 2000;130:715–718.

52. Vincent JB. The potential value and toxicity of chromium picolinate as a nutritional supplement, weight loss agent and muscle development agent. *Sports Med.* 2003;33:213–230.

53. Lukaski HC. Magnesium, zinc, and chromium nutriture and physical activity. *Am J Clin Nutr.* 2000;72(2 Suppl):585S–593S.

54. Campbell WW, Joseph LJ, Anderson RA, Davey SL, Hinton J, Evans WJ. Effects of resistive training and chromium picolinate on body composition and skeletal muscle size in older women. *Int J Sport Nutr Exerc Metab.* 2002;12:125–135.

55. Pittler MH, Stevinson C, Ernst E. Chromium picolinate for reducing body weight: meta-analysis of randomized trials. *Int J Obes Relat Metab Disord.* 2003;27:522–529.

56. Lukaski HC, Siders WA, Penland JG. Chromium picolinate supplementation in women: effects on body weight, composition, and iron status. *Nutrition.* 2007;23:187–195.

57. Volek JS, Silvestre R, Kirwan JP, Sharman MJ, Judelson DA, Spiering BA, Vingren JL, Maresh CM, Vanheest JL, Kraemer WJ. Effects of chromium supplementation on glycogen synthesis after high-intensity exercise. *Med Sci Sports Exerc.* 2006;38:2102–2109.

58. Balk EM, Tatsioni A, Lichtenstein AH, Lau J, Pittas AG. Effect of chromium supplementation on glucose metabolism and lipids: a systematic review of randomized controlled trials. *Diabetes Care.* 2007;30:2154–2163.

59. Haller CA, Duan M, Jacob P 3rd, Benowitz N. Human pharmacology of a performance-enhancing dietary supplement under resting and exercise conditions. *Br J Clin Pharmacol.* 2008;65:833–840.

60. Fugh-Berman A, Myers A. Citrus aurantium, an ingredient of dietary supplements marketed for weight loss: current status of clinical and basic research. *Exp Biol Med.* 2004;229:698–704.

61. Greenway F, de Jonge-Levitan L, Martin C, Roberts A, Grundy I, Parker C. Dietary herbal supplements with phenylephrine for weight loss. *J Med Food.* 2006;9:572–578.

62. Haaz S, Fontaine KR, Cutter G, Limdi N, Perumean-Chaney S, Allison DB. Citrus aurantium and synephrine alkaloids in the treatment of overweight and obesity: an update. *Obes Rev.* 2006;7:79–88.

63. Wang Y, Jones PJ. Dietary conjugated linoleic acid and body composition. *Am J Clin Nutr.* 2004;79(6 Suppl):1153S–1158S.

64. Tricon S, Yaqoob P. Conjugated linoleic acid and human health: a critical evaluation of the evidence. *Curr Opin Clin Nutr Metab Care.* 2006;9:105–110.

65. Campbell B, Kreider RB. Conjugated linoleic acids. *Curr Sports Med Rep.* 2008;7:237–241.

66. Kreider RB. Effects of creatine supplementation on performance and training adaptations. *Mol Cell Biochem.* 2003;244:89–94.

67. Volek JS, Rawson ES. Scientific basis and practical aspects of creatine supplementation for athletes. *Nutrition.* 2004;20:609–614.

68. Branch JD. Effect of creatine supplementation on body composition and performance: a meta-analysis. *Int J Sport Nutr Exerc Metab.* 2003;13:198–226.

69. Nissen SL, Sharp RL. Effect of dietary supplements on lean mass and strength gains with resistance exercise: a meta-analysis. *J Appl Physiol.* 2003;94:651–659.

70. Bemben MG, Lamont HS. Creatine supplementation and exercise performance: recent findings. *Sports Med.* 2005;35:107–125.

71. Tipton KD, Ferrando AA. Improving muscle mass: response of muscle metabolism to exercise, nutrition and anabolic agents. *Essays Biochem.* 2008;44:85–98.

72. Lopez RM, Casa DJ, McDermott BP, Ganio MS, Armstrong LE, Maresh CM. Does creatine supplementation hinder exercise heat tolerance or hydration status? A systematic review with meta-analyses. *J Athl Train.* 2009;44:215–223.

73. Watt KK, Garnham AP, Snow RJ. Skeletal muscle total creatine content and creatine transporter gene expression in vegetarians prior to and following creatine supplementation. *Int J Sport Nutr Exerc Metab.* 2004;14:517–531.

74. Brown GA, Vukovich M, King DS. Testosterone prohormone supplements. *Med Sci Sports Exerc.* 2006;38:1451–1461.

75. Kritz-Silverstein D, von Mühlen D, Laughlin GA, Bettencourt R. Effects of dehydroepiandrosterone supplementation on cognitive function and quality of life: the DHEA and Well-Ness (DAWN) Trial. *J Am Geriatr Soc.* 2008;56:1292–1298.

76. Food and Drug Administration. 2004. Final Rule Declaring Dietary Supplements Containing Ephedrine Alkaloids Adulterated Because They Present an Unreasonable Risk. http://www.fda.gov/oc/initiatives/ephedra/february2004/finalsummary.html. Accessed March 9, 2010.

77. Food and Drug Administration. 2000. Safety of Dietary Supplements Containing Ephedrine Alkaloids. (Transcript of a public meeting held August 8–9, 2000.) http://www.fda.gov/Food/DietarySupplements/ReportsMeetingsPresentations/ucm105925.htm. Accessed March 9, 2010.

78. CANTOX Health Services International. Safety Assessment and Determination of a Tolerable Upper Limit of Ephedra; 2000. http://www.crnusa.org. Accessed March 9, 2010.

79. Shekelle PG, Hardy ML, Morton SC, Maglione M, Mojica WA, Suttorp MJ, Rhodes SL, Jungvig L, Gagne J. Efficacy and safety of ephedra and ephedrine for weight loss and athletic performance: a meta-analysis. *JAMA.* 2003;289:1537–1545.

80. Food and Drug Administration. Evidence on the safety and effectiveness of ephedra: implications for regulation. 2003. http://www.fda.gov/ola/2003/dietarysupplements1028.html. Accessed March 9, 2010.

81. Baylis A, Cameron-Smith D, Burke LM. Inadvertent doping through supplement use by athletes: assessment and management of the risk in Australia. *Int J Sport Nutr Exerc Metab.* 2001;11:365–383.

82. Bell DG, Jacobs I, Zamecnik J. Effects of caffeine, ephedrine and their combination on time to exhaustion during high-intensity exercise. *Eur J Appl Physiol Occup Physiol.* 1998;77:427–433.

83. Bell DG, Jacobs I, McLellan TM, Zamecnik J. Reducing the dose of combined caffeine and ephedrine preserves the ergogenic effect. *Aviat Space Environ Med.* 2000;71:415–419.

84. Bell DG, Jacobs I. Combined caffeine and ephedrine ingestion improves run times of Canadian Forces Warrior Test. *Aviat Space Environ Med.* 1999;70:325–329.

85. Bell DG, Jacobs I, McLellan TM, Miyazaki M, Sabiston CM. Thermal regulation in the heat during exercise after caffeine and ephedrine ingestion. *Aviat Space Environ Med*. 1999;70:583–588.

86. Williams AD, Cribb PJ, Cooke MB, Hayes A. The effect of ephedra and caffeine on maximal strength and power in resistance-trained athletes. *J Strength Cond Res*. 2008;22:464–470.

87. Chester N, Mottram DR, Reilly T, Powell M. Elimination of ephedrines in urine following multiple dosing: the consequences for athletes, in relation to doping control. *Br J Clin Pharmacol*. 2004;57:62–67.

88. Delafuente JC. Glucosamine in the treatment of osteoarthritis. *Rheum Dis Clin North Am*. 2000;26:1–11.

89. Clegg DO, Reda DJ, Harris CL, Klein MA, O'Dell JR, Hooper MM, Bradley JD, Bingham CO, Weisman MH, Jackson CG, Lane NE, Cush JJ, Moreland LW, Schumacher HR Jr, Oddis CV, Wolfe F, Molitor JA, Yocum DE, Schnitzer TJ, Furst DE, Sawitzke AD, Shi H, Brandt KD, Moskowitz RW, Williams HJ. Glucosamine, chondroitin sulfate, and the two in combination for painful knee osteoarthritis. *N Engl J Med*. 2006;354:795–808.

90. Sawitzke AD, Shi H, Finco MF, Dunlop DD, Bingham CO 3rd, Harris CL, Singer NG, Bradley JD, Silver D, Jackson CG, Lane NE, Oddis CV, Wolfe F, Lisse J, Furst DE, Reda DJ, Moskowitz RW, Williams HJ, Clegg DO. The effect of glucosamine and/or chondroitin sulfate on the progression of knee osteoarthritis: a report from the glucosamine/chondroitin arthritis intervention trial. *Arthritis Rheum*. 2008;58:3183–3191.

91. Wandel S, Jüni P, Tendal B, Nüesch E, Villiger PM, Welton NJ, Reichenbach S, Trelle S. Effects of glucosamine, chondroitin, or placebo in patients with osteoarthritis of hip or knee: network meta-analysis. *BMJ*. 2010;341: c4675.

92. Gleeson M. Dosing and efficacy of glutamine supplementation in human exercise and sport training. *J Nutr*. 2008;138(suppl):2045S–2049S.

93. Candow DG, Chilibeck PD, Burke DG, Davison KS, Smith-Palmer T. Effect of glutamine supplementation combined with resistance training in young adults. *Eur J Appl Physiol*. 2001;86:142–149.

94. Phung OJ, Baker WL, Matthews LJ, Lanosa M, Thorne A, Coleman CI. Effect of green tea catechins with or without caffeine on anthropometric measures: a systematic review and meta-analysis. *Am J Clin Nutr*. 2010;91: 73–81.

95. Diepvens K, Westerterp KR, Westerterp-Plantenga MS. Obesity and thermogenesis related to the consumption of caffeine, ephedrine, capsaicin, and green tea. *Am J Physiol Regul Integr Comp Physiol*. 2007;292:R77–R85.

96. Molinari M, Watt KD, Kruszyna T, Nelson R, Walsh M, Huang WY, Nashan B, Peltekian K. Acute liver failure induced by green tea extracts: case report and review of the literature. *Liver Transpl*. 2006;12:1892–1895.

97. Bonkovsky HL. Hepatotoxicity associated with supplements containing Chinese green tea (Camellia sinensis). *Ann Intern Med*. 2006;144:68–71.

98. Liatsos GD, Moulakakis A, Ketikoglou I, Klonari S. Possible green tea-induced thrombotic thrombocytopenic purpura. *Am J Health Syst Pharm*. 2010;67:531–534.

99. Collier SR, Collins E, Kanaley JA. Oral arginine attenuates the growth hormone response to resistance exercise. *J Appl Physiol*. 2006;101:848–852.

100. Collier SR, Casey DP, Kanaley JA. Growth hormone responses to varying doses of oral arginine. *Growth Horm IGF Res*. 2005;15:136–139.

101. Kanaley JA. Growth hormone, arginine and exercise. *Curr Opin Clin Nutr Metab Care*. 2008;11:50–54.

102. Slater GJ, Jenkins D. Beta-hydroxy-beta-methylbutyrate (HMB) supplementation and the promotion of muscle growth and strength. *Sports Med*. 2000;30:105–116.

103. Rowlands DS, Thomson JS. Effects of beta-hydroxy-beta-methylbutyrate supplementation during resistance training on strength, body composition, and muscle damage in trained and untrained young men: a meta-analysis. *J Strength Cond Res*. 2009;23:836–846.

104. Kraemer WJ, Hatfield DL, Volek JS, Fragala MS, Vingren JL, Anderson JM, Spiering BA, Thomas GA, Ho JY, Quann EE, Izquierdo M, Häkkinen K, Maresh CM. Effects of amino acids supplement on physiological adaptations to resistance training. *Med Sci Sports Exerc*. 2009;41:1111–1121.

105. Crowe MJ, O'Connor DM, Lukins JE. The effects of beta-hydroxy-beta-methylbutyrate (HMB) and HMB/ creatine supplementation on indices of health in highly trained athletes. *Int J Sport Nutr Exerc Metab*. 2003;13: 184–197.

106. Gallagher PM, Carrithers JA, Godard MP, Schulze KE, Trappe SW. Beta-hydroxy-beta-methylbutyrate ingestion, part II: effects on hematology, hepatic and renal function. *Med Sci Sports Exerc.* 2000;32:2116–2119.

107. Horowitz JF, Klein S. Lipid metabolism during endurance exercise. *Am J Clin Nutr.* 2000;72(2 Suppl):558S–563S.

108. Hawley JA. Effect of increased fat availability on metabolism and exercise capacity. *Med Sci Sports Exerc.* 2002;34:1485–1491.

109. Jeukendrup AE, Aldred S. Fat supplementation, health, and endurance performance. *Nutrition.* 2004;20:678–688.

110. Angus DJ, Hargreaves M, Dancey J, Febbraio MA. Effect of carbohydrate or carbohydrate plus medium-chain triglyceride ingestion on cycling time trial performance. *J Appl Physiol.* 2000;88:113–119.

111. Horowitz JF, Mora-Rodriguez R, Byerley LO, Coyle EF. Preexercise medium-chain triglyceride ingestion does not alter muscle glycogen use during exercise. *J Appl Physiol.* 2000;88:219–225.

112. Goedecke JH, Clark VR, Noakes TD, Lambert EV. The effects of medium-chain triacylglycerol and carbohydrate ingestion on ultra-endurance exercise performance. *Int J Sport Nutr Exerc Metab.* 2005;15:15–27.

113. Kern M, Lagomarcino ND, Misell LM, Schuster VV. The effect of medium-chain triacylglycerols on the blood lipid profile of male endurance runners. *J Nutr Biochem.* 2000;11:288–292.

114. Marra MV, Boyar AP. Position of the American Dietetic Association: nutrient supplementation. *J Am Diet Assoc.* 2009;109:2073–2085.

115. Neuhouser ML, Wassertheil-Smoller S, Thomson C, Aragaki A, Anderson GL, Manson JE, Patterson RE, Rohan TE, van Horn L, Shikany JM, Thomas A, LaCroix A, Prentice RL. Multivitamin use and risk of cancer and cardiovascular disease in the Women's Health Initiative cohorts. *Arch Intern Med.* 2009;169:294–304.

116. NIH State-of-the-Science Conference Statement on Multivitamin/Mineral Supplements and Chronic Disease Prevention. *NIH Consens State Sci Statements.* 2006;23:1–30.

117. McCormick DB. Vitamin/mineral supplements: of questionable benefit for the general population. *Nutr Rev.* 2010;68:207–213.

118. Gornik HL, Creager MA. Arginine and endothelial and vascular health. *J Nutr.* 2004;134(suppl):2880S–2887S.

119. Gomez-Cabrera MC, Domenech E, Romagnoli M, Arduini A, Borras C, Pallardo FV, Sastre J, Viña J. Oral administration of vitamin C decreases muscle mitochondrial biogenesis and hampers training-induced adaptations in endurance performance. *Am J Clin Nutr.* 2008;87:142–149.

120. Ristow M, Zarse K, Oberbach A, Klöting N, Birringer M, Kiehntopf M, Stumvoll M, Kahn CR, Blüher M. Antioxidants prevent health-promoting effects of physical exercise in humans. *Proc Natl Acad Sci U S A.* 2009;106: 8665–8670.

121. Campbell B, Roberts M, Kerksick C, Wilborn C, Marcello B, Taylor L, Nassar E, Leutholtz B, Bowden R, Rasmussen C, Greenwood M, Kreider R. Pharmacokinetics, safety, and effects on exercise performance of L-arginine alpha-ketoglutarate in trained adult men. *Nutrition.* 2006;22:872–881.

122. Little JP, Forbes SC, Candow DG, Cornish SM, Chilibeck PD. Creatine, arginine α-ketoglutarate, amino acids, and medium-chain triglycerides and endurance and performance. *Int J Sport Nutr Exerc Metab.* 2008;18:493–508.

123. Evans RW, Fernstrom JD, Thompson J, Morris SM Jr, Kuller LH. Biochemical responses of healthy subjects during dietary supplementation with L-arginine. *J Nutr Biochem.* 2004;15:534–539.

124. Prosser JM, Majlesi N, Chan GM, Olsen D, Hoffman RS, Nelson LS. Adverse effects associated with arginine alpha-ketoglutarate containing supplements. *Hum Exp Toxicol.* 2009; 28:259–262.

125. Nieman DC, Henson DA, McAnulty SR, Jin F, Maxwell KR. n-3 polyunsaturated fatty acids do not alter immune and inflammation measures in endurance athletes. *Int J Sport Nutr Exerc Metab.* 2009;19:536–546.

126. Bloomer RJ, Larson DE, Fisher-Wellman KH, Galpin AJ, Schilling BK. Effect of eicosapentaenoic and docosahexaenoic acid on resting and exercise-induced inflammatory and oxidative stress biomarkers: a randomized, placebo controlled, cross-over study. *Lipids Health Dis.* 2009;8:36.

127. Buckley JD, Burgess S, Murphy KJ, Howe PR. DHA-rich fish oil lowers heart rate during submaximal exercise in elite Australian Rules footballers. *J Sci Med Sport.* 2009;12:503–507.

128. Raastad T, Høstmark AT, Strømme SB. Omega-3 fatty acid supplementation does not improve maximal aerobic power, anaerobic threshold and running performance in well-trained soccer players. *Scand J Med Sci Sports.* 1997;7:25–31.

129. Mickleborough TD, Lindley MR, Ionescu AA, Fly AD. Protective effect of fish oil supplementation on exercise-induced bronchoconstriction in asthma. *Chest*. 2006;129:39–49.

130. Malaguti M, Baldini M, Angeloni C, Biagi P, Hrelia S. High-protein-PUFA supplementation, red blood cell membranes, and plasma antioxidant activity in volleyball athletes. *Int J Sport Nutr Exerc Metab*. 2008;18:301–312.

131. Simopoulos AP. Omega-3 fatty acids, exercise, physical activity and athletics. *World Rev Nutr Diet*. 2008;98:23–50.

132. Rodriguez NR, DiMarco NM, Langley S; American Dietetic Association; Dietitians of Canada; American College of Sports Medicine. Position of the American Dietetic Association, Dietitians of Canada, and the American College of Sports Medicine: Nutrition and athletic performance. *J Am Diet Assoc*. 2009;109:509–527.

133. Lemon PW. Beyond the zone: protein needs of active individuals. *J Am Coll Nutr*. 2000;19:513–521.

134. Poortmans JR, Dellalieux O. Do regular high protein diets have potential health risks on kidney function in athletes? *Int J Sport Nutr Exerc Metab*. 2000;10:28–38.

135. Rozenek R, Ward P, Long S, Garhammer J. Effects of high-calorie supplements on body composition and muscular strength following resistance training. *J Sports Med Phys Fitness*. 2002;42:340–347.

136. Jonnalagadda SS, Rosenbloom CA, Skinner R. Dietary practices, attitudes, and physiological status of collegiate freshman football players. *J Strength Cond Res*. 2001;15:507–513.

137. Burke DG, Chilibeck PD, Davidson KS, Candow DG, Farthing J, Smith-Palmer T. The effect of whey protein supplementation with and without creatine monohydrate combined with resistance training on lean tissue mass and muscle strength. *Int J Sport Nutr Exerc Metab*. 2001;11:349–364.

138. Dunford M, Doyle JA. *Nutrition for Sport and Exercise*. 2nd ed. Belmont, CA: Thompson/Wadsworth; 2011.

139. Cribb P, Williams AD, Carey MF, Hates A. The effect of whey isolate and resistance training on strength, body composition, and plasma glutamine. *Int J Sport Nutr Exerc Metab*. 2006;16:494–509.

140. Candow DG, Burke NC, Smith-Palmer T, Burke DG. Effect of whey and soy protein supplementation combined with resistance training in young adults. *Int J Sport Nutr Exerc Metab*. 2006;16:233–424.

141. Tipton KD, Elliott TA, Cree MG, Wolf SE, Sanford AP, Wolfe RR. Ingestion of casein and whey proteins result in muscle anabolism after resistance exercise. *Med Sci Sports Exerc*. 2004;36:2073–2081.

142. Phillips SM. The science of muscle hypertrophy: making dietary protein count. *Proc Nutr Soc*. 2011;70:100–103.

143. Tang JE, Moore DR, Kujbida GW, Tarnopolsky MA, Phillips SM. Ingestion of whey hydrolysate, casein, or soy protein isolate: effects on mixed muscle protein synthesis at rest and following resistance exercise in young men. *J Appl Physiol*. 2009;107:987–992.

144. Cribb PJ, Hayes A. Effects of supplement timing and resistance exercise on skeletal muscle hypertrophy. *Med Sci Sports Exerc*. 2006;38:1918–1925.

145. Kreider RB, Campbell B. Protein for exercise and recovery. *Phys Sportsmed*. 2009;37:13–21.

146. Manninen AH. Hyperinsulinaemia, hyperaminoacidaemia and post-exercise muscle anabolism: the search for the optimal recovery drink. *Br J Sports Med*. 2006;40:900–905.

147. West DW, Burd NA, Coffey VG, Baker SK, Burke LM, Hawley JA, Moore DR, Stellingwerff T, Phillips SM. Rapid aminoacidemia enhances myofibrillar protein synthesis and anabolic intramuscular signaling responses after resistance exercise. *Am J Clin Nutr*. 2011;94:795–803.

148. Sukala WR. Pyruvate: beyond the marketing hype. *Int J Sport Nutr*. 1998;8:241–249.

149. Stanko RT, Robertson RJ, Spina RJ, Reilly JJ Jr, Greenawalt KD, Goss FL. Enhancement of arm exercise endurance capacity with dihydroxyacetone and pyruvate. *J Appl Physiol*. 1990;68:119–124.

150. Stanko RT, Robertson RJ, Galbreath RW, Reilly JJ Jr, Greenawalt KD, Goss FL. Enhanced leg exercise endurance with a high-carbohydrate diet and dihydroxyacetone and pyruvate. *J Appl Physiol*. 1990;69:1651–1656.

151. Morrison MA, Spriet LL, Dyck DJ. Pyruvate ingestion for 7 days does not improve aerobic performance in well-trained individuals. *J Appl Physiol*. 2000;89:549–556.

152. Stanko RT, Tietze DL, Arch JE. Body composition, energy utilization, and nitrogen metabolism with a 4.25-MJ/d low-energy diet supplemented with pyruvate. *Am J Clin Nutr*. 1992;56:630–635.

153. Stanko RT, Tietze DL, Arch JE. Body composition, energy utilization, and nitrogen metabolism with a severely restricted diet supplemented with dihydroxyacetone and pyruvate. *Am J Clin Nutr*. 1992;55:771–776.

154. Nieman DC, Henson DA, Davis JM, Angela Murphy E, Jenkins DP, Gross SJ, Carmichael MD, Quindry JC, Dumke CL, Utter AC, McAnulty SR, McAnulty LS, Triplett NT, Mayer EP. Quercetin's influence on

exercise-induced changes in plasma cytokines and muscle and leukocyte cytokine mRNA. *J Appl Physiol.* 2007;103:1728–1735.

155. Davis JM, Murphy EA, Carmichael MD. Effects of the dietary flavonoid quercetin upon performance and health. *Curr Sports Med Rep.* 2009;8:206–213.

156. Kressler J, Millard-Stafford M, Warren GL. Quercetin and endurance exercise capacity: a systematic review and meta-analysis. *Med Sci Sport Exerc.* 2011 May 20. Epub ahead of print.

157. Davis JM, Carlstedt CJ, Chen S, Carmichael MD, Murphy EA. The dietary flavonoid quercetin increases VO2max and endurance capacity. *Int J Sport Nutr Exerc Metab.* 2010;20:56–62.

158. Nieman DC, Henson DA, Maxwell KR, Williams AS, McAnulty SR, Jin F, Shanely RA, Lines TC. Effects of quercetin and EGCG on mitochondrial biogenesis and immunity. *Med Sci Sports Exerc.* 2009;41:1467–1475.

159. McAnulty SR, McAnulty LS, Nieman DC, Quindry JC, Hosick PA, Hudson MH, Still L, Henson DA, Milne GL, Morrow JD, Dumke CL, Utter AC, Triplett NT, Dibarnardi A. Chronic quercetin ingestion and exercise-induced oxidative damage and inflammation. *Appl Physiol Nutr Metab.* 2008;33:254–262.

160. Utter AC, Nieman DC, Kang J, Dumke CL, Quindry JC, McAnulty SR, McAnulty LS. Quercetin does not affect rating of perceived exertion in athletes during the Western States endurance run. *Res Sports Med.* 2009;17: 71–83.

161. Quindry JC, McAnulty SR, Hudson MB, Hosick P, Dumke C, McAnulty LS, Henson D, Morrow JD, Nieman D. Oral quercetin supplementation and blood oxidative capacity in response to ultramarathon competition. *Int J Sport Nutr Exerc Metab.* 2008;18:601–616.

162. Kreider RB, Melton C, Greenwood M, Rasmussen C, Lundberg J, Earnest C, Almada A. Effects of oral D-ribose supplementation on anaerobic capacity and selected metabolic markers in healthy males. *Int J Sport Nutr Exerc Metab.* 2003;13:76–86.

163. Dhanoa TS, Housner JA. Ribose: more than a simple sugar? *Curr Sports Med Rep.* 2007;6:254–257.

164. Jentjens RL, Jeukendrup AE. Effect of acute and short-term administration of vanadyl sulphate on insulin sensitivity in healthy active humans. *Int J Sport Nutr Exerc Metab.* 2002;12:470–479.

165. Smith DM, Pickering RM, Lewith GT. A systematic review of vanadium oral supplements for glycaemic control in type 2 diabetes mellitus. *QJM.* 2008;101:351–358.

166. Yeh GY, Eisenberg DM, Kaptchuk TJ, Phillips RS. Systematic review of herbs and dietary supplements for glycemic control in diabetes. *Diabetes Care.* 2003;26:1277–1294.

167. Yfanti C, Akerström T, Nielsen S, Nielsen AR, Mounier R, Mortensen OH, Lykkesfeldt J, Rose AJ, Fischer CP, Pedersen BK. Antioxidant supplementation does not alter endurance training adaptation. *Med Sci Sports Exerc.* 2010;42:1388–1395.

168. McGinley C, Shafat A, Donnelly AE. Does antioxidant vitamin supplementation protect against muscle damage? *Sports Med.* 2009;39:1011–1032.

169. Peake JM. Vitamin C: effects of exercise and requirements with training. *Int J Sport Nutr Exerc Metab.* 2003;13: 125–151.

170. Institute of Medicine. *Dietary Reference Intakes for Vitamin C, Vitamin E, Selenium, and Carotenoids.* Washington, DC: National Academies Press; 2000.

171. Williams SL, Strobel NA, Lexis LA, Coombes JS. Antioxidant requirements of endurance athletes: implications for health. *Nutr Rev.* 2006;64:93–108.

172. Teixeira VH, Valente HF, Casal SI, Marques AF, Moreira PA. Antioxidants do not prevent postexercise peroxidation and may delay muscle recovery. *Med Sci Sports Exerc.* 2009;41:1752–1760.

173. Douglas RM, Chalker EB, Treacy B. Vitamin C for preventing and treating the common cold. *Cochrane Database Syst Rev.* 2000:CD000980.

174. Willis KS, Peterson NJ, Larson-Meyer DE. Should we be concerned about the vitamin D status of athletes? *Int J Sport Nutr Exerc Metab.* 2008;18:204–224.

175. Cannell JJ, Hollis BW, Sorenson MB, Taft TN, Anderson JJ. Athletic performance and vitamin D. *Med Sci Sports Exerc.* 2009;41:1102–1110.

176. Institute of Medicine. *Dietary Reference Intakes for Calcium and Vitamin D.* Washington, DC: National Academies Press; 2010.

Section 2

Sports Nutrition Assessment and Energy Balance

Ask any sports dietitian and she or he will tell you that athletes want to alter their body composition. Gaining or losing weight, increasing muscle mass, decreasing body fat, or a combination of such goals are top priorities for most competitive athletes. Chapter 8 provides an understanding of the nutrition assessment component of the Nutrition Care Process, whereas Chapter 9 examines the various body composition measurement tools and summarizes the pros and cons of methods of measuring body composition to help the practitioner choose the appropriate technique. Energy balance is thoroughly explained in Chapter 10 (a new chapter for the 5th edition), and, finally, the section provides the practitioner with an understanding of the research behind recommendations on weight management (Chapter 11). These four chapters will answer many of the frequently asked questions by athletes and coaches.

Chapter 8

NUTRITION ASSESSMENT

Maria G. Boosalis, PhD, MPH, RD

Introduction

The focus of this chapter is nutrition assessment, the first step in the Nutrition Care Process (NCP) (1). The NCP is defined as a systematic problem-solving method that registered dietitians (RDs) use to critically think and make decisions to address nutrition-related problems and provide safe and effective quality nutrition care (1). It includes four distinct, interrelated steps: (*a*) nutrition assessment; (*b*) nutrition diagnosis; (*c*) nutrition intervention; and (*d*) nutrition monitoring and evaluation. Even though each step of the NCP builds upon the previous one, it is not a linear process but requires critical thinking, problem solving, and a revisiting of previous steps to revise, modify, and continuously refine and update recommendations.

Nutrition assessment is the NCP step in which all detailed information that is nutrition-related or relevant, especially regarding nutritional status, is obtained. When a thorough nutrition assessment is completed, the other steps in the NCP become evident. Following the collection of nutrition assessment data, a relevant nutrition diagnosis (ie, the identification of the nutrition-related problem that the RD will address) is documented. After this important step, the RD designs and implements an appropriate nutrition intervention to address the specific nutrition diagnosis. Once the nutrition intervention is implemented, the RD monitors progress, documents nutrition-related outcomes, and makes any necessary adjustments to the NCP.

The following sections provide a detailed overview of each of the five "A" through "E" components of a complete nutrition assessment: the Anthropometric, Biochemical, Clinical, Dietary, and Environmental components of information (2). Briefly, the "A" component (anthropometric) is the "measure of man" (or woman, child, or infant). Some may refer to anthropometrics as body composition analysis. The "B" component (biochemical) includes all laboratory assays/tests, usually done on biological fluids to determine whether they are within the normal range or limits; this includes static (direct) and functional (indirect) tests (2,3). The "C" component (clinical) encompasses past and current medical history, history of present illness, family history, physical examination findings, and a review of systems (ROS) looking for signs of disease or illness, and includes blood pressure measurement, sleep habits, and assessment of any physical limitations (2). The goal of the "D" component (dietary) is to determine and document any substance that goes into the mouth (eg, usual or unusual intake of food, beverages, prescription medicines, over-the-counter [OTC] supplements, ergogenic aids, nutraceuticals, functional foods and beverages, or alcohol). The "E" component (environmental) includes all aspects of an individual's environment/living conditions that may affect his or her ability to obtain, provide, purchase, prepare, and/or consume food and beverages (2).

What are the advantages to completing a thorough nutrition assessment of an athlete? Obtaining information across all the "A" through "E" components or parameters allows the sports dietitian to make the nutrition-related diagnosis, design the best nutrition and lifestyle intervention, as well as establish a plan to both monitor and evaluate the outcomes of that intervention, hence completing the NCP.

Anthropometric Nutrition Assessment

The two most common and routine anthropometric measures are the height and weight of an individual taken across his or her life span. (In infants, a supine length and head circumference are also routinely measured, but a discussion of this is beyond the scope of this chapter.) When recording an individual's height and weight, document whether it is reported or measured, and when it was obtained.

Another common anthropometric measure is body mass index (BMI), which is derived from an individual's measured height and weight: $BMI = Weight (kg)/Height (m)^2$. The National Heart, Lung, and Blood Institute (NHLBI) Web site provides a BMI calculator and discusses the strengths and limitations of using BMI as a screening/diagnostic tool (4). Briefly, BMI is a reliable indicator of total body fat, which, in turn, is related to the risk of disease and death. The measure is valid for men and women, but it does have some limits. One of the limitations relevant to athletes is that BMI may overestimate body fat in individuals who have a muscular build. On the other hand, it may underestimate body fat in older individuals or others who have lost muscle mass. Although there is a positive relationship between percentage of body fat and BMI, it is not a perfect direct correlation and variations exist (5).

BMI is used as a screening tool to identify whether an individual's weight puts them at increased risk for a weight-related comorbidity, such as diabetes, cardiovascular disease, or hypertension, among others (6). For adults, the lowest risk for a weight-related comorbidity is in those whose BMI is between 18.5 and 24.9. In adults 65 years of age and older, the Nutrition Screening Initiative recommends a BMI in the range of 24 to 27 (7) whereas NHLBI sets the recommended range as between 25 and 27 (8,9).

Due to continued growth, the weight-related BMI classification of youth between the ages of 2 and 20 years differs from that of adults. Although a youth's BMI is calculated using the same formula as previously described, it must be plotted on the appropriate Centers for Disease Control and Prevention (CDC) BMI-for-age growth charts (for either girls or boys) (10,11), in which a percentile for a specific BMI is derived. The terminology for these respective BMI percentile categories are as follows: < 5th percentile, underweight; 5th–84th percentile, healthy weight; 85th–94th percentile, overweight; ≥ 95th percentile, obesity; and a proposed ≥ 99th percentile as severe obesity (12).

Another valuable piece of anthropometric information is an individual's weight history, especially in individuals whose weight is of concern, whether high or low. For example, individuals should be asked if they have experienced any recent weight change. If they answer in the affirmative, additional questions about whether the weight change was intentional or unintentional are necessary, and the RD should consider whether further investigation is warranted. Potential points of inquiry include the following: What is the pattern of this weight change? What can be discerned from the pattern? How much weight does an athlete gain during the "off" season or while recovering from injury? Is there a history of extreme weight loss related to excessive physical activity or a history of large weight fluctuations and/or "yo-yo" dieting, especially to achieve some sort of "ideal" training or competition weight? In adults generally, appropriate questions include: What has been their minimum/maximum weight? In their mind, What is the "ideal" weight? How easy or difficult has it been to maintain this "ideal" weight?

In the case of adults whose BMI value classifies them as either overweight or obese, the "location" of this excess weight in the form of fat is important to the nutrition assessment. Specifically, the predominant distribution of fat around the abdomen, termed abdominal or visceral fat, is associated with a greater risk of a weight-related comorbidity. This abdominal or visceral fat is clinically most easily determined by measuring an individual's waist circumference (WC), as described by NHLBI standards (13). This measurement is taken in an individual at a horizontal line parallel to floor just above their iliac crest; NHLBI recommends men have a WC of 40 inches or less (102 cm) and women 35 inches or less (88 cm). Men and women whose WC is bigger than these cutoffs and who have a BMI between 25 and 34.9 have increased obesity-associated disease risks (13). For a detailed discussion of this measurement, see Chapter 9.

Worldwide WC percentile data are available, and measuring a WC in youth may provide another marker for success relative to weight loss (14). For example, Maffeis et al (15) reported that children with a WC more than the 90th percentile were more likely to have multiple cardiovascular risk factors compared with those with a lesser value. Moreover, this 90th percentile cutoff has been used to estimate the prevalence of metabolic syndrome in youth in various additional studies (14,16–18). This 90th percentile WC was also suggested as a standard to identify metabolic syndrome in youth by the International Diabetes Foundation in their recent consensus report (14). However, a single universal standard in youth is still being studied.

In summary, at a minimum the aforementioned anthropometric measures (with the possible exception of WC in youth) should be done routinely for the "A" component of the nutrition assessment. Chapter 9 discusses other anthropometric or body composition measurements that can also be included in this category. These other measurements are designed to assess either a two-compartment (fat vs fat-free mass) model, a three-compartment (fat, fat-free mass, bone mineral) model, and/or a four-compartment (fat, fat-free mass, bone mineral, water) model of body composition. In most cases, the two-compartment model is most frequently used. These various types of measurements include the measurement of skinfold thickness, bioelectrical impedance analysis (BIA), dual energy x-ray absorptiometry (DXA), underwater weighing, and BOD POD (air displacement plethysmography). See Chapter 9 for further details on these other anthropometric/body composition measurements.

Biochemical Nutrition Assessment

The assessment of biochemical status involves measurement of various parameters in three distinct categories: macronutrients, micronutrients, and major organ systems.

Macronutrients

Protein status is one of the prime macronutrients to assess. Generally, the status of an individual's circulating level of protein is measured to identify malnutrition and/or low protein stores. Although the level of circulating albumin is commonly measured to assess for protein-calorie malnutrition or nutrition compromise, albumin's long half-life (~18–21 days) means that it responds slowly to changes in protein intake. Thus, it serves as an indicator of long-term protein status, and does not indicate a short-term response to feeding. To assess a short-term response, transthyretin (previously known as thyroxine-binding prealbumin), with a half-life of approximately 2 days, is measured. It should also be noted that with both of these proteins, their synthesis and subsequent levels are negatively affected by inflammation and a full-blown systemic inflammatory stress response (ie, their synthesis is decreased so their circulating levels are therefore decreased). What is less known is whether extended periods of exercise (ie, repeated long-distance running, over-exercising, and/or acute or chronic sports-related injuries) has any effect on the circulating levels of these proteins because of the possible presence of a chronic or acute systemic inflammatory response (19,20) or an alteration in immune function (21). As with all levels of circulating metabolites, alterations in fluid status (overhydration or underhydration) may adversely affect circulating levels.

With respect to carbohydrate status, an individual's ability to metabolize or handle glucose is determined by checking fasting plasma glucose or hemoglobin A1C levels, or by performing an oral glucose tolerance test (OGTT). If an abnormal result is obtained in any of these measurements, further tests would be warranted to rule out glucose intolerance, glucose sensitivity, and/or type 1 or type 2 diabetes (22).

Determining lipid or fat status generally involves ruling out risk factors for cardiovascular disease. Toward that end, circulating levels of total cholesterol, high- and low-density lipoprotein cholesterol (HDL- and LDL-cholesterol, respectively), as well as circulating levels of triglycerides in the serum, are measured as biochemical indicators. On a clinical or research basis, circulating levels of high-sensitivity C-reactive protein and homocysteine levels may be measured (a discussion of these measurements is beyond the scope of this chapter). Additionally, if there are any suspicions or signs suggesting fat malabsorption, appropriate fecal fat stool tests are done (23).

Certainly not least in this category of macronutrient status is fluid and hydration status, a critical component of any athlete's assessment. A detailed discussion of this topic is found in Chapter 6.

Micronutrients

With respect to micronutrient status, individual vitamins, minerals, and/or electrolytes might be measured if any compromise in their status (deficiency or excess) is suspected. That said, the most frequently observed micronutrient deficiencies are those implicated in nutrition-related anemias, usually involving a deficit in intake, absorption, and/or metabolism of iron, folic acid, and/or vitamin B-12. Albeit rare, there is a nutrition-related anemia due to a deficiency of copper caused by excess supplementation with zinc; further supplementation with copper and a reduction (if not elimination) of excess zinc supplementation are warranted until the anemia corrects.

The most prevalent nutrition-related anemia is due to a deficiency of iron, which has numerous health consequences. At an early subclinical/clinical phase, undesirable pregnancy outcomes, delayed development in infants and children, and impairment of either cognitive function and/or physical work performance can occur, whereas the functional consequences occur later when a decrease in hemoglobin concentration is observed (24). Iron-deficiency anemia is generally hypochromic and microcytic in nature, with a decrease in hepatocyte iron as indicated by increased circulating levels of transferrin (2). In addition, circulating levels of ferritin in the serum, which reflect iron stores, are generally depressed. There are also specific stages of iron deficiency that have been described (25). Briefly, depleted iron stores is considered stage 1 and includes an absence of stainable bone marrow iron and a reduced total iron binding capacity as well as serum ferritin concentration. Early functional iron deficiency is considered stage 2 and includes a decreased transferrin saturation, an increase in free erythrocyte protoporphyrin, as well as an increase in circulating levels of transferrin receptor in the serum. The final stage, stage 3, is iron-deficiency anemia, in which a decreased concentration of hemoglobin and reduced mean cell volume is identified. Detailed tables on laboratory values, cutoff values, and diagnostic strategies to identify iron-deficiency anemia can be found in reference 26.

Athletes as a group are particularly susceptible to iron-deficiency anemia. Both men and women who regularly follow an intense exercise regimen (eg, competitive endurance and ultra-endurance sports) seem to have marginal and/or inadequate iron status (24,27–31). Reasons for this phenomenon include, but are not limited to, a greater turnover of red blood cells, elevated losses of blood via the gastrointestinal tract, and rupture of red blood cells within the foot while running (footstrike hemolysis).

Vegetarian and female athletes are at increased risk of iron depletion and/or deficiency. These athletes should pursue dietary strategies that will ensure the adequacy of their iron intake. For example, consuming foods with ascorbic acid when eating foods rich in nonheme iron will enhance the absorption of dietary iron. If dietary strategies are not sufficient to maintain adequate iron status, supplementation with iron may be needed. For example, female swimmers who took a daily supplement of 125 mg ferrous sulfate maintained adequate iron stores with no adverse gastrointestinal effects (32).

Several etiologies can result in a deficiency of folic acid and/or vitamin B-12 that can result in a nutrition-related anemia. Specifically, a deficiency of either or both of these B vitamins presents as a megaloblastic anemia that is macrocytic and generally normochromic in nature. Whatever the particular etiology, determining the status of both folic acid and vitamin B-12 is essential, generally through the measurement of their respective circulating levels. Ruling out a vitamin B-12 deficiency is critical, because if both deficiencies are present folate supplementation will correct the megaloblastic anemia but the neurological manifestations of vitamin B-12 deficiency may progress undetected and, depending on their duration, may become irreversible. These neurologic manifestations include but are not limited to sensory and motor disturbances as well as cognitive changes including memory loss/dementia (33).

Other nutrients that may be compromised in various clinical or sports-related situations include zinc, vitamin D, and calcium, possibly some of the B vitamins, and vitamin C. If malnutrition is suspected, especially as a result of disordered eating, further care must be taken to rule out a deficiency of these aforementioned nutrients along with any other suspected vitamins/minerals. In reference 2, the sports dietitian can view a table of common findings and signs/symptoms to determine whether further biochemical testing is warranted.

Organ Function

The final category of biochemical tests measures organ function, especially in those organ systems involved in the digestion, absorption, metabolism, and excretion of nutrients and their end products. Box 8.1 presents organ function tests. More information can be found in reference 34.

BOX 8.1   Organ System Review

- **Gastrointestinal tract**: Tests to measure malabsorption include fecal fat, B-12 malabsorption via Schilling test.
- **Liver**: Tests to measure liver function include ammonia, aspartate aminotransferase (AST), alanine aminotransferase (ALT), alkaline phosphatase, gamma-glutamyl transpeptidase (GGT), albumin, hepatitis virus, albumin, bilirubin, total protein, coagulation tests (eg, prothrombin time, partial thromboplastin time).
- **Pancreas**: Tests to measure pancreas function include serum amylase and serum lipase.
- **Kidneys**: Tests to measure renal function include albumin, total protein, serum creatinine, creatinine clearance, glomerular filtration rate, blood urea nitrogen, nitrogen balance, serum protein.
- **Thyroid**: Tests to measure thyroid function include thyroid stimulating hormone (TSH), T4, T3.
- **Cardiorespiratory**: Tests to measure heart and lung function include arterial blood gases, cardiac enzymes, creatine kinase, lactate dehydrogenase (LDH), aspartate aminotransferase (AST), homocysteine, lipid profile including total cholesterol, low-density lipoprotein (LDL), high-density lipoprotein (HDL), serum triglycerides.

Clinical Nutrition Assessment

The data for the clinical component of a nutrition assessment are generally collected by a member of the health care team other than the sports dietitian, such as the team physician or a certified athletic trainer. Such data include pertinent nutrition-related information regardless of which member of the health care team does the examination/interview.

The nutrition-related information in the clinical component includes, but is not limited to, the following:

- An individual's current medical history, relevant past medical history, and family history of common comorbidities and major diseases. This information is particularly important when there are no biochemical tests available to screen for presence of common comorbidities or additional disease risks in the individual.
- All prescription medications as well as nonprescription and OTC medications, nutritional and herbal supplements, ergogenic aids, vitamin and/or mineral supplements, and the determination of any possible drug-nutrient interactions or nutrient-nutrient interactions.
- Use of alcohol and recreational drugs.
- Average or usual amount of sleep (both naps and at night) and history of snoring and whether the individual wakes up at night to "catch his or her breath."
- Blood pressure measurement to screen for hypertension.
- Physical examination/review of systems (ROS):

  o General: appetite/weight change, weakness, fatigue, fever, chills, night sweats, changes in sleep pattern, edema, and/or abdominal swelling
  o Skin: rash, dry skin, acanthosis nigricans
  o Nails: breaking, koilonychia, clubbing
  o Hair: loss, changes in texture, ease of pluckability (> 8 to 10 hairs at one time), and flag sign (alternate color "bands" or stripes in hair corresponding to periods of malnutrition)
  o Neurological: confusion, memory loss, gait change, loss of position sense, numbness, paresthesia
  o Eyes: difficulty with night vision, Bitot's spots, macular degeneration, cataracts
  o Gastrointestinal symptoms/alimentary: assess "mouth to anus" (eg, abdominal pain, nausea/vomiting, diarrhea, constipation, swallowing problems, early satiety, indigestion, heartburn, mouth lesions/ulcers, tooth decay, sore tongue, gum, dentures)
  o Cardiopulmonary: shortness of breath (SOB), wheezing, asthma, arrhythmias
  o Renal: polyuria, polydipsia, difficulty/pain urinating, blood in urine, color of urine
  o Musculoskeletal: hands, back, joints, knees, feet, shoulders, neck, pain, range of motion, osteopenia, osteoporosis, arthritis

Metabolic Syndrome

Identification of metabolic syndrome in adults includes identifying the presence of three of five select or specific measures in an individual, utilizing information derived from the first three components ("A" through "C") of a complete nutrition assessment (35). In the anthropometric category, a measurement of an individual's WC is used to screen and identify abdominal obesity (35), as described previously in the anthropometric section. In the biochemical category, the presence of atherogenic dyslipidemia is used to help identify the presence of metabolic syndrome in an individual. Specifically, elevated levels of circulating triglycerides (criteria ≥ 150 mg/dL) and/or decreased circulating levels of high-density lipoprotein

(HDL) cholesterol (< 40 mg/dL in men and < 50 mg/dL in women) are used. Another biochemical measure that can be used to diagnose this syndrome is an elevated fasting blood glucose measurement (≥ 100 mg/dL using American Diabetes Association revised criteria for impaired fasting glucose) (35,36). In the clinical component, an individual's blood pressure (BP) reading is used to help identify the presence of metabolic syndrome. Toward this end, a BP reading with a systolic BP ≥ 130 mmHg or diastolic BP ≥ 85 mmHg (35) is the criteria used. To summarize, the presence of any three out of the five aforementioned criteria identifies the presence of the metabolic syndrome in an adult. The criteria for youth have not as yet been determined, although several have been suggested and reviewed (14).

Energy Requirements

The assessment or determination of energy needs of an individual can be included as part of the clinical or dietary component of a complete nutrition assessment. Wherever this information is placed, there are numerous methods that can be used to determine these needs. The reader is referred to Chapter 10 for those details. Briefly, most of the techniques involve some method of indirect instead of direct calorimetry because the latter requires a highly sophisticated chamber or specially designed suit and is used primarily in research settings. Indirect calorimetry, on the other hand, is based on the fact that energy needs as well as energy expenditure depend on oxygen utilization (VO_2) and carbon dioxide production (VCO_2) and their known relationship to the respiratory quotient (RQ) = VCO_2/VO_2. The doubly labeled water technique, for instance, uses indirect calorimetry methodology to measure energy expenditure in free-living individuals as they go about their daily life and physical activity routines (37). In fact, the Estimated Energy Requirement (EER) of the Dietary Reference Intakes was based on prediction equations for normal-weight individuals developed from data on total daily energy expenditure using the doubly labeled water technique (38).

There are also several prediction equations for calculating basal and total energy needs that are based, in some way, on an individual's height, weight, age, and sex, with additional calculations made in some cases for level of physical activity. The reader is referred to Chapter 10 for further details on predicted energy calculations.

Dietary Nutrition Assessment

The dietary component of a complete nutrition assessment is generally obtained by the sports dietitian. The overall objective of this component is to determine the total intake of food and beverages that the individual routinely consumes. In other words, everything the individual consumes, including medications, OTC supplements, all beverages, and foods needs to be documented, followed by a nutrition analysis of reported intake. In addition, any drug-nutrient and food-drug interactions need to be noted. Examples of common interactions are described in reference 39 as well as in an online drug-nutrient interaction tool run by Medscape (40).

There are several methodologies used to determine an individual's dietary intake. The primary methodologies include, but are not limited to, dietary recalls, dietary records, food frequency questionnaires (FFQ), and direct observation.

The most common dietary recall assessment method is the 24-hour recall. The advantage of this method is that it requires very little respondent burden, although it does require the respondent to have an intact memory. The respondent also must be able to accurately quantify his or her intake to determine amount of food and beverages consumed. This ability usually requires the help of a skilled interviewer to translate the individual's recall information into accurate food and beverage descriptions and portion sizes, which is critical for the accuracy of this methodology. Because the skilled interviewer, generally the sports dietitian, is asking the individual to report and quantify their dietary intake in the past 24-hour period, the data collected may not reflect long-term or usual habits of the respondent.

Another commonly used dietary assessment method is the dietary record, generally gathered over a 3-day period. The 3-day period is usually consecutive and includes 2 typical days and 1 atypical day (usually 2 weekdays and 1 weekend day). This methodology requires the individual be given prior instruction to accurately complete their records as well as a follow-up meeting with a skilled interviewer to fill in any missing pieces of information. This methodology also requires a fairly large respondent burden because individuals are instructed to record everything they have to eat and drink, including amounts and methods of preparation. Another disadvantage of this methodology is that the mere act of recording food and beverage intake can alter what the individual consumes. For instance, an individual may not eat something because he or she does not want to go to the trouble of recording it or might be anxious or embarrassed to let someone else know what was consumed. Another important consideration to determine is whether the days selected to obtain the dietary record are representative of the individual's usual intake. On the positive side, dietary records have been widely used in weight management to both increase awareness of intake and as a way to monitor and control intake.

Epidemiologic studies, due to their large number of subjects, generally use food frequency questionnaires as the primary tool to assess dietary intake of research subjects. FFQs are also available to use as part of the dietary component of a routine nutrition assessment. Although the nature of these questionnaires is not quantitative, they may be used to give an average intake over a set period of time. For example, the FFQ used to collect dietary intake for the National Health and Nutrition Examination Survey (NHANES) can be viewed online (see reference 41). Information regarding the exact methodology and interviewing techniques used to gather NHANES information is described elsewhere (42,43).

FFQs can also be designed to capture consumption for specific food sources of nutrients or nutrient types. These types of questionnaires include assessments for calcium- and vitamin D–containing foods for risk of osteoporosis; fruit and vegetables for antioxidants; whole grains and legumes for fiber; types and amounts of fat sources for cardiovascular disease; and high-sodium foods for hypertension, to name a few. FFQs are often combined with 24-hour dietary recalls or dietary records as cross-validation and/or to improve accuracy of reported intake.

The last type of general dietary assessment method involves direct observation. This methodology is as it sounds: the RD directly observes and records the food and beverage intake of an individual. This method requires minimal, if any, respondent burden, but it requires a high degree of interviewer burden. An example of this type of observation is when the sports dietitian eats with a team and notes their intake or when she or he observes intake of an individual with an eating disorder. This ability to "observe" may be difficult to establish methodologically without altering intake, and care must be taken when using this type of monitoring. On the other hand, because direct observation requires no change or input on the part of the individual and, in theory, should note usual intake without any chance of influence by methodology, it can also serve as a cross-validation to improve accuracy of dietary recalls and/or records.

Environmental Nutrition Assessment

The last component of a complete nutrition assessment involves the collection of information regarding the environment or environmental characteristics in which individuals purchase, store, prepare, and consume their food and beverages (2,44). There are several types of seemingly unrelated information gathered in this category, all of which are significant alone as well as together.

Before beginning any nutrition intervention, the individual's willingness or ability to change as well as any barriers to change need to be assessed. One common model used is the Stages of Change model (45), which is also known as the Transtheoretical Model (46). Specifically, the individual is categorized into one of these six stages of change: precontemplation, contemplation, preparation, action, maintenance, or relapse. The individual's current stage determines what type of intervention may or may not be accomplished. Following are brief descriptions of the different stages. See also reference 47 for further insight and motivational interviewing tips to encourage change in an individual.

In the precontemplation stage, the individual is not currently thinking about making any change(s) in his or her behavior. The person may be resigned and feel that he or she has no control regarding the behavior, and at times may even be in denial or not believe the situation applies to him or her. The individual also tends to believe that any consequences regarding his or her behavior(s) are not serious (ie, "ignorance is bliss"). If this is the current situation, the sports dietitian can validate the athlete's lack of readiness and reinforce that the decision whether to change is the athlete's while trying to guide him or her to develop a reason to change. Toward that end, the sports dietitian can both encourage reevaluation/self-exploration of the current decision while explaining the specific risk of inaction and making it personal to the individual's circumstance. The overall goal of this approach is to ultimately move the individual further along the change continuum. The short-term goal is to get them from "no" to "I'll think about it." In any case, the sports dietitian wants to leave the door open to have future conversations with the individual.

In the contemplation stage, the individual weighs the benefits and the costs of the behavior and/or proposed change, but is still "on the fence" regarding making any changes. If this is the current situation, the sports dietitian should continue to validate the individual's experience and acknowledge that it is still his or her decision whether to make a change. In addition, the sports dietitian should clarify the pros and cons of making the change for the individual while encouraging him or her to continue thinking about the process with self-exploration techniques (eg, would they be willing to continue listing pros and cons of the change to discuss at next visit?) The overall goal continues to be the same, to move the individual to the next stage, in this case, the preparation stage by leaving the door open to making the change.

In the preparation stage, the individual experiments with small changes (ie, "testing the waters") that he or she is willing to share. If this is the current situation, the sports dietitian can help identify obstacles and help with problem-solving scenarios for overcoming the obstacles. In addition, the sports dietitian can help the individual identify and elicit support systems and verify that the individual has the necessary skills to make appropriate changes to sustain the behavior or dietary change(s). Moreover, the sports dietitian can assist the individual to make small, initial changes to enter the next "action" stage.

In the action stage, the individual is making a definitive action to change. In this situation, the sports dietitian can continue to bolster self-efficacy and assist the individual to make the necessary behavioral or dietary changes and continue to strategize to overcome any obstacles. In addition, the sports dietitian can also focus on restructuring cues and enlist the individual's support system for maintaining and sustaining the behavioral or dietary changes to enter the next stage: maintenance.

In the maintenance stage, the individual practices the new behavior over time to prevent the last stage, relapse. In this maintenance stage, the sports dietitian, along with the individual, creates a plan for follow-up support as well as reinforcing internal rewards for sustaining these changes. In addition, the sports dietitian should discuss coping mechanisms regarding relapse.

Relapse or a resumption of previous behaviors is unfortunately a normal experience and part of the change process, but when it happens the individual usually feels demoralized. If this stage does occur, the sports dietitian helps the individual identify and evaluate the trigger for this relapse as well as reassess motivation and obstacles or barriers to the new behavioral or dietary changes. Moreover, the sports dietitian and individual design stronger strategies to handle and ideally prevent relapse from occurring in the future.

Using this model can be challenging in the sports environment because often an athlete is sent to the sports dietitian by a coach who "demands" behavior change. The sports dietitian can help determine whether the coach's goals for body weight or muscle mass are reasonable and communicate these findings to the athlete.

Once the stage is determined for an athlete, other information regarding the environment is collected. Specifically, and in no particular order, information about an individual's financial status is gathered to determine whether it is adequate to cover the cost of basic living expenses, especially food. Many athletes are on a fixed meal plan, but many are not. The sports dietitian may find it challenging to help the athlete select foods on a limited budget.

The individual's level of physical and lifestyle activity is critical to the nutrition assessment of athletes at every performance level. It determines the athlete's individual energy needs, has implications for general health and nutrition recommendations, and helps screen for any excess patterns as are sometimes found in eating disorders. As applicable, information about the specific intensity, type, and duration of exercise and training also must be collected, especially in youth and highly trained athletes. Any unusual "training rituals," especially related to food and/or beverage consumption, should also be noted. Use of laxatives, purging agents, OTC supplements, and ergogenic aids could be noted in the nutrition assessment as well.

Determining an individual's level of comprehension and/or education level is critical to gauge the type of instruction and educational materials used as well as how to design and focus the specific nutrition intervention, monitoring, and evaluation plans.

An individual's living arrangements must also be assessed in the "E" component. Any aspects of the home environment that may influence the athlete's ability to store and prepare food and beverages needs to be noted. For example, does an athlete live in a dorm or apartment? Is refrigerator or freezer space available? Does the athlete have or an oven, cooktop, or microwave oven? Is there a grocery store nearby or does the athlete shop in a convenience store near campus? Athletes who live in a dormitory may not prepare any meals. In this case, what is their intake of pre-prepared foods, fast foods, or convenience foods, which may be high in sodium, fat, sugar, and calories? Obviously, the types of food preparation facilities available to the athlete affect the types of foods and beverages purchased and consumed and the type of dietary recommendations that can be made.

Lifestyle and daily routine have a very profound effect on what the individual eats, or is even able to eat, given challenges such as time constraints (eg, when do they rise in morning; what are their class, training and conditioning or practice schedules?) An individual's psycho-social-cultural support system is another critical piece of information to obtain because it helps assess the context in which dietary changes can be made, as well as where an individual may get assistance and support in making changes. For instance, is the individual the main purchaser or preparer of food and beverages he or she consumes or is someone else responsible for those duties? If the latter is the case, then that individual must also be interviewed and counseled to assist in making the necessary dietary changes.

Cultural context and special cultural food practices can greatly influence an individual's food and beverage choices and must be considered when designing a nutrition intervention and making any dietary recommendations. In general, the more support an individual has to make necessary dietary changes, the more likely the individual will be successful. It is also important to assess to psychological influences on food consumption and exercise. For example, is this individual an emotional eater who uses the consumption of certain foods or beverages to cope with perceived or real stress in his/her life? Does the individual exercise or train excessively as an alternative way to cope with negative stressors in his or her life? Does he or she have an extremely competitive nature?

An individual's beliefs and or cultural systems are especially important to help identify dietary restrictions and practices that influence and may potentially compromise nutritional intake. It is important to respect these beliefs when designing the nutrition intervention, monitoring, and evaluation plans. For example, there are religious groups that practice fasting from meat or all animal products on certain days of the week or throughout the year, and these customs should be considered when providing nutritional counseling.

Summary

Box 8.2 illustrates how the "A" through "E" components of a nutrition assessment are used as the first step of the NCP. As described in this chapter, there is a considerable amount of information that can be obtained in each A through E component of a complete nutrition assessment. Although it is important to gather and review information within each component, it is not necessary to collect all of the information in each category. In the example in Box 8.2, heavy emphasis was rightly put in the anthropometric category on using body composition measurements to obtain valuable information. On the other hand, biochemical data were not collected or necessary in this case because there were no signs or symptoms of nutrient excesses or deficiencies uncovered in the dietary records, clinical findings, or the family history. Although considerably more information can be gathered in the clinical component of a nutrition assessment, the example in Box 8.2 used minimal data that were sufficient for this situation. Specifically, the decision to forgo collection of biochemical data is supported by the absence of a family history of chronic diseases coupled with no additional clinical findings of concern. The dietary component of this illustration provides insight to possible contributing factors to the nutrition issues and problems, and it identifies areas where changes can be made to solve the suspected problem. In this case, the discovery of increased fast-food consumption likely contributed to the athlete's higher weight and higher intake of fat. This information can give the sports dietitian a starting point for discussion and to begin the intervention. As for the last component, the assessment of the athlete's environment shows that he lives at home with supportive parents who are able financially and physically to meet his nutrition needs, which improves the chances for success in any dietary intervention or subsequent recommendation. Knowing the athlete's willingness to change also improves success of any planned intervention. In sum, Box 8.2 demonstrates the usefulness and added benefits of an A through E nutrition assessment. It leads to a successful completion of the entire NCP and a satisfactory nutrition-related outcome (48).

BOX 8.2   Nutrition Assessment as Part of Nutrition Care Process (NCP) for an Athlete

Scenario: 16-year-old male high school boxer wants to compete in a lower weight class.

Nutrition Assessment (A–E)

- **A**: Height, weight, weight history, and body composition using air displacement plethysmography collected:
  - Athlete weighs 73.2 kg (161.2 pounds), which is 6.2 pounds heavier that allowed for light middleweight boxing class.
  - Recent (past 6–8 months) increase in weight; no change in height.
  - Body composition analysis revealed the athlete had 12.7% body fat and 87.3% lean mass.
- **B**: No labs requested because no signs/symptoms of nutrient excesses and/or deficiencies via dietary records, clinical findings, and/or family history were noted or suspected.

---

continues

BOX 8.2   Nutrition Assessment as Part of Nutrition Care Process (NCP) for an Athlete (continued)

- **C**: Blood pressure within normal limits; no known allergies; Review of Systems within normal limits as per sports physical; family history negative for diabetes, heart disease, hypertension, obesity; no physical limitations, restrictions, or injuries noted. No use of prescription medicines, over-the-counter supplements, or ergogenic aids noted.
- **D**: 3-day diet and activity records were collected.
  o Analysis of diet records revealed athlete averaged 2,100 kcal/d, with 54% carbohydrate, 15% protein, and 31% fat.
  o No use of prescription medicines, over-the-counter supplements, or ergogenic aids (as noted in clinical category as well).
  o Intake of fluids appropriate for needs and activity level.
  o Frequents fast-food restaurants with friends at minimum twice a week.
- **E**: Lives at home with supportive parents; all nutrition and physical needs met; no known dietary restrictions or omissions due to financial, religious, or sociocultural reasons; he recently received driver's license and frequents fast-food restaurants with friends.

Nutrition Diagnoses
- Number 1: Excessive energy intake (problem) related to physiological need to decrease body weight to compete in light middleweight class (etiology) as evidenced by reports of excessive oral food and beverage intake (signs and symptoms).
- Number 2: Undesirable food choices (problem) related to lack of knowledge about choosing healthful meals at favorite restaurant (etiology) as evidenced by an inability to lose excess body fat and body weight as needed for weight-class sport participation (signs and symptoms).

Nutrition Intervention
- Client-centered outcomes for each nutrition diagnosis were established:
  o Overall: RD consulted American College of Sports Medicine (ACSM) position stand on weight loss safety in wrestling and these data were used for the boxer; because that athlete is 16 years old and still growing, the athlete could not get lower than 7% body fat without medical clearance.
  o Intervention for nutrition diagnosis number 1: Body weight goal of 158 pounds with 12% body fat in 1 month and 155 pounds with a 10% body fat in 2 months was established.
  o Intervention for nutrition diagnosis number 2: Fast food choices were reviewed with athlete to demonstrate healthful choices that fit with meal plan containing 1,900 kcal with 60% carbohydrate, 20% protein, and 20% fat. School lunch meals and pre- and post-workout snacks were planned as well.
- Detailed fluid plan was established.
- Food monitoring log was developed to help athlete track his food intake.

Nutrition Monitoring and Evaluation
- Progress was monitored:
  o Overall goals were set for 1 and 2 months to achieve safe weight loss with weekly follow-up by e-mail and/or telephone contact.

continues

BOX 8.2   Nutrition Assessment as Part of Nutrition Care Process (NCP) for an Athlete (continued)

○ Scheduled 3-day food records were sent via e-mail to RD for evaluation.

○ Reassessment of body composition planned at 1 month and 2 months of intervention.

○ During the 2-month intervention, the athlete lost 6.3 pounds and weighed 154.8 pounds with 11% body fat and 89% lean mass, making him eligible for the lower light middle-weight class.

○ Athlete was successful in meeting his body composition as well as his performance goals. With respect to the latter, he won the state Golden Gloves title in the light middleweight division, advanced to and won the Junior Olympic Regional. He then went on to compete at the national level, where he finished second for his weight class.

Source: Data are from reference 48.

References

1. Writing Group of the Nutrition Care Process/Standardized Language Committee. Nutrition Care Process and Model Part I: the 2008 update. *J Am Diet Assoc.* 2008;108:1113–1117.

2. Gorman LS, Boosalis MG. Nutritional assessment. In: Bishop ML, Fody EP, Schoeff LE, eds. *Clinical Chemistry Techniques, Principles, Correlations.* 6th ed. Philadelphia, PA: Lippincott, Williams & Wilkins; 2010:651–672.

3. Lee RD, Nieman DC. *Nutritional Assessment.* 3rd ed. New York, NY: McGraw Hill Higher Education; 2003:304.

4. Calculate Your Body Mass Index. National Heart, Lung and Blood Institute, National Institutes of Health. http://www.nhlbisupport.com/bmi. Accessed January 10, 2011.

5. Gallagher D, Heymsfield SB, Heo M, Jebb SA, Murgatroyd PR, Sakamoto Y. Healthy percentage body fat ranges: an approach for developing guidelines based on body mass index. *Am J Clin Nutr.* 2000;72:694–701. http://www.ajcn.org/cgi/content/abstract/72/3/694. Accessed December 27, 2010.

6. Bray GA. *Contemporary Diagnosis and Management of Obesity.* Newtown, PA: Handbooks in Health Care; 1998.

7. Nutrition Screening Initiative. Report of Nutrition Screening I: Toward a Common View. Washington, DC: Nutrition Screening Initiative. 1991. http://www.jblearning.com/samples/0763730629/Frank_Appendix10D.pdf. Accessed December 27, 2010.

8. Body Mass Index. MedlinePlus, US National Library of Medicine, National Institutes of Health. http://www.nlm.nih.gov/medlineplus/ency/article/007196.htm. Accessed January 10, 2011.

9. Cook Z, Kirk S, Lawrenson S, Sandford S. Use of BMI in the assessment of undernutrition in older subjects: reflecting on practice. *Proc Nutr Soc.* 2005;64:313–317. http://journals.cambridge.org/action/displayAbstract?fromPage=online&aid=814076. Accessed December 27, 2010.

10. Centers for Disease Control and Prevention. CDC Growth Charts: United States. Body mass index-for-age percentiles: Boys, 2 to 20 years. http://www.cdc.gov/growthcharts/data/set2/chart%2015.pdf. Accessed January 10, 2011.

11. Centers for Disease Control and Prevention. CDC Growth Charts: United States. Body mass index-for-age percentiles: Girls, 2 to 20 years. http://www.cdc.gov/growthcharts/data/set2/chart%2016.pdf. Accessed January 10, 2011.

12. Barlow SE; the Expert Committee. Expert Committee recommendations regarding the prevention, assessment, and treatment of child and adolescent overweight and obesity: summary report. *Pediatrics.* 2007;120(Suppl 4): S164–S288.

13. National Heart, Lung and Blood Institute. Classification According to Waist Circumference. Guidelines on Overweight and Obesity: Electronic Textbook. http://www.nhlbi.nih.gov/guidelines/obesity/e_txtbk/txgd/4142.htm. Accessed January 10, 2011.

14. Zimmet P, Alberti KGMM, Kaufman F, Tajima N, Silink M, Arslanian S, Wong G, Bennett P, Shaw J, Caprio S; IDF Consensus Group. The metabolic syndrome in children and adolescents: an IDF consensus report. *Pediatric Diabetes*. 2007;8:299–306. http://www3.interscience.wiley.com/cgi-bin/fulltext/118545689/HTMLSTART. Accessed December 27, 2011.

15. Maffeis C, Pietrobelli A, Grezzani A, Provera S, Tatò L. Waist circumference and cardiovascular risk factors in prepubertal children. *Obes Res*. 2001;9:179–187.

16. Weiss R, Dziura J, Burgert TS, Tamporlane WV, Taksali SE, Yeckel CW, Allen K, Lopes M, Savoye M, Morrison J, Sherwin RS, Caprio S. Obesity and the metabolic syndrome in children and adolescents. *N Engl J Med*. 2004;350:2362–2374.

17. Cook S, Weitzman M, Auinger P, Nguyen M, Dietz WH. Prevalence of a metabolic syndrome phenotype in adolescents: findings from the third National Health and Nutrition Examination Survey, 1988–1994. *Arch Pediatr Adolesc Med*. 2003;157:821–827.

18. Ford ES, Ajani UA, Mokdad AH. The metabolic syndrome and concentrations of C-reactive protein among U.S. youth. *Diabetes Care*. 2005;28:878–881.

19. Angeli A, Minetto M, Dovio A, Paccotti P. The overtraining syndrome in athletes: a stress-related disorder. *J Endocrinol Invest*. 2004;27:603–612.

20. Smith LL. Cytokine hypothesis of overtraining: a physiological adaptation to excessive stress? *Med Sci Sports Exerc*. 2000;32:317–331.

21. Mackinnon LT. Chronic exercise training effects on immune function. *Med Sci Sports Exerc*. 2000;32(suppl): S369–S376.

22. Diagnosis and classification of diabetes mellitus. *Diabetes Care*. 2010;33(suppl):S62–S69.

23. Fody EP. Pancreatic function and gastrointestinal function. In: Bishop ML, Fody EP, Schoeff LE, eds. *Clinical Chemistry Techniques, Principles, Correlations*. 6th ed. Philadelphia, PA: Lippincott, Williams & Wilkins; 2010:651–672.

24. Institute of Medicine. *Dietary Reference Intakes for Vitamin A, Vitamin K, Arsenic, Boron, Chromium, Copper, Iodine, Iron, Manganese, Molybdenum, Nickel, Silicon, Vanadium, and Zinc*. Washington, DC: National Academies Press; 2001.

25. Table 9-2: Laboratory Measurements Commonly Used in the Evaluation of Iron Status. In: Institute of Medicine. *Dietary Reference Intakes for Vitamin A, Vitamin K, Arsenic, Boron, Chromium, Copper, Iodine, Iron, Manganese, Molybdenum, Nickel, Silicon, Vanadium, and Zinc*. Washington, DC: National Academies Press:302. http://www.nap.edu/openbook.php?record_id=10026&page=302#p2000560c9960302001 Accessed January 10, 2011.

26. Killip S, Bennett JM, Chambers MD. Iron deficiency anemia. *Am Fam Physician*. 2007;75:671–678. http://www.aafp.org/afp/2007/0301/p671.html. Accessed December 27, 2011.

27. Clarkson PM, Haymes EM. Exercise and mineral status of athletes: calcium, magnesium, phosphorus, and iron. *Med Sci Sports Exerc*. 1995;27:831–843.

28. Raunikar RA, Sabio H. Anemia in the adolescent athlete. *Am J Dis Child*. 1992;146:1201–1205.

29. Lampe JW, Slavin JL, Apple FS. Iron status of active women and the effect of running a marathon on bowel function and gastrointestinal blood loss. *Int J Sports Med*. 1991;12:173–179.

30. Fogelholm M. Inadequate iron status in athletes: an exaggerated problem? In: *Sports Nutrition: Minerals and Electrolytes*. Boca Raton, FL: CRC Press, 1995;81–95.

31. Beard J, Tobin B. Iron status and exercise. *Am J Clin Nutr*. 2000;72(suppl):594S–597S.

32. Brigham DE, Beard JL, Krimmel RS, Kenney WL. Changes in iron status during competitive season in female collegiate swimmers. *Nutrition*. 1993;9:418–422.

33. Institute of Medicine. *Dietary Reference Intakes for Thiamin, Riboflavin, Niacin, Vitamin B6, Folate, Vitamin B12, Pantothenic Acid, Biotin, and Choline*. Washington, DC: National Academies Press; 1998.

34. Bishop ML, Fody EP, Schoeff LE, eds. *Clinical Chemistry Techniques, Principles, Correlations*. 6th ed. Philadelphia, PA: Lippincott, Williams & Wilkins; 2010.

35. Grundy SM, Brewer HB Jr, Cleeman JI, Smith SC Jr, Lenfant C; American Heart Association; National Heart, Lung, and Blood Institute. Definition of metabolic syndrome: report of the National Heart, Lung, and Blood Institute/American Heart Association Conference on Scientific Issues Related to Definition. *Circulation.* 2004;109: 433–438. http://circ.ahajournals.org/cgi/content-nw/full/109/3/433/TBL1. Accessed December 27, 2010.

36. National Diabetes Information Clearinghouse (NDIC), National Institute of Diabetes and Digestive and Kidney Diseases (NIDDK), National Institutes of Health. Insulin Resistance and Prediabetes. http://www.diabetes.niddk .nih.gov/dm/pubs/insulinresistance. Accessed January 10, 2011.

37. Schoeller DA. Measurement of energy expenditure in free-living humans by using doubly labeled water. *J Nutr.* 1988;118:1278–1289.

38. Institute of Medicine. *Dietary Reference Intakes for Energy, Carbohydrate, Fiber, Fat, Fatty Acids, Cholesterol, Protein, and Amino Acids (Macronutrients).* Washington, DC: National Academies Pres; 2005. http://www.nap .edu/openbook.php?record_id=10490&page=107. Accessed January 10, 2011.

39. Hermann J. Drug-Nutrient Interactions Fact Sheet. Oklahoma Cooperative Extension Service T-3120, Division of Agricultural Sciences and Natural Resources. Oklahoma State University. http://pods.dasnr.okstate.edu/docushare/ dsweb/Get/Document-2458/T-3120web.pdf. Accessed January 10, 2011.

40. Drug Interaction Checker. Medscape Reference: Drugs, Diseases, and Procedures. http://reference.medscape .com/drug-interactionchecker. Accessed July 12, 2011.

41. NHANES Food Questionnaire. National Cancer Institute. http://riskfactor.cancer.gov/diet/FFQ.English.June0304 .pdf. Accessed January 10, 2011.

42. Dwyer J, Picciano MF, Raiten DJ, et al. Collection of food and dietary supplement intake data: what we eat in America. *J Nutr.* 2003;133(suppl):590S–600S. http://jn.nutrition.org/cgi/reprint/133/2/590S.pdf. Accessed January 10, 2011.

43. Dietary Interview. 24-hour Dietary Recall Interview. Centers for Disease Control and Prevention. National Center Health Statistics, NHANES. http://www.cdc.gov/nchs/data/nhanes/dietary.pdf. Accessed January 10, 2011.

44. Sebastian JG, Boosalis MG. Nutritional aspects of home health care. In: Martinson IN, Widmer AG, Protillo CJ, eds. *Home Health Care Nursing.* 2nd ed. Philadelphia, PA: WB Saunders, 2002:140–179.

45. Zimmerman GL, Olsen CG, Bosworth MF. A "stages of change" approach to helping patients change behavior. *Am Fam Physician.* 2000;61:1409–1416.

46. Spahn JM, Reeves RS, Kiem KS, LaQuatra I, Kellogg M, Jortberg B, Clark NA. State of the evidence regarding behavior change theories and strategies in nutrition counseling to facilitate health and food behavior change. *J Am Diet Assoc.* 2010;110:879–891.

47. Prochaska and DiClemente's Stages of Change Model. University of California Los Angeles (UCLA) Center for Human Nutrition. http://www.cellinteractive.com/ucla/physcian_ed/stages_change.html. Accessed January 10, 2011.

48. Rosenbloom C. Sports nutrition: applying ADA's Nutrition Care Process and Model to achieve quality care and outcomes for athletes. *SCAN'S PULSE.* 2005;24:10–17.

Chapter 9

ASSESSMENT OF BODY SIZE AND COMPOSITION

CHRISTOPHER M. MODLESKY, PhD

Introduction

The body is an elaborate structure consisting of many components that change with growth, development, physical activity, and aging. Monitoring these changes assists health professionals in their assessment of nutritional status, physical fitness, and disease risk. Specifically, measurement of body size allows for tracking the changes in the physical dimensions of the body, whereas measurement of body composition allows for following changes in its gross chemical composition (ie, bone, fat-free soft tissue, and fat mass). Excess body weight, especially body fat, often reflects high energy intake, reduced levels of physical activity, or a combination thereof, and can contribute to poor nutritional status and physical performance. Adiposity is also believed to increase disease risk because it is positively associated with cardiovascular disease, diabetes mellitus, and other chronic diseases (1). Extremely low body weight and low body fat reflect disease states associated with undernutrition, such as anorexia nervosa and diseases associated with poor musculoskeletal status, such as osteoporosis. The purposes of this chapter are to (*a*) review the application of body size and body composition measurement in adults, and (*b*) describe the most common and the most accurate measurement techniques.

Assessment of Body Size

With respect to physical performance, there are advantages and disadvantages associated with being a particular body size, which are evident in different sports. Taller people tend to be successful in sports in which reaching a level high above the ground is required, such as basketball and volleyball. Shorter people have an advantage in sports that require rotation of the body around an axis, such as gymnastics. Within team sports a particular position may dictate a size advantage. In football a large body mass is advantageous to offensive linemen, giving them the size and power to move players in their path. Conversely, wide receivers tend to be much lighter and to have a lower percentage of body fat than linemen, allowing them to run at great speeds.

With the exception of very low body weight, disease risk increases with body weight at a given height (2). This adverse relationship between body weight and disease has led to the search for an ideal or desirable body weight.

Height-Weight Tables

Insurance companies initially developed height-weight tables to provide, for given heights, gross weight ranges associated with the greatest longevity and lowest mortality rate (3). Although they are widely used, these tables have been scrutinized because the data collection procedures were flawed and the sample used to create the tables was not representative of the general population (4,5). Moreover, a weight for height gives no insight into a person's body composition or body fat distribution (5). In some instances, healthy individuals who are highly muscular might be considered overweight and at risk for disease, whereas individuals with a high proportion of body fat but a body weight in the desirable range would be considered at low risk for disease. Despite their flaws, height-weight tables may be useful if used in conjunction with other markers of disease risk—such as diet, blood lipid profile, and anthropometric measurements—to identify individuals at risk for chronic disease.

Body Mass Index

Body mass index (BMI) is a measure of body size (based on height and weight) that is used to assess disease risk. In people with a BMI more than 20, morbidity increases as BMI increases (2). In contrast, a very low BMI (< 18.5) is associated with undernutrition, anemia, menstrual irregularities, and a higher risk for skeletal fracture (6). Furthermore, it may be a sign that someone suffers from anorexia nervosa. Similar to height-weight tables, there are several versions of BMI that are commonly used. The most widely accepted BMI is the Quetelet Index in which weight (kg) is divided by height squared (m^2). BMI can also be calculated as follows:

$$BMI = [weight\ (lb)/height\ (in)^2] \times 704.5$$

BMI is used more frequently than height-weight tables to assess disease risk in the general population for the following reasons:

- BMI is moderately correlated with body fat percentage ($r = 0.58$) (7).
- BMI is readily used for comparisons among men, women, children, and individuals of different heights.
- BMI reflects health status, with high and very low values associated with health detriments.

However, similar to height-weight tables, BMI is insensitive to varying degrees of fat mass, fat-free mass, and fat distribution (3). This can be a particular problem in athletes. For example, a very large physically fit male athlete measuring 76 inches (1.93 meters) in height and weighing 250 lb (113.6 kg) with a lean body (< 15% fat) has a BMI of 30.5. Such a value would be considered overweight or obese by any BMI recommendations currently available. On the other hand, a sedentary woman with a poor diet, measuring 65 inches (1.65 meters) in height, and weighing 140 lb (63.4 kg), with a high percentage of body fat (40%) by any standard would have an optimal BMI of 23.4.

Several BMI ranges have been proposed to identify healthy and at-risk individuals (8,9). However, some factors, such as age and race, make it difficult to define a desirable BMI range. Some studies suggest the recommended BMI ranges should increase with age (10–12) and should be higher in African Americans than in whites (13,14). After a careful review of the scientific literature, the National Heart, Lung, and Blood Institute (NHLBI) Obesity Education Initiative Expert Panel on the Identification, Evaluation, and Treatment of Overweight and Obesity in Adults (2) has recommended the following BMI ranges:

- Underweight: < 18.5
- Normal: 18.5–24.9
- Overweight: 25.0–29.9
- Class I obesity: 30.0–34.9
- Class II obesity: 35–39.9
- Extreme obesity: ≥ 40

Moreover, the panel recommended that BMI should not be used alone, but instead evaluated in conjunction with other markers such as fat distribution, when assessing health risk and making weight loss or weight gain recommendations (2).

Waist Circumference and Waist-to-Hip Ratio

Fat distribution has been identified as an important marker of disease risk (15,16). For instance, individuals exhibiting a larger proportion of fat in the upper half of the body (android obesity or apple shape) are at greater risk for health complications than individuals having a larger proportion of fat in the lower half (gynoid obesity or pear shape). More specifically, deep abdominal (visceral) fat is a strong independent predictor of disease (15,16). Diseases associated with android obesity include hypertension, hypercholesterolemia, diabetes, cardiovascular disease, metabolic syndrome, and gallbladder disease (17,18), with women also having a greater risk for oligomenorrhea (8) and breast cancer (9).

One of the easiest ways to assess upper-body fat distribution and obesity type is to measure waist circumference. The girth of the abdomen is highly correlated ($r = 0.77$ to 0.87) with deep abdominal fat measured using computed tomography, an expensive technique that provides precise measurement of deep and subcutaneous adipose tissue (15,16). Another approach is to combine waist circumference with hip circumference to calculate waist-to-hip ratio. A higher waist-to-hip ratio reflects android obesity and is associated with greater disease risk. Risk increases steeply when waist-to-hip ratio is more than 0.95 in men or more than 0.8 in women (19). However, because waist circumference provides a better measure of deep abdominal fat than waist-to-hip ratio (15,16), measurement of waist circumference is preferred when assessing risk of disease (2,16).

Federal Clinical Guidelines

Although height-weight tables, BMI, and waist circumference each give some insight into disease risk, a combined approach can provide more definitive information. Accordingly, the NHLBI released guidelines for the identification, evaluation, and treatment of overweight and obesity in adults (2). These guidelines were developed based on a careful assessment of the obesity-related scientific literature. Assessment of overweight and obesity involves three important measures: BMI, waist circumference, and risk factors for diseases and conditions associated with obesity. All individuals 18 years of age and older with a BMI of 25 or more are considered at risk for several chronic diseases. Treatment is recommended for individuals who are classified as overweight (BMI = 25–29.9) or obese (BMI ≥ 30) who have two or more risk factors (see Box 9.1) (2,20). Treatment is also recommended for men with a waist circumference more than 40 inches

BOX 9.1   Risk Factors to Consider Before Recommending Obesity Treatment

Disease Conditions
- Established coronary disease
- Other atherosclerotic diseases (peripheral artery disease, abdominal aortic aneurysm, symptomatic carotid artery disease)
- Type 2 diabetes mellitus
- Sleep apnea

Other Obesity-Related Diseases
- Gynecological abnormalities
- Osteoarthritis
- Gallstones and their complications
- Stress incontinence

Cardiovascular Risk Factors
- Cigarette smoking
- Hypertension (systolic blood pressure $\geq$ 140 mmHg or diastolic blood pressure $\geq$ 90 mmHg, or patient is taking antihypertensive agents)
- High-risk low-density lipoprotein cholesterol ($\geq$ 160 mg/dL)
- Low high-density lipoprotein cholesterol (< 40 mg/dL)*
- Impaired fasting glucose (110 to 125 mg/dL)
- Family history of premature coronary heart disease (definite myocardial infarction or sudden death in father or other male first-degree relative $\leq$ 55 years of age, or in mother or other female first-degree relative $\leq$ 65 years of age)
- Age (men $\geq$ 45 years; women $\geq$ 55 years or postmenopausal)

Other Risk Factors
- Physical inactivity
- High serum triglycerides (> 200 mg/dL)

Source: Adapted from National Heart, Lung, and Blood Institute. *Clinical Guidelines on the Identification, Evaluation, and Treatment of Overweight and Obesity in Adults: The Evidence Report.* Bethesda, MD: National Institutes of Health; 1998. Data marked with * are from the National Heart, Lung, and Blood Institute. *Third Report of the National Cholesterol Education Program (NCEP) Expert Panel on Detection, Evaluation, and Treatment of High Blood Cholesterol in Adults (Adult Treatment Panel III).* Bethesda, MD: National Heart, Lung, and Blood Institute; 2001.

(102 cm) and women with a waist circumference more than 35 inches (88 cm). Because waist circumference cutpoints lose their predictive power in clients with a BMI of 35 or more, the latter guidelines are appropriate only for those with a BMI ranging from 25 to 34.9 (2).

Although overweight and obesity have received substantial attention, being underweight (BMI < 18.5) is also a substantial problem. Athletes involved in sports that have an aesthetic component (21) or athletes involved in endurance sports that require translocation of the body are most susceptible to weight-restriction practices and low body weight (22). Although low body weight is associated with optimal health and may enhance performance in certain sports, a body weight that is too low is associated with nutritional deficiency, menstrual irregularities (ie, amenorrhea), anemia, and low bone mass (22,23). Osteopenia, an early stage of osteoporosis, is fairly prevalent in athletes involved in sports with a marked emphasis on body weight (24,25). Hence, avoiding very low body weight (BMI < 18.5) is a reasonable recommendation.

Body Size Measurement Techniques

Standing Height

Standing height is one of the most fundamental physical measures used to quantify body size. In addition to being used in combination with body weight to screen for disease risk, it is used to detect growth deficiencies in children and skeletal diseases, such as osteoporosis, that lead to a significant reduction in standing height in the elderly.

Equipment

A stadiometer (a vertical measurement board or rod with a horizontal headpiece) may be used to measure standing height using this procedure (26):

1. The client is measured while standing on a flat horizontal surface that is at a right angle to the stadiometer.
2. The client should wear as little clothing as possible to facilitate optimal body position, and should be barefoot or wearing thin socks.
3. The head, upper back (or shoulder blades), buttocks, and heels should be positioned against the vertical board or rod of the stadiometer. If a reasonable natural stance cannot be maintained while these body parts are touching the vertical board, the person can be positioned so that only the buttocks and heels or head are touching the board.
4. Weight should be distributed evenly on both feet with heels together, arms to the side, palms facing the thighs, legs straight, and the head in the Frankfort Horizontal Plane (ie, looking straight ahead).
5. Before measurement, a deep breath should be taken and held until the headpiece is pressed against the head (enough to compress the hair) and measurement is attained.
6. Measurement should be made to the nearest 0.5 cm or 0.125 inch while viewing the measure at eye level to the headboard.

Measuring height using a tape measure against the wall is not recommended. If it is done, a wall that does not have a baseboard and is not in contact with a carpeted floor should be used (26).

Body Weight

Body weight is another fundamental physical measurement used to quantify body size. Periodic measurement of body weight is important because extremes are associated with nutritional, metabolic, and cardiovascular disorders. Body weight is also used to estimate energy expenditure and body composition.

Equipment

A beam-balance scale with movable weights may be used to measure body weight using this procedure (26):

1. The scale should be on a hard, flat, horizontal surface.
2. Before measurement, the scale should be calibrated to zero.

3. It is important to calibrate the scale monthly or quarterly, and whenever the scale is moved. Measurement accuracy can be verified using standard weights.
4. Ideally, weight should be measured before consumption of the first meal and after the bladder has been emptied.
5. When being measured, the client should wear as little clothing as possible.
6. The client should stand still over the center of the scale platform with weight evenly distributed between both feet.
7. Weight is determined to the nearest 0.5 lb or 0.2 kg using the movable beam. Body weight in pounds divided by 2.2 yields weight in kilograms (1 kg = 2.2 lb).

A calibrated digital scale can also be used to assess body weight.

If the person being measured cannot stand without assistance, a beam chair scale or a bed scale can be used. When measuring an infant, a leveled pan scale with a pan at least 100 cm in length is recommended (26).

Body Circumference

Body circumference measurements are used to estimate muscularity (27), fat patterning (28), nutritional status, changes in the physical dimensions of a child during growth, and changes in adults during weight-loss or weight-gain programs. When combined with measurements of skinfold thickness, circumference measurements can also estimate adipose tissue and the underlying muscle and bone (29).

Equipment
A flexible but inelastic tape measure may be used to measure body circumference using this procedure (28):

1. The zero end of the tape measure is held in one hand while the other end of the tape is held in the other hand.
2. The areas being measured should be free of clothing or covered by as little clothing as possible.
3. All circumference measurements, other than the head and neck, should be taken with the plane of the tape around the body part perpendicular to the long axis of the segment being measured.
4. When measuring the head, the tape should compress the hair and the soft tissue of the scalp. For all circumference measurements other than the head, the tape should be snug but not tight enough to compress the soft tissue.
5. Measurements should be recorded to the nearest 0.5 cm or 0.125 inch.

Locations for circumference measurements of the head, neck, mid-upper arm, wrist, chest, waist, hips, and thigh are found in Figures 9.1 through 9.10.

Body Breadth

Body breadth measurements are useful in the determination of body type and frame size (29). Somatotyping is one body-typing technique in which body breadths, along with circumference measures, are used to categorize individuals into three distinct categories (27):

- Endomorphy: relative fatness and leanness
- Mesomorphy: relative musculoskeletal development per unit of height
- Ectomorphy: relative linearity

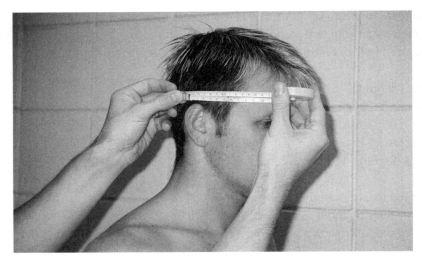

FIGURE 9.1   Head circumference is taken just above the eyebrows and posteriorly so that maximum circumference is measured.

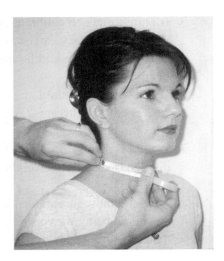

FIGURE 9.2   Neck circumference is measured just below the laryngeal prominence (Adam's apple) with the head in the Frankfort Horizontal Plane (looking straight ahead).

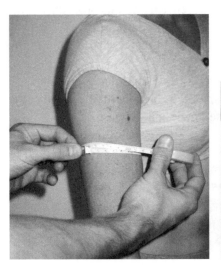

FIGURE 9.3   Mid-arm circumference of the upper arm is measured midway between the acromion process of the scapula and the olecranon process of the ulna.

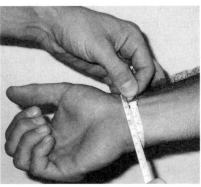

FIGURE 9.4   Wrist circumference is measured just distal to the styloid processes of the radius and ulna.

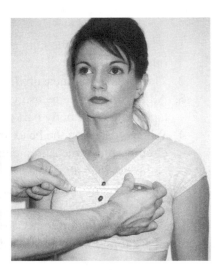

FIGURE 9.5   Chest circumference is measured horizontally at the 4th costosternal joints (at the level of the 6th ribs), after normal expiration.

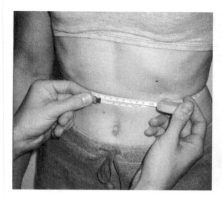

FIGURE 9.6 Waist circumference is measured just above the uppermost border of the iliac crests (ie, hip bones).

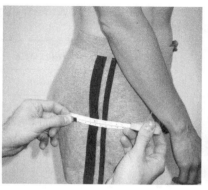

FIGURE 9.7 Hip (buttocks) circumference is measured over the maximal circumference of the buttocks.

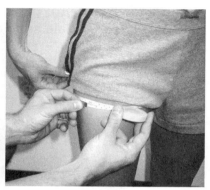

FIGURE 9.8 Proximal thigh circumference is measured horizontally, just distal to the gluteal fold.

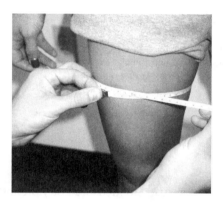

FIGURE 9.9 Mid-thigh circumference is measured midway between the inguinal crease and the proximal border of the patella.

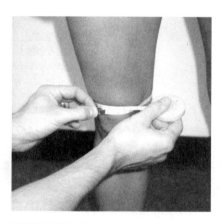

FIGURE 9.10 Distal thigh circumference is measured just proximal to the femoral epicondyles.

Specific somatotypes associated with athletic success have been identified for some, but not all, sports. For instance, a higher degree of endomorphy has been linked to lower performance scores in elite female gymnasts (30) and moderately trained distance runners (31). Unfortunately, there are no somatotype guidelines for specific athletic groups. On the other hand, assessing frame size can help determine a desirable weight for a given height and can help determine appropriate lean weight gains in athletes and in malnourished individuals. Frame size can be categorized using Table 9.1, which was developed based on the first and second National Health and Nutrition Examination Survey data sets (32).

TABLE 9.1 Frame Size by Elbow Breadth (cm) of US Male and Female Adults[a]

| Age, y | Frame Size | | |
	Small	Medium	Large
Males			
18–24	≤ 6.6	> 6.6 and < 7.7	≥ 7.7
25–34	≤ 6.7	> 6.7 and < 7.9	≥ 7.9
35–44	≤ 6.7	> 6.7 and < 8.0	≥ 8.0
45–54	≤ 6.7	> 6.7 and < 8.1	≥ 8.1
55–64	≤ 6.7	> 6.7 and < 8.1	≥ 8.1
65–74	≤ 6.7	> 6.7 and < 8.1	≥ 8.1
Females			
18–24	≤ 5.6	> 5.6 and < 6.5	≥ 6.5
25–34	≤ 5.7	> 5.7 and < 6.8	≥ 6.8
35–44	≤ 5.7	> 5.7 and < 7.1	≥ 7.1
45–54	≤ 5.7	> 5.7 and < 7.2	≥ 7.2
55–64	≤ 5.8	> 5.8 and < 7.2	≥ 7.2
65–74	≤ 5.8	> 5.8 and < 7.2	≥ 7.2

[a]Derived from NHANES I and II combined data sets.
Source: Reprinted with permission from Frisancho R. New standards of weight and body composition by frame size and height for assessment of nutritional status of adults and the elderly. *Am J Clin Nutr.* 1984;40:806–819. Copyright © *Am J Clin Nutr.* American Society for Nutrition.

Procedure

A standard anthropometer, sliding caliper, or spreading caliper may be used to measure body breadths using this procedure (29):

1. The client being measured should wear as little clothing as possible to facilitate identification of measurement sites.
2. Using the tips of the fingers, identify the bony landmarks of the area to be measured.
3. Using both hands, hold the anthropometer or caliper so that the tips of the index fingers are adjacent to the projecting blades.
4. Position the blades of the anthropometer or sliding caliper at the bony landmarks.
5. Apply enough pressure to the blades so that the underlying skin, fat, and muscle contribute minimally to the measurement.
6. Measurements are made to the nearest 0.1 cm or 0.125 inch.

To minimize experimenter bias, measurements should be made sequentially, such that all sites are measured once and then the sequence is repeated until a minimum of three measurements are made at each site. The mean measurement at each site is recorded.

Proper measurement of the elbow and ankle breadth is demonstrated in Figures 9.11 and 9.12. Elbow breadth, regarded as the best marker of frame size, can also be measured using a Frameter (5) (see Figure 9.13) (29).

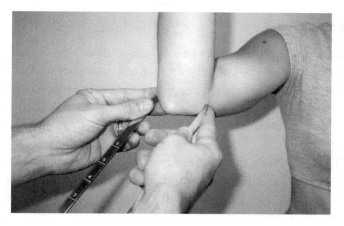

FIGURE 9.11 Measurement of elbow breadth using a standard anthropometer. The measurement is taken at the epicondyles of the humerus.

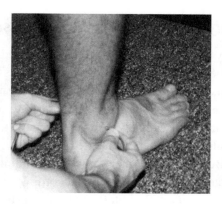

FIGURE 9.12 Measurement of ankle breadth, using a spreading caliper, taken at the maximum distance between the most medial extension of the medial malleolus and the most lateral extension of the lateral malleolus in the same horizontal plane.

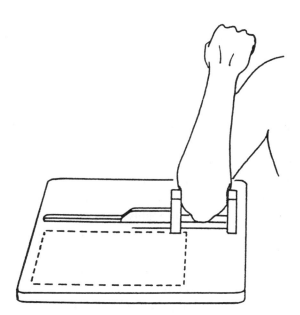

FIGURE 9.13 Elbow breadth measured using a Frameter. Reprinted with permission from Lohman TG, Roche AF, Martorell R, eds. *Anthropometric Standardization Reference Manual.* Champaign, IL: Human Kinetics; 1988, by permission of TG Lohman.

Assessment of Body Composition

Although height-weight and BMI charts are used to determine appropriate weights and to assess disease risk, they have poor sensitivity for classifying body composition (5,33). Body composition is more closely tied to disease risk than are anthropometric measurements (33), with a higher body fat percentage related to increased risk of metabolic and cardiovascular diseases (34).

Body Composition and Disease Risk

Many of the adverse conditions associated with obesity are linked to excess amounts of total body fatness, but the actual contribution of body fatness to disease risk has yet to be determined. Our poor understanding of this complex issue is attributed to a paucity of large, prospective, epidemiological randomized studies that use the most accurate techniques to assess body composition (33). Further, causal associations with chronic diseases likely take years to detect, making it unclear whether changes in body composition precede or follow the onset of disease (33).

Because of the uncertainty surrounding the role of total body fatness in disease risk, the development of standards has been difficult. According to Lohman (35), the mean body fat percentage is 15% in men and 25% in women. Body fat values of 10% to 22% in men and 20% to 32% in women are generally considered satisfactory (35). However, the data supporting these values have not been clearly defined (2). Furthermore, the most accessible methods used to assess body fat are generally limited. Until more research examining the relationship between body composition and disease risk is conducted, the use of body fat percentage as a marker of disease risk should be viewed with caution.

An increasing amount of evidence suggests the distribution rather than the absolute amount of fat in the body is more predictive of disease risk, with a higher concentration of fat in the intra-abdominal region associated with a higher risk for metabolic and cardiovascular diseases (36). Moreover, a higher concentration of fat within and around skeletal muscle is an independent predictor of type 2 diabetes (37,38). Although it is important to assess the distribution of body fat, the most accurate methods (ie, magnetic resonance imaging and computed tomography) are expensive, have limited availability, and require tedious processing procedures.

Body Composition and Performance

Body composition is related to athletic performance, especially in sports that require translocation of the body horizontally (ie, running) or vertically (ie, jumping) (39). Excess body fat is detrimental because it adds to the load carried by the body (ie, body mass) without contributing to the body's force-producing capacity. Furthermore, a greater metabolic cost is incurred, limiting prolonged performance (40–42).

Specific body composition recommendations for athletes have yet to be determined, although ranges for different sports have been published (43). Because each athlete probably has a fat percentage and body weight at which he or she performs best, it may be more appropriate to use the ranges as a guide but identify specific levels of fat and fat-free mass that are optimal for a particular athlete.

Body composition can also be used to monitor the health of an athlete and to track compositional changes after weight loss or gain during training. Often, when an athlete is trying to lose weight during a training program that incorporates resistance training, body weight may not change but an increase in fat-free mass and a decrease in fat mass are likely. Unless body composition is accurately assessed, these positive changes may go unnoticed. Even if body composition is assessed, small changes may not be detected using the most widely available techniques (44,45), and large changes may be detected but the amount of change may be inaccurate (46,47).

Body composition differs from one athlete to another, but some athletes believe that extremely low levels of body fat are necessary for success in their sport. On the contrary, very low body fat levels can have deleterious effects on health and physical performance. Minimum levels have not been clearly defined for most sports, but body fat percentages less than 5% in men and less than 12% in women are generally not recommended (43). When considering minimum body fat percentage values, it is important to note that error is associated with all methods of assessment. Under the best conditions, most methods still have an error of 3% to 4% body mass (34,48,49). Therefore, a body fat percentage may actually be less or more than reported. For example, a body fat of 13% may actually be 9% to 10% or even less, which is a dangerously low level in females. The margin of error associated with body composition assessment techniques must be explained to athletes. To account for the error and to safeguard against reaching a body fat percentage that is too low, a more conservative approach would be to increase the lower limit a few percentage points. For example, instead of a lower limit of 5% fat, a limit of 8% would be a safer recommendation.

Body Composition Measurement Techniques

The composition of the human body can be described using several different classification systems, such as those based on body tissue (muscle, adipose, nervous, connective, etc) and chemical (fat, water, protein, mineral, etc) makeup. Methods that produce the most accurate measures of tissue or chemical composition tend to have poor accessibility, a high expense, and extensive processing procedures. Methods that are more accessible, inexpensive, and require little analysis time are generally less accurate. The following section reviews some of the different methods used to assess body composition, including their advantages and disadvantages.

Criterion Methods of Body Composition

Providing the most accurate estimates of human body components are criterion (or gold standard) methods of body composition assessment, against which other methods are compared. Three techniques regarded as criterion methods of body composition assessment are magnetic resonance imaging (MRI), computed tomography (CT), and multicomponent models.

Magnetic Resonance Imaging and Computed Tomography

MRI and CT are imaging techniques used to estimate whole-body and regional adipose, muscle, bone, and nervous tissue (50). Magnetic resonance is based on the interaction among nuclei of hydrogen atoms, which are abundant in all biological tissues, and the magnetic fields generated and controlled by MRI instrumentation (51). CT uses x-ray to produce images of the different tissues in the body. Although both techniques have been shown to provide accurate and reliable estimates of body composition (52), their high expense, limited availability, and tedious processing procedures, as well as the high radiation exposure associated with CT, limits their use to research and clinical studies.

Multicomponent Models

There are basically two types of multicomponent models: (*a*) elaborate models based on in vivo measurement of the elemental constituents within the body, using in vivo neutron activation analysis (IVNAA); and (*b*) simpler, less expensive chemical models based on the in vivo measurement of water and/or mineral (bone) and body density.

Although IVNAA is the most accurate body composition technique, yielding measurements of body fat percentage within 1% body mass (53), its extreme expense and radiation exposure limit its use and availability. The simpler chemical multicomponent models are slightly less accurate than the IVNAA model, but they are acceptable criterion methods. The four-component (ie, water, mineral, protein, and fat) chemical model, in which body water, mineral, and density are assessed, measures body fat percentage within 1.5% body mass (53). Although a three-component model, in which body water and density are assessed, involves measurement of one less body component than the four-component model (ie, body mineral is not

TABLE 9.2   Percent Body Fat Equations Based on Two-, Three-, and Four-Component Models

No. of Components (Source)	Equation
2—body density (Siri [56])	% Body fat = $(495/D_b) - 450$
2—body density (Brozek et al [57])	% Body fat = $(457/D_b) - 414.2$
2—body water	% Body fat = [water (kg)/weight (kg)]/0.73
3 (Modlesky et al [55])	% Body fat = $(2.1176/D_b) - 0.78W - 1.351$
4 (Lohman [58])	% Body fat = $(2.747/D_b) - (0.714W) + (1.146M) - 2.0503$

Abbreviations: D_b, body density (g/cm^3); M, mineral fraction of body mass; W, water fraction of body mass.

measured), the loss in accuracy is minimal (54,55). Three- and four-component models are frequently used by scientists to accurately assess body composition and to validate simpler, more accessible body composition techniques. Percentage fat equations based on the three- and four-component models are presented in Table 9.2 (55–58).

Despite the advances with multicomponent models, a paucity of studies have used them to assess the accuracy of the simpler, less expensive, and more accessible body composition techniques (55,59–63). The accuracy of the simpler techniques will remain limited until they are validated against the criterion methods.

Dual-energy X-ray Absorptiometry

Dual-energy x-ray absorptiometry (DXA), derived from single and dual photon absorptiometry, was originally developed to assess the bone mineral content and areal density. The technology is based on the x-ray energy attenuation properties of bone mineral and soft tissue (64). X-ray energy transmitted through the client is attenuated (lost) in proportion to the material's composition and thickness, and thickness of the components within the material. Bone mineral, because it has a much higher density, attenuates an x-ray beam to a greater degree than soft tissue. Similarly, soft tissue is differentiated into fat and fat-free tissue based on their different attenuation properties. Measurements are made while the client is lying supine on the DXA table. Low dose x-rays are passed through the client in the posterior to anterior position. Older pencil-beam systems pass a thin x-ray beam through the body side to side, traveling head to toe in 0.6- to 1.0-cm increments (65). Pencil-beam instruments usually scan the body in 12 to 15 minutes. Newer fan-beam systems pass an x-ray beam across a larger area and, thus, can scan the entire body in as little as 2½ minutes. Most total body scans require between 2½ to 15 minutes, depending on the instrumentation. Up to 30 minutes may be required with larger subjects when they are scanned on older pencil-beam instruments and a slower scan mode is used.

Accuracy

Compared with a four-component model, the accuracy of body fat assessment from DXA seems to be as good as or slightly better than hydrodensitometry in college-aged athletes and nonathletes (less than ± 3% body fat percentage points) (66), but it is questionable in children (59,60) (unless child-specific software is used [67]) and in the elderly (59,61).

Advantages

DXA is a fairly quick, comfortable, and noninvasive procedure that has good accuracy for assessing body fat in athletes and in the general population. It provides measurements of three body components (bone mineral, fat-free soft tissue, and fat masses) vs two components from most other methods (fat and fat-free masses). Moreover, it provides regional estimates of body composition (arms, legs, head, and trunk).

Disadvantages

Although the cost of a single DXA scan is somewhat reasonable (approximately $85 to $115 depending on the region of the country), the cost of a DXA system is very expensive, ranging in price between $60,000 and $200,000. Furthermore, many states require a licensed x-ray technician or technician with a limited scope x-ray license to perform the tests and appropriate medical supervision. In addition to these major limitations, the instrument is not portable or mobile.

Hydrodensitometry (Underwater Weighing)

This densitometric technique for body composition assessment relies on a two-component model, in which the body is divided into fat and fat-free components. Assuming the density of the fat component (~0.9 g/cm^3), fat-free component (~1.1 g/cm^3), and the total body are known, the contribution of each component to the total can be calculated. The assumed density of fat is derived from 20 subcutaneous and abdominal adipose tissue samples taken from three men and two women (68), whereas the density of the fat-free component is based on the dissection of animals (69,70), three male human cadavers (57), and the assumed densities of fat, mineral, protein, and water (56). Researchers and clinicians can determine body density by dividing body weight measured on land by body volume measured using underwater weighing (ie, water displacement) or plethysmography (ie, air displacement) techniques. Based on these assumptions and the measurement of total body density, percentage body fat can be calculated using equations developed by Siri (56) or Brozek et al (57) found in Table 9.2. Percentage body fat equations based on more advanced three- and four-component models are also reported in Table 9.2 (55,58).

Until approximately 20 years ago, underwater weighing was considered one of the gold standard techniques of body composition assessment against which all other methods were compared. Although measurements of body composition have become more sophisticated with multiple body components (ie water, mineral, protein, and fat) or body tissues (ie, muscle, adipose, and bone) being examined, underwater weighing alone is an acceptable method of body composition assessment. The technique is based on Archimedes's principle that a body immersed in a fluid is acted on by a buoyancy force equal to the volume of the fluid displaced (71). Because fat is less dense than fat-free tissue, a greater proportion of body fat will cause a person to be more buoyant (float) and weigh less in water. Conversely, a greater proportion of fat-free tissue will cause the person to be less buoyant (sink) and weigh more in water. This contrast is demonstrated in Figure 9.14 (72). The clients are the same height and weight, but the client on the left has a higher body density and a lower percentage body fat.

Equipment

The following equipment is needed for hydrodensitometry:

1. Underwater weighing tank, pool, or hot tub 4 to 5 feet deep
2. 9-kg Chatillion autopsy scale or a digital scale with 10-g increments (A 15-kg scale with 25-g increments may be necessary for very obese subjects.)
3. Overhead beam or diving board from which the scale can hang

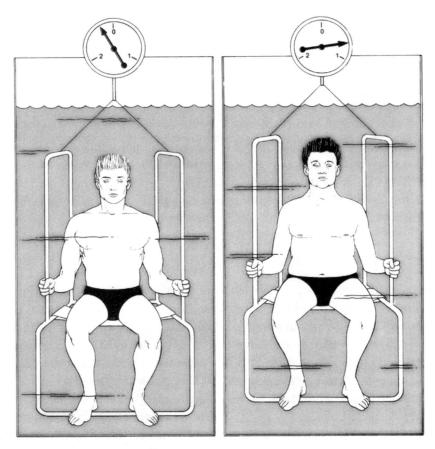

FIGURE 9.14   Underwater weighing of two men who have the same height and weight but different degrees of density and fatness. The man on the left has a greater body density and lower percentage body fat. Reprinted from Powers SK, Howley HT. *Exercise Physiology: Theory and Application to Fitness and Performance.* Dubuque, IA: William C. Brown Publishers; 1990, with permission from The McGraw Hill Companies. All rights reserved.

4. Chair (32 inches wide with a back height of 24 inches) made from ¾- to 1-inch plastic pipe with holes drilled in the pipe to avoid air entrapment and a belt secured to the chair to keep the individual in the chair while submerged under water. This is especially important for obese subjects. Because the density of fat is less than the density of water, subjects with a high body fat percentage will have a tendency to float in the water.
5. Weights to give the chair a minimum weight in the water of 3 kg (4 to 6 kg with the obese)
6. Thermometer to record the temperature of the water during measurement

Procedure

The procedure for hydrodensitometry is as follows (73):

1. The chair, weights, and belt secured to the chair hang from the scale into the tank.
2. The water in the tank should be filtered, chlorinated, 89° to 95° F (~32° to 35° C), and range from shoulder to chin height when the client is sitting in the chair.

3. When placed in the water, the weight of the chair minus the weight of the client should be at least 3 kg. A higher weight (4 to 6 kg) may be required for obese people. These weights can be obtained by adding weights to the chair.

4. Hydrodensitometry should be done after a 2- to 3-hour fast of food and drink. Foods that can cause an excess amount of intestinal gas should be avoided approximately 12 hours before the measurement.

5. After a bowel movement and urinary void (if necessary), the person is weighed on land while wearing only a bathing suit.

7. The client enters the tank of water and submerges up to the chin without touching the chair. The weight of the chair, any attached weights, and the belt that is secured to the chair is then recorded.

8. The person is instructed to sit in the chair that is suspended from the scale and to secure himself or herself to the chair via the belt. The feet should be positioned on the front bar of the chair, which serves as a foot rest.

9. Just as a maximal exhalation is being completed, full submersion under the water is accomplished by slowly leaning forward. Upon submersion, the person must remain still in the chair with feet on the foot rest and hands on the side rails of the chair.

10. While the subject is underwater, the measurer should keep one hand on the scale to steady it and observe the weight of the person underwater to the nearest 10 g.

11. The test should be repeated 10 times and the final three trials averaged (73).

12. During each trial, temperature of the water should be recorded.

13. The density of the water during measurement can be determined using Table 9.3 (74,75).

14. Because some air remains in the lungs after forced exhalation, the residual lung volume of air (RLV, in liters) must be measured or estimated (measurement is preferred). The RLV can be measured using nitrogen washout, oxygen dilution, or helium dilution techniques before, after, or during the underwater weighing procedure. Measurement during the procedure is preferred. Residual lung volume can be estimated using the following equations (76):

$$RLV_{males} = (0.017 \times Age) + (0.06858 \times Ht) - 3.447$$

$$RLV_{females} = (0.009 \times Age) + (0.08128 \times Ht) - 3.9$$

Where: Age = age in years and Ht = height in inches.

TABLE 9.3 Water Density at Different Temperatures

Water Temperature, °Celsius	Water Density, g/cm³
28	0.996264
29	0.995976
30	0.995678
31	0.995372
32	0.995057
33	0.994734
34	0.994403
35	0.994063

Source: Data are from references 74 and 75.

15. Body density (D_b) is calculated using the following equation:

$$D_b = \frac{W_a}{\dfrac{(W_a - W_w)}{D_w} - (RLV + GV)}$$

Where: W_a = weight in air (kg); W_w = weight of the person, chair, belt, and weights in the water (kg) minus the weight of the chair, belt, and weights recorded in step 6 (kg); D_w = density of the water at the time of measurement (kg/L); GV = an estimate of gastrointestinal volume during underwater weighing (assumed to be 0.1 liter).

16. Body fat percentage is calculated using the Siri (56) or Brozek et al (57) equation (see Table 9.2), which yield almost identical estimates of percentage body fat (ie, within 1% body fat), except in individuals who are obese (ie, % fat > 30%) and very lean (ie, % fat < 5%).

Accuracy

The accuracy of percentage body fat from underwater weighing is approximately ± 4% in the general population (56) and ± 2.7% in the population from which the Siri and Brozek et al equations were developed (young white males) (77). Thus, in the general population, a 20% estimate of fat from underwater weighing typically varies between 16% and 24%.

Advantages

Underwater weighing is an established technique for assessing body composition and it has good accuracy.

Disadvantages

The equations typically used to estimate percentage fat from body density yield reasonably accurate measurements, especially in young white males. However, the density of the fat-free mass can stray markedly in population groups other than young white males and result in larger error. For instance, a lower density of the fat-free mass has been reported in men with extreme muscularity (55,78). Other equations have been proposed for African Americans (79) and women (34); however, there is evidence that the Siri and Brozek et al equations are appropriate for these groups (78,80,81).

Air Displacement Plethysmography

Air displacement plethysmography is another technique used to assess body composition by body density. The BOD POD Body Composition System, an air-displacement plethysmograph, seems to have overcome many of the problems experienced with its predecessors. The BOD POD determines body volume from air displacement and body fat percentage is calculated using the Siri (56) or Brozek et al (57) equations (see Table 9.2).

Accuracy

Fields et al evaluated the accuracy of body composition estimates from the BOD POD (82). The few studies that compared body composition estimates from the BOD POD with estimates from a four-component model suggested that the BOD POD underestimates percentage body fat by 2% to 3% in adults and children; however, Fields et al concluded that the BOD POD provides valid and reliable estimates of body composition in the general population.

Advantages

Assessment of body composition via the BOD POD is comfortable and involves very little stress (no submersion in water or pinching is required). Moreover, the procedure is fairly quick, requiring only approximately 10 minutes.

Disadvantages

The cost of a single body composition assessment using the BOD POD is reasonable (between $20 and $100), but the cost of a system is expensive, ranging between $28,000 and $44,000. There is also an infant model (PeaPod) that costs just less than $100,000. It also lacks portability, requiring a small space to house the chamber and other system components.

Hydrometry

Hydrometry is another technique for body composition assessment. Until the early 1990s, it was considered a gold standard in body composition assessment. This technique also involves a two-component model in which water is assumed to represent approximately 73% of the body's fat-free component. Thus, a higher amount of body water indicates a higher amount of fat-free tissue. Total body water is measured by the dilution of a known quantity of nonmetabolizable tracer (eg, deuterium oxide). A lower concentration of tracer after ingestion and equilibration (~3 to 4 hours) reflects a higher amount of body water and vice versa. Tracer concentration can be assessed in a variety of body fluids such as blood, urine, and saliva.

Accuracy

The accuracy associated with hydrometry is similar to that of underwater weighing (approximately ± 4% in the general population and ± 2.7% in groups in which body fat is assessed using an equation developed specifically for that population (55).

Advantages

The advantage of using body water to assess body composition is that it provides a good measure of body fatness in the general population. Body water is primarily used in research settings in combination with other body measures using a multicomponent approach to assessing body composition.

Disadvantages

The disadvantages of hydrometry are the tedious analysis procedures and exposure to body fluids. Furthermore, because the water concentration of the fat-free component may vary from the assumed 73%, population-specific equations should be developed for groups with different concentrations of water in the fat-free component.

Bioelectrical Impedance Analysis

Bioelectrical impedance analysis (BIA) is commonly used to assess body composition in field settings. The technique is based on the conductive and dielectric properties of different tissues within the body at different frequencies. Tissues that contain large amounts of fluid and electrolytes, such as blood, have high conductivity, whereas fat, bone, and lungs have high resistance or are dielectric (83,84). A small alternating current that is passed through the body flows predominantly through tissue with higher conductivities. BIA determines the resistance to flow (impedance) of the current as it passes through the body.

Procedure

A bioelectrical impedance analyzer and the tetrapolar (ie, four-electrode) technique are described here (83,84):

1. The subject must remove shoes, socks, and metallic jewelry.
2. Measurement occurs while the client is lying supine on a flat surface that is nonconductive, such as a bed or cot free of metal framing. It is recommended that the measurement is taken after the client is lying supine for 10 minutes to allow for fluid shifts that occur after one moves from the standing position to the supine position (85). Measurement in individuals restricted to bed rest for several hours may lead to errors of 1.0 to 1.5 liters in estimated body water (86).
3. The client's head should be flat or supported by a thin pillow.
4. The arms are abducted slightly so they do not touch the trunk.
5. Legs are separated so that the ankles are at least 20 cm apart and the thighs are not touching.
6. The client and analyzer should be at least 50 cm from metallic objects and electronic equipment.
7. The skin at each site is cleaned with alcohol before application of the electrodes.
8. Placement of electrodes is demonstrated in Figure 9.15. Electrodes are attached to the wrist (midway between the styloid processes), hand (at least 5 cm distal to the wrist electrode), ankle (midway between the malleoli), and foot (at least 5 cm distal to the ankle electrode).
9. The source cable (black) is attached to the electrodes on the hand and foot. The source cable introduces the current to the client.
10. The sensing cable (red) is attached to the electrodes on the wrist and ankle.
11. An excitation current ranging from 500 to 800 μA at a frequency of 50 kHz is transmitted by the electrolytes within body fluids and impeded by the resistive tissues.
12. The electrical impedance of the tissues provides an estimate of total body water, from which fat-free and fat components are determined.

Accuracy

The standard error estimate for body water from BIA is typically less than 2 liters (84). Although body fat estimates from BIA can vary by as much as 10% of body mass because of differences in instrumentation and methodologies, most prediction errors for young adults are 5% or less. It is generally recommended that

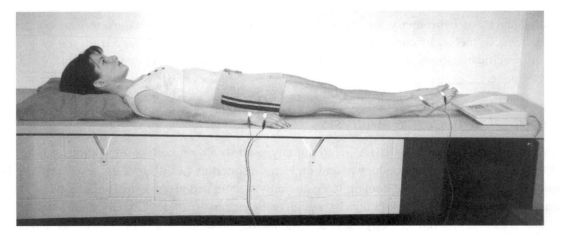

FIGURE 9.15   Position of electrodes when assessing body composition using bioelectrical impedance analysis.

BOX 9.2   Equation to Estimate Body Composition from Bioelectrical Impedance Analysis in Elderly Men and Women

FFM = (0.28 Height^2/Resistance) + 0.27 Weight + 4.5 Sex + 0.31 (Thigh circumference) − 1.732

Where: FFM = fat-free mass measured in kg; Height is measured in cm; Resistance is measured in ohms; Weight is measured in kg; Sex = 1 for male and 0 for female; Thigh circumference is measured in cm.

Source: Formula is from reference 87.

---

population-specific equations be used to reduce potential error associated with the BIA technique. Although population-specific equations are available (75), very few population-specific equations have been validated against accepted criterion techniques. Population-specific equations that have been validated using multi-component models are reported in Box 9.2 (34,87).

In addition to the technique described earlier, body composition can be estimated using BIA systems that are handheld or stood on (scale). The added advantage of the scale systems is the simultaneous assessment of body weight. Recent studies suggest that the handheld systems need improvement before they can be widely adopted because they yield estimates of body composition that do not agree well with more established methods (88–90). Studies evaluating the accuracy of body composition estimates by leg-to-leg BIA systems are mixed. Some studies suggest the systems provide valid estimates of fat mass and fat-free mass in the obese (91) and accurately track body composition changes associated with weight loss or weight gain (92,93). Conversely, other studies suggest that the accuracy is limited (94–96), especially in athletes involved in weight-control sports. More research examining the accuracy of body composition measures from BIA vs measures from multicomponent models are needed. Box 9.3 describes the use of leg-to-leg BIA in weight-control sports.

Advantages

The advantages of using BIA to assess body composition are its convenience, ease of use, reliable measurement, and relatively low expense. The regional versions can be purchased for as little as $30.

Disadvantages

The primary disadvantage of BIA is that many studies report considerable variability in its estimates of fat and fat-free mass when compared to more established techniques (94–96). This is particularly problematic when small differences in body composition must be detected. A second disadvantage is that the accuracy of body fat assessment may be compromised in very muscular athletes with disproportionately high concentrations of water in the fat-free mass; amputees; and those suffering from unilateral hemiparesis, edema, or tissue atrophy (84). Lastly, few population-specific equations have been validated using a criterion method of body composition assessment.

Skinfold Thickness

Skinfold thickness measurement is one of the most commonly used field methods for assessing body composition. The method is based on the assumptions that subcutaneous fat represents a certain proportion of

BOX 9.3   Leg-to-Leg BIA Systems and Weight Control Sports

Body composition is often used as a gauge for athletic success and health. However, finding a practical method that provides accurate measurement of fat and fat-free mass in the field can be difficult. Many professionals have turned to bioelectrical impedance analysis (BIA) systems that are handheld or stood on (leg-to-leg) because they are portable, require no specialized training, and provide quick results (94). An additional advantage of the scale systems is the simultaneous assessment of body weight. In weight-control sports such as wrestling, minimum body fat values are being used to determine the minimum weight at which an athlete can compete at the middle school, high school, and collegiate level. Therefore, the accuracy of the body composition method used is critical. If minimum weight is underestimated, it may support the use of unhealthy weight loss practices. Conversely, an overestimation of minimum weight can put an athlete in a higher weight class and at a competitive disadvantage (94).

Unfortunately, the use of leg-to-leg BIA systems in weight-control sports has been questioned (94,95). In a study of collegiate athletes, minimum weight estimates from a four-component model (ie, criterion method) were not different from estimates from underwater weighing, skinfolds, dual-energy x-ray absorptiometry (DXA), and a leg-to-leg BIA system (94). However, standard deviation (SD) of the difference between minimum weight estimates from the criterion method and estimates from the BIA system was more highly variable from subject to subject than the other measurement methods. For comparison, minimum weight was predicted within ± 2.2 kg (or 4.8 lb) in 89% of the athletes when the underwater weighing method was used, but in only 47% of the athletes when the BIA system was used. A similar finding was observed in a study of collegiate wrestlers (95). Despite the limited precision of the leg-to-leg BIA systems, they are widely available and marketed for use in the sport of wrestling. Although the leg-to-leg BIA method for assessing is practical for assessing body composition, until the precision is improved, using it to determine minimum weight in weight-control sports is questionable.

the total body fat, and total subcutaneous fat can be accurately determined by measuring skinfold thickness at a few specific sites on the body.

Procedure

Skinfold calipers that apply a constant pressure of 10 g/mm^2 are often used. Harpenden and Lange calipers are preferred. The following procedure is used (97):

1. Using anatomical landmarks and a tape measure when necessary, carefully identify the site to be measured.
2. Those with little experience may mark the site with a black felt pen.
3. Common skinfold measurement sites include the chest (Figure 9.16), abdomen (Figure 9.17), mid-thigh (Figure 9.18), triceps (Figure 9.19), suprailium (Figure 9.20), and subscapula (Figure 9.21).
4. The skinfold is grabbed and elevated by the thumb and index finger of the left hand. The amount of tissue being grabbed must form a fold with sides being approximately parallel.
5. Hold skinfold calipers in the right hand, with the heads perpendicular to the site being measured and the dial facing up. After opening the caliper arms with pressure, the caliper heads are applied to the fold and pressure is gradually released. The heads should be applied where the sides of the fold are parallel, approximately midway between the body site where the skinfold originates and the crest of the skinfold.

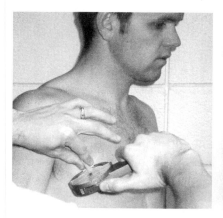

FIGURE 9.16 Chest skinfold measured with the long axis of the fold directed to the nipple.

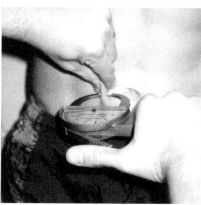

FIGURE 9.17 Abdomen skinfold measured immediately lateral of the umbilicus.

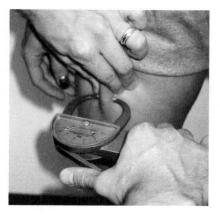

FIGURE 9.18 Mid-thigh skinfold measured midway between the inguinal crease and the proximal border of the patella.

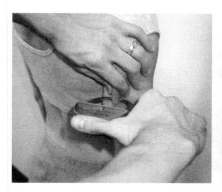

FIGURE 9.19 Triceps skinfold measured on the midline posterior surface of the arm over the triceps muscle, at the midpoint between the acromion process of the scapula and the olecranon process of the ulna.

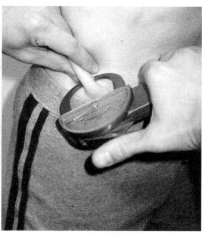

FIGURE 9.20 Suprailiac skinfold measured on the midaxillary line just superior to the iliac crest.

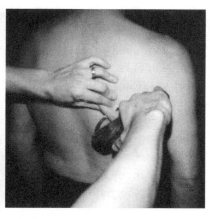

FIGURE 9.21 Subscapular skinfold measured at an approximately 45-degree angle just inferior to the inferior angle of the scapula.

6. Read the dial to the nearest 1 mm approximately 4 seconds after the caliper has been applied to the site. Waiting longer to observe the measurement causes smaller readings because fluids are forced from the tissues at the site.

7. After the measurement is read the calipers should be opened and then removed from the site.

8. A minimum of two measurements should be taken for each site. If the first two measurements vary by more than 1 mm, additional measurements should be taken until consistency is established. A minimum of 15 seconds should be allowed between measurements. It is recommended that all sites are measured before the second set of measurements is made.

9. In the obese, it may be necessary to grab the skinfold with two hands while a partner measures the skinfold thickness. If the fold is too thick to apply the calipers, an alternative body composition method is necessary.

10. Sites should not be measured when the skin is moist (to avoid grabbing excess skin and increasing skinfold measures), or immediately after exercise (because body fluid shifts may increase the skinfold size).
11. When all sites have been measured, adult body fat percentage can be determined using Tables 9.4 and 9.5 (98), derived using skinfold equations developed by Jackson et al (99,100).

Accuracy

Several factors can influence the accuracy of body fat estimates from skinfolds, such as the equation used to calculate body fat percentage. When population-specific equations are used, the accuracy of skinfold estimates of percentage body fat is generally 3% to 4% body weight (77). Population-specific equations can be found in other publications (75). Unfortunately, few studies have examined the applicability of different skinfold equations using a criterion method. A recent study that used a four-component model as a criterion method (101) suggested skinfolds provide accurate estimates of body fat in collegiate wrestlers when the following equation, published by Lohman (77), is used:

$$D_b = 1.0982[0.000815 \, (SFT + SFS + SFA)] + [0.00000084(SFT + SFS + SFA)^2]$$

Where: SFT, SFS, and SFA represent skinfold thickness of the thigh, subscapula, and abdomen, respectively, and D_b indicates body density.

On the other hand, equations developed specifically for boys and girls (102) have been found to yield percentage fat estimates 3.5% less than estimates from a four-component model (67).

Another factor that can affect body fat estimates is the technician measuring skinfold thickness. Lohman et al (103) found that up to 17% of the variability in skinfold thickness measurement can be attributed to the technician, even if the technician is trained.

The type of caliper can also have a substantial effect on body fat estimates. For instance, the inexpensive Adipometer caliper yields mean estimates of body fat that are similar to the expensive Harpenden caliper (103,104). Conversely, the expensive Lange caliper has been found to give body fat estimates 3.5 percentage points higher than the Harpenden caliper (103). The discrepancy between investigators and calipers is greater for the abdomen, suprailiac, and thigh than for the subscapula and triceps.

Advantages

Some advantages of using skinfolds to assess body composition include low expense, little space required to store the equipment, quick measurement, and reasonably accurate estimates of percentage body fat.

Disadvantages

Disadvantages of using skinfold calipers are the considerable effect on accuracy of the skill of the technician measuring skinfold thickness, the caliper used, and the equation used on body fat estimates. Although population-specific equations are available, few equations have been validated using a criterion method of body composition assessment.

Near-Infrared Interactance

Near-infrared interactance (NIR) is based on the principles of light absorption and reflection. The method was originally developed to determine the amount of protein, water, and fat in agriculture products, which are assumed to have different bands of light absorption (105). The commercially available portable NIR device produced by Futrex, Inc uses a light probe with a silicon detector, two near-infrared diodes that emit light at a wavelength of 940 nm, and two near-infrared diodes that emit light at a wavelength of 950 nm.

TABLE 9.4 Percent Fat Estimate for Men: Sum of Chest, Abdomen, and Thigh Skinfolds

Sum of Skinfolds, mm	Age to Last Year								
	Under 22	23–27	28–32	33–37	38–42	43–47	48–52	53–57	Over 57
8–10	1.3	1.8	2.3	2.9	3.4	3.9	4.5	5.0	5.5
11–13	2.2	2.8	3.3	3.9	4.4	4.9	5.5	6.0	6.5
14–16	3.2	3.8	4.3	4.8	5.4	5.9	6.4	7.0	7.5
17–19	4.2	4.7	5.3	5.8	6.3	6.9	7.4	8.0	8.5
20–22	5.1	5.7	6.2	6.8	7.3	7.9	8.4	8.9	9.5
23–25	6.1	6.6	7.2	7.7	8.3	8.8	9.4	9.9	10.5
26–28	7.0	7.6	8.1	8.7	9.2	9.8	10.3	10.9	11.4
29–31	8.0	8.5	9.1	9.6	10.2	10.7	11.3	11.8	12.4
32–34	8.9	9.4	10.0	10.5	11.1	11.6	12.2	12.8	13.3
35–37	9.8	10.4	10.9	11.5	12.0	12.6	13.1	13.7	14.3
38–40	10.7	11.3	11.8	12.4	12.9	13.5	14.1	14.6	15.2
41–43	11.6	12.2	12.7	13.3	13.8	14.4	15.0	15.5	16.1
44–46	12.5	13.1	13.6	14.2	14.7	15.3	15.9	16.4	17.0
47–49	13.4	13.9	14.5	15.1	15.6	16.2	16.8	17.3	17.9
50–52	14.3	14.8	15.4	15.9	16.5	17.1	17.6	18.2	18.8
53–55	15.1	15.7	16.2	16.8	17.4	17.9	18.5	19.1	19.7
56–58	16.0	16.5	17.1	17.7	18.2	18.8	19.4	20.0	20.5
59–61	16.9	17.4	17.9	18.5	19.1	19.7	20.2	20.8	21.4
62–64	17.6	18.2	18.8	19.4	19.9	20.5	21.1	21.7	22.2
65–67	18.5	19.0	19.6	20.2	20.8	21.3	21.9	22.5	23.1
68–70	19.3	19.9	20.4	21.0	21.6	22.2	22.7	23.3	23.9
71–73	20.1	20.7	21.2	21.8	22.4	23.0	23.6	24.1	24.7
74–76	20.9	21.5	22.0	22.6	23.2	23.8	24.4	25.0	25.5
77–79	21.7	22.2	22.8	23.4	24.0	24.6	25.2	25.8	26.3
80–82	22.4	23.0	23.6	24.2	24.8	25.4	25.9	26.5	27.1
83–85	23.2	23.8	24.4	25.0	25.5	26.1	26.7	27.3	27.9
86–88	24.0	24.5	25.1	25.7	26.3	26.9	27.5	28.1	28.7
89–91	24.7	25.3	25.9	26.5	27.1	27.6	28.2	28.8	29.4
92–94	25.4	26.0	26.6	27.2	27.8	28.4	29.0	29.6	30.2
95–97	26.1	26.7	27.3	27.9	28.5	29.1	29.7	30.3	30.9
98–100	26.9	27.4	28.0	28.6	29.2	29.8	30.4	31.0	31.6
101–103	27.5	28.1	28.7	29.3	29.9	30.5	31.1	31.7	32.3
104–106	28.2	28.8	29.4	30.0	30.6	31.2	31.8	32.4	33.0
107–109	28.9	29.5	30.1	30.7	31.3	31.9	32.5	33.1	33.7
110–112	29.6	30.2	30.8	31.4	32.0	32.6	33.2	33.8	34.4
113–115	30.2	30.8	31.4	32.0	32.6	33.2	33.8	34.5	35.1
116–118	30.9	31.5	32.1	32.7	33.3	33.9	34.5	35.1	35.7
119–121	31.5	32.1	32.7	33.3	33.9	34.5	35.1	35.7	36.4
122–124	32.1	32.7	33.3	33.9	34.5	35.1	35.8	36.4	37.0
125–127	32.7	33.3	33.9	34.5	35.1	35.8	36.4	37.0	37.6

Source: Table 5 (Percent Fat Estimate for Men) from Jackson AS, Pollock ML. Practical assessment of body composition. *Phys Sportsmed.* 1985;13:85. Copyright © 1985. Reprinted with permission from JTE Multimedia.

TABLE 9.5 Percent Fat Estimate for Women: Sum of Triceps, Suprailium, and Thigh Skinfolds

Sum of Skinfolds, mm	Age to Last Year								
	Under 22	23–27	28–32	33–37	38–42	43–47	48–52	53–57	Over 57
23–25	9.7	9.9	10.2	10.4	10.7	10.9	11.2	11.4	11.7
26–28	11.0	11.2	11.5	11.7	12.0	12.3	12.5	12.7	13.0
29–31	12.3	12.5	12.8	13.0	13.3	13.5	13.8	14.0	14.3
32–34	13.6	13.8	14.0	14.3	14.5	14.8	15.0	15.3	15.5
35–37	14.8	15.0	15.3	15.5	15.8	16.0	16.3	16.5	16.8
38–40	16.0	16.3	16.5	16.7	17.0	17.2	17.5	17.7	18.0
41–43	17.2	17.4	17.7	17.9	18.2	18.4	18.7	18.9	19.2
44–46	18.3	18.6	18.8	19.1	19.3	19.6	19.8	20.1	20.3
47–49	19.5	19.7	20.0	20.2	20.5	20.7	21.0	21.2	21.5
50–52	20.6	20.8	21.1	21.3	21.6	21.8	22.1	22.3	22.6
53–55	21.7	21.9	22.1	22.4	22.6	22.9	23.1	23.4	23.6
56–58	22.7	23.0	23.2	23.4	23.7	23.9	24.2	24.4	24.7
59–61	23.7	24.0	24.2	24.5	24.7	25.0	25.2	25.5	25.7
62–64	24.7	25.0	25.2	25.5	25.7	26.0	26.7	26.4	26.7
65–67	25.7	25.9	26.2	26.4	26.7	26.9	27.2	27.4	27.7
68–70	26.6	26.9	27.1	27.4	27.6	27.9	28.1	28.4	28.6
71–73	27.5	27.8	28.0	28.3	28.5	28.8	29.0	29.3	29.5
74–76	28.4	28.7	28.9	29.2	29.4	29.7	29.9	30.2	30.4
77–79	29.3	29.5	29.8	30.0	30.3	30.5	30.8	31.0	31.3
80–82	30.1	30.4	30.6	30.9	31.1	31.4	31.6	31.9	32.1
83–85	30.9	31.2	31.4	31.7	31.9	32.2	32.4	32.7	32.9
86–88	31.7	32.0	32.2	32.5	32.7	32.9	33.2	33.4	33.7
89–91	32.5	32.7	33.0	33.2	33.5	33.7	33.9	34.2	34.4
92–94	33.2	33.4	33.7	33.9	34.2	34.4	34.7	34.9	35.2
95–97	33.9	34.1	34.4	34.6	34.9	35.1	35.4	35.6	35.9
98–100	34.6	34.8	35.1	35.3	35.5	35.8	36.0	36.3	36.5
101–103	35.3	35.4	35.7	35.9	36.2	36.4	36.7	36.9	37.2
104–106	35.8	36.1	36.3	36.6	36.8	37.1	37.3	37.5	37.8
107–109	36.4	36.7	36.9	37.1	37.4	37.6	37.9	38.1	38.4
110–112	37.0	37.2	37.5	37.7	38.0	38.2	38.5	38.7	38.9
113–115	37.5	37.8	38.0	38.2	38.5	38.7	39.0	39.2	39.5
116–118	38.0	38.3	38.5	38.8	39.0	39.3	39.5	39.7	40.0
119–121	38.5	38.7	39.0	39.2	39.5	39.7	40.0	40.2	40.5
122–124	39.0	39.2	39.4	39.7	39.9	40.2	40.4	40.7	40.9
125–127	39.4	39.6	39.9	40.1	40.4	40.6	40.9	41.1	41.4
128–130	39.8	40.0	40.3	40.5	40.8	41.0	41.3	41.5	41.8

Source: Table 6 (Percent Fat Estimate for Women) from Jackson AS, Pollock ML: Practical assessment of body composition. *Phys Sportsmed.* 1985;13:86. Copyright © 1985. Reprinted with permission from JTE Multimedia.

At a measurement site, typically the bicep, the intensity of light or optical density emitted at the different wavelengths is determined. The machine estimates body fat using the optical density at the two different wavelengths, body weight, height, sex, and activity level.

Assessment of the accuracy of NIR, using underwater weighing as the criterion, has yielded conflicting results. Although a few studies suggest that NIR has reasonable accuracy (106), others suggest its use is problematic in children and adolescents (107), women (108), the obese (109,110), and collegiate football players (111). Discrepancies have also been found when different models of the instrument were used (112). Furthermore, the ability of NIR to detect changes in fat and fat-free mass has not been determined. In conclusion, NIR may be a promising method for assessing body composition, but research to date suggests that further development of this technology is needed before it can be used with confidence.

Summary

The methods for assessing body size are straightforward and firmly established. Several methods have been developed for assessing body composition. The use of the most accurate methods (ie, CT, MRI, and multicomponent models) are restricted by their expense, processing procedures, and limited availability. Although less-expensive methods are available, their accuracy is limited, especially when the outcome is dependent on age, sex, and race. Age-, sex-, and race-specific equations have been developed, but studies assessing their validity against a criterion method are generally lacking. General tips to help accurately measure in body composition are presented in Box 9.4.

Federal guidelines (2) have been developed to identify those at risk for disease using simple anthropometric measurements. Although assessment of body composition would likely aid in the assessment of the individual's disease risk, appropriate guidelines are needed. A useful application of body composition assessment would be to track change during a training program; however, large changes are probably needed before they are detected. Even then, the accuracy of the change is limited in the noncriterion methods. The limitations of body composition assessment methods must be recognized when used in the field.

BOX 9.4   Tips for Measuring Body Composition

- Clients should not exercise several hours before measurement.
- For many measurement techniques, clients should be adequately hydrated before measurement.
- Measurements that are included in the assessment, such as height and weight, should be done as precisely and accurately as possible.
- When assessing changes in body composition, the same measurer should do the assessment using the same technique and instrumentation.
- Error associated with many methods of body composition assessment can be substantially reduced if done by a trained and experienced measurer.
- Clients need to be educated about accuracy limitations because they often think body fat percentage numbers are as accurate as scale weights. Most methods for estimating body fat have an error range of 3% to 4% or more under the best circumstances.
- Use population-specific equations to determine body fat when appropriate, especially equations that have been validated against a multicomponent model.

References

1. Bray GA. Complications of obesity. *Ann Intern Med.* 1985;103:1052–1062.
2. National Heart, Lung, and Blood Institute. *Clinical Guidelines on the Identification, Evaluation, and Treatment of Overweight and Obesity in Adults: The Evidence Report.* Bethesda, MD: National Institutes of Health; 1998.
3. Robinett-Weiss N, Hixson ML, Keir B, Sieberg J. The metropolitan height-weight tables: perspectives for use. *J Am Diet Assoc.* 1984;84:1480–1481.
4. Knapp TR. A methodological critique of the "ideal weight" concept. *JAMA.* 1983;250:506–510.
5. Frisancho RF. Nutritional anthropometry. *J Am Diet Assoc.* 1988;88:553–555.
6. van der Voort DJ, Geusens PP, Dinant GJ. Risk factors for osteoporosis related to their outcome: fractures. *Osteoporos Int.* 2001;12:630–638.
7. Revicki DA, Israel RG. Relationship between body mass indices and measures of body adiposity. *Am J Public Health.* 1986;76:992–994.
8. Rimm AA, Hartz AJ, Fischer ME. A weight shape index for assessing risk of disease in 44,820 women. *J Clin Epidemiol.* 1988;41:459–465.
9. Shapira DV, Kumar NB, Lyman GH, Cox CE. Abdominal obesity and breast cancer risk. *Ann Intern Med.* 1990; 112:182–186.
10. Andres R, Elahi D, Tobin JD, Muller DC, Brant L. Impact of age on weight goals. *Ann Intern Med.* 1985;103: 1030–1033.
11. Sichieri R, Everhart JE, Hubbard VS. Relative weight classifications in the assessment of underweight and overweight in the United States. *Int J Obes Relat Metab Disord.* 1992;16:303–312.
12. Lew EA, Garfinkel L. Variations in mortality by weight among 750,000 men and women. *J Chronic Dis.* 1979; 32:563–576.
13. Wienpahl J, Ragland DR, Sidney S. Body mass index and 15-year mortality in a cohort of black men and women. *J Clin Epidemiol.* 1990;43:949–960.
14. Durazo-Arvizu R, Cooper RS, Luke A, Prewitt TE, Liao Y, McGee DL. Relative weight and mortality in U.S. blacks and whites: findings from representative national population samples. *Ann Epidemiol.* 1997;7:383–395.
15. Despres JP, Prud'homme D, Pouliot MC, Tremblay A, Bouchard C. Estimation of deep abdominal adipose-tissue accumulation from simple anthropometric measurements in men. *Am J Clin Nutr.* 1991;54:471–477.
16. Pouliot MC, Despres JP, Lemieux S, Moorjani S, Bouchard C, Tremblay A, Nadeau A, Lupien PJ. Waist circumference and abdominal sagittal diameter: best simple anthropometric indexes of abdominal visceral adipose tissue accumulation and related cardiovascular risk in men and women. *Am J Cardiol.* 1994;73:460–468.
17. Larsson B, Svardsunn K, Welin L, Wilhelmsen L, Bjorntorp P, Tibblin G. Abdominal adipose tissue distribution, obesity, and risk of cardiovascular disease and death: 13 year follow up of participants in the study of men born in 1913. *BMJ.* 1984;288:1401–1404.
18. Wannamethee G, Shaper AG. Body weight and mortality in middle aged British men: impact of smoking. *BMJ.* 1989;299:1497–1502.
19. Ducimetiere RP, Cambien F, Avons P, Jacqueson A. Relationships between adiposity measurements and the incidence of coronary heart disease in a middle-aged male population: the Paris Prospective Study I. In: Vague J, Bjorntorp P, GuyGrand M, Rebuffe-Scrive M, Vague P, eds. *Metabolic Complications of Human Obesities.* Amsterdam, The Netherlands: Elsevier; 1985:31–38.
20. National Heart, Lung, and Blood Institute. *Third Report of the National Cholesterol Education Program (NCEP) Expert Panel on Detection, Evaluation, and Treatment of High Blood Cholesterol in Adults (Adult Treatment Panel III).* Bethesda, MD: National Heart, Lung, and Blood Institute; 2001.
21. Byrne S, McLean N. Elite athletes: effects of the pressure to be thin. *J Sci Med Sport.* 2002;5:80–94.
22. Otis CL, Drinkwater B, Johnson M, Loucks A, Wilmore J. American College of Sports Medicine position stand. The Female Athlete Triad [see comments]. *Med Sci Sports Exerc.* 1997;29:i–ix.
23. Coin A, Sergi G, Beninca P, Lupoli L, Cinti G, Ferrara L, Benedetti G, Tomasi G, Pisent C, Enzi G. Bone mineral density and body composition in underweight and normal elderly subjects. *Osteoporos Int.* 2000;11:1043–1050.

24. Bennell KL, Malcolm SA, Wark JD, Brukner PD. Skeletal effects of menstrual disturbances in athletes. *Scand J Med Sci Sports.* 1997;71:261–273.

25. Khan KM, Liu-Ambrose T, Sran MM, Ashe MC, Donaldson MG, Wark JD. New criteria for female athlete triad syndrome? As osteoporosis is rare, should osteopenia be among the criteria for defining the female athlete triad syndrome? *Br J Sports Med.* 2002;36:10–13.

26. Gordon CC, Chumlea WC, Roche AF. Stature, recumbent length, and weight. In: Lohman TG, Roche AF, Martorell R, eds. *Anthropometric Standardization Reference Manual.* Champaign, IL: Human Kinetics; 1988:3–8.

27. Carter JEL, Heath BH. *Somatotyping: Development and Applications.* Cambridge, England: Cambridge University Press; 1990.

28. Callaway CW, Chumlea WC, Bouchard C, Himes JH, Lohman TG, Martin AD, Mitchell CD Mueller WH, Roche A, Seefeldt VD. Circumferences. In: Lohman TG, Roche AF, Martorell R, eds. *Anthropometric Standardization Reference Manual.* Champaign, IL: Human Kinetics; 1988:39–54.

29. Wilmore JH, Frisancho RA, Gordon CC, Himes JH, Martin AD, Martorell R, Seefeldt VD. Body breadth equipment and measurement techniques. In: Lohman TG, Roche AF, Martorell R, eds. *Anthropometric Standardization Reference Manual.* Champaign, IL: Human Kinetics; 1988:27–38.

30. Claessens AL, Lefevre J, Beunen G, Malina RM. The contribution of anthropometric characteristics to performance scores in elite female gymnasts. *J Sports Med Phys Fitness.* 1999;39:355–360.

31. Berg K, Latin RW, Coffey C. Relationship of somatotype and physical characteristics to distance running performance in middle age runners. *J Sports Med Phys Fitness.* 1998;38:253–257.

32. Frisancho R. New standards of weight and body composition by frame size and height for assessment of nutritional status of adults and the elderly. *Am J Clin Nutr.* 1984;40:806–819.

33. Baumgartner RN, Heymsfield SB, Roche AF. Human body composition and the epidemiology of chronic disease. *Obesity Res.* 1995;3:73–95.

34. Lohman TG. *Advances in Body Composition Assessment.* Champaign, IL: Human Kinetics; 1992.

35. Lohman TG. Body composition methodology in sports medicine. *Phys Sportsmed.* 1982;10:47–58.

36. Bjorntorp P. "Portal" adipose tissue as a generator of risk factors for cardiovascular disease and diabetes. *Arteriosclerosis.* 1990;10:493–496.

37. Goodpaster BH, Thaete FL, Kelley DE. Thigh adipose tissue distribution is associated with insulin resistance in obesity and in type 2 diabetes mellitus. *Am J Clin Nutr.* 2000;71:885–892.

38. Goodpaster BH, Thaete FL, Simoneau JA, Kelley DE. Subcutaneous abdominal fat and thigh muscle composition predict insulin sensitivity independently of visceral fat. *Diabetes.* 1997;46:1579–1585.

39. Beunen G, Malina RM, Ostyn M, Renson R, Simons J, Van Gerven D. Fatness, growth, and motor fitness of Belgian boys 12 through 20 years of age. *Hum Biol.* 1983;55:599–613.

40. Cureton KJ, Sparling PB, Evans BW, Johnson SM, Kong UD, Purvis JW. Effect of experimental alterations in excess weight on aerobic capacity and distance running performance. *Med Sci Sports Exerc.* 1978;15:218–223.

41. Cureton KJ, Sparling PB. Distance running performance and metabolic responses to running in men and women with excess weight experimentally equated. *Med Sci Sports Exerc.* 1980;12:288–294.

42. Buskirk ER, Taylor HL. Maximal oxygen intake and its relation to body composition, with special reference to chronic physical activity and obesity. *J Appl Physiol.* 1957;11:72–78.

43. Houtkooper LB, Going SB. Body composition: how should it be measured? Does it affect performance? *Sports Sci Exch.* 1994;7(5).

44. Evans EM, Saunders MJ, Spano MA, Arngrimsson SA, Lewis RD, Cureton KJ. Body composition changes with diet and exercise in obese women: a comparison of estimates from clinical methods and four-component model. *Am J Clin Nutr.* 1999;70:5–12.

45. Evans EM, Saunders MJ, Spano MA, Arngrimsson SA, Lewis RD, Cureton KJ. Effects of diet and exercise on the density and composition of the fat-free mass in obese women. *Med Sci Sports Exerc.* 1999;31:1778–1787.

46. Fogelholm GM, Sievanen HT, van Marken Lichtenbelt WD, Westerterp KR. Assessment of fat-mass loss during weight reduction in obese women. *Metabolism.* 1997;46:968–975.

47. Albu J, Smolowitz J, Lichtman S, Heymsfield SB, Wang J, Pierson RN Jr, Pi-Sunyer FX. Composition of weight loss in severely obese women: a new look at old methods. *Metabolism.* 1992;41:1068–1074.

48. American College of Sports Medicine. ACSM position stand on weight loss in wrestlers. *Med Sci Sports Exerc.* 1996;28:ix–xii.

49. Lukaski HC. Methods for the assessment of human body composition: traditional and new. *Am J Clin Nutr.* 1987;46:537–556.

50. Ross R, Goodpaster B, Kelley D, Boada F. Magnetic resonance imaging in human body composition research. From quantitative to qualitative tissue measurement. *Ann N Y Acad Sci.* 2000;904:12–17.

51. Ross R. Magnetic resonance imaging provides new insights into the characterization of adipose and lean tissue distribution. *Can J Physiol Pharmacol.* 1996;74:778–785.

52. Mitsiopoulos N, Baumgartner RN, Heymsfield SB, Lyons W, Gallagher D, Ross R. Cadaver validation of skeletal muscle measurement by magnetic resonance imaging and computerized tomography. *J Appl Physiol.* 1998;85:115–122.

53. Heymsfield SB, Lichtman S, Baumgartner RN, Wang J, Kamen Y, Aliprantis A, Pierson RN Jr. Body composition of humans: comparison of two improved four-component models that differ in expense, technical complexity, and radiation exposure. *Am J Clin Nutr.* 1990;52:52–58.

54. Withers RT, LaForgia J, Pillans RK, Shipp NJ, Chatterton BE, Schultz CG, Leaney F. Comparisons of two-, three-, and four-compartment models of body composition analysis in men and women. *J Appl Physiol.* 1998;85:238–245.

55. Modlesky CM, Cureton KJ, Lewis RD, Prior BM, Sloniger MA, Rowe DA. Density of the fat-free mass and estimates of body composition in male weight trainers. *J Appl Physiol.* 1996;80:2085–2096.

56. Siri WE. Body composition from fluid spaces and density: analysis of methods. In: Brozek J, Henschel A, eds. *Techniques for Measuring Body Composition.* Washington, DC: National Academy of Sciences National Research Council; 1961:223–244.

57. Brozek J, Grande F, Anderson JT, Keys A. Densitometric analysis of body composition: revision of some quantitative assumptions. *Ann N Y Acad Sci.* 1963;110:113–140.

58. Lohman TG. Applicability of body composition techniques and constant for children and youths. In: Pandolf K, ed. *Exercise and Sports Science Reviews.* 14th ed. New York, NY: Macmillan; 1986:325–357.

59. Bergsma-Kadijk JA, Baumeister B, Deurenberg P. Measurement of body fat in young and elderly women: comparison between a four-compartment model and widely used reference methods. *Br J Nutr.* 1996;75:649–657.

60. Roemmich JN, Clark PA, Weltman A, Rogol AD. Alterations in growth and body composition during puberty. I. Comparing multicompartment body composition models. *J Appl Physiol.* 1997;83:927–935.

61. Clasey JL, Hartman ML, Kanaley J, Wideman L, Teates CD, Bouchard C, Weltman A. Body composition by DEXA in older adults: accuracy and influence of scan mode. *Med Sci Sports Exerc.* 1997;29:560–567.

62. Cote KD, Adams WC. Effect of bone density on body composition estimates in young adult black and white women. *Med Sci Sports Exerc.* 1993;25:290–296.

63. Ortiz O, Russell M, Daley TL, Baumgartner RN, Waki M, Lichtman S, Wang J, Pierson RN Jr, Heymsfield SB. Differences in skeletal muscle and bone mineral mass between black and white females and their relevance to estimates of body composition. *Am J Clin Nutr.* 1992;55:8–13.

64. Lukaski HC. Soft tissue composition and bone mineral status: evaluation by dual energy x-ray absorptiometry. *J Nutr.* 1993;123:438–443.

65. Lohman TG. Dual-energy X-ray absorptiometry. In: Roche AF, Heymsfield SB, Lohman TG, eds. *Human Body Composition.* Champaign, IL: Human Kinetics; 1996:63–78.

66. Prior BM, Cureton KJ, Modlesky CM, Evans EM, Sloniger MA, Saunders M, Lewis RD. In vivo validation of whole-body composition estimates from dual-energy X-ray absorptiometry. *J Appl Physiol.* 1997;83:623–630.

67. Wells JCK, Fuller NJ, Dewit O, Fewtrell MS, Elia M, Cole TJ. Four-component model of body composition in children: density and hydration of fat-free mass and comparison with simpler models. *Am J Clin Nutr.* 1999;69:904–912.

68. Fidanza F, Keys A, Anderson JT. Density of body fat in man and other mammals. *J Appl Physiol.* 1953;6:252–256.

69. Morales MF, Rathbun EN, Smith RE, Pace N. Theoretical considerations regarding the major body tissue components, with suggestions for application to man. *J Biol Chem.* 1945;158:677–684.

70. Rathbun EN, Pace N. The determination of total body fat by means of the body specific gravity. *J Biol Chem.* 1945;158:667–676.

71. Behnke AR. Comment of the determination of whole body density and a resume of body composition data. In: Brozek J, Henschel A, eds. *Techniques for Measuring Body Composition.* Washington, DC: National Academy of Sciences National Research Council; 1961:118–133.

72. Powers SK, Howley HT. *Exercise Physiology: Theory and Application to Fitness and Performance.* Dubuque, IA: William C. Brown Publishers; 1990.

73. Going SB. Densitometry. In: Roche AF, Heymsfield SB, Lohman TG, eds. *Human Body Composition.* 3rd ed. Champaign, IL: Human Kinetics; 1996:3–23.

74. *Handbook of Physical Chemistry.* Cleveland, OH: Chemical Rubber Company; 1967.

75. Heyward VH, Stolarczyk LM. *Applied Body Composition Assessment.* Champaign, IL: Human Kinetics; 1996.

76. Goldman HI, Becklake MR. Respiratory function tests; normal values at median altitudes and the prediction of normal results. *Am Rev Tuberc.* 1959;79:457–467.

77. Lohman TG. Skinfolds and body density and their relation to body fatness: a review. *Hum Biol.* 1981;53:181–225.

78. Prior BM, Modlesky CM, Evans EM, Sloniger MA, Saunders MJ, Lewis RD, Cureton KJ. Muscularity and the density of the fat-free mass in athletes. *J Appl Physiol.* 2001;90:1523–1531.

79. Schutte JE, Townsend EJ, Hugg J, Shoup RF, Malina RM, Blomqvist CG. Density of lean body mass is greater in blacks than in whites. *J Appl Physiol.* 1984;56:1647–1649.

80. Millard-Stafford ML, Collins MA, Modlesky CM, Snow TK, Rosskopf LB. Effect of race and resistance training status on the density of fat-free mass and percent fat estimates. *J Appl Physiol.* 2001;91:1259–1268.

81. Visser M, Gallagher D, Deurenberg P, Wang J, Pierson RN Jr, Heymsfield SB. Density of fat-free body mass: relationship with race, age, and level of body fatness. *Am J Physiol.* 1997;272:E781–E787.

82. Fields DA, Goran MI, McCrory MA. Body-composition assessment via air-displacement plethysmography in adults and children: a review. *Am J Clin Nutr.* 2002;75:453–467.

83. Baumgartner RN. Electrical impedance and total body electrical conductivity. In: Roche AF, Heymsfield SB, Lohman TG, eds. *Human Body Composition.* Champaign, IL: Human Kinetics; 1996:79–107.

84. Bioelectrical impedance analysis in body composition measurement. *NIH Technol Assess Statement.* 1996;(Dec 12–14):1–35.

85. Ellis KJ, Bell SJ, Chertow GM, Chumlea WC, Knox TA, Kotler DF, Lukaski HC, Schoeller DA. Bioelectrical impedance methods in clinical research: a follow-up to the NIH Technology Assessment Conference. *Nutrition.* 1999;15:874–880.

86. Kushner RF, Gudivaka R, Schoeller DA. Clinical characteristics influencing bioelectrical impedance analysis measurements. *Am J Clin Nutr.* 1996;64(suppl):423S–427S.

87. Houtkooper LB, Going SB, Lohman TG, Roche AF, Van Loan M. Bioelectrical impedance estimation of fat-free body mass in children and youth: a cross-validation study. *J Appl Physiol.* 1992;72:366–373.

88. Lukaski HC, Siders WA. Validity and accuracy of regional bioelectrical impedance devices to determine whole-body fatness. *Nutrition.* 2003;19:851–857.

89. Gartner A, Dioum A, Delpeuch F, Maire B, Schutz Y. Use of hand-to-hand impedancemetry to predict body composition of African women as measured by air displacement plethysmography. *Eur J Clin Nutr.* 2004;58:523–531.

90. Varady KA, Santosa S, Jones PJH. Validation of hand-held bioelectrical impedance analysis with magnetic resonance imaging for the assessment of body composition in overweight women. *Am J Hum Biol.* 2007;19: 429–433.

91. Strain GW, Wang J, Gagner M, Pomp A, Inabnet WB, Heymsfield SB. Bioimpedance for severe obesity: comparing research methods for total body water and resting energy expenditure. *Obesity.* 2008;16:1953–1956.

92. Jebb SA, Siervo M, Murgatroyd PR, Evans S, Fruhbeck G, Prentice AM. Validity of the leg-to-leg bioimpedance to estimate changes in body fat during weight loss and regain in overweight women: a comparison with multi-compartment models. *Int J Obes.* 2007;31:756–762.

93. Thomson R, Brinkworth GD, Buckley JD, Noakes M, Clifton PM. Good agreement between bioelectrical impedance and dual-energy X-ray absorptiometry for estimating changes in body composition during weight loss in overweight young women. *Clin Nutr.* 2007;26:771–777.

94. Clark RR, Bartok C, Sullivan JC, Schoeller DA. Minimum weight prediction methods cross-validated by the four-component model. *Med Sci Sports Exerc.* 2004;36:639–647.

95. Clark RR, Bartok C, Sullivan JC, Schoeller DA. Is leg-to-leg BIA valid for predicting minimum weight in wrestlers? *Med Sci Sports Exerc.* 2005;37:1061–1068.

96. Swartz AM, Evans MJ, King GA, Thompson DL. Evaluation of a foot-to-foot bioelectrical impedance analyser in highly active, moderately active and less active young men. *Br J Nutr.* 2002;88:205–210.

97. Harrison GC, Buskirk ER, Carter JEL, Johnston FE, Lohman TG, Pollack ML, Roche AF, Wilmore J. Skinfold thicknesses and measurement technique. In: Lohman TG, Roche AF, Martorell R, eds. *Anthropometric Standardization Reference Manual.* Champaign, IL: Human Kinetics; 1988:55–70.

98. Jackson AS, Pollock ML. Practical assessment of body composition. *Phys Sportsmed.* 1985;13:76–90.

99. Jackson AS, Pollock ML. Generalized equations for predicting body density of men. *Br J Nutr.* 1978;40:497–504.

100. Jackson AS, Pollock ML, Ward A. Generalized equations for predicting body density of women. *Med Sci Sports Exerc.* 1980;12:175–182.

101. Clark RR, Bartok C, Sullivan JC, Schoeller DA. Minimum weight prediction methods cross-validated by the four-component model. *Med Sci Sports Exerc.* 2004;36:639–647.

102. Slaughter MH, Lohman TG, Boileau RA, Horswill CA, Stillman RJ, Van Loan MD, Bemben DA. Skinfold equations for estimation of body fatness in children and youth. *Hum Biol.* 1988;60:709–723.

103. Lohman TG, Pollock ML, Slaughter MH, Brandon L, Boileau RA. Methodological factors and the prediction of body fat in female athletes. *Med Sci Sports Exerc.* 1984;16:92–96.

104. Léger LA, Lambert J, Martin P. Validity of plastic caliper measurements. *Hum Biol.* 1982;54:667–675.

105. Lanza E. Determination of moisture, protein, fat and calories in raw pork and beef by near infrared spectroscopy. *J Food Sci.* 1983;48:471–474.

106. Nielsen DH, Cassady SL, Wacker LM, Wessels AK, Wheelock BJ, Oppliger RA. Validation of Futrex 5000 near-infrared spectrophotometer analyzer for assessment of body composition. *J Orthop Sports Phys Ther.* 1992;16: 281–287.

107. Cassady SL, Nielsen DH, Janz KF, Wu Y, Cook JS, Hansen JR. Validity of near infrared body composition analysis in children and adolescents. *Med Sci Sports Exerc.* 1993;25:1185–1191.

108. Eaton AW, Israel RG, O'Brien KF, Hortobagyi T, McCammon MR. Comparison of four methods to assess body composition in women. *Eur J Clin Nutr.* 1993;47:353–360.

109. Heyward VH, Cook KL, Hicks VL, Jenkins KA, Quatrochi JA, Wilson WL. Predictive accuracy of three field methods for estimating relative body fatness of nonobese and obese women. *Int J Sport Nutr.* 1992;2:75–86.

110. Wilmore KM, McBride PJ, Wilmore JH. Comparison of bioelectric impedance and near-infrared interactance for body composition assessment in a population of self-perceived overweight adults. *Int J Obes Relat Metab Disord.* 1994;18:375–381.

111. Houmard JA, Israel RG, McCammon MR, O'Brien KF, Omer J, Zamora BS. Validity of a near-infrared device for estimating body composition in a college football team. *J Appl Sport Sci Res.* 1991;5:53–59.

112. Smith DB, Johnson GO, Stout JR, Housh TJ, Housh DJ, Evetovich TK. Validity of near-infrared interactance for estimating relative body fat in female high school gymnasts. *Int J Sports Med.* 1997;18:531–537.

Chapter 10

ENERGY BALANCE

CHRISTOPHER MELBY, DRPH

Introduction

The rapid increase in the prevalence of obesity in the United States has spawned a weight-loss industry that is fraught with quick-fix approaches, diet gimmicks, misinformation, and confusion for the public. Athletes and other active individuals attempting to lose body weight for reasons of health, metabolic fitness, and sports performance are not immune to such marketing. Similarly, athletes attempting to gain weight are also faced with a barrage of often conflicting information about how to best achieve their goals. Given these scenarios, a firm understanding of the factors that affect energy balance will enable health practitioners to provide their clients with the most accurate scientific approaches possible, and can help them sort through the vast amounts of misinformation clamoring for their attention. In this chapter, the foundational principles of energy balance will be examined, which will set the stage for Chapter 11 on dietary approaches to body weight regulation. The concepts presented in this chapter have relevance to athletes attempting to alter body weight and composition, as well as nonathletes initiating diet and exercise changes. It is important to recognize the dynamic nature of energy balance, wherein changes in one side of the equation can result in changes in the other side, which can have substantial effects on body weight regulation. Box 10.1 defines some of the terms that will be used throughout this chapter.

Foundational Principles of Bioenergetics

The foundational principles for body weight regulation come from the field of bioenergetics. Energy is defined as the capacity to do work, and in the case of the human body, this work is of a biologic and physical nature, which includes a variety of cellular processes such as transport of ions against their concentration gradient, the synthesis of various compounds such as glycogen and proteins, and, of course, skeletal muscle contraction for physical activity.

Figures 10.1 and 10.2 provide a schematic overview of several fundamental aspects of energy metabolism in the human body. Energy contained in the chemical bonds of the adenosine triphosphate molecule is the primary "currency" of energy used for biologic work. Upon hydrolysis of ATP to ADP and inorganic phosphate (Pi), energy is released (exergonic process), which is used for vital cellular processes. The daily ATP requirement is met, not by tapping into a large reservoir of stored ATP, but rather primarily by rapidly resynthesizing ATP from ADP and Pi in the mitochondria. This process of ATP synthesis is highly endergonic, with the necessary energy input provided indirectly from the oxidation of macronutrients, including carbohydrates, fats, and deaminated amino acids. In oxidation reactions catalyzed by dehydrogenase enzymes, hydrogen atoms are removed from macronutrient intermediates by the coenzymes nicotinamide adenine dinucleotide (NAD+) and flavin adenine dinucleotide (FAD), resulting in the reduction of these molecules to NADH and FADH$_2$. These reduced coenzymes in turn undergo oxidation in the electron transport system, with the electrons being passed between conjugate redox pairs in the respiratory chain to ultimately reduce oxygen to form water. These oxidation/reduction reactions result in protons being pumped from the mitochondrial matrix across the inner mitochondrial membrane, resulting in the generation of a membrane potential and a pH gradient. This potential energy is then used to drive the endergonic process of ATP synthesis from ADP and Pi as the hydrogen ions (protons) move back across the inner mitochondrial membrane by way of a specific conductance pathway associated with ATP synthase. In this way, oxidation reactions are coupled to phosphorylation of ADP, hence the term *oxidative phosphorylation* to describe the

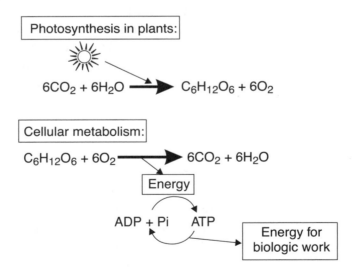

FIGURE 10.1   The synthesis of glucose in plants via photosynthesis provides chemical energy for the human body. The metabolism of glucose shows how the exergonic process of glucose oxidation in cellular respiration provides the energy required for ATP synthesis. Lipids and proteins (amino acids) also undergo oxidation to provide the necessary energy for ATP synthesis.

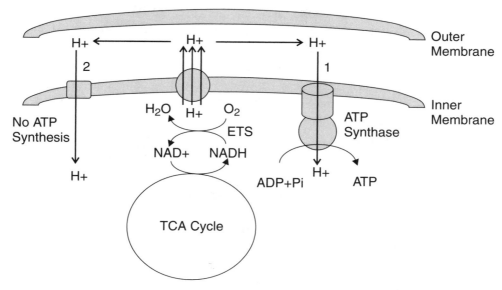

FIGURE 10.2   Simplified mitochondrial bioenergetics. In the tricarboxylic acid cycle (TCA or Kreb's cycle) oxidation reactions catalyzed by dehydrogenase enzymes result in hydrogen atoms being removed from substrates by the coenzymes nicotinamide adenine dinucleotide (NAD+) and flavin adenine dinucleotide (FAD; not shown in diagram) resulting in the reduction of these molecules to NADH and $FADH_2$. These reduced coenzymes in turn undergo oxidation in the electron transport system, with the electrons being passed between conjugate redox pairs in the respiratory chain to ultimately reduce oxygen to form water. These oxidation/reduction reactions result in protons being pumped from the mitochondrial matrix across the inner mitochondrial membrane, resulting in the generation of a membrane potential and a pH gradient. As shown in **arrow 1**, this energy is then used to drive the endergonic process of ATP synthesis from ADP and Pi as the hydrogen ions (protons) move back across the inner mitochondrial membrane by way of a specific conductance pathway associated with ATP synthase. If protons "leak" back into the matrix by conduction pathways not linked to ATP synthase shown by **arrow 2** (eg, by uncoupling proteins found in highly thermogenic brown adipose tissue [BAT]), the coupling efficiency of oxidation and phosphorylation is reduced, and more heat and fewer ATP molecules are synthesized relative to the amount of oxygen consumed. (For more information, see reference 1.)

synthesis of ATP inside the mitochondria. Given the importance of oxygen as the final oxidizing agent in the electron transport chain, determining the rate of oxygen consumption and carbon dioxide production via indirect calorimetry provides an accurate measure of whole-body energy expenditure except when substantial amounts of ATP are produced anaerobically.

Metabolic Efficiency

The second law of thermodynamics dictates that the cellular reactions that generate ATP are less than perfectly efficient—that is, at least a portion of the energy released from the oxidation of macronutrients will be lost as heat rather than conserving all of the available energy in the phosphoanhydride bonds of ATP molecules. Note that even under normal conditions, the cellular oxidation of glucose results in greater amounts of heat production than energy conserved as ATP. The more heat produced and the fewer ATP molecules synthesized relative to the potential energy in a macronutrient, the more energetically inefficient is the process.

Returning to our discussion of mitochondrial bioenergetics, if protons "leak" back into the matrix by conduction pathways not linked to ATP synthase (eg, by uncoupling proteins found in highly thermogenic brown adipose tissue (BAT), the coupling efficiency of oxidation and phosphorylation is reduced, and more heat and fewer ATP molecules are synthesized relative to the amount of oxygen consumed. A person who produces more heat and fewer ATP per mole of substrate would thus be less energetically efficient compared to an individual who produces more ATP relative to the amount of substrate oxidized. It follows then, that energetic inefficiency is characterized by more substrate required to synthesize a given amount of ATP, which in turn will require more oxygen consumption (reduction of oxygen to water) in the mitochondria. There is considerable research interest in variable efficiency rates of cellular energy transduction, which could theoretically help explain susceptibility and resistance to obesity among humans living in the same obesigenic environment (1). The commonly observed phenomenon that individuals subjected to the same magnitude of energy deficit or surplus do not all lose or gain the same amount of weight, respectively, has been suggested to be at least partly due to individual differences in energy efficiency in response to dieting or overeating (2). The recently published observations of variable amounts of brown fat depots in human adults (3) and the observation that the amount of brown fat in adults is inversely correlated with BMI (4) provide credible evidence for human differences in metabolic efficiency.

As we examine the energy balance equation it will be important to remember four specific principles: (*a*) the laws of thermodynamics are inviolable; (*b*) the large variation in human responses to similar diet and/or exercise changes likely results, at least in part, from differences in energetic efficiency linked to genetic and epigenetic variation; (*c*) changing one side of the energy balance scale will usually result in metabolic and/or behavioral changes in the other side; and (*d*) human responses to diet and exercise that seem contrary to our understanding of bioenergetics (eg, individuals losing far less weight than predicted based on their purported decreases in energy intake and increases in exercise) cannot be violations of the laws of thermodynamics. These are due instead to substantial limitations in our ability to accurately measure energy intake and total energy expenditure and its individual components as well as our limited ability to measure changes in energetic efficiency in response to external perturbations such as changes in diet and exercise.

The Energy Balance Equation

The first law of thermodynamics states that energy is neither created nor destroyed, but it is transformed from one form to another. Because we must account for the energy we consume (macronutrients) and the energy we expend in carrying out the processes vital to life, the energy balance equation is based on this law. Succinctly stated, this equation dictates that energy consumed in excess of expenditure will result in increased energy stores, and that body energy stores will decrease if energy consumed is less than expenditure. Despite the perceptions of some individuals who seem readily susceptible to weight gain, it is impossible to increase body energy stores without energy intake exceeding energy expenditure. We simply cannot defy the first law of thermodynamics in an attempt to explain why some individuals are more prone to weight gain than others. An understanding of the various determinants of both sides of the balance—energy expenditure and intake—will enable us to appreciate the many nuances and complexities of this equation, which will help ensure its proper use (Figure 10.3).

Neuroendocrine Regulation of Energy Balance

Both energy intake and expenditure can be readily modified by voluntary behavior—after all, the amount and types of food we eat and our level of physical activity are choices we make. However, over the past several

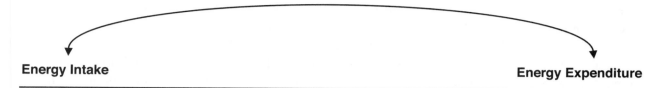

Energy Intake	Energy Expenditure
• Food availability	• Resting metabolic rate
• Serving sizes	• Body size—respiring mass
• Macronutrient composition	• Lean body mass
• Energy density	• Internal organs—liver, heart, brain, lungs
• Hedonic qualities—taste, texture, etc.	• Thyroid hormones
• Personal preferences	• Gender
• Dietary fiber	• Thermic effect of food
• Hunger signals	• Meal size
• Ghrelin	• Macronutrient composition of meal
• Neuropeptide Y and other neuropeptides	• Obligatory thermogenesis—digestion, absorption, assimilation, synthesis
• Transient decrease in blood glucose	• Facultative thermogenesis—sympathetic nervous system
• Satiety signals	• Hormonal response—insulin
• Cholecystokinin, leptin, insulin	• Physical activity energy expenditure
• Sociocultural norms	• Exercise energy expenditure—mode, intensity, duration, frequency
• Socioeconomic status	• Excess postexercise energy expenditure
• Psychological factors	• Non-exercise activity thermogenesis (NEAT)
• Emotions—anger, stress, anxiety, etc.	• Activities of daily living
• Coping responses	• Fidgeting
• Living environment	• Posture
• Cooking skills	• Energy efficiency—adaptive thermogenesis, mitochondrial proton leaks, futile cycles, etc

FIGURE 10.3   The dynamic or interactive energy balance equation predicts that body energy stores are a function of energy intake and energy expenditure, both of which are influenced by a multitude of factors. Sizable changes in energy intake usually evoke compensatory behavioral and metabolic changes in energy expenditure that defend the initial body weight. Conversely, sizable changes in energy expenditure may evoke changes in energy intake. These compensatory changes vary substantially between individuals and are related to neuroendocrine adjustments and cognitive factors.

decades considerable evidence has emerged showing that energy balance is regulated by a host of neuroendocrine factors. This notion is summarized by Jeffrey Friedman, MD, PhD, an internationally recognized scientist known for his work in molecular genetics, energy regulation, and obesity, states: "The simplistic notion that weight can be controlled by 'deciding' to eat less and exercise more is at odds with substantial scientific evidence illuminating a precise and powerful biologic system that maintains body weight within a relatively narrow range" (5). Although his view of the magnitude of genetic control over body weight is not shared by all scientists, it does highlight the fact that regulatory controls of body weight do exist. The hypothalamus integrates a host of signals from the liver, gut, and adipose tissue to regulate energy expenditure and the initiation, termination, and frequency of eating. A discussion of the variety of afferent signals including insulin, leptin, and ghrelin is beyond the scope of this chapter, but it should be understood that a powerful homeostatic regulation of food intake occurs such that severe energy restriction leading to weight loss typically results in a strong internal drive to eat, whereas an overabundance of food intake and weight gain is often followed by a reduction in food intake. These homeostatic compensatory responses have been observed in both animals and humans and are part of the "set point" theory, wherein deviations from a biologically determined weight are met with metabolic and feeding changes that alter energy expenditure and intake in an effort to defend the "set point" and to return body weight to its preestablished level (6). For example, as adipose tissue expands, the adiposity-related signals insulin and leptin increase in circulation (7–9). Through their effect on specific hypothalamic neurons, they stimulate increased energy expenditure and a sense of satiety leading to decreased food intake. A loss of body fat reduces these signals, leading to decreased energy expenditure and increased food intake (8,9). This communication between adipose tissue and the brain suggests that the control of body weight extends beyond volitional behavior.

The rapid increase in human obesity may seem to be at odds with the set point theory because "corrective internal actions" would seem to be lacking in a substantial portion of the population in the face of our current obesigenic environment. However, it may be that the obesity-prone person regulates body weight, but simply at a higher "set point" than the obesity-resistant individual (8). It is also possible that impairments in regulation occur such that the brain becomes "resistant" to peripheral signals such as leptin and insulin. There is also the possibility that most humans exhibit a stronger, more powerful defense against weight loss than against weight gain. Regardless, it is evident that compensatory changes in energy intake occur in both obese and nonobese individuals (including athletes) in response to energy excesses or deficiencies (10,11). The magnitude of these compensatory responses is probably under both genetic control and environmental influences. The contributions of genes vs voluntary behavior in ultimately determining an individual's body weight are unknown. The "either-or" debate (genetic/biologic determinism vs voluntary choices) is not particularly helpful in dealing with individual clients. What is important is to seek understanding of the behavioral and metabolic features of the individual client or athlete, with the aim of developing the most effective personalized approach to achieving a healthy and competitive body weight and composition.

Energy Expenditure

There are four components of total daily energy expenditure (TDEE) that make up one side of the energy balance scale: resting metabolic rate (RMR), the thermic effect of food (TEF), nonexercise activity thermogenesis (NEAT), and exercise energy expenditure (ExEE) (Figure 10.3). A brief discussion of each of the four components follows.

Resting Metabolic Rate

RMR is the energy expended by an individual for cellular processes necessary to maintain life while lying supine in a postabsorptive, awakened state (12). For sedentary individuals, the RMR accounts for approximately 70% to75% of daily energy expenditure (13). There are many factors that influence RMR, the most pronounced being body size (especially lean body mass), with greater respiring tissue mass accounting for greater energy expenditure. Among adults, RMR is generally lower in women than men, mostly due to differences in lean body mass. It decreases with advancing age, primarily resulting from age-related declines in lean mass. It has been estimated that RMR decreases approximately 2% per decade in healthy adult women, and approximately 3% per decade in healthy adult men (14). Although skeletal muscle accounts for a sizable portion of lean tissue, the internal organs including the liver, heart, brain, kidneys, and lungs together expend far more energy *at rest* than does skeletal muscle. Numerous hormones affect RMR as well, especially the thyroid hormone tri-iodothyronine (T_3). Individuals with a hypoactive thyroid gland have lower metabolic rates than their body size would predict and they tend to readily gain weight and experience profound fatigue until the condition is corrected. On the other hand, a hyperactive thyroid gland leads to decreased energy efficiency characterized by increased RMR and weight loss.

Measurement of RMR

Typically RMR is measured for 30 to 60 minutes in the early morning approximately 10 to 12 hours after the previous evening's meal while lying quietly in a recumbent position in a thermoneutral environment (12). Most often RMR is measured via indirect calorimetry, a process involving the measurement of respiratory gases. Because oxygen utilization in the mitochondria is directly tied to ATP synthesis and heat production, the measurement of oxygen consumption (and carbon dioxide production) is used to accurately quantify energy expenditure. A ventilatory mask, mouthpiece, or canopy is used in conjunction with a metabolic cart equipped with a flow meter and CO_2 and O_2 analyzers. Based on the oxygen consumption per minute and the energy equivalent per liter of oxygen, energy expenditure per minute is determined, which is then extrapolated to a 24-hour period. Some handheld measurement devices are also available. These are less expensive and provide reasonably accurate measurements of RMR, but they are generally not capable of measuring the energy costs of exercise when ventilation rates are much higher than during rest.

Estimation of RMR by Prediction Equations

Because indirect calorimetry is not accessible by all athletes, many RMR prediction equations have been developed. These typically include such variables as body size, age, and sex, with more sophisticated equations including some measure of lean and fat mass as well. Some commonly used equations are provided in Box 10.2 (15–19). Unfortunately, the development of RMR equations for athletes has lagged behind those established for the general population, and it is possible that the accuracy of the common equations overestimate RMR values in obese individuals, owing to their lower lean-to-fat mass ratio, while these same equations may underestimate RMR in athletes, who typically exhibit a higher lean-to-fat mass ratio than characteristic of the general population.

Effect of Exercise on RMR

In a number of studies, endurance-trained athletes have been found to exhibit higher RMR than nonathletes. However, this phenomenon does not seem to result from any adaptations to exercise training. It is more likely that the combination of high exercise energy expenditure and high energy intake (high flux) in these athletes can temporarily, but not permanently, increase their RMR when measured the next morning after exercise (20). However, there is little evidence that the amount of physical activity done for health maintenance and weight control by recreational exercisers will produce any increases in RMR, with the possible exception of such exercise in older individuals (21).

Some fitness enthusiasts have promoted the idea that because regular weightlifting can increase skeletal muscle mass, such exercise will substantially increase RMR. Although this may be an attractive notion, this increased muscle mass is likely to occur only for the individual who becomes a serious weightlifter. The contribution of each pound of muscle mass to *resting* energy expenditure is far less than that of a similar mass of such internal organs as liver, heart, etc, so one would have to substantially increase muscle mass to increase RMR. Most people who lift weights for health rather than for bodybuilding or sports competition will not increase their muscle mass enough to produce more than a small increase in RMR. For the serious weight trainer, a single prolonged strenuous bout of weight lifting may increase RMR when measured the following morning (22). Nevertheless, it is clear that for both athletes and nonathletes, young and old, the *major* impact of both endurance and resistance exercise on total daily energy expenditure occurs during the activity itself, and not from any substantial increases in RMR.

BOX 10.2   Equations for Estimating Resting Metabolic Rate (RMR)

There is likely not a single best equation for all athletes, because there is substantial diversity in body composition among athletes competing in different sports. If fat-free mass (FFM) can be accurately determined, the Cunningham equation often works well, but as the amount of body fat increases in athletes, its contribution to RMR will increase, which is not accounted for in this particular equation. For female athletes, the Owen equation is often used, as it was derived specifically from the study of elite female athletes. However, the number of female athletes studied to derive this equation was quite small (n = 8). The example in this box uses the Mifflin-St. Jeor equation, but the reader is encouraged to use each of the equations for the sample athlete to identify the range of predicted RMR values.

Harris-Benedict Equation (15)

Males: RMR (kcal/d) = 66.4730 + 13.7516W + 5.0033H − 6.7750A

Females: RMR (kcal/d) = 665.0955 + 9.5634W + 1.8496H − 4.6756A

Where: W = weight (kg); H = height (cm); A = age (y).

Cunningham Equation (16)

Males: RMR (kcal/d) = 370 + 21.6FFM

Females: RMR (kcal/d) = 370 + 21.6FFM

Where: FFM = fat-free mass

Owen Equation (17,18)

Males: RMR (kcal/d) = 879 + 10.2W

Females: RMR (kcal/d) = 795 + 7.18W

Female athletes: RMR (kcal/d) = 50.4 + 21.1W

Where: W = weight (kg)

Mifflin-St. Jeor Equation (19)

Males: RMR (kcal/d) = 10W + 6.25H − 5A + 5

Females: RMR (kcal/d) = 10W + 6.25H − 5A − 161

Where: W = weight (kg); H = height (cm); A = age (y)

Example

30-year-old male endurance athlete (very active) who is 1.75 m tall (5 ft, 9 in) and weighs 73 kg (160.6 lb). Using the Mifflin-St. Jeor equation:

RMR = (10 × 73) + (6.25 × 175) − (5 × 30) + 5 = 1,679 kcal/d

Source: Data are from references 15–19.

Thermic Effect of Food

TEF is defined as the increase in energy expenditure above RMR in response to the ingestion of food. This increase in energy expenditure is attributable to obligatory components that include digestion, absorption, transport, and assimilation of the food we eat, as well as a facultative component. The latter is the portion of TEF that results from the increase in sympathetic nervous system activity that accompanies food consumption.

Measurement of TEF

The TEF is usually measured in the same way as RMR, ie, via indirect calorimetry. A meal of known macronutrient and calorie content is provided and the increase in energy expenditure above RMR is measured over a 3- to 6-hour period, with more accurate determinations made over at least 5 to 6 hours (13). The average TEF for a mixed meal accounts for approximately 10% of energy ingested. The thermic effect of the individual macronutrients varies considerably, with fat having the lowest at approximately 3% of ingested fat calories, followed by carbohydrates at 5% to 10% of ingested carbohydrate energy, and proteins having the highest thermic effect at 20% to 30% of protein calories (23).

Physical Activity Energy Expenditure (PAEE)

The PAEE is the energy expenditure above resting values that results from skeletal muscle contraction, including that required for movement, balance, and maintenance of posture. This component can be further divided into the ExEE and NEAT.

Exercise Energy Expenditure (ExEE)

Exercise is defined as volitional movement done for the purpose of improving or maintaining one or more features of either health- or performance-related physical fitness (24). Exercise is typically the most variable component of daily energy expenditure, and for the athlete attempting to modify body weight and composition, it is obviously the component under the most volitional control. The energetic cost of daily exercise is based on the frequency, duration, intensity, and mode of exercise, and on a given day can range from zero calories for the nonexerciser, to several thousand calories for an individual who participates in a long-distance endurance event such as a marathon. Athletes who participate in regular strenuous and prolonged exercise training have very high TDEE values, which may require conscientious efforts on their part to obtain adequate energy intake. For example, in a previous study, it was estimated the energy requirements in competitive cyclists to be approximately 4,300 kcal/d while in training, and less than 2,400 kcal on very sedentary days (20).

The energy expended for a given exercise bout are usually determined by indirect calorimetry done in a laboratory and then extrapolated to a free-living situation with adjustments made for body size. A compendium of the energy expenditure values for many modes, durations, and intensities of exercise has been published by the American College of Sports Medicine (25). These values are useful in helping determine the contribution of PAEE to TDEE and energy balance. Often the energetic cost of exercise is expressed in metabolic equivalents, or METs, which are multiples of RMR. For example, if an individual expends 1.25 kcal/min at rest, and during a given training session has an exercise energy expenditure of 17.5 kcal/min, his exercise intensity is: 17.5 kcal/min ÷ 1.25 kcal/min = 14 METs. Energy expenditure is elevated for a period following exercise, and this excess postexercise energy expenditure should be considered part of the total ExEE.

Nonexercise Activity Thermogenesis (NEAT)

NEAT is the energy expenditure resulting from physical activity that is not considered exercise, such as activities of daily living and fidgeting. This component of TDEE is difficult to measure, and often is determined by default after measuring the other three components and subtracting them from TDEE, or by using light weight sensors to detect posture and motion. Primarily owing to the work of James Levine at the Mayo Clinic, NEAT is now widely recognized as an important and highly variable component of TDEE (26,27). Maintaining body posture is also part of NEAT. Obese individuals have been shown to spend more time sitting during the day than do nonobese individuals (28). Sitting energy expenditure is lower than standing, as the latter requires muscle contractions necessary to maintain balance.

Determination of TDEE

The accurate determination of TDEE, which is used to identify a person's energy requirements, is difficult at best. Whole-room calorimeters are used by some scientists, but are not available for most people, and even when used by scientists their use typically underestimates TDEE because ambulation is limited within the small chamber. The use of stable isotopes of hydrogen and oxygen (ie, doubly labeled water) provides accurate measures of TDEE in a free-living environment, but use of this approach is impractical apart from access to a major research institution. The factorial method involves measurement of the individual components of TDEE and then summing these up to determine TDEE. However, this approach is very labor intensive and impractical. Pedometers, accelerometers, and heart rate monitors can be useful in quantifying the amount of physical activity, especially when accompanied by activity diaries. However, conversion of data from steps walked, accelerometer counts, or changes in heart rate to precise energy expenditure values can be problematic. In light of these issues, TDEE is commonly estimated by multiplying either estimated or measured RMR by a specified physical activity level (PAL), which is a factor based on estimated PAEE. For a sedentary person, the estimates are likely to be more accurate, owing to a small contribution of physical activity to TDEE. However, for athletes there is substantial room for error based on the significant contribution of ExEE to TDEE. The PAL values have been derived from a variety of methods, including the factorial approach and the use of doubly labeled water. Table 10.1 (29) provides the values for PALs established by the Institute of Medicine based on a compilation of doubly labeled water values in free-living

TABLE 10.1   Institute of Medicine Physical Activity Levels (PAL)

PAL Category	Mean PAL Value (Range)	Example
Sedentary	1.25 (1.1–1.39)	A person with a sedentary occupation who spends his entire day sitting.
Low level of physical activity	1.50 (1.40–1.59)	An office worker who sits most of the day other than the walking necessary to perform tasks of daily living.
Active	1.75 (1.60–1.89)	Athlete who exercises approximately 1 h/d or a person with an active vocation equivalent to walking 6–8 mile/d.
Very active	2.20 (1.90–2.50)	Competitive athlete engaging in several hours of vigorous exercise training.

Source: Data are from reference 29.

TABLE 10.2 Estimated Energy Requirements for Adults (≥ Age 19 y) Based on Predicted Total Daily Energy Expenditure

Sex	Estimated Energy Requirement,[a] kcal/d	Physical Activity (PA) Coefficients
Male	$662 - 9.53A + [PA \times (15.9W + 540H)]$	• 1.00: Sedentary • 1.11: Low active • 1.25: Active • 1.48: Very active
Female	$354 - 6.91A + [PA \times (9.36W + 726H)]$	• 1.00: Sedentary • 1.12: Low active • 1.27: Active • 1.45: Very active

[a] A = age (y); W = weight (kg); H = height (m)
Source: Data are from reference 29.

individuals. The PALs range from 1.25 for an extremely sedentary person with limited opportunity to be ambulatory to more than 2.5 for an athlete who spends hours per day in exercise training. For example, in the study mentioned earlier (20), the competitive cyclists had resting metabolic rates of approximately 1,800 kcal/d and estimated TDEE values of 4,300 kcal/d, with a calculated PAL of 4,300 kcal/1,800 kcal = approximately 2.4. Interestingly, on sedentary days, these same athletes exhibited TDEE reflective of a PAL of approximately 1.42.

Another means of estimating TDEE has been provided by the Institute of Medicine. An expert panel of scientists under contract from the US Department of Health and Human Services was convened to develop estimates of daily energy intake commensurate with good nutrition (29). Based on studies using doubly labeled water to quantify TDEE in free-living individuals, the panel established mathematically derived equations that use age, height, body weight, and physical activity factors to estimate TDEE. These male- and female-specific equations are provided in Table10.2 (29). Note that the physical activity (PA) coefficients used in these equations are not the same as PALs. Box 10.3 provides a comparison of two estimations of an athlete's energy requirements, one using the Mifflin-St Jeor formula and the other using the Institute of Medicine equation. As can be seen in these calculations, TDEE for this person varied by several hundred calories, demonstrating the difficulty in accurately determining TDEE.

Energy Intake

There are many factors that affect energy intake among active individuals, including the availability and palatability of food, macronutrient composition, social norms, peer pressure, economics, and psychological and emotional factors, to name a few (Figure 10.3). These external and internal factors interact with neuroendocrine signals to affect food intake. While it is beyond the scope of this chapter to provide a thorough discussion of all of these factors, the potential for dietary composition to affect energy intake and energy balance warrants some discussion.

Effect of Dietary Composition on Energy Intake

There is evidence that habitual intake of high-fat, mixed meals promote higher energy intake than lower fat meals (30). It seems that the higher energy content of the former is less well "noticed," a phenomenon termed *passive overconsumption.* Given the higher energy intake and the fact that, of the three macronutrients,

---

BOX 10.3   Sample Calculations of Total Daily Energy Expenditure

Athlete Profile
A 30-year-old male endurance athlete (very active) is 1.75 m tall (5 ft 9 in) and weighs 73 kg (160.6 lb). Estimated PAL for this athlete is 2.2. Estimated PA is 1.48.

Example 1: Estimate Using Mifflin-St. Jeor Equation and PAL

$$RMR\ (kcal/d) = 10W + 6.25H - 5A + 5$$

Where: W = weight (kg); H = height (cm); A = age (y).

$$RMR = (10 \times 73) + (6.25 \times 175) - (5 \times 30) + 5 = 1{,}679\ kcal/d$$

$$TDEE = RMR \times PAL$$

$$TDEE = 1679 \times 2.2 = 3{,}694\ kcal/d$$

Example 2: Estimate Using Estimated Energy Requirement

$$EER = 662 - 9.53A + [PA \times (15.9W + 540H)]$$

Where: A = age (y); W = weight (kg); H = height (m).

$$EER = 662 - (9.53 \times 30) + 1.48\ [(15.9 \times 73) + (540 \times 1.75)] = 3{,}493\ kcal/d$$

---

dietary fat is the weakest at promoting its own oxidation, one can envision why overfeeding and fat deposition can so readily occur when the dietary composition is high in fat.

Measurement of Energy Intake

Just like the measurement of energy expenditure, the accurate determination of one's energy intake is also fraught with difficulties. Self-reported energy intake can be derived from diet recalls, diet records, and food frequency questionnaires using computer software with the US Department of Agriculture database for nutrient composition of foods. However, self-reported intake often substantially underestimates actual energy intake (31,32). Inaccuracies in dietary self-report severely limit their use in attempting to accurately quantify energy intake.

If an individual's body weight and body composition are stable, energy intake and energy expenditure will be similar over time. Estimating energy expenditure by using an appropriate PAL or equation in Table 10.2 is likely to provide a more accurate estimate of energy intake than will the self-reported dietary intake method. However, self-reported levels of physical activity used to establish an appropriate PAL (Table 10.1) or PA coefficient (Table 10.2) are often overestimated, and one must consider this possibility when there is a large mismatch between self-reported dietary intake and estimated energy requirements.

Complexities of the Energy Balance Equation

An overly simplistic view of the energy balance equation may lead to projections or even promises of the magnitude of weight loss or weight gain that an athlete should achieve based on his or her diet or exercise changes. However, these projections often assume that all other factors that affect the energy balance equation remain the same. Such a static equation fails to account for homeostatic behavioral and metabolic adjustments in response to perturbations in energy intake and expenditure that render the static energy balance equation inadequate to accurately depict the reality of the human experience. Less than predicted changes in body weight and composition can lead to both athlete and counselor discouragement and frustration.

Dietary-Induced Changes in Energy Balance

Energy Deficit Leading to Weight Loss

It is clear from many studies that during the dynamic phase of weight loss (active weight loss), a hypoenergetic diet results in a decrease in RMR and TDEE. The decreases in energy expenditure with active weight loss can be attributed to a loss of respiring body mass as well as a decrease in energy expenditure per unit body mass, the latter reflecting an increase in energy efficiency. However, there is considerable controversy about whether this increased energy efficiency persists when the individual has maintained this lost weight for a considerable time period. If the increased energy efficiency persists in the reduced weight state, this could help explain the inability of so many individuals to maintain the lost weight, and the reported high levels of exercise and calorie-counting that are required of many individuals to maintain long-term weight loss (33). A recent well-controlled inpatient study (34) sheds some important light on this controversy. Not surprisingly, the investigators found that individuals who lost 10% or more of their body weights over a 5- to 8-week period had a reduced TDEE that was greater than what could be accounted for by loss of body mass when measured within a few weeks of the weight loss. In the same study, another cohort of individuals that had maintained 10% or more weight loss for a minimum of 1 year was examined. The TDEE of this group was also significantly lower than predicted by their metabolic body size. The authors concluded that weight loss produces an increased energy efficiency (lower energy requirements) that persists long-term in those individuals who are able to maintain the weight loss. In an attempt to explain their findings, in a separate study the same research group found weight loss was associated with an increased skeletal muscle work efficiency at very low exercise intensities (eg, pedaling a bicycle at 10 to 25 watts of power) (35).

Given the aforementioned issues, the following scenario describes inappropriate use of the energy balance equation to identify the amount of weight to be lost by a dieting client. Suppose the health practitioner and client agree that a 17-pound weight loss would improve the athlete's sports performance. They set a goal of reducing her energy intake by 500 kcal per day, with the specific daily food reductions identified after a comprehensive dietary assessment. Given that a pound of fat is equivalent to approximately 3,500 kcal, they might conclude that the dietary change would lead to a loss of 1 pound of fat per week (500 kcal/d × 7 days = 3,500 kcal), which over a 4-month period (17 weeks) would result in a 17-pound decrease in body fat. However, the eventual weight loss is far less than predicted, and both client and professional are disappointed and frustrated. In reality, one should not use such a static equation because changes in food intake can result in metabolic and behavioral changes in factors that influence energy expenditure. Owing to the hypocaloric state, RMR will decrease to an extent greater than explained by loss of respiring tissue mass, ie, metabolic efficiency increases. Also, compared to the pre-diet state, the energy cost of any particular weight-bearing movement decreases as body mass is lost, and TEF is reduced as less food is consumed. Thus, an initial 500 kcal deficit shrinks over time with subsequent reduction in the velocity of weight loss. Additionally, not all weight loss is body fat (typically about 75% fat loss, 25% lean), and the energy content of fat and lean tissue are not the same. One can see that given the dynamics induced by an energy deficit, the specific amount of weight lost in a given period is not readily predictable. Adding to this complexity are the difficulties in accurately reducing energy intake by 500 kcal, the possible changes in exercise energy expenditure that can occur when dieting, and the considerable interindividual variation in changes in BMR and PAEE that can occur in response to a reduction in energy intake over a number of months.

Energy Excess Leading to Weight Gain

For the active individual attempting to gain weight (including athletes wanting to increase lean body mass), an increase in energy intake is crucial. However, the increased energy consumption may be offset by compensatory changes in metabolism, such that TDEE energy expenditure will increase and thus attenuate increases in lean body mass. These compensatory changes in energy expenditure are highly variable, as are the magnitude of weight gain and increases in lean mass and body fat. For example, in several studies (36,37) in which individuals were overfed an additional 1,000 kcal/d for several months, there were 3- to 5-fold differences in the magnitude of weight gain between the highest and lowest gainers. In a study from the Mayo Clinic, there was a 10-fold difference in the amount of body fat deposition between the highest and lowest gainers, despite the same magnitude of overfeeding between study participants (1,000 kcal in excess of maintenance requirements) (36). Overfeeding increases RMR in most individuals beyond what would be expected by their changes in body size; ie, overfeeding results in decreased energy efficiency. Also, increases in TEF and the energy cost of movement contribute to an increase in TDEE. Adding to the complexity is the dramatic changes in NEAT that can occur in some individuals. In the Mayo Clinic study, an increase in NEAT was a much stronger predictor of attenuated weight gain than were increases in RMR and TEF (36).

Exercise-Induced Changes in Energy Balance

Just as a change in energy intake can influence energy expenditure, an increase in PAEE can also influence energy intake. Although physical activity is obviously the best means of increasing energy expenditure, the effects on weight loss of exercise alone typically reveal modest results (38) unless substantial increases in ExEE occur without compensatory increases in energy intake (39). The reasons why an exercise-only approach to weight loss produces such small losses of body weight for many individuals is worthy of discussion (see Box 10.4).

The magnitude of an exercise-induced energy deficit and weight loss can be affected by more than just the energy cost of the exercise, as compensatory changes in both NEAT and energy intake may occur. Just as occurs with dieting and overfeeding, there is substantial individual variability in the amount of weight loss due to exercise, as is highlighted by a recent study by King et al (40). In this experimental investigation, overweight and obese individuals underwent prescribed and supervised exercise (500 kcal/session) for 5 days per week for 12 weeks. The average weight loss was 3.7 kg (8.1 lb), which was similar to that predicted using the static energy balance equation, suggesting no metabolic or compensatory changes. However, there was a very large individual response, with four of the 30 study participants actually gaining weight, and in the remaining 26 subjects the weight loss ranged from 1 kg (2.2 lb) to 14.7 kg (32.3 lb). This occurred despite rigorous control and supervision of the exercise program so that all individuals were achieving the same energy cost of exercise. The major predictor of the magnitude of weight change was the change in energy intake that accompanied the exercise. These findings suggest that in response to initiating sizable weekly energy expenditure in exercise, some individuals increase, whereas other individuals actually reduce their energy intakes. Why there is a difference in response is not understood, but it is clear that there are very large differences in body weight and composition changes in response to the same amount of exercise (41).

It is also possible that in response to an increase in exercise energy expenditure, compensatory decreases in NEAT could offset the impact on energy balance. In a study at the University of Vermont,

---

BOX 10.4   The Limited Potential for Substantial Weight Loss from Exercise in a Previously Sedentary Person

Suppose that a sedentary individual attempting to lose some weight decides to do so by starting an exercise program. He establishes a goal of walking for 40 minutes a day, 5 days per week. Based on our understanding of energy balance issues, how much weight might this individual expect to lose over the course of several weeks and months if he tenaciously sticks to his new exercise regimen? The following information provided about this individual will be helpful to our discussion:

- Resting energy expenditure = 1.25 kcal/min = 1,800 kcal/d
- Sitting/standing energy expenditure = 1.5 kcal/min
- Exercise characteristics:
  - Duration: 40 min/exercise session
  - Frequency: 5 times/wk
  - Intensity: 5 METs = 6.25 kcal/min
- *Gross* daily energy cost of 40 min exercise: 6.25 kcal/min × 40 min = 250 kcal/d
- *Net* energy cost of exercise: 250 kcal − (40 min × 1.5) = 190 kcal/d
- Net energy cost of exercise per week: 190 kcal × 5 d/wk = 950 kcal/wk

These data show that while the gross energy cost of the walking exercise is 250 kcal for the 40 minutes, the net energy cost is 60 kcal less, owing to the fact that even if the person had not exercised, he would have expended at least 60 kcal during the 40 minutes while sitting/standing. Without any compensatory changes in dietary intake or other components of energy expenditure, the projected energy deficit over the course of a single month would be less than 4,000 kcal, equivalent to a monthly weight loss of slightly more than 1 lb, assuming no other metabolic or behavioral compensations, which is highly unlikely. This weight loss is far less than one might expect from a monthlong diet. A head-to-head comparison of the amount of weight loss achieved by exercise only vs diet only is somewhat unfair, as the magnitude of energy deficit created by a hypocaloric diet is usually far greater than that created by starting an exercise program.

---

elderly individuals who initiated an endurance exercise training program failed to significantly increase their TDEE, presumably because of a compensatory decline in NEAT during the nonexercise portion of the day (42). However, there remains the possibility that the reverse could be true in some individuals—that is, their NEAT may increase with improved physical fitness (see Figure 10.4).

Effect of Acute Exercise on Postexercise Energy Expenditure

Based on studies done almost 50 years ago, there was a common belief that upon completion of an exercise bout, individuals would continue to expend energy at an excess rate for a prolonged period of time, possibly up to 24 hours. This excess postexercise energy expenditure was thought to be a substantial contributor to TDEE in those who exercised. However, based on more carefully controlled studies, it is apparent that this is usually not the case. Although research has clearly shown that energy expenditure remains increased to more than pre-exercise resting baseline levels immediately after exercise, the magnitude of this postexercise elevation of energy expenditure is almost always quite small unless the exercise bout is of high intensity and prolonged duration. Endurance exercise of the intensity and duration commonly done by

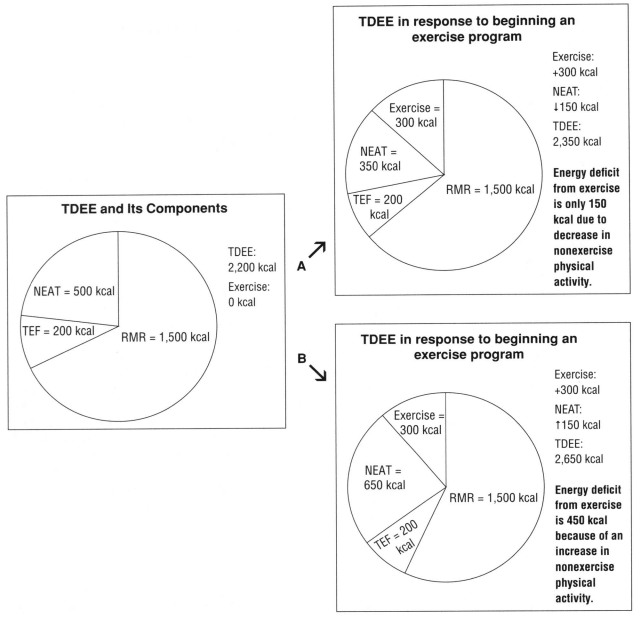

FIGURE 10.4 Two possible scenarios depicting the change in energy balance of a sedentary individual who begins an exercise program to create an energy deficit. Initially the person is in energy balance with a total daily energy expenditure (TDEE) of 2,200 kcal (PAL = 1.47), based on a resting metabolic rate (RMR) of 1,500 kcal, a thermic effect of food (TEF) of 200 kcal, and nonexercise activity thermogenesis (NEAT) of 500 kcal. The person begins an exercise program and adds a net 300 kcal to the energy expenditure side of his energy balance equation. However, as can be seen in scenario A, the person compensates by reducing her activities of daily living, so the net change in energy expenditure is not 300 kcal, but only 150 kcal (see references 41 and 42). In scenario B, in addition to the increase in exercise energy expenditure, the person actually increases NEAT by 150 kcal, and the net increase in TDEE is 450 kcal. Note that any change in energy intake as a result of a change in exercise must also be considered when considering the overall impact on energy balance of beginning an exercise program.

recreational exercisers (for example, walking for 30 to 60 minutes or jogging at a pace of 8 to10 minutes per mile for 30 minutes) typically results in a return to baseline of energy expenditure well within the first hour of recovery (43). The postexercise energy bonus for this type of exercise probably accounts for only about 10 to 30 additional calories expended beyond the exercise bout itself (44). In athletes performing high-intensity, long-duration exercise, the postexercise energy expenditure may remain elevated for a longer period and could contribute a bit more to TDEE (20,43). As discussed earlier in this chapter, endurance athletes who are in a state of high energy flux (high energy intake and expenditure) may have postexercise elevations detectable the morning after exercise (20), but it is the rare individual who can regularly achieve this state of high flux. The average person who does considerably less strenuous exercise will likely experience little meaningful contribution of this postexercise bonus to his or her total daily energy expenditure.

Several studies suggest that vigorous weightlifting exercise may increase energy expenditure to more than usual resting values for several hours and possibly even until the morning of the following day (22,45). However, the average person at the gym who spends more time socializing than exercising will not experience a prolonged elevation of postexercise energy expenditure after a bout of resistance exercise. The possibility remains that, for both endurance and resistance exercise, the accumulation of even modest excess postexercise energy expenditure over the course of months and years can substantially impact energy expenditure. However, it is clear that the vast majority of energy expenditure occurs during the exercise itself rather than after.

Summary

Individual behavioral and metabolic characteristics affect acute and chronic energy balance and fundamentally explain the various body shapes and sizes present within the human population, including athletes. Energy balance is at the core a simple concept—if energy intake exceeds expenditure, the excess energy will be stored in the body primarily as fat, unless concomitant exercise or physical maturation favors greater storage as lean body mass; if energy expenditure exceeds intake, body energy stores will be lost. However, energy balance is best understood as a dynamic, rather than a static, equation wherein changes on one side of the scale can produce unintentional compensatory metabolic and behavioral changes on the other side of the scale. Because body weight is regulated by a host of neuroendocrine factors, because adaptative changes to energy intake and expenditure can modify energy balance and energy efficiency, and because there are considerable difficulties in accurately quantifying both intake and expenditure, the simplicity of this concept gives way to considerable complexity. Even with intact regulatory systems, it seems that in the face of our current obesigenic environment, the regulatory systems of many humans are poorly equipped to adequately protect against excess body weight and fat gain. Maintaining relatively high daily energy expenditure via ExEE and NEAT can help protect against unhealthy weight gain in the face of our current abundance of highly palatable food. Although body fat stores can be reduced by creating an energy deficit, severe energy restriction by dieting can result in metabolic adaptations that sabotage maintenance of lost weight. Increases in physical activity can contribute to increased energy expenditure, but the magnitude of this increase is often quite small for the beginning exerciser. Realistic expectations regarding energy intake and expenditure and their effects on body weight and composition must replace the often mythical promises marketed to hopeful consumers by advertisements, gimmickry, and fad diets. Understanding the behavioral and metabolic features of the elite or recreational athlete are important in developing the most effective individualized approaches to facilitate their achievement of a healthy and competitive body weight and composition.

References

1. Harper ME, Green K, Brand MD. The efficiency of cellular energy transduction and its implications for obesity. *Annu Rev Nutr.* 2008;28:13–33.

2. Leibel RL, Rosenbaum M, Hirsch J. Changes in energy expenditure resulting from altered body weight. *N Engl J Med.* 1995,332:621–628.

3. Virtanen KA, Lidell ME, Orava J, Heglind M, Westergren R, Niemi T, Taittonen M, Laine J, Savisto NJ, Enerback S, Nuutila P. Functional brown adipose tissue in healthy adults. *N Engl J Med.* 2009;360:1518–1525.

4. Cypess AM, Lehman S, Williams G, Tal I, Rodman D, Goldfine AB, Kuo FC, Palmer EL, Tseng YH, Doria A, Kolodny GM, Kahn CR. Identification and importance of brown adipose tissue in adult humans. *N Engl J Med.* 2009;360:1509–1517.

5. Friedman JM. Modern science versus the stigma of obesity. *Nat Med.* 2004;10:563–569.

6. Keesey RE, Powley TL. Body energy homeostasis. *Appetite.* 2008;51:442–445.

7. Schwartz MW, Baskin DG, Kaiyala KJ, Woods SC. Model for the regulation of energy balance and adiposity by the central nervous system. *Am J Clin Nutr.* 1999;69:584–596.

8. Schwartz MW, Niswender KD. Adiposity signaling and biological defense against weight gain: absence of protection or central hormone resistance? *J Clin Endocrinol Metab.* 2004;89:5889–5897.

9. Niswender KD, Baskin DG, Schwartz MW. Insulin and its evolving partnership with leptin in the hypothalamic control of energy homeostasis. *Trends Endocrinol Metab.* 2004;15:362–369.

10. Major GC, Doucet E, Trayhurn P, Astrup A, Tremblay A. Clinical significance of adaptive thermogenesis. *Int J Obes (Lond).* 2007;31:204–212.

11. Melby CL, Schmidt WD, Corrigan D. Resting metabolic rate in weight-cycling collegiate wrestlers compared with physically active, noncycling control subjects. *Am J Clin Nutr.* 1990;52:409–414.

12. Bullough RC, Melby CL. Effect of inpatient versus outpatient measurement protocol on resting metabolic rate and respiratory exchange ratio. *Ann Nutr Metab.* 1993;37:24–32.

13. Levine JA. Measurement of energy expenditure. *Public Health Nutr.* 2005;8:1123–1132.

14. Roberts SB, Dallal GE. Energy requirements and aging. *Public Health Nutr.* 2005;8:1028–1036.

15. Harris JA, Benedict FG. *A Biometric Study of Basal Metabolism in Man.* Publication no. 279. Washington, DC: Carnegie Institution of Washington; 1919.

16. Cunningham JJ. Body composition as a determinant of energy expenditure: a synthetic review and a proposed general prediction equation. *Am J Clin Nutr.* 1991;54:963–969.

17. Owen OE, Holup JL, D'Alessio DA, Craig ES, Polansky M, Smalley KJ, Kavle EC, Bushman MC, Owen LR, Mozzoli MA, Kendrick ZV, Boden GH. A reappraisal of the caloric requirements of men. *Am J Clin Nutr.* 1987;46:875–885.

18. Owen OE, Kavle E, Owen RS, Polansky M, Caprio S, Mozzoli MA, Kendrick ZV, Bushman MC, Boden G. A reappraisal of caloric requirements in healthy women. *Am J Clin Nutr.* 1986;44:1–19.

19. Mifflin MD, St Jeor ST, Hill LA, Scott BJ, Daugherty SA, Koh YO. A new predictive equation for resting energy expenditure in healthy individuals. *Am J Clin Nutr.* 1990;51:241–247.

20. Bullough RC, Gillette CA, Harris MA, Melby CL. Interaction of acute changes in exercise energy expenditure and energy intake on resting metabolic rate. *Am J Clin Nutr.* 1995;61:473–481.

21. Bell C, Day DS, Jones PP, Christou DD, Petitt DS, Osterberg K, Melby CL, Seals DR. High energy flux mediates the tonically augmented beta-adrenergic support of resting metabolic rate in habitually exercising older adults. *J Clin Endocrinol Metab.* 2004;89:3573–3578.

22. Melby C, Scholl C, Edwards G, Bullough R. Effect of acute resistance exercise on postexercise energy expenditure and resting metabolic rate. *J Appl Physiol.* 1993;75:1847–1853.

23. van Baak MA. Meal-induced activation of the sympathetic nervous system and its cardiovascular and thermogenic effects in man. *Physiol Behav.* 2008;94:178–186.

24. Caspersen CJ, Powell KE, Christenson GM. Physical activity, exercise, and physical fitness: definitions and distinctions for health-related research. *Public Health Rep.* 1985;100:126–131.

25. Ainsworth BE, Haskell WL, Whitt MC, Irwin ML, Swartz AM, Strath SJ, O'Brien WL, Bassett DR Jr, Schmitz KH, Emplaincourt PO, Jacobs DR Jr, Leon AS. Compendium of physical activities: an update of activity codes and MET intensities. *Med Sci Sports Exerc.* 2000;32(9 Suppl):S498–S504.

26. Levine JA. Nonexercise activity thermogenesis—liberating the life-force. *J Intern Med.* 2007;262:273–287.

27. Levine JA, Vander Weg MW, Hill JO, Klesges RC. Non-exercise activity thermogenesis: the crouching tiger hidden dragon of societal weight gain. *Arterioscler Thromb Vasc Biol.* 2006;26:729–736.

28. Levine JA, Lanningham-Foster LM, McCrady SK, Krizan AC, Olson LR, Kane PH, Jensen MD, Clark MM. Interindividual variation in posture allocation: possible role in human obesity. *Science.* 2005;307:584–586.

29. Brooks GA, Butte NF, Rand WM, Flatt JP, Caballero B. Chronicle of the Institute of Medicine physical activity recommendation: how a physical activity recommendation came to be among dietary recommendations. *Am J Clin Nutr.* 2004;79(suppl):921S–930S.

30. Stubbs RJ, Harbron CG, Murgatroyd PR, Prentice AM. Covert manipulation of dietary fat and energy density: effect on substrate flux and food intake in men eating ad libitum. *Am J Clin Nutr.* 1995;62:316–329.

31. Goldberg GR, Black AE, Jebb SA, Cole TJ, Murgatroyd PR, Coward WA, Prentice AM. Critical evaluation of energy intake data using fundamental principles of energy physiology: 1. derivation of cut-off limits to identify under-recording. *Eur J Clin Nutr.* 1991;45:569–581.

32. Melby CL, Ho RC, Jeckel K, Beal L, Goran M, Donahoo WT. Comparison of risk factors for obesity in young, nonobese African-American and Caucasian women. *Int J Obes Relat Metab Disord.* 2000;24:1514–1522.

33. Wing RR, Hill JO. Successful weight loss maintenance. *Annu Rev Nutr.* 2001;21:323–341.

34. Rosenbaum M, Hirsch J, Gallagher DA, Leibel RL. Long-term persistence of adaptive thermogenesis in subjects who have maintained a reduced body weight. *Am J Clin Nutr.* 2008;88:906–912.

35. Goldsmith R, Joanisse DR, Gallagher D, Pavlovich K, Shamoon E, Leibel RL, Rosenbaum M. Effects of experimental weight perturbation on skeletal muscle work efficiency, fuel utilization, and biochemistry in human subjects. *Am J Physiol Regul Integr Comp Physiol.* 2010;298:R79–R88.

36. Levine JA, Eberhardt NL, Jensen MD. Role of nonexercise activity thermogenesis in resistance to fat gain in humans. *Science.* 1999;283:212–214.

37. Bouchard C, Tremblay A, Despres JP, Nadeau A, Lupien PJ, Theriault G, Dussault J, Moorjani S, Pinault S, Fournier G. The response to long-term overfeeding in identical twins. *N Engl J Med.* 1990;322:1477–1482.

38. Christiansen T, Paulsen SK, Bruun JM, Ploug T, Pedersen SB, Richelsen B. Diet-induced weight loss and exercise alone and in combination enhance the expression of adiponectin receptors in adipose tissue and skeletal muscle, but only diet-induced weight loss enhanced circulating adiponectin. *J Clin Endocrinol Metab.* 2010;95:911–919.

39. Bouchard C, Tremblay A, Nadeau A, Dussault J, Despres JP, Theriault G, Lupien PJ, Serresse O, Boulay MR, Fournier G. Long-term exercise training with constant energy intake. 1: effect on body composition and selected metabolic variables. *Int J Obes.* 1990;14:57–73.

40. King NA, Hopkins M, Caudwell P, Stubbs RJ, Blundell JE. Individual variability following 12 weeks of supervised exercise: identification and characterization of compensation for exercise-induced weight loss. *Int J Obes (Lond).* 2008;32:177–184.

41. Donnelly JE, Hill JO, Jacobsen DJ, Potteiger J, Sullivan DK, Johnson SL, Heelan K, Hise M, Fennessey PV, Sonko B, Sharp T, Jakicic JM, Blair SN, Tran ZV, Mayo M, Gibson, C, Washburn RA. Effects of a 16-month randomized controlled exercise trial on body weight and composition in young, overweight men and women: the Midwest Exercise Trial. *Arch Intern Med.* 2003;163:1343–1350.

42. Goran MI, Poehlman ET. Endurance training does not enhance total energy expenditure in healthy elderly persons. *Am J Physiol.* 1992;263:E950–E957.

43. Phelain JF, Reinke E, Harris MA, Melby CL. Postexercise energy expenditure and substrate oxidation in young women resulting from exercise bouts of different intensity. *J Am Coll Nutr.* 1997;16:140–146.

44. Sedlock DA, Fissinger JA, Melby CL. Effect of exercise intensity and duration on postexercise energy expenditure. *Med Sci Sports Exerc.* 1989;21:662–666.

45. Osterberg KL, Melby CL. Effect of acute resistance exercise on postexercise oxygen consumption and resting metabolic rate in young women. *Int J Sport Nutr Exerc Metab.* 2000;10:71–81.

Chapter 11

WEIGHT MANAGEMENT

Marie Dunford, PhD, RD, and Michele A. Macedonio, MS, RD, CSSD

Introduction

Many athletes look for a performance edge by changing weight and body composition. Changing the amount of weight, skeletal muscle, or body fat has potential performance advantages if goals are set appropriately. Unfortunately, athletes may set inappropriate weight and body composition goals or try to achieve their goals too quickly or during the wrong part of the competitive season. Such changes may be detrimental to performance and negatively impact health (1).

A sports dietitian can help an athlete assess his or her current weight and body composition and compare it to successful athletes in their sport. This allows the athlete to set weight range and body composition goals that support performance without negatively affecting training, recovery, and health. Once appropriate goals are established, the sports dietitian also helps the athlete develop an eating plan that is well matched to his or her sport, training schedule, and food preferences. This chapter reviews the factors that need to be considered when establishing weight and body composition goals, and a case study illustrates how to practically apply this information.

Weight Management Goals of Athletes

Depending on the individual, the athlete may want to: (*a*) increase skeletal muscle mass; (*b*) increase skeletal muscle mass and slightly increase body fat; (*c*) increase skeletal muscle mass and decrease body fat simultaneously; (*d*) decrease body fat; or (*e*) increase body fat. As shown in Table 11.1, these changes may result in increased size, strength, power, speed, or cardiovascular endurance, which may improve performance (2,3).

Most athletes engage in some form of resistance training to maintain or increase muscular strength, power, and endurance. It is often beneficial for novice athletes or those moving to more demanding levels of competition (eg, high school to college, college to professional) to substantially increase skeletal muscle size, which usually also increases strength and muscle endurance. However, for many athletes muscular strength and endurance are more important than increased size because too much muscle can result in decreased speed or perceived decreases in flexibility or agility.

Changes in body fat can also substantially influence performance. Excess body fat is detrimental for many athletes because it reduces speed (2). Decreasing excess body fat may have a positive effect on performance.

TABLE 11.1   Weight Goals and Expected Performance Outcomes

Goal	Expected Performance Outcomes	Examples
Increase skeletal muscle mass	Increase strength and power	Sprinters, bodybuilders
Increase skeletal muscle mass and slightly increase body fat	Increase size and strength; be better matched physically to opponents	Athletes in contact sports, especially as they progress to elite levels
Increase skeletal muscle mass and decrease body fat simultaneously	Increase strength and power; increase power-to-weight ratio	Athletes in "ball" sports, cyclists, rowers, wrestlers
Decrease body fat	Increase speed; improve vertical or horizontal distance	Long-distance runners, gymnasts, figure skaters, high-jumpers
Increase body fat	Increase size (mass)	Powerlifters, sumo wrestlers

However, trying to achieve an ever-lower percentage of body fat is a performance disadvantage because of health problems that can develop, such as disrupted hormonal balance or disordered eating behaviors (4).

Although it is not mentioned as frequently as fat loss, some athletes may need to gain body fat. Physical size alone can be a performance advantage, especially in contact sports, and some additional body fat may help the athlete to be better matched to his or her opponents.

Determining Optimal Performance Weight and Body Composition Ranges

Optimal performance weight and body composition are unique to each individual, so genetic predisposition and individual characteristics should always be kept in mind. However, a comparison needs to be made between the physical characteristics that are associated with success in the sport and the individual's current physical characteristics. Factors to consider when determining an optimal performance weight range are listed in Box 11.1 and discussed in this chapter, but not all may apply to the particular athlete.

Sport-Related Characteristics

Certain physical characteristics are associated with success in particular sports. For example, all competitive bodybuilders have a high percentage of skeletal muscle mass and a low percentage of body fat. Conversely,

---

BOX 11.1   Factors to Consider in Setting Weight-Management Goals

Sport-related Characteristics
- Sport
- Position
- Relative need for power and endurance
- Power-to-weight ratio
- Relative need for speed, flexibility, agility, and mobility

Physique-related Characteristics
- Body weight
- Body composition
- Body size
- Body build
- Body appearance

sumo wrestlers are large-bodied with a considerable amount of body fat. Elite distance runners tend to be lightweight, light-boned, and have a relatively low percentage of body fat because these characteristics are associated with efficiently moving the body a long distance as quickly as possible. Appearance may be a factor in scoring, such as in women's gymnastics and figure skating. Thus, some sports have greater physical uniformity among competitors, especially at the elite levels of competition (see Box 11.2). However, successful athletes in individual, noncontact sports, such as tennis or golf, are of many different body weights.

In contact sports, being physically well-matched to one's opponents is often a key to success, but physical size alone is not the determining factor in most sports. The relative need for power, speed, or endurance and the need to be agile, flexible, or mobile may be particularly important and a key to the individual's success. The physical characteristics of successful athletes in the sport should be considered as a guideline, but in many sports there is room for tremendous individual variability.

Position Played

Physical uniformity may be associated with position. For example, a football lineman tends to be physically similar to other linemen, but different in weight and body composition when compared to running backs and receivers. Particularly in contact sports, the position played may dictate the need for a particular size, weight, or body composition.

In many team sports, there are a range of weights and body compositions for a given position. For example, in soccer some defenders are more muscular and heavier in weight while others are lighter in weight with comparatively less muscle, yet each can be successful as a defender. Weight and body composition vary in baseball outfielders, in part because of their offensive skills. Some hit for power while others hit to get on base, steal bases, and score on base hits. Power hitters benefit from greater body weight whereas fast base runners are likely to have a body composition associated with speed (eg, relatively low percentage of body fat). Sports in which position plays a major role include baseball, basketball, football, ice and field hockey, lacrosse, rugby, soccer, and softball.

Relative Need for Power and Endurance

Athletes are often characterized as strength/power or endurance athletes (see Figure 11.1). For example, short-distance runners such as 100-meter and 200-meter runners depend primarily on explosive power. They have substantial upper and lower body skeletal muscle mass and a relatively heavy body weight.

BOX 11.2   Weight and Body Composition Uniformity Among Athletes

More Uniformity
- Baseball catchers
- Basketball centers
- Bodybuilders
- Figure skaters
- Football linemen
- Gymnasts
- Long-distance cyclists
- Long-distance runners
- Powerlifters
- Rhythmic gymnasts

Less Uniformity
- Baseball pitchers
- Divers
- Golfers
- Recreational triathletes
- Tennis players

Power   **Endurance**

Archery	Baseball	Downhill skiing	Basketball	Cross-country skiing
Bodybuilding	Golf	Fencing	Boxing	Distance cycling
Discus	Gymnastics, floor	Figure skating	Handball	Distance running
Gymnastics, vault	exercise	Rowing	Kickboxing	Distance swimming
Pole-vault	Volleyball	Wrestling	Lacrosse	Duathlon
Powerlifting			Racquetball	Triathlon
Rifle			Rugby	Ultradistance racing
Shot put			Soccer	
Sprints			Tennis	
			Water polo	

FIGURE 11.1   The power-endurance continuum. Some sports depend predominantly on power as shown on the left side of the continuum, whereas others depend to a large degree on endurance capacity, as shown on the right. Many sports require a blend of power and endurance. It may be helpful to determine the relative position of the athlete's sport or position on the continuum so that realistic weight and body composition goals can be established.

As the distance increases to the middle distances (eg, 1,500 meters), body composition begins to change as the race favors endurance rather than power. The 1,500-meter runner is less muscular and lighter in weight than the 100-meter runner. Long-distance runners, such as marathon runners, tend to be light in weight and have a relatively low percentage of body fat because these characteristics are associated with efficiently moving the body quickly over a long distance. Cycling and swimming are other sports in which the distance covered influences the relative need for power and endurance, and therefore, weight and body composition.

Those who rely only on strength or explosive power include bodybuilders, powerlifters, and certain field athletes such as shot putters and discus, hammer, and javelin throwers. Powerlifters and "throwers" benefit from being large-bodied and strong. Body fat adds to total body weight, which can be a performance advantage because it adds mass. However, too high a percentage of body fat can be a health disadvantage, particularly if the excess fat is abdominal fat.

Most sports require a combination of power and endurance. For example, basketball and soccer require intermittent short bursts of power (eg, fast break, breakaway play) as well as cardiovascular endurance. Body weight and composition must be fine-tuned for the athlete to be able to do both well. Particularly challenging are those sports that require several power and endurance events, such as decathlon. Decathletes must have a body composition that is not too muscular (a disadvantage when running the 1,500-meter race) or too low in weight (a disadvantage when shot putting).

Body composition is also a factor in cardiovascular conditioning. Reducing excess body fat may improve cardiovascular endurance and allow athletes to continue to perform well near the end of the game. This is especially important in sports with overtime periods, such as basketball and soccer. Although conditioning is important for all athletes, improved cardiovascular endurance may be the primary goal for performance-focused recreational athletes and older players who are competing for playing time with younger players. Such players often try to reduce excess body fat as a way to improve endurance and performance.

Power-to-Weight Ratio

Power-to-weight ratio refers to the amount of power (ie, explosive skeletal muscle strength) that can be generated per pound or kilogram of body weight. A high power-to-weight ratio is a performance advantage in many sports and is a result of a relatively low percentage of body fat and a relatively high percentage of skeletal muscle for the total amount of body weight. For example, male professional distance cyclists tend to have approximately 7% to 10% body fat with well-developed upper- and lower-body muscle mass. Excess body fat is "dead weight" because it must be moved but it does not contribute to muscle power.

Examples of sports that benefit from a high power-to-weight ratio include boxing, wrestling, martial arts, rowing (crew), high-jumping, pole-vaulting, distance running, swimming, and cycling. A high power-to-weight ratio is also advantageous for athletes in positions that cover a large area of the field, rink, or court and depend on speed, such as many basketball, ice hockey, lacrosse, rugby, and soccer positions.

Power-to-weight ratio can be changed in two ways—increasing power by increasing skeletal muscle mass and decreasing weight by decreasing body fat. Unless an athlete has a large amount of excess body fat, maximizing power by increasing muscle mass is more likely to benefit performance than minimizing body fat. Athletes need to be aware that extreme changes in either direction can be detrimental to performance. For example, increasing skeletal muscle mass to too great a degree can cause too large of an increase in body weight, which can reduce speed. Conversely, decreasing body fat to too great a degree can be detrimental to performance due to a lack of sufficient body fat to support rigorous training and competition. There can also be health-related problems brought on by these changes, such as joint problems or changes in hormone concentrations.

Relative Need for Speed, Mobility, Flexibility, and Agility

The need for speed and mobility is an influence on body weight and composition goals. Some athletes may benefit from an increase in lower-body muscle mass and a decrease in body fat to increase sprint speed. Others may benefit from maintenance of muscle mass but a decrease in excess body fat. Because speed is easily measured, the impact of weight and body composition changes on speed can be easily assessed. Some athletes state that too much muscle reduces their flexibility and agility.

Weight Certification Requirements

Boxing, wrestling, some of the martial arts, and lightweight crew (rowing) are examples of sports with weight categories. Weight-regulated sports put considerable emphasis on scale weight because the athlete cannot compete until weight is certified. There is a theoretical performance advantage to being at the top rather than the bottom of the weight category and this may influence the athlete to choose to compete in a weight category that is below a biologically comfortable weight.

The need to have weight certified cannot be overlooked as a significant factor in the athlete's preparation for competition. Unfortunately, the fastest way to manipulate scale weight is to reduce body water. To do so, athletes restrict water intake, lose excessive amounts through sweating, and take diuretics. These are dangerous practices, especially when they are combined, because body temperature can be elevated to a medically unsafe and sometimes fatal level.

In the past, wrestling was the poster child for hazardous practices used to "make weight" or "cut weight," terms used to describe large and rapid loses in scale weight through extraordinary measures (eg, starvation, severe dehydration, excessive exercise). Some wrestlers died from these practices and wrestling now has rules that require the establishment of a minimum weight category before the beginning of the season based on body composition and proper hydration. However, not all weight-regulated sports have adopted such rule changes, and athletes in those sports remain at risk for potential medical problems and detrimental performance outcomes (eg, fainting, lack of concentration).

Physique-Related Characteristics

The challenge for both the athletes and the professionals who work with them is to determine ranges for weight and body composition that are compatible with excellent performance *and* the individual's genetic potential and unique characteristics.

Body Weight

Weight is usually expressed as a single number, although it should be stated as a weight range. Using a weight range helps to account for the error that is inherent in any form of measurement, and it helps to prevent misinterpretations due to natural day-to-day fluctuations in body weight, especially in water weight. A baseline weight is one of the first assessment measures taken, but an appropriate weight range cannot be established until information is known about the individual athlete's height, body build, and body composition, as well as the sport and position played.

Body Composition

Body composition assessment is necessary to set an appropriate weight range and to monitor changes in lean body mass and storage fat. An accurate assessment is critical, as explained in Chapter 9. However, the most accurate measures are not readily accessible or affordable to most athletes. Many have access to only one method, which will need to be repeated over time to track any changes.

Body composition cannot predict success in any sport, but it can affect optimal performance (3). Table 11.2 lists the body composition of competitive athletes in some sports as reported in the scientific literature (1,4). These figures are only a guideline and should be used cautiously.

Body Size

Size refers to height, weight, and body build. Body size has increased in many sports over the past 50 years, including football, basketball, ice hockey, baseball, and tennis (5,6). A dramatic increase has been seen in the weight of football linemen at every level, from professional to youth. Some of this weight has been an increase in abdominal fat, a known health risk and a likely performance disadvantage due to a lack of fitness and speed (7,8).

Although there are exceptions, many athletes need to increase body size as they step up to the next level of competition (eg, high school to college, college to professional). In many cases, this means an increase in skeletal muscle mass and body weight. It may also mean a small increase in body fat. Although size can be manipulated, it is ultimately determined by genetics. It is important to note that during adolescence there is wide variability in when an athlete achieves full physical maturity.

Body Build

Body build, also referred to as *somatotype,* may be useful when discussing the influence of genetic predisposition on body composition. Classification is based on three categories: endomorphic, mesomorphic, or ectomorphic. Endomorphs tend to be stocky with wide hips and at risk for easily gaining body fat, particularly in the abdominal area. Mesomorphs tend to gain skeletal muscle mass relatively easily and generally do not gain excessive amounts of body fat. Ectomorphs appear to be thin. Some individuals clearly fall into one of the three categories, but many reflect more than one somatotype.

Body build is associated with certain sports. For example, shot putters tend to be endomorphs, bodybuilders tend to be mesomorphs, and distance runners tend to be ectomorphs. Visual appraisal does not quantify body dimensions but is a way to draw general observations about successful performance related to physique. Until an individual reaches full physical maturity, it may be difficult to accurately assess physique.

TABLE 11.2   Estimated Body Composition of Selected Well-Trained Athletes

Sport	Position or Distance	% Body Fat
Males		
Baseball, college	All positions	11–17
Baseball, professional	All positions	8.5–12
Basketball, professional	Centers	9–20
	Forwards	7–14
	Guards	7–13
Cycling, road, professional	Long distance	7–10
Football (American), college (NCAA Division I)	Defensive backs	7–14.5
	Receivers	9–16.5
	Quarterbacks	14–22
	Linebackers	12.5–23.5
	Defensive linemen	14.5–25
	Offensive linemen	18.5–28.5
Judo, national team	All weight classes	8.5–19
Rugby, professional	All positions	9–20
Soccer, professional or college	All positions	7.5–18
Tennis, elite		8–18
Water polo, national team		6.5–17.5
Wrestling, college		6.5–16
Running, elite	Middle distance	8–16.5
	Long distance	12–18
Soccer, college	All positions	13–19
Swimming or diving, college	Middle distance or diving	17–30
	Long distance	20–34
Tennis, elite		15–25
Females		
Running, elite	Middle distance	8–16.5
	Long distance	12–18
Soccer, college	All positions	13–19
Swimming or diving, college	Middle distance or diving	17–30
Swimming or diving, masters	Long distance	20–34
Tennis, elite		15–25

Body Appearance

Body appearance cannot be overlooked as a factor when setting weight and body composition goals. Body-builders are scored on body appearance, and weight as well as body composition are part of the subjective scoring of other aesthetic sports, such as women's gymnastics and figure skating. Dissatisfaction with weight, body shape, or body image can lead to disordered eating and eating disorders in both men and women.

For most athletes, body appearance is not part of the scoring. However, popular athletes featured in visual media may feel pressure to attain and maintain an athletic physique. Some sports, such as women's high-jump, pole-vaulting, and beach volleyball, feature tight-fitting clothing that reveals the body's contour. In general, female athletes are more concerned than males with physical appearance, particularly fatness, and are more likely to restrict energy intake and use weight-loss supplements (9). Appearance is one reason that athletes use anabolic steroids. Interestingly, an athletic appearance is so socially powerful that some high school nonathletes use anabolic steroids to achieve a body composition that is associated with rigorous athletic training (10).

Four-Step Process for Achieving Weight and Body Composition Goals

The goal for the athlete is an optimal performance weight range that reflects a healthy body composition. Although the specific goals will depend on the individual, the process used to achieve the goals is universal. Four steps are critical:

- Assessment
- Goal setting
- Action plan
- Evaluation and reassessment

Assessment

No two athletes are the same. Assessment is the starting point for any successful plan designed to achieve body weight and body composition goals. A proper assessment creates a picture of an individual athlete's current status, providing baseline information that is used for setting realistic and achievable goals for where an athlete wants to be. This baseline information also becomes the basis for individual action plans designed to reach desired weight and body composition ranges and serves as a point of comparison. The more information that an assessment provides the better able an athlete is to create a successful action plan and to gauge progress. Box 11.3 summarizes the assessment measurements used to create an individualized and targeted nutrition plan geared to help athletes set target goals, design effective action plans, and evaluate and reassess progress.

BOX 11.3   Assessment Measurements

Physical Assessment Measures
- Height
- Weight
- Girth measurements
- Predominant somatotype (body build)
- Body composition (% lean mass, % body fat)

Physiological Assessment Measures
- Physical exam (including laboratory tests)
- Health history
- Diet analysis ($\geq$ 3 days)
- Resting metabolic rate (measured or estimated)
- Energy expenditure analysis (including intensity and duration of exercise)
- Performance measurements (eg, relative peak power, running speed)

Physical Assessment

Height and weight measurements are easy to do and are necessary to determine optimal performance weight. Athletes in some sports and positions are often of similar height and weight. Height measurements are necessary when assessing weight because many formulas include height as a factor. Stadiometers provide the most accurate height measurement and make measuring quick and simple. However, in the absence of a stadiometer, height can be measured by having the athlete stand barefoot on a hard surface and against a wall looking straight ahead with head, shoulders, buttocks, and heels touching the wall. The athlete should stand as tall and straight as possible. With a ruler or other flat straight edge placed on the head of the athlete, the wall is marked at the underside of 90-degree angle where the ruler meets the wall. Then, the distance from the ground to the marking on the wall is measured.

Optimal weight is relative to height. Weight-class sports specify weight categories with specific weight ranges, so weight is a key issue for these athletes. To some degree, body weight is an important factor for all athletes. For those athletes who strive for a low body weight and a low body fat, body mass index (BMI) may also be a necessary assessment measure as an indication of health status. Weight measurements should be taken in the morning after urinating and before eating or drinking, using the same properly calibrated scale, with the athlete wearing minimal clothing. Note that one weight measurement does not tell the whole story. To most accurately assess progress toward one's goal, serial weights should be taken regularly and in a uniform manner. Regular weights also help an athlete keep tabs on hydration status and provide athletes with a basis for rehydration strategies.

Girth measurements provide a tool for measuring body size and proportion. Although not a direct measure of body composition, measuring the girth, or circumference, at six sites is helpful in tracking change in body composition over time. Girth measurements are inexpensive and easy to take. For the most accuracy, a metal tape measure is used to measure circumference, typically at the waist, hips, thighs, calves, arms, and chest. Changes in girth measurements can be an indicator that the current plan is working. Somatotype can be visually determined.

Body composition is an important factor in determining optimal performance weight. An accurate body composition measurement is necessary for a comprehensive nutrition assessment because body weight is only part of the picture. The composition of that weight is often the more important part. For practical purposes, the body is divided into two major compartments: fat and lean. Body fat is either essential fat or storage fat. Essential fat, present in heart, lungs, liver, spleen, and lipid-rich tissues of the central nervous system, is necessary for normal physiological functioning. In women, there is additional sex-specific essential fat that has biological functions for reproduction and other hormonal functions. Essential fat in women is approximately four times that of men. Storage fat is primarily in adipose tissue, including visceral fat that protects organs from trauma and fat beneath the skin. To maintain health and normal body function, lower limits for body fat percentage are set at 3% for males and 12% for females.

Fat-free mass (FFM) and lean body mass (LBM), although often used interchangeably, are not the same. Lean body mass contains a small percentage of non–sex-specific essential fat (approximately 3% of body mass), whereas fat-free mass contains no fat (FFM = body mass – fat mass). In fully hydrated, healthy adults, the main difference between FFM and LBM is essential fat. *Lean body mass* is generally the term used in body composition measurement. The percentage of LBM is often part of equations used to determine energy needs.

Obtaining an accurate body composition measure is not as easy as measuring body weight, height, and girth. For a detailed explanation of body composition methods, their strengths and weaknesses, refer to Chapter 9.

Physiological Assessment

Physiological measurements that provide valuable baseline information about the athlete include those obtained at a physical exam, such as biochemical assays and clinical examination, and measurements of metabolic rate, nutrient intake, and exercise expenditure. For a detailed explanation on how to conduct a comprehensive sports nutrition assessment, refer to Chapter 8.

When available, laboratory tests allow the sports dietitian to evaluate the nutritional status of the athlete by ascertaining whether biochemical parameters are within healthful ranges. Once this information is collected it can be used as a target for dietary modifications and as a measure of progress. A clinical examination includes past and present medical history, family history, signs of disease or illness, and habits that may affect health, such as sleep patterns.

A detailed 3- to 5-day diet record and nutrient analysis is an indispensable part of a comprehensive assessment. The diet assessment provides a view of the athlete's usual eating patterns, as well as a measure of the quantity and the quality of the food intake. This information provides the basis for a nutrition plan designed to help the athlete reach body weight and body composition goals. Dietary intake studies reveal that people routinely underestimate portions when recording food intake. Therefore, it is crucial to instruct athletes to eat as they usually do and to record portions as accurately and completely as possible so that the information reflects usual food intake and meal patterns. Nutrient analysis software can be used to analyze the nutrient content of a food record, but it is only as good as the database on which the program is based. For the most complete information, the USDA Nutrient Database (www.ars.usda.gov/main/site_main .htm?modecode=12-35-45-00) should form the foundation for the nutrient analysis program.

Knowledge of metabolic rate provides an energy baseline that forms the foundation for a targeted, realistic, and effective weight-management plan. Resting metabolic rate (RMR) refers to the energy requirement needed for all metabolic processes of the active cell mass required to maintain normal regulatory balance and body functions at rest. As explained in Chapter 10, RMR can be estimated by measuring oxygen consumption via indirect calorimetry or by using prediction equations (see Box 10.2 in Chapter 10).

Physical activity, also referred to as exercise energy expenditure (ExEE), has a profound effect on total daily energy expenditure (TDEE). For athletes, the energy needed for training, conditioning, and performance represents a substantial proportion of total daily energy needs. World-class athletes, for instance, can almost double their TDEE with 3 to 4 hours of intense training. It is important that athletes record daily exercise and note both the intensity and the duration of the exercise. An accurate determination of TDEE is difficult because of the variability of the contribution of physical exercise. Refer to Chapter 10 for information on how best to estimate TDEE.

Performance measurements, such as running speed or relative peak power, allow athletes to determine a baseline and track improvements in performance. Running speed is easy to measure. Relative peak power (RPP) is a measurement to determine power-to-weight ratio. The 30-second Wingate test measures both average and peak power of the lower body. Upper-body power can be measured by using a modified Wingate test or an arm ergometer (11).

Goal Setting

Careful interpretation of the assessment measures will determine if the athlete's current weight and body composition are appropriate. Begin by determining whether body composition is well matched to the sport (see Table 11.2) and the athlete's genetic predisposition for leanness.

Although the athlete may want to focus only on weight or body composition goals, it is important that athletes set at least three related goals. A minimum of one goal should be set in each area—performance, weight and body composition, and health. Performance-based goals may range from simply finishing an event such as a marathon or triathlon to very specific goals such as decreasing performance time by 10 seconds. A weight range should be set to reflect a body composition range that is appropriate. As shown in Box 11.4, a formula can be used to help set the weight range. For many athletes, the health goal may be continued good health, but some may need to set specific goals, such as continuing to menstruate, decreasing

---

BOX 11.4   Calculating Target Weight

The following formula, calculated using both a lower and higher percentage body fat, is used to establish a weight range. To use this formula, an assessment of body composition must be done because fat-free mass must be known.

Target Body Weight = Current Fat-free Mass/(1 – % Desired Body Fat)

Example
A long-distance cyclist currently weighs 187 lb. His body composition is 87% fat-free mass (163 lb) and 13% body fat. His goal is 8% to 10% body fat with no change in lean mass. An appropriate weight range to reflect this body composition goal is 177 to 181 lb (assuming all weight is lost from adipose tissue).

Target Body Weight = 163 lb/(1 – 0.08) = 163 lb/0.92 = 177 lb

Target Body Weight = 163 lb/(1 – 0.1) = 163 lb/0.9 = 181 lb

This same formula may be used no matter how the athlete wants to change body composition. For example, if this cyclist wanted to increase muscle mass by 5 lb to 168 lb and decrease body fat at the same time, his estimated weight range would be 183 to 187 lb (168 lb/0.92 and 168 lb/0.9).

---

abdominal fat, or bringing a biochemical parameter into a healthful range. In each case, goals need to be SMART. SMART, an acronym that athletes can easily remember, signifies the essential qualities of effective goals: **S**pecific, **M**easurable, **A**chievable, **R**ealistic, and **T**ime-driven.

Action Plan

The fundamental features of an effective action plan include the following:

- Appropriate energy intake
- Adequate amounts of protein, carbohydrate, and fat
- Proper macronutrient proportions
- Appropriate training plan and daily physical activity
- Personal food preferences, cost, and convenience

The number of calories needed daily cannot be predicted with precision, but an assessment of RMR and usual physical activity can help to establish an estimate. For those who wish to gain weight by increasing skeletal muscle mass, a rule of thumb guideline for males is baseline calorie intake plus 400 to 500 kcal daily. For females, an addition of 300 to 400 kcal more than baseline is recommended. However, individuals vary to a great degree and recommended daily energy intake must be individualized.

To reduce weight by reducing body fat, a guideline is baseline intake minus 300 to 500 kcal/d for males and minus 200 to 300 kcal/d for females. Greater reductions in daily energy intake may leave the athlete unable to maintain or increase energy output from physical activity and exercise. To gain skeletal muscle mass and lose body fat simultaneously, energy intake must be as precise as possible. A starting point for daily intake is baseline requirements plus 300 kcal/d for males and plus 200 kcal/d for females. However, close monitoring is needed and total energy intake may need to be adjusted by 50- to 100-kcal increments daily until the desired outcome is reached. For those who wish to increase body fat, energy intake more than baseline is necessary.

The Academy of Nutrition and Dietetics (formerly American Dietetic Association), Dietitians of Canada, and the American College of Sports Medicine (3) recommend that endurance and strength athletes consume at least 1.2 g of protein per kg of body weight daily. Athletes who are trying to lose body fat may consume protein at approximately1.5 g/kg/d, in an effort to protect against the loss of lean body mass when calories are restricted. The recommended protein intake to increase skeletal muscle mass in strength athletes is typically approximately 1.7 g/kg/d. Carbohydrate should be sufficient to resynthesize muscle glycogen stores daily (~5 to 8 g/kg). Fat restriction should be moderate. A rule of thumb calculation for moderate fat intake is approximately 1 g/kg/d or about 25% to 30% of total energy intake. Restricting fat intake to less than 20% of total energy intake is not recommended. Current body weight is typically used to make g/kg/d calculations. As body weight decreases, especially to a large degree, recalculations are necessary to reflect the athlete's current (now lower) body weight.

Most athletes are encouraged to eat three meals and two or three snacks daily. This distribution of calories and nutrients helps athletes be adequately fueled before exercise and to fully recover after exercise. Some postexercise carbohydrate and protein are necessary for the adequate resynthesis of muscle glycogen and the repair and synthesis of skeletal muscle. Food intake and training must be coordinated. Each diet plan must be individualized, incorporating personal food preferences, religious beliefs, convenience, and cost.

Evaluation and Reassessment

Even the plan that seems perfect on paper needs evaluation. Evaluation allows the athlete to determine if goals are being met. If progress is too slow or too fast, adjustments can be made before there is an impact on training, performance, or health. Reassessment of many of the original assessment measures is invaluable for tracking progress and, at times, adjusting the original goals. A case study illustrating a comprehensive plan of a linebacker in the National Football League (NFL) is found in Box 11.5.

A common question asked by health professionals is, should athletes use a high-protein diet when attempting weight loss? It is well known that low-calorie diets in humans can lead to negative nitrogen balance and a significant loss of lean body mass. Research has shown that when rats receive a high-protein, low-energy diet they can achieve positive nitrogen balance. Research in humans is not as clear. However, several studies in overweight and obese women have shown that the loss of lean body mass can be reduced (but not prevented entirely) with higher protein diets (12,13).

Researchers are now beginning to study the use of high-protein, low-calorie diets by athletes as a way to protect against the loss of lean body mass to the extent possible. Mettler and colleagues (14) studied 20 resistance-trained athletes. The experimental group consumed a high-protein (~ 2.3 g/kg or ~35% of total energy intake) weight-loss diet whereas the control group consumed a moderate protein (~ 1 g/kg or ~15% of total energy intake) weight-loss diet. Both groups consumed 60% less than their usual energy intake for 14 days and lost the same amount of fat mass (a little more than 1 kg or ~2.5 lb). However, the high-protein diet group lost significantly less lean body mass than the control group (~0.3 kg vs ~1.6 kg). The authors note that the athletes in the high-protein diet group reported more fatigue and a lesser sense of well-being than the control group. These feelings did not impact their ability to maintain the required volume and intensity of training during the 14-day study, but it is not known if carbohydrate intake would be too low to support training if the diet were extended more than 2 weeks.

Because protection of lean body mass is critical to most athletes, a high-protein, low-calorie diet is often recommended to athletes who want to lose weight primarily from body fat. Unfortunately, the amount of

---

BOX 11.5   Case Study of a Linebacker in the National Football League

An outside linebacker who is 6 feet 1 inch (1.85 meters) and weighs 226 lb (102.7 kg), with 19% body fat (43 lb [19.5 kg]) and 183 lb (83.2 kg) of lean mass, wants to be "ripped" by training camp. During his first 2 years in the NFL, this athlete struggled to maintain his weight during the season. He lives alone and prepares his own meals. During the season the team provides breakfast and lunch but he often finds he is too tired after a day of intense training to prepare a full dinner meal and he is concerned that his nutrition may be lacking.

The athlete's goal is to earn a starting linebacker position in the upcoming season. To do this he needs to gain strength and increase speed and agility. Wanting to be in peak condition when he reports to the team for conditioning, this athlete is engaged in an intense 6-hour workout 4 days a week at a high-level training facility during the break between the end of the season and off-season workouts.

Together the athlete and the sports dietitian collected the necessary nutrition assessment data, set realistic achievable goals, planned an effective nutrition strategy to support his training regimen, and set benchmarks for evaluation and reassessment.

Step 1: Assessment
In the assessment, the sports dietitian collected the following data:
- Height: 6 ft 1 in (1.85 m)
- Weight: 226 lb (102.7 kg)
- Somatotype: Mesomorph/ectomorph
- Body composition (BOD POD):
  o ~19% body fat
  o ~43 lb (19.5 kg) body fat
  o ~183 lb (83.2 kg) lean mass
- Metabolic rate: 2,510 kcal
- Dietary intake: 2,805 kcal
- Average daily physical activity: 1,828 kcal

The assessment of height and weight indicates that the athlete's current size is sufficient to play in the NFL, but his weight and percentage of lean body mass are lower than those of many of his competitors. His mesomorphic/ectomorphic body build suggests that he can gain skeletal mass, but perhaps not as easily as a true mesomorph. A detailed 3-day record of dietary intake reveals that his average daily energy intake is 2,805 kcal.

Due to his large body size and large amount of skeletal muscle mass, the energy needed to support his resting metabolic rate is substantial, approximately 2,500 kcal/d. In addition, he expends more than 1,800 kcal/d, in large part due to his rigorous workouts. It is quickly apparent that his current intake does not meet the predicted amount of calories he needs daily to maintain current weight and body composition. This is predominantly due to his fatigue after hours of working out and his lack of cooking skills. However, he likes to eat and enjoys a wide variety of foods. He will need to consume substantially more calories if he wishes to increase skeletal muscle mass.

Step 2: Goal Setting
When asked, the athlete could quickly list his goal: earn a starting position by being stronger and quicker than the other linebackers on the team. But he was not able to translate this goal into measurable objectives. For example, when the sports dietitian asked him how much he

continues

BOX 11.5   Case Study of a Linebacker in the National Football League (continued)

thought he should weigh or how quickly he expected to gain skeletal muscle mass, his answers suggested weight and body composition goals that were unrealistic. The sports dietitian helped him establish some realistic goals and an appropriate time frame in which to meet them (see following chart). For example, he wanted to increase body mass as well as lean mass for greater bulk and strength. A goal weight of 230 to 233 lb was established by calculating a realistic gain of lean mass (0.5–0.75 lb gain over 8 weeks) and adding it to his current weight. In working with the sports dietitian, he was able to establish goals that were SMART—specific, measurable, achievable, realistic, and time-driven.

Goal

- Earn a starting position

- Gain strength to become the strongest

- Gain speed and agility to become the quickest linebacker on the team by camp

Objective

- Gain 0.75 lb/wk. After 8 weeks reach goal weight range of 230–233 lb.

- Gain 0.5–0.75 lb lean mass per week. After 8 linebacker on the team by camp weeks, increase lean mass by 6 lb.

- After 8 weeks, achieve a body fat of 18%–19%.

Step 3: Action Plan

The athlete's action plan had four basic objectives:

- Increase calorie intake.
- Consume a high-carbohydrate, moderate-protein, moderate-fat diet.
- Distribute food intake over the course of the day to fuel activity and reduce fatigue.
- Consume a recovery snack immediately after exercise.

The athlete's initial meal plan of 4,800 kcal/d was based on his total energy expenditure of approximately 4,338 kcal plus an additional 500 kcal to cover the metabolic cost of building additional skeletal muscle tissue. Macronutrient distribution was based on 1.7 g protein per kg body weight and 8 g carbohydrate per kg body weight. The 4,800 kcal were distributed in a meal pattern of three meals plus two snacks. Pre-exercise meals and postexercise snacks were designed to insure adequate fuel, sufficient high-quality protein, and proper rehydration, and to support maximum muscle growth.

Using the 3-day food records, the sports dietitian made suggestions for increasing portion sizes of certain foods and incorporating ready-to-eat or easy to prepare foods into meals and snacks. A supermarket tour proved helpful, as did a few basic cooking classes.

Step 4: Evaluation and Reassessment

The evaluation and reassessment step involved the following tasks:

- Keep food intake record and evaluate for energy intake, macronutrient balance, and nutrient adequacy.
- Record weight weekly.
- Measure body composition after 4 and 8 weeks; compare strength, power, and performance before and after 8-week program.

The effectiveness of the initial meal plan was determined by monitoring weight, and after 2 weeks it was decided that an additional 200 kcal/d might be needed to achieve the target weekly weight gain. When the additional calories were added, weekly weight gain stayed on target. At the end

continues

BOX 11.5   Case Study of a Linebacker in the National Football League (continued)

of 8 weeks, this athlete had reached his body weight goal of 232 lb (105.5 kg). A reassessment of his body composition indicated 18% body fat and a gain of 6 lb (2.7 kg) in lean body mass. Having reached his preseason goals, this athlete followed a modified plan during the season and, for the first time in his NFL career, he was able to maintain his target weight throughout the season. In addition, this was an injury-free season in which he started 16 games at weakside linebacker and was ranked first on the team with a career-high 143 tackles. He moved from weakside to middle linebacker, where he started the final eight games of the season.

Follow-up

Two years later, the linebacker suffered a severe knee sprain midway through the season and was placed on injured reserve. He was committed to arriving at off-season workouts in peak condition. At the end of the season, he once again engaged in a rigorous strength and conditioning program, 6 hours a day, 4 days a week, at the same training facility where he trained 2 years prior. During the time that he was placed on injured reserve, his weight dropped to 229 lb (104.1 kg). A body composition assessment determined that he was 19% body fat and 185.5 lb (84.3 kg) of lean body mass. During the 8-week conditioning program, his goal was to increase total weight to 232 lb (105.5 kg) with 18% body fat. With his starting weight of 229 lb (104.1 kg), this meant a gain of 3.5 lb (1.6 kg) lean mass and a loss of 0.5 lb (0.23 kg) of body fat. Because he needed to slightly trim body fat and slowly gain muscle, his meal plan was modified to a 4,800-kcal meal plan with 1.9 g protein per kg body weight and 8 g carbohydrate per kg body weight. Weekly monitoring of weight of indicated just less than ½-lb gain per week. By the end of the conditioning program, this athlete had reached his goals.

---

protein in a "high-protein" diet is often not clearly defined. The study by Mettler and colleagues used a diet containing protein at a high level (~2.3 g/kg) for a very short period of time (2 weeks), and it is not known if other levels of protein or time frames are equally effective (14). Obviously, more research is needed.

The major concern about high-protein, calorie-reduced diets is that the carbohydrate content may not be sufficient to restore muscle glycogen and support training and performance over many weeks or months. It is prudent for athletes who are attempting to lose weight, protect against the loss of lean body mass, maintain their level of training, and maintain or improve their performance to work with a sports dietitian to achieve their goals. The amount of protein needed to achieve all of these goals is likely to require some trial and error. The other macronutrients, carbohydrate and fat, will also need to be fine-tuned.

Summary

Weight management goals and plans must be highly individualized. Factors that determine optimal weight and body composition ranges include sports-related characteristics, such as position played, relative need for power and endurance, and the need for speed, mobility, flexibility, and agility. Physique-related characteristics, such as body size, build, weight, composition, and appearance, must also be considered. Achieving optimal weight and body composition goals requires assessment, goal setting, an action plan, and evaluation and reassessment.

References

1. Macedonio M, Dunford M. *The Athlete's Guide to Making Weight*. Champaign, IL: Human Kinetics; 2009.
2. Wilmore JH, Costill DL, Kinney WL. *Physiology of Sport and Exercise*. 4th ed. Champaign, IL: Human Kinetics; 2008.
3. Rodriguez NR, Di Marco NM, Langley S. American Dietetic Association; Dietitians of Canada; American College of Sports Medicine position stand. Nutrition and athletic performance. *J Am Diet Assoc*. 2009;109:509–527.
4. Dunford M, Doyle JA. *Nutrition for Sport and Exercise*. Belmont, CA: Thomson Wadsworth; 2008.
5. Yamamoto JB, Yamamoto BE, Yamamoto PP, Yamamoto LG. Epidemiology of college athlete sizes, 1950s to current. *Res Sports Med*. 2008;16:111–127.
6. Montgomery DL. Physiological profile of professional hockey players—a longitudinal comparison. *Appl Physiol Nutr Metab*. 2006;31:181–185.
7. Laurson KR, Eisenmann JC. Prevalence of overweight among high school football linemen. *JAMA*. 2007;297:363–364.
8. Malina RM, Morano PJ, Barron M, Miller SJ, Cumming SP, Kontos AP, Little BB. Overweight and obesity among youth participants in American football. *J Pediatr*. 2007;151:378–382.
9. Muller SM, Gorrow TR, Schneider SR. Enhancing appearance and sports performance: are female collegiate athletes behaving more like males? *J Am Coll Health*. 2009;57:513–520.
10. Calfee R, Fadale P. Popular ergogenic drugs and supplements in young athletes. *Pediatrics*. 2006;117:e577–e589.
11. Hill DW. The critical power concept. A review. *Sports Med*. 1993;16:237–254.
12. Millward DJ. Macronutrient intakes as determinants of dietary protein and amino acid adequacy. *J Nutr*. 2004;134(suppl):1588S–1596S.
13. Millward DJ. Protein and amino acid requirements of adults: current controversies. *Can J Appl Physiol*. 2001;26(suppl):S130–S140.
14. Mettler S, Mitchell N, Tipton KD. Increased protein intake reduces lean body mass loss during weight loss in athletes. *Med Sci Sports Exerc*. 2010;42:326–337.

Section 3

Sports Nutrition Across the Life Cycle and for Special Populations

Athletics is not restricted to the young elite or the professional athlete. Today, children participate in competitive sports as do older adults. This section provides the sports dietitian with insight into the physiological and health-related issues of diverse populations. Understanding the unique needs of these populations will help the sports dietitian develop plans to meet the needs of each athlete, whether it is a collegiate athlete who is challenged by lack of cooking skills or an athlete with diabetes who needs medical nutrition therapy. In this section, life cycle issues are discussed in chapters dealing with youth, college-age, and older athletes (Chapters 12, 13, and 14, respectively). A chapter on elite athletes (Chapter 15) is included to highlight the opportunities and challenges faced by the sports dietitian when planning nutrition strategies for high-performing athletes. The unique nutritional needs of vegetarian athletes, pregnant women, athletes with disordered eating, and those with type 1 and type 2 diabetes are also included in this section (Chapters 16 through 20).

Chapter 12

CHILD AND ADOLESCENT ATHLETES

Pamela M. Nisevich Bede, MS, RD, CSSD

Introduction

Pediatric athletes have unique nutritional needs and although various principles of sports nutrition are similar for young and old alike, there are some important differences in energy expenditure, substrate utilization, and thermoregulation in youth during exercise. Studies and recommendations on fueling and counseling adult athletes are widely available, but the same is not true for children and adolescent athletes. Research trials involving young athletes are understandably limited. So, although much of the information provided in this chapter is based on research studies involving children and adolescents, to fully understand the impact of nutrition on the performance and health of young athletes, some extrapolation must come from high-quality studies on adult athletes.

Participation of Youth in Sport

Participation in sports throughout the world continues to increase. In the United States alone, childhood and youth sports are gaining in both popularity and participation; between 1998 and 2007 participation in organized sports by youth ages 7 to 17 years increased by 9.3% (1). Currently in the United States, more than 38 million children participate in sports each year (2), with 57% of all high school students playing on formal sports teams (3). In Europe, depending on country, between 53% to 98% of youth are involved in sports.

Trends in recent decades include increased numbers of female participants, increased duration and intensity of training, increased participation in "extreme" sports (such as BMX racing, skateboarding, and mountain climbing), earlier specialization and consequently year-round training, and increased difficulty of skills practiced.

Ironically, despite ever-increasing numbers of youth participating in sports, the epidemic of pediatric obesity continues. This crisis is at the top of many public health and nutrition intervention agendas; therefore, a special section on pediatric obesity is included within this chapter.

Benefits and Drawbacks of Youth Participation in Sports

There are both positive and negative aspects associated with the increasing popularity of participation in youth sports. The positives include overall improved physical fitness that includes both cardiorespiratory fitness and muscular strength, reduced body fat levels, decreased risk for cardiovascular and metabolic diseases, enhanced bone health, reduction of the symptoms of depression and anxiety (4), and increased self-esteem and emotional well-being (5). In addition, research has shown that adolescent athletes maintain healthier nutritional habits than nonathletic peers (5,6). Conversely, the negative aspects of participating in sports include the risk of injury, including overuse injury, and the mindset of "win at all costs," which may lead to unhealthy behaviors such as drug use, violence in sports, disordered eating, and an increased risk for injury (3,4,7).

According to the National Center for Sports Safety, more than 3.5 million children ages 14 and younger receive medical treatment for sports injuries each year (8). Additional data from the Centers for Disease Control and Prevention (CDC) reported that nearly 1.9 million children younger than the age of 15 years were treated in emergency departments in 2001 for sports-related injuries. The most common injuries included sprains and strains, growth plate injuries, repetitive motion injuries (ie, overuse injuries), and heat-related illnesses, including dehydration and heat stroke (2,7). In fact, injuries associated with participation in sports and recreational activities account for 21% of all traumatic brain injuries among children in the United States (8). The sports dietitian can aid in reducing some of the negative aspects of sports participation by working with athletes, coaches, and parents to discuss proper nutrition for recovery from exercise and guidelines for adequate hydration to help alleviate the incidence of heat-related illness.

Differences Between Child and Adolescent Athletes and Adults

Young athletes are not mini-adults. Each young athlete grows and matures at his or her own rate. Many factors affect the rate of maturation, including genetics and metabolic and hormonal responses to exercise. Substantial differences exist between adult athletes and young athletes, including the following:

- Children have an immature anaerobic metabolic system and their substrate utilization during activity may vary depending on their age and pubertal status (9).
- Anaerobic glycolytic ATP rephosphorylation may be reduced in young individuals during high-intensity exercise (9).
- Prepubertal children may also have reduced activity of phosphofructokinase-1 and lactate dehydrogenase enzymes. All of these factors may be related to the reduced sympathetic response to exhaustive resistance exercise in young athletes.
- Data suggest that children rely more on fat oxidation for energy during exercise than do adults. This finding is age-dependent; glycolytic activity tends to increase with age. Furthermore, this hypothesis is supported by findings that children have increased free fatty acid mobilization, glycerol release, and growth hormone levels during exercise. Children and adolescents are less able than adults to achieve ATP rephosphorylation by anaerobic metabolic pathways during high-intensity exercise (9).
- The period of adolescent development involves anatomic, physiological, and metabolic changes and is characterized by a faster rate of growth than during any other period of life (10). This rapid growth and development results in increased requirements for energy and nutrients, as evidenced by the age-specific Dietary Reference Intake (DRI) recommendations.

- Children have lower muscle strength, which is related to altered muscle fiber growth and results in lower anaerobic capacity. Introducing young athletes to strenuous activity must be done cautiously (9).
- The limited data and research on young athletes in comparison with adult athletes are often attributed to ethical concerns and methodological constraints (9). Much of the research that does exist involves very small samples, and study designs are often indirect, relatively noninvasive, and carry little or no risk to the young subject (9).

Growth and Development

The growth pattern of an individual child or adolescent is often neither stable nor predictable. Annual growth evaluations using the standardized percentile charts from the National Center for Health Statistics (11–14) are helpful when evaluating growth patterns. These charts are available at the CDC Web site (www.cdc.gov/growthcharts). The body mass index (BMI) charts are helpful in assessing risk of underweight, overweight, and obese status. However, growth charts should not be relied on alone; there is potential for error when interpreting BMI without some assessment of body composition (lean body mass and bone density). Because of great fluctuations in patterns of growth, the energy needs of young athletes are not stable and may be difficult for the sports dietitian to estimate. To best determine if the energy intake of an athlete is adequate to maintain growth, development, health, and performance, nutrition professionals should monitor growth, body mass trends, and other anthropometric variables of the athlete (15). In addition, periods of rapid growth may lead to unexpected periods of lethargy, poor coordination and movement efficiency, and result in considerable fluctuations in energy needs.

Childhood

Childhood is a time of steady and slow growth during preschool and school years, but this growth can at times be quite erratic in individual children. Growth spurts are often accompanied by changes in appetite and food consumption (16). Growth during childhood is slow compared to growth in infancy and adolescence. On average, weight increases approximately 2 to 3 kg (0.9 to 1.4 lb) per year until the child is 9 to 10 years of age. At this point the rate of weight gain increases, signaling the approach of puberty and adolescence. Increases in height average between 6 to 8 cm (2.4 to 3.2 inches) per year from age 2 years until puberty begins.

There is limited information on the effect of intense exercise on the growth of young athletes. This is likely due to the fact that sport specificity, body type, and self-induced energy deficits are confounding variables that require more study (17,18). Although current research does not suggest that high levels of training will decrease growth potential, delays in growth have been documented in athletes in sports such as dance and gymnastics (19). These delays in growth are thought to be related to inadequate nutritional practices vs excessive training. In addition, studies have found that once training load was decreased (thereby allowing energy available for growth), "catch-up" growth was achieved (15).

Adolescence

Adolescence is period of life accompanied by a multitude of changes, including physical, cognitive, emotional, and social changes, all of which provide challenges and opportunities to both sports dietitians and athletes. Adolescence is a nutritionally vulnerable time of life (20) as it is a time of rapid yet fluctuating growth, accompanied by changes in body composition and patterns of eating.

Growth spurts in adolescents typically occur between the ages of 10 and 12 years for females and 2 years later for males (20). In females, this growth is accompanied by an increase in the proportion of body fat to muscle mass; in males, growth is accompanied by increases in lean body mass and increased blood volume. On average, males who participate in sports have normal growth rates and maturation compared to their nonathletic peers. In addition, some athletic males are seemingly advanced in maturation as their increased muscle mass favors power and performance (21). During adolescence, outwardly accelerated gains in height are achieved, and it is estimated that pubescent adolescents accrue 15% of their final adult height and 45% of their maximal skeletal mass during adolescence (20). On average, during puberty, girls grow 25 cm (10 in) and gain 24 kg (53 lb) whereas boys grow 28 cm (11 in) and gain 32 kg (70 lb) (22). The growth pattern and velocity may be related to genetics but can be influenced by many factors, including energy balance (17,22).

Despite accelerated growth and increased nutrient requirements, research involving this age group has found that adolescents do not adhere to the Dietary Guidelines for Americans and consequently do not consume adequate amounts of fruits, vegetables, calcium-rich foods, and many micronutrients. Conversely, this age group tends to have an excessive intake of total fat, saturated fat, cholesterol, sodium, and sugar (23,24). The sports dietitian should also recognize that adolescents are more likely than their younger and adult counterparts to engage in unsafe weight-loss methods, and adolescence (and slightly older) is a prime age for development of eating disorders. By being aware of these tendencies, the nutrition professional can aid adolescent athletes in making healthy food choices and developing appropriate attitudes about food and nutrition.

Nutrition Assessment and Nutrient Recommendations

Active children require a sufficient energy intake to support optimal growth and development as well as to meet the increased energy demands associated with training and physical activity. Involvement in sports has the potential to negatively influence nutrient intakes through time constraints, travel, and sport-specific eating-related attitudes (5). The sports dietitian can assist young athletes by helping them develop an appropriate eating pattern and schedule and making recommendations to ensure that their meal patterns are well balanced and adequate.

Energy Needs, Energy Balance, and Energy Intake

Although limited, research involving young athletes has found that participation in sport at any level generally increases nutrient requirements. Young athletes need energy to fuel training and competition while also meeting needs for growth, health, body mass maintenance, and daily physical activities. Should these elevated energy requirements consistently be unmet, the results may include short stature, delayed puberty, menstrual irregularities, poor bone health, and increased risk of injuries. Concerning overall total energy requirements, some estimates for energy expenditure in young athletes are extrapolated from adult data; however, this approach is flawed because children are less metabolically efficient (15,25). Consequently, children's energy requirements (per kilogram of body weight) during walking and running can be as much as 30% higher than adults. When undergoing strenuous training, young athletes are likely to compensate for the elevated energy expenditure by conserving energy via increased sedentary behaviors the remainder of the day (26).

Given all of the factors mentioned, it is difficult to determine a DRI for energy in young athletes. Researchers Eisenmann and Wickel reviewed research regarding the total daily energy expenditure (TDEE) of young athletes and categorized energy needs based on age groups (27). For child and adolescent athletes participating in a wide range of sports, TDEE ranged from as low as 2,457 kcal to as high as 4,022 kcal for males and from 2,184 kcal to as high as 2,886 kcal for females. For studies that provided TDEE as a measure of kcal/kg, the TDEE ranged from as low as 44 kcal/kg across sexes to as high as 57 kcal/kg for males and as high as 51 kcal/kg for female athletes (27). The researchers were quick to suggest that direct comparisons between research studies involving young athletes should be made with caution because the available data vary by age and body size of the subjects, sport, level of competition, and overall methods of assessing TDEE. For best evaluation of a young athlete's energy needs, careful monitoring of growth, body mass, and other anthropometric values can help health professionals determine whether energy intake is adequate for a young athlete to maintain growth, development, and performance (15).

Food Records and Recalls as Tools for Evaluating a Young Athlete's Nutrition Profile

Much of the scientific research involving young athletes is understandably noninvasive and uses diet records and recalls. These records and recalls are relied on heavily as a tool to aid the nutrition professional in evaluating the adequacy of an athlete's diet and energy needs.

Accurate food records can provide the practitioner with a wealth of information, but working with young athletes often presents a challenge in obtaining an accurate food recall. Practitioners report that very young athletes may fail to provide accurate information because of a lack of knowledge or forgetfulness, whereas the older athlete may purposely underreport or overreport intake to please a parent, coach, athletic trainer, or sports dietitian. To avoid the inaccuracies presented by young test subjects' food records, research findings suggest that parents can be a reliable source for recording and reporting accurate energy intake of younger athletes (28).

Bandini and colleagues examined whether the accuracy of reported energy intake fluctuated as females moved from middle school to high school (29). The researchers examined energy intake (EI) and energy expenditure (EE) of 26 females ages 10, 12, and 15 years old. The researchers measured EI via use of 7-day diet records and relied on doubly labeled water to determine EE (29). The authors found that as the girls aged, they tended to report EI less accurately; the average accuracy at 10 years was 88% ± 13%, 77% ± 21% at 12 years, and 68% ± 17% at age 15 years. Based on this study and others (29,30), it may be necessary for the sports dietitian working with female adolescent athletes to keep in mind that as children age, their diet records may substantially underestimate their intakes.

Although some studies question the validity of diet records, multiple well-designed studies have found that, on the whole, young athletes tend to eat more healthfully than their nonathletic counterparts. Recently, the Project EAT (Eating Among Teens) Student Survey, which included 4,746 students ages 11 to 18 years, revealed that among females, breakfast was eaten more often among weight-related sport participants than either team-sport athletes or nonathletes. Additionally, weight-related sport participants reported eating dinner and snacks more frequently than other youths. Male subjects involved in sports also reported eating breakfast and lunch more frequently than their less athletic counterparts (dinner and snack frequencies were similar across groups).

When considering all data from the survey, the researchers concluded that although there were few substantial differences between athletes participating in team sports vs weight-related sports, statistically significant differences existed between youth involved in sports and youth not involved in sports (6). Based on this study and other similar studies, sports dietitians can assume that active youth consume breakfast more frequently and have greater intakes of protein, calcium, iron, and zinc.

Multiple factors influence a young athlete's nutrient needs, and whereas the DRIs aim to ensure adequate energy for growth, development, and maturation, the DRIs do not take into account the increased nutritional needs of very active child or adolescent athletes. Indeed, it is difficult to develop a standardized recommendation for energy intake for this group because of large individual variability. Therefore, the practitioner should calculate an athlete's estimated energy requirement using equations that consider the individual's age, height, body weight, and physical activity classification (sedentary, moderately active, active, and very active) (26).

When Energy Intake Becomes Excessive: The Pediatric Obesity Crisis

The steady increase in obesity in the United States and around the globe has also affected child and adolescent athletes. There is likely no one factor to blame for the obesity crisis; this epidemic is probably a result of a hypercaloric diet coupled with a multitude of factors including, but not limited to, reduced physical activity in everyday tasks as well as reduced leisure-time exercise (31).

The number of school-age children who are overweight or obese seems to be increasing in all areas of the world, but comparisons are difficult to make because of different criteria for defining overweight and obesity. For our purposes, we will rely on a set of gender and age-adjusted cutoff points for BMI that are equivalent to adult BMIs of 25 (overweight) and 30 (obese), and which were developed by an expert committee convened by the International Obesity Task Force (IOTF) (32). BMI can be used as a tool to evaluate the weight status of children ages 2 to 18 years. A child's weight status is determined based on an age- and sex-specific percentile for BMI rather than by the BMI categories used for adults. Classifications of overweight and obesity for children and adolescents are age- and sex-specific because children's body composition varies as they age and varies between boys and girls (33). The cutoffs developed for children are divided into 6-month increments and used in growth-chart format. For children and adolescents (ages 2 to 19 years), the BMI value is plotted on the CDC gender-specific growth charts to determine the corresponding BMI-for-age percentile (11,13).

Individuals with BMI values that plot at or more than the 85th percentile and less than the 95th percentile are classified as overweight (formerly classified as "at risk for overweight"). Individuals with a BMI that plots at or more than the 95th percentile are classified as obese (formerly classified as "overweight"). These definitions are based on the 2000 CDC Growth Charts for the United States and the 2007 Expert Committee recommendations (34).

Results from the National Health and Nutrition Examination Survey (NHANES) conducted in 1999–2000 and 2003–2004 indicate that the prevalence of pediatric overweight and obesity is increasing. In 1999–2000, approximately 29% of youth ages 6 to 17 years were classified as having BMIs more than the IOTF cutoffs for overweight; 10% of these youth were clinically obese. By 2003–2004, 35% of youth ages 6 to17 years were overweight, whereas more than 13% were obese (35). Additional data from a more recent NHANES survey (2007–2008) indicate that an estimated 17% of children and adolescents ages 2 to 19 years are obese. Between 1976–1980 and 1999–2000, the prevalence of obesity clearly increased. Between 1999–2000 and 2007–2008 there was no significant trend in obesity prevalence across the age group of 2 to 19 years. However, there was a marked increase in the prevalence of obesity in the very young; the rate of obesity in children ages 2 to 5 years increased from 5% to 10.4% between 1976–1980 and 2007–2008. In children ages 6 to 11 years, the rate was even more accelerated: this age group experienced an increase from 5% to 19.6% between 1976–1980 and 2007–2008.

These alarming results indicate a continuing and accelerated trend in the prevalence of overweight and obesity among children and adolescents in the United States. Obese children and adolescents are at risk for health problems during their youth and as adults. These early-onset risk factors include cardiovascular disease (such as high blood pressure, high cholesterol), type 2 diabetes, and metabolic syndrome (36) among others. Evidence also shows that overweight and obese children are more likely to be made fun of and have lower levels of self-esteem compared with normal weight peers.

Obese children and adolescents are more likely than normal weight youth to become obese adults (37,38). For example, one study found that approximately 80% of children who were overweight at ages 10 to 15 years were obese adults at age 25 years (37). Another study found that 25% of obese adults were overweight as children. The latter study also found that if overweight begins before 8 years of age, obesity in adulthood is likely to be more severe (37,38). Later in life, overweight athletes are at an increased risk of hypercholesterolemia, gallbladder disease, cardiovascular disease, hypertension, and type 2 diabetes mellitus.

When overweight and obese children and adolescents participate in sports, the sports dietitian, as well as coaches, certified athletic trainers, and parents, should be aware of some of the effects that excessive weight has on an athlete's performance:

- Increased body weight is associated with a decrease in postural stability, and weight loss in obese athletes has been linked to an improvement in balance control (39).
- There seems to be a higher incidence of injuries in young athletes who are obese vs not obese (40,41). The increased risk of injury associated with being overweight or obese may in part be due to these athletes' overall reduced physical activity level (41).
- At the societal level, promoting physical activity for children and improving dietary habits are key strategies for reducing the incidence of overweight and obesity (41).
- Athletes who gain weight at an accelerated pace in an effort to "bulk up" for their sport may accrue excess fat, which may result in reduced speed, endurance, agility, and work efficiency, as well as poor acclimation to heat (42).

Due to increased risk for injury and even death, caution is essential when introducing overweight and obese young athletes to physical activity (43). Once an athlete is medically cleared for activity, the sports dietitian is in the unique position to aid young overweight and obese athletes in the desire to improve both performance and weight. The advisability of substantial weight loss depends on the severity of obesity, the athlete's age and potential for growth, and potential underlying medical conditions.

Not all overweight or even obese athletes need to lose weight. Often it is recommended that they maintain weight until height increases, thereby bringing the athlete's BMI to a healthy level. However, an increase in height alone is unlikely to bring a severely obese child's BMI to within the optimal range. Athletes who would benefit from weight loss should be counseled on the harmful effects of extreme or inappropriate weight-loss practices. The young athlete should be informed that when weight is lost too rapid or is a result of substantial reduction in energy intake, lean muscle mass will be lost, which can negatively affect performance. Therefore, when weight loss is necessary, the loss should be gradual (not exceeding 1.5% of total body weight each week) and should be monitored not only for total body weight lost but also for positive changes in body composition. The information in Table 12.1, which is based on the 2007 Expert Committee recommendations regarding the prevention, assessment, and treatment of child and adolescent overweight and obesity, can be helpful in determining whether a young athlete requires weight maintenance or weight loss (34).

When working with youth who need to lose weight, the Evidence Analysis Library of the Academy of Nutrition and Dietetics (formerly American Dietetic Association) recommends that the weight-management program involve multiple components, including a nutrition prescription translated into a specific eating plan. The appropriate nutrition intervention should be based on an individualized nutrition prescription, detailing macronutrient and micronutrient needs, because research demonstrates improvement in weight status in children and adolescents is more successful when an individualized nutrition prescription is included, and less successful when an individualized nutrition prescription is not included (44).

To determine the nutrition prescription, the sports dietitian must consider the young athlete's age, growth parameters, body composition, potential need for weight loss, and physical activity. The equations

TABLE 12.1   Recommendations from the Expert Committee Regarding the Prevention, Assessment, and Treatment of Child and Adolescent Overweight and Obesity

Age, y	BMI Status	Recommended Treatment
2–5	BMI = 85th–94th percentile	Weight maintenance until BMI is < 85th percentile or slowing of weight gain is indicated by a downward deflection in the BMI curve.
	BMI ≥ 95th percentile	Weight maintenance until BMI is < 85th percentile; however, if weight loss occurs with a healthy adequate diet, then it should not exceed 1 lb/mo.[a]
	BMI > 21 or 22 (rare; very high)	Gradual weight loss, not to exceed 1 lb/mo.[a]
6–11	BMI = 85th–94th percentile	Weight maintenance until BMI is < 85th percentile or slowing of weight gain is indicated by a downward deflection in the BMI curve.
	BMI = 95th–98th percentile	Weight maintenance until BMI is < 85th percentile or gradual weight loss of 1 lb/mo.[a]
	BMI ≥ 99th percentile	Weight loss not to exceed an average of 2 lb/wk.[a]
12–18	BMI = 85th–94th percentile	Weight maintenance until BMI is < 85th percentile or slowing of weight gain is indicated by a downward deflection in the BMI curve.
	BMI = 95th–98th percentile	Weight loss until BMI is < 85th percentile, with no more than an average of 2 lb/wk.[a]
	BMI ≥ 99th percentile	Weight loss not to exceed an average of 2 lb/wk.[a]

[a]If greater loss (than what is recommended) is noted, the patient should be monitored for causes of excessive weight loss.
Source: Data are from reference 34.

listed in Box 12.1 (44) assist in determining energy needs for overweight youth ages 3 to 18 years. Once the athlete's overall energy needs are determined, the sports dietitian and the athlete can work together to develop an acceptable and well-balanced diet plan to promote both health and sport.

Carbohydrate Intake

Requirements

As in adult athletes, carbohydrate intake is of utmost importance to the young athlete. Although young children are thought to lack the full development of glycolytic capacity and consequently may rely more on fat to fuel activity, this seems to be resolved in adolescence. Whether young athletes fully benefit from a high-carbohydrate diet has yet to be established. Due to a lack of research, it is unclear whether young athletes need the same carbohydrate intake as adult athletes (15,45). However, research by Riddell and colleagues found that during heavy exercise, total carbohydrate utilization in adolescents may be as high as 1.0 to 1.5 g/kg/h (46). Carbohydrate is undeniably an important fuel to optimize athletic performance and recovery in young athletes. Although carbohydrate-loading is not recommended for young athletes, they still stand to benefit from a well-balanced diet rich in whole grains, fruits, vegetables, and low-fat dairy because these foods provide energy, nutrients, and fiber. In general, it is recommended that young athletes consume at least 50% of total daily energy intake as carbohydrate (26). According to Burke and colleagues (45), the use of refined carbohydrates (ie, sport drinks, gels, and energy bars) during training and competition can be helpful. Additional research suggests that young athletes, like adults, tolerate a concentration of 6% to 8% carbohydrate solutions (47). However, it should be noted that overuse of these items may increase the risk for childhood obesity (15).

BOX 12.1 Determining Energy Needs in Overweight Children and Adolescents

According to the *Dietary Reference Intakes for Energy, Carbohydrate, Fiber, Fat, Fatty Acids, Cholesterol, Protein, and Amino Acids (Macronutrients)*, Total Energy Expenditure (TEE) in overweight youth (ages 3 to 18 years) in a weight maintenance situation should be calculated using the following equations:

Overweight Boys Ages 3–18 Years

$$TEE = 114 - (50.9 \times \text{Age [y]}) + PA \times (19.5 \times \text{Weight [kg]} + 1161.4 \times \text{Height [m]})$$

Where PA is the physical activity coefficient:

- PA = 1.00 if physical activity level (PAL) is estimated to be ≥ 1.0 < 1.4 (sedentary)
- PA = 1.12 if PAL is estimated to be ≥ 1.4 < 1.6 (low active)
- PA = 1.24 if PAL is estimated to be ≥ 1.6 < 1.9 (active)
- PA = 1.45 if PAL is estimated to be ≥ 1.9 < 2.5 (very active)

Overweight Girls Ages 3–18 Years

$$TEE = 389 - (41.2 \times \text{Age [y]}) + PA \times (15.0 \times \text{Weight [kg]} + 701.6 \times \text{Height [m]})$$

Where PA is the physical activity coefficient:

- PA = 1.00 if PAL is estimated to be ≥ 1.0 < 1.4 (sedentary)
- PA = 1.18 if PAL is estimated to be ≥ 1.4 < 1.6 (low active)
- PA = 1.35 if PAL is estimated to be ≥ 1.6 < 1.9 (active)
- PA = 1.60 if PAL is estimated to be ≥ 1.9 < 2.5 (very active)

Source: Data are from reference 44.

Sources of Carbohydrate Commonly Consumed by Young Athletes

Most young athletes frequently consume carbohydrates, but they may need to be encouraged to reduce consumption of snack foods and sugar-laden beverages. The intake of simple sugars in adolescents is likely to be higher than what is recommended. For example, sweetened beverages such as sports drinks, energy drinks, and soft drinks rank fourth out of the top 25 sources of energy in the diet of Americans over the age of 2 (48). The high intake of sugars in the younger population suggests a preference for sweet foods, which may lead to food patterns that are not conducive to high levels of performance. Many young athletes are not aware of the wide range of carbohydrate sources in the food system and they need to be encouraged to expand their palate. The sports dietitian can facilitate diet changes in this group by identifying which flavors and textures an athlete prefers and recommend a healthier, more appropriate option.

Protein Intake

Requirements

Rapid growth and development during childhood and adolescence increase the requirements for energy and nutrients; any restriction in overall energy intake coupled with a high level of physical activity could alter protein metabolism and impair growth and maturation (10,19,49). The dietary protein recommendation is 0.8 to 1.0 g/kg/d in adolescents, but this recommendation is based on nonactive adolescents rather than those involved in regular training (49). An upper limit of 1.7 g/kg/d has been found to be appropriate for adult athletes in training, and this amount is expected to be applicable for children and adolescents as well (50).

Boisseau and colleagues examined whether regular intensive exercise training affects protein turnover in young gymnasts (19). The authors studied 10 pre- and early-pubertal athletes and 10 age-matched sedentary control subjects. Using 7-day diet records and the noninvasive end-product method with [15N]-glycine, the researchers determined that although the young athletes ingested less than the recommended dietary allowance, the difference between the two groups was not significant and the results suggested that these young athletes do not need more protein to meet the needs of growth, maturation, and exercise (19).

The requirement for protein relative to energy intake needs clarification for athletes in whom energy balance may be compromised due to growth spurts, excess energy expenditure due to a high volume of training, or energy intake restriction for a weight-class sport (26). Many studies suggest that young athletes require more protein per kilogram than their nonactive peers (19,49). Although this is true, the sports dietitian should not be quick to add a large quantity of protein to an athlete's typical intake; assessments of protein intake in young athletes have shown that on average and per kilogram of body weight, most athletes already ingest adequate protein and easily meet estimated higher needs (32).

Sources of Protein Commonly Consumed by Young Athletes

Younger children tend to have a limited palate. Very young children may be hesitant to add more animal products to their diet (aside from dairy products), and observations from practitioners suggest that many young children prefer carbohydrate- and fat-rich foods over protein. Many adolescent athletes often have an adequate intake of protein but should be encouraged to select lean protein choices over the more commonly consumed burgers, bacon, sausages, high-fat dairy, and fried foods. Some protein-rich and nutrient-dense snack and meal choices are shown in Table 12.2.

Fat Intake

Requirements

Although there is no Recommended Dietary Allowance (RDA) or Adequate Intake (AI) set for fat, AIs have been established for the essential fatty acids: linoleic acid and linolenic acid. The recommended intake of total fat established by the Acceptable Macronutrient Distribution Range (AMDR) suggests 20% to 35% of daily energy intake should come from fat (16,26). Young athletes desiring weight control may reduce overall dietary fat to create an energy deficit (without sacrificing carbohydrate or protein intake). Although children use proportionately more fat as a substrate during exercise, there is no evidence that young athletes involved in endurance activities will benefit from a higher fat content in their diet (45). Although no one has yet investigated the impact of adjusting fat intake on performance in this age group (9,19), researchers have found that ingestion of high-fat foods before exercise may reduce the magnitude of growth hormone secretion during exercise (51). In theory, if growth hormone increase during exercise is important to muscle adaptation and growth, then a high-fat intake (prior to exercise) may have a negative effect on performance (15).

Sources of Fat Commonly Consumed by Young Athletes

Over the past quarter century, trends in children's food choices showed a decrease in the consumption of fat from milk as well as from fats/oils, pork, mixed meats, eggs, and desserts. However, the percentage of fat from poultry, cheese, and snacks increased. The percentage of energy intake from total fats and saturated fats fell, but total fat intakes did not decrease because total energy intake did not decrease (23). In addition,

TABLE 12.2   Protein-Rich Snacks and Meals for Young Athletes

Meal or Snack	Energy, kcal	Carbohydrate, g	Protein, g	Fat, g
2 slices whole wheat bread, toasted; 2 tsp light cream cheese spread; 1 egg, cooked; ½ cup fresh baby spinach; 1 navel orange	445	61	18	17
1 English muffin, toasted; 1 slice low-fat (2%) American cheese; 1 cup low-fat fruit-on-the-bottom yogurt; 1 serving of fresh fruit	450	78	17	8
Shake made from 2 Tbsp whey protein powder, any flavor; 1 medium banana; 2 Tbsp fat-free chocolate syrup; 8 oz fat-free milk; ½ cup crushed ice	420	77	19	4
3 mini bagels topped with 1 Tbsp low-fat cream cheese; 1 cup fresh berries; water to drink	365	73	10.6	5
1 cup grapes; 1 oz pretzels dipped in 1 Tbsp peanut butter	360	44	18	11.5
½ cup fat-free fruit sorbet topped with 2 Tbsp ground nuts; 1 cup fresh blueberries; 1 slice angel food cake	350	65	9	6
8 oz light yogurt mixed with ½ sliced kiwi fruit and ½ cup low-fat granola	335	55	13	7
Grilled sandwich: 2 slices whole grain bread topped with 1 slice low-fat (2%) American cheese and 1 oz each of deli roast beef, chicken, and lean ham	290	27	26	8
1 whole grain bagel topped with ⅓ cup marinara sauce and 1 oz low-fat mozzarella cheese, broiled	260	37	15.3	6
8 oz low-fat chocolate milk; 1 cup fresh apple or pear	230	45	8.3	3
3 oz grilled, nonbreaded chicken fingers (made from chicken breast tenders); 2 Tbsp barbeque sauce for dipping	180	9	27	3

Source of nutrient information: Nutritionist Pro Version 4.4.0. Copyright 2010 Axxya Systems.

a snapshot of NHANES data from 2005–2006 showed that on average children ages 2 to 5 years consumed approximately 31% of energy from total fat and 11.3% to 11.5% of total energy from saturated fat; children ages 6 to 11 years consumed approximately 33.9% of energy from total fat and 12% to 12.2% of total energy from saturated fat; adolescents ages 12 to 19 years consumed approximately 30% of energy from total fat and 11.5% to 11.6% of total energy from saturated fat (23,24).

Many athletes could benefit from education on appropriate intake and sources of fat. Many athletes ingest more fat than they realize by consuming items labeled as "crispy," "pan-fried," "broasted," "creamed," and others. Additionally, young athletes should be encouraged to obtain less than 10% of their total daily energy from saturated fat (26) and to keep *trans* fat intake to a minimum. Consequently, the young athlete may need assistance with healthfully filling the energy void left by chips, crackers, cookies, cakes, candy, and fried foods while transitioning to a more healthful pattern of eating. Athletes restricting overall fat intake in an attempt to reduce energy consumption should be counseled on the importance of and sources of essential fatty acids.

Fluids and Hydration

Requirements

Limited research using tracer methodology has been done regarding fluid turnover and fluid needs for active children. However, it is vital for the young athlete to monitor and maintain adequate fluid balance to prevent dehydration to sustain normal cardiovascular and thermoregulatory functions required for exercise performance (26). Fluids are of utmost importance to the young athlete because children have a greater ratio of surface area to body mass and also absorb environmental heat more readily than adults (52). Consequently, children are at a greater risk for experiencing heat stress when exercising in hot environments. Nonathletic children have a faster metabolic rate and generate greater heat production than adults working at the same volume. In addition, children not only have higher thresholds before even beginning to sweat, their sweating capacity is considerably lower, reducing their ability to dissipate body heat by evaporation (42). Based on these findings, it is critical to provide information on proper hydration to all children and especially to those who are new to an activity or climate because children take longer to acclimate to hot, humid environments (2 weeks vs 1 week), which increases their risk of heat-related injury (42).

As children mature, there seems to be an increase in sweat rate when adjusting for body surface area. An increase in electrolyte loss often follows an increase in sweat rate in both children and adolescent athletes. Encouraging young athletes to replenish electrolytes by using sport drinks helps the athlete replace fluids and as well as carbohydrates. Research has shown that when children or adolescents are provided water to drink, they do not replace their fluid losses as completely as when they are offered a flavored drink or a flavored sport beverage (containing both carbohydrate and electrolytes). Conveniently, the presence of sodium in the beverage not only replaces losses but also heightens the desire to drink more, resulting in better recovery of optimal hydration (53).

In adults, loss of 2% of body weight due to dehydration has been shown to have detrimental effects on performance. The same is true for children, but the negative side effects of fluid loss (decreased performance, increases in core temperature [42]) begin to occur at a 1% decrease in body weight (53). Whereas nonathletic children tend to produce greater amounts of heat during activity, older adolescents tend to sweat more than younger adolescents. Similar to the effects of dehydration on adults, it can be assumed that dehydration in children leads to decreased endurance and performance by negatively affecting the cardiovascular system, thermoregulation, and central fatigue or perceived exhaustion (26).

Practical Advice on Hydration for Young Athletes

Regardless of age, athletes whose sweat loss exceeds fluid intake become dehydrated during activity. Dehydration of 1% may impair performance in children, and greater percentages of dehydration can lead to disturbances in physiological function and increase the risk for heat illness (52). To prevent dehydration and promote euhydration in young athletes, the sports dietitian can offer the following advice from the National Athletic Trainers' Association Position Statement: Fluid Replacement for Athletes (54) as well as recommendations from the American Academy of Pediatrics (AAP) (42). Chapter 21 provides additional hydration guidelines for working with youth participating in high-intensity intermittent sports. The recommendations are as follows:

- Establish a hydration protocol for young athletes, including a rehydration strategy that considers the athlete's sweat rate, sport dynamics (such as rest breaks, time-outs, fluid access, etc), availability of fluids (and reminder to bring fluids to all practice sessions and games), environmental factors, level of fitness, exercise duration and intensity, and individual preferences.

- Be aware that hypohydration and dehydration practices are used by athletes who participate in weight-sensitive sports in an attempt to lose weight or appear leaner. Voluntary dehydration practices to watch out for (and discourage) include fluid restriction, spitting, use of laxatives and diuretics, rubber suits, steam baths, and saunas.
- Ensure that fluids are easily accessible to all athletes. Young athletes often forget their water bottle and coaches and parents should be encouraged to ensure that there is fluid provided at each practice and game.
- Encourage athletes to begin a practice session or competition well hydrated and drink electrolyte-containing fluids throughout the training session. Athletes can be instructed to observe the color of their urine and continue drinking fluids until the urine is light yellow to clear in color.
- Emphasize that after exercise young athletes should focus on correcting fluid losses accumulated during the event. Young athletes may become more aware of their personal sweat rate and loss of fluids by monitoring hydration status by weighing before and after exercise sessions. Chapter 6 provides more information on hydration status. Additionally, young athletes should be encouraged to attain euhydration status within 2 hours after activity and via use of carbohydrate- and electrolyte-containing beverages.

Micronutrient Intake

Minerals represent approximately 4% to 5% of a young athlete's body weight (16). Minerals and vitamins are necessary for normal growth and development, and insufficient intake can result in impaired growth and diseases associated with deficiencies (16). Micronutrients play the same roles in athletes as in nonathletes. These roles include the synthesis and formation of body tissues, maintenance of fluid balance within specific compartments, and acting as cofactors for facilitating metabolic reactions regulated by enzymes (26).

Research on the dietary intakes of young athletes indicates that they consume vitamin levels at or close to the DRIs while surpassing the intake of their nonactive peers (26). In addition, there is no current research suggesting that the vitamin needs of athletic youth are higher than their sedentary counterparts.

Although there is limited research available on the mineral losses of youth in sports, adult data suggest that, aside from those minerals lost in sweat and feces, elevated metabolism through exercise does not increase mineral requirements. However, in the diets of children and adolescents, two micronutrients (iron and calcium) deserve attention because they are frequently identified as being deficient and can affect overall health and performance.

In adolescents, puberty increases the requirement for iron because of increases in hemoglobin mass, tissue deposition, growth spurt, and onset of menstruation in females (26). Iron depletion and deficiency have been documented in endurance athletes, athletes restricting dietary intake, and female athletes (26). Some studies show that as many as 40% to 50% of female athletes have low ferritin stores (55). Although low iron intake may not necessarily result in anemia, it may lead to impaired muscle metabolism and cognitive function (15). Cause of low iron stores may be related to the following (16,26,56–58):

- Increased growth and physical demands
- Menstruation in females or bleeding disorders in either sex
- Poor absorption
- Sports-related hemolysis and blood loss
- Poor overall intake (self-imposed restriction or imbalanced diet pattern)

- Heavy sweat loss
- Poor socioeconomic status and food insecurity

Inadequate intake of calcium, when coupled with heavy, intense training, can have a detrimental effect on bone health in maturing children (26). Although exercise itself does not increase the need for calcium, the body of an amenorrheic female athlete may require more calcium than those with normal menses. In amenorrheic females, an intake closer to 1,500 mg/d of calcium may be necessary (45). In all athletes, there is a threshold for calcium intake beyond which any additional intake does not result in retention. When calcium intake is low during childhood and adolescence, higher calcium retention partially compensates for the deficit (59). However, chronic low calcium intake (< 400 mg/d) is detrimental to bone development and overall health (60).

Because iron deficiency, low levels of iron, and poor intake of iron and calcium commonly occur in young athletes, it may be helpful for the sports dietitian to discuss optimal intake and food sources of iron and calcium. Low intakes can be ameliorated by providing young athletes with strategies for increasing dietary iron and calcium and discussing forms of each nutrient that are readily absorbable. A candid discussion on the side effects and consequences of inadequate micronutrient intake would be of benefit to the athlete who is at risk for a deficiency. Sometimes, medically supervised supplementation may be warranted (15). Table 12.3 lists good sources of calcium for young athletes.

Sport-Specific Nutrition

Nutrition recommendations often vary from sport to sport. This section will briefly discuss some differences among sports of varying intensities.

TABLE 12.3 Good Sources of Calcium[a] for Young Athletes

Food, Standard Amount	Calcium, mg	Energy, kcal
Plain yogurt, nonfat (13 g protein/8 oz), 8 oz	452	127
Plain yogurt, low-fat (12 g protein/8 oz), 8 oz	415	143
Soy beverage, calcium-fortified, 1 cup	368	98
Fruit yogurt, low-fat (10 g protein/8 oz), 8 oz	345	232
Sardines, Atlantic, in oil, drained, 3 oz	325	177
Mozzarella cheese, part-skim, 1.5 oz	311	129
Fat-free (skim) milk, 1 cup	306	83
Low-fat (1%) milk, 1 cup	290	102
Low-fat chocolate milk (1%), 1 cup	288	158
Reduced-fat (2%) milk, 1 cup	285	122
Fortified ready-to-eat cereals (various), 1 oz	236–1043	88–106
Spinach, cooked from frozen, ½ cup	146	30
Soybeans, green, cooked, ½ cup	130	127

[a]A good source of calcium provides at least 100 mg of calcium per serving, which is 10% of the Daily Value for calcium (1,000 mg).
Source: Nutrient values from Agricultural Research Service (ARS) Nutrient Database for Standard Reference, Release 17. Foods are from ARS single nutrient reports, sorted in descending order by nutrient content in terms of common household measures. Food items and weights in the single nutrient reports are adapted from those in 2002 revision of USDA Home and Garden Bulletin No. 72, Nutritive Value of Foods. Mixed dishes and multiple preparations of the same food item have been omitted from this table.

Endurance Sports

Children and adolescents are well adapted to prolonged (endurance) exercise of moderate intensity (9). However, activity lasting longer than 1 hour and done at an intensity equating to approximately 70% of VO_{2max} is limited by carbohydrate stores. Carbohydrate stores or muscle glycogen content may be lower in children compared to adults. Therefore, arriving at an activity well fueled and with full glycogen stores is important. To remain fueled during activity, athletes should be counseled to plan ahead and consume carbohydrate-rich and easily digestible foods and drinks prior to practice or an event.

Strength, Weight-Class, and Speed Sports

Strength and weight-class sports are defined by repeated bouts of high-intensity or maximal exercise, typically lasting from a few seconds to 3 minutes (26). These sports include sprinting, jumping, power lifting, wrestling, rowing, and others. Because these sports are anaerobic in nature, the majority of energy needed to perform activity is derived from the ATP/creatine phosphate system and from the breakdown of glycogen stores used for anaerobic glycolysis.

Various studies have reported that training may increase ATP, phosphocreatine (PCr), and glycogen muscle stores in children (9). These increases are related to elevated muscle and blood lactate levels during maximal exercise, which suggests that strength training in youth enhances glycolytic activity. Additionally, muscle ATP and PCr levels have been found to be similar when at rest, in both child/adolescent and adult subjects, suggesting that the capacity for physical activity of young athletes is not impaired as long as the duration of activity is very short. Therefore, the young athlete is likely to excel at sports such as short-distance running, swimming, and jumping (9).

Although young athletes have the physiological capacity for power sports, their nutrient needs remain high to perform optimally. Protein is necessary for the development of muscle that is needed to excel in power and strength sports (26). In addition, when carbohydrate intake is inadequate, the young body will rely on protein stores for energy. This catabolic action can be prevented by assuring that the young athlete has adequate energy intake prior to the start of activity.

Sports Focused on Body Image and/or Weight

According to the AAP, children and adolescents are becoming more involved in sports in which weight control is perceived to be advantageous for an individual or team (42). Weight control is not only practiced in sports such as ballet, gymnastics, figure skating, and dance (sports in which females are the primary competitors), but also in a wide variety of sports that promote the perceived need for weight control. According to an AAP policy statement, these sports include, but are not limited to, bodybuilding, cheerleading, dancing, endurance sports, diving, rowing, swimming, and wrestling because these sports, at times, emphasize leanness, thinness, and competing at the lowest possible weight. Other sports, such as football, rugby, basketball, and power lifting promote gaining lean body mass.

In an attempt to lose weight and body fat or gain muscle, some athletes resort to unhealthy weight-control practices. Although the aim of this chapter is not to fully explore the causes and consequences of eating disorders among athletes, no chapter on child and adolescent nutrition would be complete without mention of disordered eating (see also Chapter 18). Practices used by young athletes to reduce weight are not unlike the practices used by adult athletes. These practices include food restriction (most common method), vomiting, overexercising, diet-pill use, inappropriate use of stimulants, skipping insulin required for diabetes management, nicotine use, and voluntary dehydration (42).

Because of unhealthy weight-control practices, the nutrient intake of athletes in various body image–focused sports is often less than optimal (5,61). Studies involving young female dancers, elite figure skaters, and gymnasts found that average energy intakes were 50% to 80% of recommended energy intake and average intakes of the micronutrients calcium, zinc, and magnesium ranged from 35% to 95% of recommendations. Additionally, research has found that iron depletion is common, occurring in 30% to 50% of female athletes (62).

According to Weimann and colleagues, elite, young female gymnasts in heavy training tend to have delayed pubertal development, minimal body fat stores, and failure to obtain full familial height (63). Conversely, male gymnasts exhibited normal growth and pubertal status. There are many potential factors that may influence those outcomes, including natural selection (in theory, small female gymnasts who have a slow pubertal development may be more successful in competition and continue their training to higher levels), but one can argue that proper nutrition may offset these height losses and other chronic conditions (such as altered bone density, delayed menarche, and stress fractures) experienced by these elite athletes.

When reviewing athletes' diets, researchers determined that the female gymnast's average nutrition intake of the following vitamins was less than 50% of the RDA: vitamins A, D, and B-complex, and the minerals magnesium, calcium, and iodine. In comparison, the male gymnasts in the study had an intake less than 50% the RDA for vitamins A and D, iodine, and carbohydrate. It should be noted that corresponding laboratory values showed no significant deficiencies in any of the aforementioned nutrients. The researchers concluded that the athletes may have been underreporting their intake, and the risk for nutrient deficiency in this population may be smaller than it seems. However, a restricted energy intake by female gymnasts is not unusual, and the risk for malnutrition should be on the forefront of the sports dietitian's mind because undernutrition, if not corrected, can lead to increased risk of injuries during pubertal growth phases (63).

Additionally, gymnasts, ballet dancers, and athletes who participate in sports in which leanness and body image are of importance are at higher risk for eating disorders (61,63). It has been reported that eating disorders are associated with sport-specific training beginning at a young age. Females as young as 5 to 7 years old competing in aesthetic sports (such as those mentioned earlier) have reported more weight concerns than girls in nonaesthetic sports and their peers who are not involved in sports (64). Although eating disorders in sports have traditionally been attributed to sports with heavy female participation, male athletes are not immune. It has been reported that 10% to 15% of high school males who participate in "weight-sensitive" sports admit to practicing unhealthful weight-loss behaviors (42).

Athletes may practice weight-control methods during the sports season or year-round, and these practices can be detrimental to the young athlete's health, well-being, growth, and performance. Athletes may benefit from a discussion led by an objective member of the health care team; coaches of most sports should not discuss weight with an athlete, whether weight gain or weight loss. Many coaches inappropriately focus on weight instead of body composition and performance and most do not have adequate nutrition background to counsel an athlete about weight (42). A sports dietitian should instead led the discussion on healthful weight-control practices to promote healthy body weight. The use of BMI values is not recommended for athletes; however, if used in young athletes, the athlete's BMI should be between the 50th and 75th percentile for BMI (42). BMI is not typically recommended for athletes because BMI can be falsely elevated in an athlete (or a nonathlete with a muscular build) as well as individuals with a high torso-to-leg ratio (65). According to the AAP, neither weight nor BMI is a good measure of athletic performance or of body fat in athletes (66). Rather than using BMI to determine the physical status of a young athlete, practitioners might choose to use body-composition measurements (body fat and lean body mass). However, even the most accurate body composition measurements have their limits. These markers, such as skinfold measurements and hydrostatic weighing, may be more accurate at providing ranges of body fat content when compared with BMI, but optimal body composition measures have not been determined for this young population. Instead, measurements of performance (speed, agility, etc) are far better gauges than body composition when it comes to determining optimal body weight for a particular athlete (66). In essence, achieving a specific percentage of body fat is not recommended for an individual athlete, but instead the athlete should focus on a range that is realistic and appropriate. Body composition methods are discussed in detail in Chapter 9.

Registered dietitians (RDs), parents, and all involved in the care of an athlete should be aware of some of the common signs that may indicate an eating disorder or disordered eating, including prolonged periods of dieting, an unusual (and unhealthy) preoccupation with nutrition and body weight, frequent weight fluctuations, and sudden increases in training intensity (61,63). More information on eating disorders can be found in Chapter 18.

Team Sports

Team sports are often characterized by high-intensity, intermittent efforts that are repeated over the duration of a game. Competition duration ranges from approximately 30 minutes to longer than 90 minutes, depending on sport and level of competition (26). Team sports often require a combination of power, agility, coordination, speed, and endurance to maintain high levels of performance.

There are fewer studies in the literature detailing the nutrient intakes among young athletes participating in team sports such as soccer, American football, baseball, softball, and hockey (5), but it is speculated that few nutrient deficiencies exist. This may be related to the nature of the sport; team sports often place an emphasis on skill and teamwork vs appearance.

When working with young athletes who participate in team sports, the sports dietitian should counsel team members about the importance of adequate macronutrient intake and replenishment of fluid to prevent energy depletion and dehydration. Adequate nutrition before, during (depending on the length of competition), and after activity will promote recovery and maintenance of the lean body mass that is critical to optimal performance in team sports (26).

Tournament Feeding

During tournaments, the young athlete may be required to participate in multiple games or matches throughout the day. Parents and coaches often struggle with what to feed the athletes during tournaments. After a game, many young athletes often turn to fast-food because of convenience, popularity, and wide availability. Although appropriate choices can be obtained from many fast-food restaurants, the young athlete often makes poor choices. High-fat, calorically dense, and nutrient-poor foods are unlikely to benefit the young athlete during future games. Rather, a lower fat, moderate-protein, and carbohydrate-rich meal is a better choice and less likely to promote feelings of sluggishness and malaise during an upcoming match. For tournament-day meal and snack ideas that are appropriate for young athletes, see Table 12.4.

Additionally, time between matches is an excellent period for recovery of lost fluids. Parents and coaches should encourage young athletes to consume adequate fluids (while leaving enough time before the upcoming match for use of the restroom). Fluids such as sport drinks will not only provide much-needed fluid and energy, but for those athletes exercising in a warm and humid environment, these beverages also replace electrolytes lost in sweat.

TABLE 12.4 Energy-Packed Snack and Meal Ideas for Tournament Days

Meal or Snack	Energy, kcal	Carbohydrate, g	Protein, g	Fat, g
Energizing milkshake: 1 cup fat-free milk blended with 2 Tbsp fat-free chocolate syrup, 1Tbsp peanut butter, 1 medium banana, and 1 cup of crushed ice.	410	68	14	9
Lunch on the go #1: 1 whole wheat pita stuffed with 2 oz lean luncheon meat (such as lean roast beef, turkey, or chicken), ½ cup shredded lettuce, 2 slices tomato, 1 tsp mustard and served with 1 oz baked potato chips.	385	62	18	8
Lunch on the go #2: 2 slices whole grain bread toasted and topped with 2 Tbsp low-fat cream cheese and mixture of 1 cup shredded, mixed vegetables (carrots, peppers, etc).	340	50	12	10
Carb-rich lunch: 1 cup of pasta tossed with tomato sauce and topped with ½ cup vegetables and 2 Tbsp grated parmesan cheese.	350	60	14	6
Bagel to go: 1 medium bagel (3.5-inch diameter) toasted and topped with 1 Tbsp apple butter and 2 Tbsp low-fat cream cheese.	350	63	10	6.5
Pudding treat: 1 cup of fat-free pudding topped with ½ cup each of blueberries, raspberries, and blackberries.	330	72	7	1.5
Nature snack: 15 animal crackers dipped in 1 Tbsp peanut butter and served with ½ cup canned fruit.	315	45	6	12
Breakfast option: 1 cup of apple-cinnamon flavored Os cereal topped with 1 cup fat-free milk and 1 medium sliced banana.	300	62	11	2
Energizing oatmeal (perfect for game-day breakfast): ⅓ cup steel cut oats mixed with ½ cup fat-free milk. Cook according to package directions and add water to reach desired consistency. Top with 2 Tbsp raisins or dried fruit.	300	56	12	3
Easy to eat snack: 2 oz pretzels (approx 40 small braided) dipped in 6 oz light, low-fat yogurt.	275	56	11	1
Pita pocket to go: 1 whole grain pita pocket stuffed with 2 Tbsp hummus, ½ cup shredded lettuce, and ½ cup sliced cucumber.	250	40	7	6.5
Snack on the run: 1 soft chocolate-chip granola bar, ½ cup unsweetened applesauce, 8 oz sport drink.	230	49	4	3
Lighter option milkshake: 6 oz light, low-fat yogurt blended with 1 cup sliced strawberries, 1 cup blueberries, ½ cup fat-free milk, and 1 cup crushed ice.	230	48	11	1

Source of nutrient information: Nutritionist Pro Version 4.4.0. Copyright 2010 Axxya Systems.

Ergogenic Aids and Dietary Supplements

Ergogenic aids are substances that are used to enhance athletic performance (see Chapter 7). Success in sports involves obtaining an "edge" over the competition, and children and adolescents may be uniquely vulnerable to the lure of supplements (67). The pressure to "win at all costs," extensive coverage in lay publications, and influential advertisements from manufacturers with exciting and emotive claims all play a role in the use of supplements by young athletes. Additionally, the knowledge that famous athletes and other role models use or promote these supplements often adds to the allure.

It is not uncommon for young athletes to use supplements, and their pattern of use is often unhealthy and chaotic (67). The poor regulation of supplements and sport foods in many countries allows young, easily influenced athletes to be the target of marketing campaigns based on exaggerated claims and hype rather than documented benefits.

The AAP policy statement on the use of performance enhancing substances (68) condemns the use of ergogenic aids, including various dietary supplements by children and adolescents. Additionally, the American College of Sports Medicine recommends that creatine not be used by children younger than 18 years of age (69). These policies are based on the unknown but potentially adverse health consequences of some supplements and considerations about the ethical use of supplements in young athletes.

According to Burke and colleagues (67), there is an ever-increasing range of supplements and sport foods that are easily accessible to athletes and coaches. Although various sport food and supplements might aid a young athlete in their training, athletes need to have a global understanding of the regulation of dietary supplements because regular travel and modern conveniences such as mail order and the Internet provide easy access to products that fall outside the scrutiny of the Food and Drug Administration (FDA) (67).

In addition, because of the popularity and availability of supplements, it is necessary for the sports nutrition professional to have a thorough working knowledge of the various products to provide sound advice about appropriate situations of use, possible benefits, potential side effects, and risks associated with use. When working with young athletes, sports dietitians should keep in mind that young athletes are easily influenced by their peers, their sports heroes, and by the media. It is important to educate the young athlete as well as the coaches and parents of young athletes about the benefits and potential risks of using supplements.

Commonly used supplements by young athletes include anabolic-androgenic steroids, steroid precursors or *prohormones,* growth hormone, creatine, and ephedrine (70–72). Creatine monohydrate in particular is a very popular supplement among young athletes. As noted previously, use is not recommended. Regardless, in a survey of 1,103 young athletes, 5.6% reported using the supplement (73). Use was more common among boys (8.8%) than girls (1.8%) and supplementation was reported by athletes in every sport, with use being more widespread among strength-dependent athletes (such as football players, wrestlers, gymnasts, and hockey players) (17). Additional supplements are discussed in detail in Chapter 7.

Reaching the Young Athlete

The impressionable young athlete is primed to digest nutrition information, and this population greatly benefits from working with an RD. Although very few high schools, middle schools, grade schools, and club teams can afford a full-time sports dietitian, sports dietitians can work as paid or volunteer consultants, providing occasional talks and also meeting with team members, parents, and coaches. When working with teams, schools, and individual youth, the sports dietitian should consider the following:

- Some young athletes are hungry for information regarding sports nutrition recommendations and are more than willing to listen to suggestions as well as change their eating patterns. Conversely, other young athletes are unwilling or not yet ready for change.
- Young athletes, like adults, often desire quick fixes and cures. Many do not want to hear about the necessity of healthy eating to improve performance and health. However, they will appreciate up-to-date handouts, information, and media links that may aid them in their quest for optimal performance.
- Young athletes, and often their parents, are looking for the next supplement that will give them an edge over their competitors. It is to the benefit of all parties to discuss the risks of various ergogenic aids and also the benefits of the "real" ergogenic aids: carbohydrate, protein, and fat.
- In hopes of securing a scholarship or simply for achievement, many parents are willing to do anything and pay any amount to give their children an edge over their peers. Enter sports nutrition. Although many schools may balk at the idea of paying for nutrition advice, sports dietitians should not undervalue their expertise regarding presentations for teams and counseling for individuals. Many schools may request a discount, but keep in mind that schools often participate in fund-raisers to cover speakers, and many parents may be more than willing to financially support a lecture or team seminar.

Young athletes are impressionable and often more up-to-date with popular trends than medical professionals and adults. Therefore, it is important for the sports dietitian to keep current on fad diets and supplements that may be tried by their young clients.

Sports dietitians must recognize that the young athletes are majorly influenced by their parents, coaches, athletic trainers, and personal trainers (when applicable). Before recommending changes, it will benefit all involved if the sports dietitian first develops a rapport with these individuals and listens to their reasoning

---

BOX 12.2   Unhealthy Weight Practices in Sport

The world of youth sports is no stranger to unhealthy weight-control practices. However, for the sport of wrestling, traditionally dominated by male participation, the percentage of athletes losing weight during the season is astounding. Numerous studies have found that the vast majority of wrestlers (80% in one study) participate in weight-loss practices each season while another study found that nearly half (45%) of wrestlers are at risk for developing an eating disorder (42). In addition, these extreme techniques (such as severe energy restriction and voluntary dehydration practices) resulted in 16 deaths of high school wrestlers over a 20-year period (1982 to 2002) (8). Because of the unhealthy and occasionally catastrophic weight-loss practices used by wrestlers, the National Collegiate Athletic Association (NCAA), the National Federation of High Schools, and the National Wrestling Coaches Federation were compelled to incorporate mandatory calculation of minimal safe wrestling weight using body-fat measurements. This program now includes the following components (42):

- Hydration testing: evaluating urine specific gravity by refractometer or urometer
- Body-composition assessment (used to determine minimal allowable weight): assessed using skinfold calipers, bioimpedance, air displacement, and or hydrostatic weighing.
- Calculation of lowest allowable weight class for each wrestler (calculator available at www.nwcacalculator.com/certification)
- Development of a weight-loss program (if appropriate)
- Nutrition education program specific to wrestling

behind the common practices they use. When making changes to a team's regimen, it may be necessary to do so gradually and with all major players—parents, coaches, trainers, managers, and, of course, the athletes—on board.

Summary

It is no secret that some of today's child athletes are the stars of tomorrow. Although children develop and progress at varying rates, all young athletes aspire to high levels in their sport. Young athletes may require more encouragement and support than their adult counterparts to reach their full athletic potential. Along with sport-specific training, coaching, and emotional support, athletic children and adolescents require nutritional guidance while on the path to success. The sports dietitian is well equipped to help them with sound nutrition strategies and guiding healthful weight for sport. Box 12.2 describes one success story in combating unhealthy weight practices (8,42).

References

1. National Sporting Goods Association. 2007 Youth participation in selected sports with comparisons to 1998. http://www.nsga.org/files/public/2006YouthParticipationInSelectedSportsWithComparisons.pdf. Accessed April 1, 2010.
2. National Institute of Arthritis and Musculoskeletal and Skin Diseases. Childhood sports injuries and their prevention: a guide for parents with ideas for kids. July 2009. NIH publication 09-4821. http://www.niams.nih.gov/Health_Info/Sports_Injuries/child_sports_injuries.asp. Accessed March 30, 2010.
3. Calfee R, Fadale P. Popular ergogenic drugs and supplements in young athletes. *Pediatrics*. 2006;117:e577–e589.
4. Caine DJ. Are kids having a rough time of it in sports? *Br J Sports Med*. 2010;44:1–3.
5. Croll JK, Neumark-Sztainer D, Story M, Wall M, Perry C, Harnack L. Adolescents involved in weight-related and power team sports have better eating patterns and nutrients intakes than non-sport-involved adolescents. *J Am Diet Assoc*. 2006;106:709–717.
6. Cavadini C, Decarli B, Grin J, Narring F, Michaud P-A. Food habits and sport activity during adolescence: differences between athletic and non-athletic teenagers in Switzerland. *Eur J Clin Nutr*. 2000;54(suppl):S16–S20.
7. Brenner JS; Council on Sports Medicine and Fitness. Overuse injuries, overtraining, and burnout in child and adolescent athletes. *Pediatrics*. 2007;119:1242–1245.
8. National Center for Sports Safety. Sports Injury Facts. http://www.sportssafety.org/sports-injury-facts. Accessed January 5, 2011.
9. Boisseau N, Delamarche P. Metabolic and hormonal responses to exercise in children and adolescents. *Sports Med*. 2000;30:405–422.
10. Rogol AD, Clark PA, Roemmich JN. Growth development in children and adolescents: effects of diet and physical activity. *Am J Clin Nutr*. 1990;72(suppl):521S–528S.
11. National Center for Health Statistics. 2000 Boys BMI-for-Age Growth Charts. http://www.cdc.gov/growthcharts/data/set1clinical/cj411023.pdf. Accessed March, 30, 2010.
12. National Center for Health Statistics. 2000 2–20 Years: Boys Stature-for-Age and Weight-for-Age Growth Charts. http://www.cdc.gov/growthcharts/data/set1clinical/cj411021.pdf. Accessed March 30, 2010.
13. National Center for Health Statistics. 2000 Girls BMI-for-Age Growth Charts. http://www.cdc.gov/growthcharts/data/set1clinical/cj411024.pdf. Accessed March, 30, 2010.
14. National Center for Health Statistics. 2000 2–20 Years: Girls Stature-for-Age and Weight-for-Age Growth Charts. http://www.cdc.gov/growthcharts/data/set1clinical/cj411022.pdf. Accessed March 30, 2010.
15. Meyer F, O'Connor H, Shirreffs SM. Nutrition for the young athlete. *J Sports Sci*. 2007; 25(Suppl 1):S73–S82.

16. Lucas BL. Nutrition in childhood. In: Mahan K, Escott-Stump S, eds. *Krause's Food, Nutrition, and Diet Therapy.* 11th ed. Philadelphia, PA: Saunders; 2004:259–283.

17. Naughton G, Farpour-Lambert NJ, Carlson J, Bradney M, Praagh EV. Physiological issues surrounding the performance of adolescent athletes. *Sports Med.* 2000;30:309–325.

18. Guest JE, Lewis NL, Guest JR. Assessment of growth in child athletes. In: Driskell JR, Wolinsky I, eds. *Nutritional Assessments of Athletes.* Boca Raton, FL: CRC Press; 2002:91–114.

19. Boisseau N, Persaud C, Jackson AA, Poortmans JR. Training does not affect protein turnover in pre- and early pubertal female gymnasts. *Eur J Appl Physiol.* 2005;94:262–267.

20. Holt K. Nutrition assessment of adolescents. In: Nevin-Folino N, ed. *Pediatric Manual of Clinical Dietetics.* 2nd ed. Chicago, IL: American Dietetic Association; 2003:163–171.

21. Malina RM. Physical activity and training: effects on stature and the adolescent growth spurt. *Med Sci Sports Exerc.* 1994a;26:759–766.

22. Mitchell KM. Nutrition during adolescence. In: Mitchell MK, ed. *Nutrition Across the Lifespan.* 2nd ed. Philadelphia, PA: WB Saunders; 2003:341–381.

23. Position of the American Dietetic Association: dietary guidance for healthy children ages 2 to 11 years. *J Am Diet Assoc.* 2004;104:660–677.

24. US Department of Agriculture, Agricultural Research Service. Nutrient Intakes from Food: Mean Amounts and Percentages of Calories from Protein, Carbohydrate, Fat, and Alcohol, One Day, 2005–2006. 2008. http://www.ars.usda.gov/ba/bhnrc/fsrg. Accessed June 16, 2010.

25. Bar-Or O. Nutritional considerations for the child athlete. *Can J Appl Physiol.* 2001;26(suppl):S186–S191.

26. Petrie HJ, Stover EA, Horswill CA. Nutritional concerns for the child and adolescent athlete. *Nutrition.* 2004; 20:620–631.

27. Eisenmann JC, Wickel EE. Estimated energy expenditure and physical activity patterns of adolescent distance runners. *Int J Sport Nutr Exerc Metab.* 2007;17:178–188.

28. Soric M, Misigoj-Durakovic M, Pedisic Z. Dietary intake and body composition of prepubescent female aesthetic athletes. *Int J Sport Nutr Exerc Metab.* 2008;18:343–354.

29. Bandini LG, Must A, Cyr H, Anderson SE, Spadano JL, Dietz WH. Longitudinal changes in the accuracy of reported energy intake in girls 10–15 y of age. *Am J Clin Nutr.* 2003;78:480–484.

30. Livingstone MBE, Prentice AM, Coward WA. Validation of estimates of energy intake by weighed dietary record and diet history in children and adolescents. *Am J Clin Nutr.* 1992;56:29–35

31. Leyk D, Rohde U, Gorges W, Ridder D, Wunderlich M, Dinklage C, Sievert A, Ruther T, Essfeld D. Physical performance, body weight and BMI of young adults in Germany 2000–2004: results of the Physical-Fitness-Test study. *Int J Sports Med.* 2006;27:642–647.

32. Cole TJ, Bellizzi MC, Flegal KM, Dietz WH. Establishing a standard definition for child overweight and obesity worldwide: international survey. *BMJ.* 2000;320:1240–1245.

33. Centers for Disease Control and Prevention. Defining childhood overweight and obesity. http://www.cdc.gov/obesity/childhood/defining.html. Accessed March 28, 2010.

34. Barlow SE; Expert Committee. Expert Committee recommendations regarding the prevention, assessment, and treatment of child and adolescent overweight and obesity: summary report. *Pediatrics* 2007;120(Suppl 4): S164–S192.

35. Lobstein T, Jackson-Leach R. Child overweight and obesity in the USA: Prevalence rates according to IOTF definitions. *Int J Pediatr Obes.* 2007;2:62–64.

36. Freedman DS, Mei Z, Srinivasan SR, Berenson GS, Dietz WH. Cardiovascular risk factors and excess adiposity among overweight children and adolescents: the Bogalusa Heart Study. *J Pediatr.* 2007;150:12–17.e2.

37. Whitaker RC, Wright JA, Pepe MS, Seidel KD, Dietz WH. Predicting obesity in young adulthood from childhood and parental obesity. *N Engl J Med.* 1997;37:869–873.

38. Serdula MK, Ivery D, Coates RJ, Freedman DS, Williamson DF, Byers T. Do obese children become obese adults? A review of the literature. *Prev Med.* 1993;22:167–177.

39. D'Hondt E, Deforche B, Bourdeaudhuij I, Lenoir M. Childhood obesity affects fine motor skill performance under different postural constraints. *Neurosci Lett.* 2008;440:72–75.

40. Bazelmans C, Coppieters Y, Godin I, Parent F, Berghmans L, Dramaix M. Is obesity associated with injuries among young people? *Eur J Epidemiol*. 2004;19:1037–1042.

41. McHugh MP. Oversized young athletes: a weight concern. *Br J Sports Med*. 2010;44:45–49.

42. American Academy of Pediatrics Committee on Sports Medicine and Fitness. Policy statement: promotion of healthy weight-control practices in young athletes. *Pediatrics*. 2005;116:1557–1564.

43. American Dietetic Association Evidence Analysis Library. Pediatric Weight Management (PWM) Nutrition Prescription in the Treatment of Pediatric Obesity: Recommendation Summary. http://www.adaevidencelibrary.com/template.cfm?template=guide_summary&key=1555. Accessed June 5, 2010.

44. American Dietetic Association Evidence Analysis Library. Determining Energy Needs in Overweight Children and Adolescents. http://www.adaevidencelibrary.com/topic.cfm?cat=3060. Accessed June 5, 2010.

45. Burke L, Millet G. Tarnopolsky MA. Nutrition for distance events. *J Sports Sci*. 2007; 25(suppl):S29–S38.

46. Riddell MC, Bar-Or O, Schwarcz HP, Heigenhauser GJ. Substrate utilization in boys during exercise with [13C]-glucose ingestion. *Eur J Appl Physiol*. 2000;83:441–448.

47. Shi X, Horn MK, Osterberg KL, Stofan JR, Zachwieja JJ, Horswill CA. Gastrointestinal discomfort during intermittent high-intensity exercise: Effect of carbohydrate-electrolyte beverage. *Int J Sport Nutr Exerc Metab*. 2004;14:673–683.

48. US Department of Agriculture, US Department of Health and Human Services. Dietary Guidelines for Americans, 2010. www.health.gov/dietaryguidelines/dga2010/DietaryGuidelines2010.pdf. Accessed October 4, 2011.

49. Boisseau N, Vermorel M, Rance M, Duche P, Patureau-Mirand P. Protein requirements in male adolescent soccer players. *Eur J Appl Physiol*. 2007;100:27–33.

50. Tipton KD, Jeukendrup AE, Hespel P. Nutrition for the sprinter. *J Sports Sci*. 2007;25(suppl):S5–S15.

51. Galassetti P, Larson J, Iwanaga K, Salsberg SL, Eliakim A, Pontello A. Effect of a high-fat meal on the growth and hormone response to exercise in children. *J Pediatr Endocrinol Metab*. 2006;19:777–786.

52. American Academy of Pediatrics. Climatic heat stress and the exercising child and adolescent. *Pediatrics*. 2000; 106:158.

53. Sawka MN, Burke LM, Eichner ER, Maughan RJ, Montain SJ, Stachenfeld NS. American College of Sports Medicine position stand: exercise and fluid replacement. *Med Sci Sports Exerc*. 2007;39:377–390.

54. Casa DJ, Armstrong LE, Hillman SK, Montain SJ, Reiff RV, Rich BRE, Roberts WO, Stone JA. National athletic trainers' association position statement: fluid replacement for athletes. *J Athl Train*. 2000;35:212–224.

55. Rowland TW, Stagg L, Kelleher JF. Iron deficiency in adolescent girls: are athletes at increased risk? *J Adolesc Health*. 1991;12:22–25.

56. Constantini NW, Eliakim A, Zigel L, Yaaron M, Falk B. Iron status of highly active adolescents: evidence of depleted iron stores in gymnasts. *Int J Sport Nutr Exerc Metab*. 2000;10:62–70.

57. Spodaryk K. Iron metabolism in boys involved in intensive physical training. *Physiol Behav*. 2002;75:201–206.

58. Felesky-Hunt S. Nutrition for runners. *Clin Podiatr Med Surg*. 2001;18:337.

59. Abrams SA, Grusak MA, Stuff J, O'Brien KO. Calcium and magnesium balance in 9–14 y-old children. *Am J Clin Nutr*. 1997;66:1172–1177.

60. Lanou AJ, Berkow SE, Bernard ND. Calcium, dairy products, and bone health in children and young adults: a reevaluation of the evidence. *Pediatrics*. 2005;115:7736–7743.

61. Sundgot-Borgen J. Prevalence of eating disorders in elite female gymnasts. *Int J Sports Nutr*. 1993;3:29–40.

62. Volpe S. Vitamins and minerals for active people. In: Dunford M, ed. *Sports Nutrition: A Practice Manual for Professionals*. 4th ed. Chicago, IL: American Dietetic Association; 2000:61–93.

63. Weimann E, Witzel C, Schwidergall S, Bohles HJ. Peripubertal perturbations in elite gymnasts caused by sport specific training regimes and inadequate nutritional intake. *Int J Sports Med*. 2000;21:210–215.

64. Davidson KK, Earnest MB, Birch LL. Participation in aesthetic sports and girls weight concerns at ages 5 and 7 years. *Int J Eat Disord*. 2002;31:312–317.

65. Roberts SB, Dallal GE. The new childhood growth charts. *Nutr Rev*. 2001;59:31–36.

66. American Academy of Pediatrics Committee on Nutrition. Sports nutrition. In: Kleinman RE, ed. *Pediatric Nutrition Handbook*. 6th ed. Elk Grove Village, IL: American Academy of Pediatrics; 2009:225–247.

67. Burke L, Cort M, Cox G, Crawford R, Desbrow B, Farthing L, Minehan M, Shaw N, Warnes O. Supplements and sports foods. In: Burke L, Deakin V, eds. *Clinical Sports Nutrition*. 3rd ed. Sidney, Australia: McGraw-Hill Australia; 2006:485–580.

68. American Academy of Pediatrics Committee on Sports Medicine and Fitness. Position on use of performance-enhancing substances. *Pediatrics*. 2005;115:1103–1106.

69. American College of Sports Medicine. Roundtable: the physiological and health effects of oral creatine supplementation. *Med Sci Sports Exerc*. 2000;32:706–717.

70. Reeder BM, Rai A, Patel DR, Cucos D, Smith F. The prevalence of nutritional supplement use among high school students: a pilot study. *Med Sci Sports Exerc*. 2002;34(suppl 1):S193.

71. Rickert VI, Pawlak-Morello C, Sheppard V, Jay VS. Human growth hormone: a new substance of abuse among adolescents? *Clin Pediatr*. 1992;31:723–736.

72. Kayton S, Cullen RW, Memken JA, Rutter R. Supplement and ergogenic aid use by competitive male and female high school athletes. *Med Sci Sports Exerc*. 2002;35(suppl):S193.

73. Metzel JD, Small E, Levine SR, Gershel JC. Creatine use among young athletes. *Pediatrics*. 2001;108:421–425.

Chapter 13

COLLEGE ATHLETES

Jennifer Ketterly, MS, RD, CSSD, and Caroline Mandel, MS, RD, CSSD

Introduction

Today there are more than 400,000 student-athletes participating in 23 different sports at more than 1,000 National Collegiate Athletic Association (NCAA) member institutions (Table 13.1) (1). Because of the rigorous demands of athletic participation, academic pressures, and the realities of college life, student-athletes are at nutritional risk. College athletes may be predisposed to poor nutrition, fatigue, and injury due to poor eating habits, lack of resources, and/or rigid training diets. Over the past 20 years, interest and investment in sports dietetics at university athletic departments have increased dramatically, starting with the United States' first collegiate sports dietitian, Kristine Clark at Penn State in 1991. What followed was a surge in the recognition of the role that sports nutrition plays in the health and success of the student-athlete. In 1994, Dr. Clark wrote an article detailing the scope of her practice, remarking. "Athletic departments in colleges and universities are beginning to recognize the role a sports nutrition professional plays in providing both clinical nutrition services to athletes and nutrition education programs to teams, coaches, and trainers" (2). At last count, there were 31 full-time, 42 on-campus, and 55 consultant registered dietitians (RDs) providing nutrition service to Division I Athletic Departments in the United States.

Collegiate Sports Dietitians

The collegiate sports dietitian is not an entry-level practitioner, but rather a specialty or advanced practitioner who is experienced in clinical nutrition, counseling, medical nutrition therapy (MNT), exercise physiology, and administration. Box 13.1 defines the specialty practitioner and advanced practitioner in sports dietetics (3). These types of positions require a food and nutrition professional with experience working in a clinical setting as part of a multidisciplinary team, counseling athletes on nutrition concerns ranging from everyday eating to performance nutrition and facilitating educational seminars to diverse groups. What makes this position unique is that the sports dietitian's role goes beyond clinical responsibilities and includes the administering and coordinating of services that encompass the top-to-bottom nutritional needs that are compliant with NCAA guidelines. An advanced degree is helpful. Many collegiate sports dietitians working with collegiate student-athletes have achieved the Certified Specialist in Sports Dietetics (CSSD) credential.

TABLE 13.1   Division I, II, and III National Collegiate Athletic Associate Member Institutions

	Division I (Private/Public)	Division II (Private/Public)	Division III (Private/Public)
Members: 1,070	333 (113/220)	291 (137/154)	446 (357/89)
Average male athlete participation/institution	266	188	219
Average female athlete participation/institution	223	128	155
Total athletes: 421,597[a]	162,837	91,956	166,804

[a]Based on institutional averages.
Source: Data are from reference 1.

BOX 13.1   Definitions of Specialty and Advanced Practitioner from the Academy of Nutrition and Dietetics Standards of Practice and Standards of Professional Performance for Registered Dietitians in Sports Dietetics

- **Specialty practitioner:** an individual who concentrates on one aspect of the profession of dietetics and may or may not have a credential or additional certification, but often has expanded roles beyond entry-level practice.
- **Advanced practitioner:** an individual who has acquired the expert knowledge base, complex decision-making skills, and competencies for expanded practice, the characteristics of which are shaped by the context in which he or she practices. Advanced practitioners may have expanded or specialty roles or both. Advanced practice may or may not include additional certification. Generally, the practice is more complex, and the practitioner has a higher degree of professional autonomy and responsibility. In addition, it is recognized that sports dietetics care is most effectively undertaken with a multidisciplinary focus and at a level beyond that practiced by an entry-level registered dietitian.

Source: Data are from reference 3.

Collegiate sports dietitians provide nutrition counseling and education to student-athletes in at least 20 different sports. This counseling and education enhances adaptation to training and can have the following benefits:

- Improved health and exercise performance
- Reduced risk of injury and illness
- Achievement and maintenance of appropriate body weight and body composition
- Improved recovery from strenuous exercise
- Optimization of hydration status
- Compliance with NCAA rules regarding sport foods, drinks, and dietary supplements

The sports dietitian therefore needs to be knowledgeable about what energy systems are used in each sport, athletes' training schedules throughout the year, as well as the sport's terminology and team culture. While emphasizing sports nutrition strategies to enhance athletic performance, the sports dietitian is also a "jack-of-all-trades" in that he or she counsels athletes about making good choices in the dining hall, at training table meals, at the grocery store, and also teaches cooking skills for off-campus living and provides MNT for diagnoses such as type 1 diabetes, celiac disease/gluten sensitivity, food allergies, gastrointestinal complaints, and eating disorders. In addition to educating student-athletes, the collegiate sports dietitian educates coaches, athletic trainers, and other department personnel on the use of sport foods, drinks, and dietary supplements that are in compliance with the rules and bylaws of the NCAA (4) as well as the International Olympic Committee (IOC) (5) for those athletes involved in Olympic sports.

Each athletic department is unique, and the role of the sports dietitian will therefore vary. However, the collegiate sports dietitian typically wears many hats, including clinician, educator, administrator, and academician.

Clinical Responsibilities

In the clinical role, the sports dietitian provides individualized nutrition education and counseling to the student-athlete. This may be done by self-referral or referral by another member of the athletic department. The reasons that a student-athlete may be referred to the sports dietitian include fatigue, poor eating habits, weight management, body composition testing, iron deficiency, disordered eating, supplement questions, history of chronic dieting, food allergies, vegan or vegetarian meal planning, gastrointestinal complaints, or medical diagnoses such as diabetes or hypertension. Also, the sports dietitian can refer individuals to the appropriate member of the athletic medicine team, campus resources, or off-campus resources such as an eating disorder support group, as necessary. The sports dietitian assesses the student-athlete's dietary intake patterns and then educates and counsels the athlete on an appropriate training diet to help him or her reach desired health and performance goals. The sports dietitian works to develop rapport with the student-athlete and uses various counseling strategies such as goal setting, behavior modification, relapse prevention, cognitive-behavioral therapy, and motivational interviewing. The sports dietitian has an arsenal of tools at his or her disposal, including evidence-based sports nutrition guidelines, MNT protocols for nutrition diagnoses, and best practice as determined by extensive practical experience in sports dietetics.

The sports dietitian participates in student-athlete pre-participation physicals in a variety of ways. Many sports dietitians have developed nutrition needs assessment tools to identify athletes at risk for poor eating habits and need for individualized nutrition counseling. Screening questions cover weight history, meal patterns, shopping habits and cooking skills, restaurant frequency, and frequently consumed foods. The sports dietitian works closely with the athletic medicine staff to screen for nutrition-related issues such as iron-deficiency anemia, disordered eating, the female athlete triad, inappropriate supplement use, and weight-management concerns. See Table 13.2 for validated eating disorders screening tools used in collegiate athletic settings (6–11) and Box 13.2 for questions to ask to screen for the female athlete triad (12). More information about eating disorders is found in Chapter 18.

Nutrition Education Responsibilities

As an educator, the collegiate sports dietitian develops and conducts sports nutrition seminars for teams, coaches, and athletic medicine staff including athletic trainers, team physicians, physical therapists, and sports counselors. Providing sports nutrition education for coaches and athletic medicine staff helps to make sure everyone is on the same page and providing a consistent nutrition message to the student-athlete. Smith-Rockwell et al (13) assessed nutrition knowledge, opinions, and practices of coaches and athletic trainers from 21 sports at an NCAA Division I institution. Participants responded correctly to 67% of nutrition knowledge questions. Coaches and athletic trainers from women's sports tended to give more correct

TABLE 13.2 Eating Disorders Screening Tools for Use with Collegiate Athletes

Screening Tool (Reference)	Description
Female Athlete Screening Tool (FAST) (6)	A self-administered 33-question screening tool that has been validated to identify eating pathology in female athletes.
SCOFF Questionnaire (7)	A simple, memorable screening instrument for use by a nonspecialist to initially screen for an eating disorder before rigorous clinic assessment is administered.
Eating Disorders Inventory 2 (EDI-2) (8)	Standardized 91-item self-report questionnaire designed to measure cognitive and behavioral characteristics of anorexia nervosa and bulimia nervosa in males and females older than 12 years of age.
Eating Disorders Inventory 3 (EDI-3) (9)	Enhanced revision of the EDI for use with females ages 13 to 53 years. Contains 91 items divided into 12 subscales that yield 6 composite scores: Eating disorders risk; Ineffectiveness; Interpersonal problems; Affective problems; Overcontrol; Psychological maladjustment.
Eating Attitudes Test-26 (EAT-26) (10)	The EAT-26 is a self-administered inventory that consists of three subscales that evaluate food preoccupation, oral control, and bulimic tendencies by measuring restrictive eating, fear of weight changes, weight-restricting activities, maladaptive thought processes, and body dissatisfaction.
Athletic Milieu Direct Questionnaire (AMDQ) (11)	19-item screening instrument for identification of eating disorders/disordered eating in NCAA Division I female athletes. A variety of response categories are used, including a 4- to 6-point Likert scale as well as multiple and dichotomous responses.

Source: Data are from references 6–11.

responses as compared to those who worked with male athletes. Those coaches and athletic trainers who had 15 or more years of experience gave more correct responses as compared to participants with fewer years of experience (14). See Table 13.3 for suggestions of sports nutrition education topics by group and facilitation strategies (12,14–16).

Other educational approaches range from low- to high-tech and include the development of handouts and fact sheets, table tents, bulletin boards, newsletters, Web sites, blogs and use of social media. Handouts and fact sheets are great tools to use for team nutrition seminars, at training tables, and in weight rooms, training rooms, and athletic medicine waiting rooms. Some collegiate sports dietitians develop their own handouts based on the needs of their student-athlete population, whereas other sports dietitians purchase or download fact sheets from the Internet. It is crucial to review all purchased or downloaded materials for credibility and appropriateness of the message for the college student-athlete population. Fact sheets developed by registered dietitians and approved by the Academy of Nutrition and Dietetics (formerly American Dietetic Association) are available from the Sports, Cardiovascular, and Wellness Nutrition dietetic practice group (www.scandpg.org).

Posting a nutrition theme periodically on a bulletin board in a training room, weight room, or medical clinic waiting area is another way to highlight relevant sports nutrition information. Posting recipes, resources, interactive quizzes, and contact information for the sports dietitian serves a dual purpose of educating student-athletes and staff as well as marketing services. Bulletin board topics that are timely and relevant to the student-athlete population are highlighted in Box 13.3. Placing table tents on dining tables at the training table is a great way to capture the student-athletes' attention when they are focused on food and nutrition. Box 13.4 lists suggested table tent topics for training tables.

BOX 13.2   The Female Athlete Triad: Questions to Ask at Pre-Participation Physical

Food
- How do you feel about food? Do you have a "relaxed" relationship with food?
- What is your eating pattern?
- How many meals do you eat per day?
- Do you have any sort of food you try to avoid?
- What did you eat and drink yesterday?
- Have you ever purged (vomiting, laxatives, extra exercise) to reduce body weight? What methods have you used? Do you currently purge?

Weight
- What has been your highest and lowest weight during the last year?
- What do you consider to be your competition weight?
- Have you tried to lose weight lately? How?
- Are you satisfied with your present weight?
- Do other persons have opinions about your weight?

Menstruation
- When did you start to menstruate?
- Has your menstrual cycle been regular after menarche?
- When did you have your last menstrual period?
- How do you feel about your menstrual cycle?
- Do you use or have you used oral contraceptives?

Training/Injuries
- Have you changed your training regimen (type, load, intensity)?
- Do you do other forms of training than that related to your sport?
- Have you experienced a stress fracture or a regular fracture?

Source: Adapted with permission from Sangenis, P, Drinkwater BL, Loucks A, Sherman RT, Sundgot-Borgen J, Thompson RA. International Olympic Committee Position Stand: The Female Athlete Triad. 2005. www.olympic.org/Assets/ImportedNews/Documents/en_report_917.pdf. Accessed March 17, 2010.

Many sports dietitians have turned low-tech handouts and bulletin boards into electronic newsletters or blog topics. Posting information about sports nutrition services, hours, contact information, and sports nutrition fact sheets on departmental Web sites are great ways to take advantage of the technology that college student-athletes use today. Videos of supermarket tours and cooking demos can also be included. Some schools have password-protected Web services available for their student athletes; for other schools, this information will be available to student-athletes as well as the general population who may be browsing the school's Web site. Allowing public access to these materials can be a useful recruiting tool.

Administrative Responsibilities

In addition to being a clinician and educator, the sports dietitian often assumes many administrative duties. The RD may plan, implement, and operate an outpatient sports nutrition clinic. To manage this practice,

TABLE 13.3   Sports Nutrition Education Topics

Audience	Topic	Seminar Suggestion
Student athletes	Hydration	Weigh athletes privately before and after exercise. Inform athletes of their weight change during training, discussing sweat rate and daily fluid requirements and replacement goals. Review ways to monitor hydration status such as urine color and weight change during exercise.
	Dining out	Bring menus and nutrition info for the team's top restaurant choices (at home and while traveling) and talk about how to select the best carbohydrates and specific meal options.
Athletic trainers	Nutritional supplements	Review most recent National Collegiate Athletic Association (NCAA) Banned Substances List and NCAA Bylaw 16.5.2.2 for list of permissible supplement categories and impermissible ingredients. Bring sample products to evaluate including some that are banned, impermissible, and permissible.
	Athletes with type 1 diabetes	Review American Diabetes Association Standards of Care (14) and National Athletic Trainers' Association Position Statement (15). Apply to athlete case studies: the athlete's diabetes care plan, supplies for athletic training kits, preparticipation physical examination (PPE); recognition, treatment, and prevention of hypoglycemia and hyperglycemia, insulin administration, travel recommendations; and athletic injury and glycemic control.
Coaches	Recovery nutrition	Present evidence on recovery. Show examples of foods as well as permissible sports foods that provide adequate carbohydrate, protein and fluid for postexercise recovery.
	Weight management	Review departmental policies: how to refer to sports dietitian, what athletes can expect when working with sports dietitian on weight loss/ weight gain strategies, how to identify athletes at risk for disordered eating.
Physicians	Iron testing protocol	Review which teams to test and at what time of year. Discuss iron level cutoffs and optimal nutrition plans and supplementation dosage recommendations. Plan student-athlete follow-up and communication strategies.
Sports counselors/ eating disorders team	Female athlete triad	Review current literature on the triad, including position statements from American College of Sports Medicine (16) and International Olympics Committee (12). Discuss ways to integrate nutrition, counseling, and medical services as a multidisciplinary team.

one typically needs to set clinic schedules, develop efficient appointment procedures, determine initial and follow-up consultations, develop forms, implement appropriate documentation, and ensure Standards of Practice (SOP) and confidentiality are followed. The collegiate outpatient practice can take place in a variety of university and athletic department facilities. For example, campus health sports medicine clinics and athletic training rooms are two common sports nutrition service locations. In any setting, it is important to market nutrition services to student-athletes and other support personnel. Services are used more often when athletes know where to find the sports dietitian, when services are offered at convenient times, and when it is easy to schedule an appointment. It's important to consider/review class schedule variances

> **BOX 13.3 Suggested Bulletin Board Topics by Semester**
>
> **Fall**
> - The Freshman 15: Is it real?
> - Meal Planning for Off-Campus Living
> - Nutrition for Pre-Exercise Meals
> - Dining Out
>
> **Winter**
> - What's New for the New Year?
> - Eating Disorders Awareness Week
> - March is National Nutrition Month
> - Nutrition for Recovery
>
> **Spring/Summer**
> - Sports Foods and Supplements
> - Breakfast Is for Champions
> - Frequently Asked Questions
> - Quick and Easy Meal Solutions

> **BOX 13.4 Table Tent Topics for Training Table**
>
> - Making Best Choices at Training Table
> - Are You Hydrated?
> - The Athlete's Plate
> - Hot Topics in Sports Nutrition
> - Snack Attack: How to Fill Nutrition Gaps
> - Get the Carbohydrate Edge
> - 10 Tips for Eating like a Champion
> - Alcohol & Performance Do Not Mix
> - Fast Food Facts
> - Dining Out—World Cuisine
> - Caffeine and Athletic Performance
> - Sports Nutrition Myths

through the week, typical treatment and practice times, and the athlete's footpath through campus when making a schedule. Also, using an appointment phone line or Web-based scheduling through campus health services electronic medical record system, sports medicine clinic, or other services with administrative support personnel will make scheduling efficient for all parties.

Another administrative role for the sports dietitian is in negotiating and managing contracts. For example, the dietitian may develop a relationship with the local pharmacy to negotiate a purchasing procedure for vitamin and mineral supplements at contracted bid prices or discounted costs. There may be potential for similar relationships and negotiations with lab services to test for iron deficiency, Grocery stores may be contacted to provide pre- and postworkout fruit, nuts, bagels, or other foods or products, and distributors or a nutritional supplement company may provide practice and game-time hydration and recovery products. Being able to negotiate cost-effective purchasing allows the sports dietitian to offer added value to the athletic department and nutrition services.

Multidisciplinary and Foodservice Responsibilities

Along with clinics and contracts, sports dietitians often develop and administer policies, procedures, and protocols; create and facilitate multidisciplinary treatment teams; work with foodservice staff; and function as an athletic department representative. Policies, procedures, and protocols for the following situations are often necessary and helpful, adding value to the sports dietitian position in a collegiate athletic setting:

- Referrals to the sports dietitian
- Eating disorders care and treatment
- Nutritional supplement purchasing, evaluation, and distribution
- Weight and body composition analysis
- Iron-deficiency screening
- Female athlete triad screening and monitoring
- Other nutrition-related sports medicine protocols, such as cramping and stress fracture prevention and postsurgical rehabilitation support

Multidisciplinary treatment and performance teams can help enhance communication among providers and other support personnel to facilitate care for the student-athlete. Eating disorders treatment teams are crucial to managing the multidisciplinary nature of these diseases. Creating performance teams with the athletic training staff and the strength and conditioning staff can be an effective way to communicate about an athlete's goals and progress while fostering respect for each discipline involved in the athlete's care. A body composition team may also be useful in some situations and with select teams.

Working with foodservice staff is a natural part of working in a collegiate environment. The *training table,* a phrase referring to the meal served to only student-athletes in a closed setting (this meal can be catered, in an on-site athletic facility, or in a residence dining hall), is an ideal place for the sports dietitian to deliver nutrition messages and help athletes select performance foods. Examples of roles that a sports dietitian can have in the foodservice environment include the following:

- Assist in negotiating fair and appropriate meal costs for the training table
- Assist with outlining food-quality standards
- Advocate for adequate staffing patterns to allow for optimal service
- Encourage food-related data collection and forecasting models to achieve cost-effective operations
- Develop and/or review cycle menus and suggest alternate preparation methods or items to meet sports nutrition needs and requirements
- Provide nutrition analysis of menu items and develop a format for posting nutrient information at point-of-purchase and/or online

Team travel and hotel stays are opportunities for the sports dietitian to offer expertise in planning and coordinating foodservice needs. Teams will often stay in hotels with foodservice availability (for both home games as well as when the team travels). A perfect liaison between the team and hotel, the sports dietitian can effectively plan the meals and communicate with the hotel staff on food-quality standards, preparation method, buffet arrangement, and budgetary limitations to ensure that the meal is appropriate, convenient, time-efficient, and conducive to the travel itinerary.

Lastly, the collegiate sports dietitian often functions as an athletic department representative on a variety of occasions. Recruiting events, campus committees, and community-sponsored functions are examples in which the sports dietitian may be asked to participate and represent the athletic department. Serving as an ambassador for the department in a professional and courteous manner provides an opportunity to develop relationships within the department and further the respect for the sports dietitian.

Academic Responsibilities

In addition to being a clinician, educator, and administrator, the dietitian working on a college campus has a unique opportunity to serve as a teacher and academician. The sports dietitian is often invited to provide guest lectures or teach a class for credit. Establishing working relationships with academic departments on campus can yield opportunities for sports nutrition research and publication as well as collaborative equipment purchases (eg, BOD POD or dual energy x-ray absorptiometry (DXA) machines for body composition analysis). Additional academic opportunities include serving as a preceptor for students in dietetics or athletic training curriculums, medical students in orthopedic rotations or sports medicine fellowships, and other sports medicine–related practicum experiences.

The Student Athlete

Collegiate athletes are a diverse group of men and women ranging in age between 17 and 24 years. They are considered to be postadolescents, young adults, or "emerging adults" (17). Research suggests that this age group is still developing mentally and physically. They are known for being more risk-taking, self-centered, and vulnerable to addiction, but less insightful or concerned about consequences than are adults (18). The student-athlete population at any NCAA institution is typically diverse in terms of gender, race, culture, religion, nutrition knowledge, and socioeconomic status. Student athletes are required to be full-time students during their years of athletic eligibility, but not all are awarded a full athletic scholarship that includes money for food and many do not have access to a sports dietitian. Nutritional needs are constantly changing throughout the student-athlete's college career. Box 13.5 lists examples of typical nutritional concerns based on year in school. In addition to learning about their sports nutrition requirements to augment training and improve athletic performance, many student-athletes learn valuable life skills regarding meal planning, grocery shopping, proper food handling, and storage, as well as nutrition guidelines for wellness and the prevention of chronic disease.

Nutrition Knowledge and Sources of Information

College athletes are a captive audience, meaning that they typically use the sports medicine and nutrition services offered to them through the athletic department or campus health services. For many, these services are unlimited and available to them at no cost for the duration of their eligibility.

Not all college student-athletes have access to a sports dietitian to provide guidance on their performance training diet and a healthy lifestyle. Rosenbloom et al (19) assessed the nutrition knowledge of athletes at one NCAA Division I institution and found that many collegiate athletes have misconceptions about the roles of specific nutrients such as carbohydrates, protein, vitamins, minerals, and supplements in sports performance. The students reported their sources of sports nutrition information included coaches, athletic trainers, strength and conditioning staff, physicians, teammates, nutrition classes, sports dietitians, parents, and popular media. They concluded that if athletes make food choices based on inaccurate nutrition information, it could have negative consequences for sports performance.

Personal Concerns

Student-athletes have a variety of personal, athletic, and health concerns that can affect their nutritional status and, in turn, their success as college students. Personal concerns include transitioning to college life, struggling with the increased time demands of collegiate academics and athletics; finances (depending on scholarship status and family resources); managing multiple relationships with coaches, teammates, teachers, family, and friends; and lack of sleep. Access to food and cooking skills may be limited. Acclimating to dining hall food choices as a freshman and moving off campus into a house or apartment and having

---

BOX 13.5   Nutrition-Related Concerns of College Student Athletes by Year of Eligibility

Freshman
- Transition to college life (dining hall meal plan, alcohol, stress, time management)
- Adapt to new team and training program
- The "freshman 15" (weight management, body image)
- Finding your social identity
- Increased competitiveness of collegiate sports
- Continued physical growth and development
- Emotional maturity and developing confidence

Sophomore
- Transition to off-campus living (shopping and cooking skills)
- Prevention of overtraining
- Training and nutritional periodization for year-round training and competition
- Balance sports with school and social life
- Perfect the taper for endurance sports

Junior
- Move out of dorms into house or apartment
- Prevention of boredom, staleness
- Nutritional variety and interest for the long haul
- Consistency with habits for continued success
- Growing demands of academic major

Senior/5th Year
- Transition from collegiate athlete to professional athlete or recreational exerciser
- Increased focus on healthful eating for a lifetime

---

to manage meal planning, grocery shopping, meal preparation, and food handling and storage for the first time as a sophomore or junior may impact an athlete's nutritional status. Athletes who live off campus but do not have transportation may have decreased access to food, which can make it challenging to follow a sound training diet. Social pressures to use alcohol and drugs can jeopardize a student-athlete's athletic performance, health, and team status.

Alcohol and drug use by college athletes is a major concern for athletic departments. Individuals involved in athletics are more likely to engage in a wide range of risky behaviors than are nonathletes [20]. Table 13.4 reports NCAA findings regarding alcohol use by student athletes from 1993 to 2005 [21] and Table 13.5 provides data on alcohol use by college student from the American College Health Association (ACHA) National College Health Assessment (NCHA) [22]. Although the NCAA study found that the overall use of alcohol by student-athletes has decreased over previous reports across all ethnic groups and in both men's and women's sports, the number of student-athletes drinking more than five drinks in a sitting has increased substantially. Most NCAA student-athletes reported that initial use of alcohol occurred in high school or earlier.

The NCAA study reported that almost 60% of student-athletes continue to believe that their use of alcoholic beverages has no effect on athletic performance or on their general health despite a push for educational programming provided to this population on the known risks of alcohol use on athletic performance and health [21]. Box 13.6 describes the consequences of alcohol use on athletic performance [23].

TABLE 13.4   Alcohol Use by NCAA Student Athletes (n = 19,676): 1993–2005

NCAA Division	Student Athletes Using Alcohol, %			
	1993	1997	2001	2005
Division I	86.3	79.2	80.5	74.4
Division II	89.1	79.7	78.8	74.5
Division III	93.2	82.6	83.3	81.5

Source: Data are from reference 21.

TABLE 13.5   Prevalence of Alcohol Use Among College Students (n = 80,121)

Frequency of Alcohol Use in Past 30 Days	Male, %	Female, %	Total, %
Never Used	18.0	17.0	17.4
Used, but not in last 30 d	11.2	15.0	13.7
Used 1–9 d	51.5	55.6	54.1
Used 10–29 d	18.5	12.1	14.4
Used all 30 d	0.80	0.20	0.40

Source: Data are from reference 22.

BOX 13.6   Consequences of Alcohol Use on Athletic Performance

- **Aerobic performance:** Alcohol is a powerful diuretic that leads to dehydration, which weakens the pumping force of the heart, impairs temperature regulation, and accelerates fatigue, all contributing to decreased aerobic and overall performance. Increased health risks during prolonged exercise in hot environments are also a concern.
- **Motor skills:** Alcohol slows reaction time and impairs precision, equilibrium, hand-eye coordination, accuracy, balance, judgment, information processing, focus, stamina, strength, power, and speed; impairments can last up to 72 hours after alcohol intake.
- **Strength, power, and sprint performance:** Alcohol leads to decreased strength, power, and sprint performance (eg, running and cycling times); decreased grip strength; decreased jump height; and faster time to fatigue during high-intensity exercise.
- **Recovery:** Alcohol is a poor source of nutrients and may replace carbohydrates in the pre- and posttraining times, leading to poor training and recovery.
- **Risk of illness and injury:** Athletes who drink alcohol have an elevated risk of injury. Regular alcohol consumption depresses immune function, increases swelling upon injury, and contributes to delayed healing.
- **Body composition/weight management:** Body fat accumulation due to ethanol storage as fat and alcohol's appetite stimulant effect may lead to negative body composition changes and overall weight gain.
- **Long-term health:** Long-term excessive alcohol consumption can cause pathological changes in liver, heart, brain, and muscle that can lead to disability; nutritional deficiencies; altered digestion, absorption, and metabolism of nutrients; muscle damage, wasting, and weakness; and impaired ability to gain muscle mass and strength.

Source: Data are from reference 23.

TABLE 13.6   College Athletes: Prevalence of Substance Use by Sport

Sport	Binge Drinking, %[a]	Marijuana, %	Illicit Drugs, %[b]
Male athletes			
Baseball	64.6	19.1	12.8
Basketball	50.2	19.1	8.6
Football	58.4	26.3	14.6
Hockey	75.4	38.5	18.8
Running	40.9	16.3	10.1
Soccer	47.1	24.9	16.0
Swimming/diving	54.0	30.2	11.3
Female athletes			
Basketball	36.5	23.2	8.9
Running	26.6	23.7	12.1
Soccer	46.9	37.8	23.0
Softball	38.2	26.5	11.9
Swimming/diving	29.4	16.5	4.9
Volleyball	39.7	25.0	11.7

[a]*Binge-drinking* is defined as five or more drinks in a row within the past 2 weeks.
[b]Illicit drugs = cocaine, crack, barbiturates, amphetamines, tranquilizers, heroin/opiates, LSD/psychedelics, and ecstasy.
Source: Data are from reference 20.

Most student-athletes reported that they do not drink or drink less during the season for their sport, but most drink after practice and/or competition (21). Collegiate student-athletes reported choosing to use alcohol for recreational and social use because it feels good and/or it helps deal with the stress of college life and collegiate athletics (21). Athletes attributed abstaining from alcohol to concerns about health, avoidance of alcohol's negative effects, or personal belief systems (21). Table 13.6 shows how alcohol and substance use differs by team for both male and female collegiate student-athletes (20).

The hazards of tobacco use are well known. The ACHA-NCHA Reference Group Summary (22) reported that 18.8% of college students had used cigarettes in the last 30 days. Cigarette use among Division I student-athletes decreased from 21.3% to 12.3% between 2001 and 2005 (21). Chewing or spit tobacco use is a common practice among college athletes despite the National Collegiate Athletic Association (NCAA) ban on the use of smokeless tobacco products. The NCAA study found that smokeless tobacco use had decreased from 22.5% to 16.2% of all Division I college athletes since 1997 (21). The same study found that use among male athletes playing specific sports is alarmingly high. For example, more than 20% of male football, golf, and lacrosse players, and more than 30% of male baseball, hockey, and wrestlers report using smokeless tobacco products. In the same study, use of smokeless tobacco by female student-athletes ranged from 0.9% (field hockey, track and field) to 19.5% (ice hockey). Smokeless tobacco can lead to periodontal disease, loss of tooth structure, tooth staining, bad breath, and gum disease as well as lead to an increased risk of oral cancer and leukoplakia (24).

Performance Concerns

College athletes are concerned about nutrition for performance enhancement, use of dietary supplements, prevention of fatigue, illness and injury, recovery from training, weight management, and altering or maintaining body composition (25). Working with student athletes to educate them about the nutritional demands of sport at the collegiate level is paramount. Their collegiate training regimen may be vastly different than it was during high school, resulting in altered nutrition requirements.

Performance Enhancement/Supplements

Although many athletes understand the relationship between optimal nutrition and athletic performance, the pressure to use sport foods and supplements is overwhelming and can lead to choosing these products instead of food and fluid intake. Many athletes use dietary supplements to enhance athletic performance. The NCAA 2009 Survey of Member Institution's Drug-Education and Drug-Testing Programs reported that 22% of Division I, II, and III institutions provide nutritional supplements to their student-athletes, with 82% Division I football schools providing nutritional supplements (26). Froiland et al reported on nutritional supplement use among 203 college athletes (115 male and 88 female) and their sources of information (27). Eighty-nine percent of the student-athletes had or were currently using nutrition supplements. By sex, females were more likely to take calcium and multivitamins and males had significant intake for ginseng, amino acids, glutamine, beta-hydroxy beta-methylbutyric acid (HMB), weight gainers, whey protein, and Juven (Abbott Nutrition). The most frequently used supplements were energy drinks (73%), calorie replacement products (61.4%), multivitamins (47.3%), creatine (37.2%), and vitamin C (32.4%). Females were more likely to obtain information from family members, and males reported seeking information from a store "nutritionist," fellow athletes, friends, or a coach. Female athletes were more likely to take supplements for their health or to make up for an inadequate diet; males took supplements to improve speed and agility, strength and power, or for weight/muscle gain (27). In the 2005 NCAA survey, 41% of student-athletes reported the use of nutritional supplements. The most commonly reported use was for creatine, protein and amino acid products, and thermogenics for weight loss. The most cited reasons for use were to improve athletic performance, for general good health, and for weight loss/weight gain (21).

Fatigue Prevention

Nutritional causes of fatigue in athletes include inadequate energy intake, glycogen depletion, dehydration, and poor iron status. Although iron deficiency can occur in both male and female athletes, it has been estimated that approximately 60% of female college athletes are affected by iron deficiency (28). Factors that contribute to iron loss in female athletes include menstruation, inadequate dietary iron intake, gastrointestinal bleeding, foot-strike hemolysis, sweat loss, and iron malabsorption. The consequences of iron deficiency are impaired athletic performance, immune function, and cognitive function. Cowell et al reported that 44% (n = 24) of 55 NCAA Division I institutions screen their female athletes for iron deficiency (28). Twenty-two of the 24 institutions who screen for iron deficiency provide nutrition advice to those female student-athletes who are iron-deficient. A great deal of variability existed among the institutions in terms of diagnostic criteria, treatment protocols, and follow-up procedures. The authors concluded that a need exists to develop standardized protocols for assessment and treatment of iron-deficiency for female college athletes (28). The following is a suggested protocol from Eichner (29):

- Serum ferritin > 40 ng/mL: Warrants no action
- Serum ferritin between 20–40 ng/mL: daily multivitamin with 27 mg elemental iron
- Serum ferritin < 20 ng/mL: 325 mg ferrous sulfate once daily; follow up after 100 tablets

Illness/Injury Prevention/Rehabilitation

In 1982, the NATA and the NCAA created an ongoing collegiate sports injury database called the NCAA Injury Surveillance System (NCAA-ISS) (30). Between 1988 and 2004, more than half of all athletic injuries to collegiate athletes were to the lower extremities. Preseason practice injury rates were two to three times higher than injury rates recorded during the regular seasons and more injuries were reported to occur during competition than practice. Concussions and anterior cruciate ligaments (ACL) injury rates increased significantly between 1988 and 2004, likely due in part to improved reporting and identification. Several sports showed decreased competition injury rates, including women's gymnastics, basketball, and field hockey. Spring football and women's basketball practice injury rates also decreased. Sports involving collision and contact, such as football and wrestling, had the highest injury rates in both games and practice; whereas men's baseball had the lowest rate of injuries in practice and women's softball had the lowest rate in games. Sports considered "noncontact," such as men's and women's soccer and basketball, still have a substantial number of injuries caused by player contact. Female athletes are at greater risk than male athletes of noncontact ACL injuries in basketball and soccer (30). Special nutritional consideration must be paid to the injured athlete, including altered energy needs, nutritional requirements pre- and postsurgery, and discontinuation of select dietary supplements presurgery. Additionally, the injured athlete may have increased concern about weight and body composition during periods of inactivity and rehabilitation.

Recovery
Emphasis on strategies for nutritional recovery from training and competition has increased. *Recovery* is a term applied to the refueling and rehydration strategies in the immediate postexercise period to gain training adaptations and prevent fatigue in the next exercise sessions (25). It takes approximately 24 hours for the body to recover from a bout of training. For athletes training at low-intensity once a day, no special recovery recommendations are required. However, for those athletes engaged in training for more than 90 minutes a day or with multiple training sessions or competitions, consuming carbohydrate (1.0–1.5 g per kg body weight) plus 10 to 20 g of protein with adequate rehydration in the immediate postexercise period (within 30 minutes) improves glycogen resynthesis and muscle rebuilding and repair (25).

Weight Management
Many student-athletes will see the sports dietitian for weight management: gain or loss. This is a great opportunity to evaluate the student-athlete's nutritional status and identify areas of need for sports nutrition education while counseling the athlete on appropriate weight management strategies. The following is the position of the Academy of Nutrition and Dietetics and the American College of Sports Medicine (25):

Body weight and composition should not be the sole criterion for participation in sports; daily weigh-ins are discouraged. Optimal body fat levels depend on the sex, age and heredity of the athlete and may be sport-specific. Body fat assessment techniques have inherent variability and limitations. Preferably weight loss (fat loss) should take place in the off-season or begin before the competitive season and involve a qualified sports dietitian.

For weight loss, the sports dietitian must assure adequate nutrient intake, provide a meal plan that minimizes loss of lean mass, and evaluate the student-athlete for risk of disordered eating. For weight gain, special care must be taken to help the athlete find ways to increase energy intake with calorically dense foods, assure adequate nutrient intake, and avoid foods high in saturated fat and cholesterol that may increase risk of chronic disease.

Body Composition
Body composition is a measure of the ratio of lean to fat mass. For a review of body composition techniques, see Chapter 9. Methods that have been used in the collegiate setting include hydrostatic weighing, skinfold measurements, air displacement plethysmography, bioelectrical impedance analysis (BIA), and

DXA. All methods have a degree of error associated with them that must be considered when interpreting results. Although the assessment of body composition can be a useful tool in helping the student athlete track the changes that occur because of modifications in nutrition and training, the NCAA Sports Medicine Handbook 2009–2010 (31) points out the following factors to consider:

- The weight on the scale does not tell an athlete what changes are occurring to his or her lean and fat mass.
- Comparing body composition with other athletes is not useful due to differences in age, weight, height, sex, and genetics and may lead to unhealthy nutrition and exercise practices.
- While achieving a body composition that helps a student athlete achieve his or her best athletic performance, a very low body fat has serious consequences on health and performance. Minimum body composition standards exist for both male and female athletes.
- Changes in body composition occur slowly over time, and reassessment twice per year is sufficient except in rare circumstances.

There is no ideal body composition of any one athlete or sport. Providing athletes with goal ranges for body composition for their particular gender and sport as well as tracking changes in lean and fat mass over time can be useful. Many collegiate athletic departments have developed weight and body composition policies outlining who will do the measurements, how results will be presented to the athlete, who will have access to the data, how these data will be used, and how often measurements are repeated. These policies help to ensure that the data will not be abused or used punitively and that the health and safety of the athlete is assured.

Health Concerns

Health concerns for the student-athlete include gastrointestinal disorders, development of cardiovascular disease risk factors, diabetes, disordered eating/eating disorders, and the female athlete triad. Although specific health assessment data on college athletes do not exist, health data reported in Table 13.7 from the National College Health Assessment (22) can help the collegiate sports RD understand the variety of health problems experienced by college students, many of which are tied to nutritional status.

Gastrointestinal Disorders

Student-athletes may present with gastrointestinal issues including gastroesophageal reflux, gastritis, nausea, constipation, diarrhea, irritable bowel syndrome, and inflammatory bowel diseases such as Crohn's disease and ulcerative colitis. The sports dietitian needs to be knowledgeable about MNT for these disorders and how to balance an adequate training diet with the rigors of an academic and athletic training schedule.

Cardiovascular Disease Risk Factors

Although cardiovascular disease (CVD) risk factors such as high cholesterol, high blood pressure, and diabetes are not the first topic on the collegiate student-athlete's mind, it is well documented that heart disease is the number one cause of morbidity and mortality for all Americans (32). Emerging science suggests that increased CVD risk is a reality for some collegiate student-athletes. Muñoz et al studied 135 NCAA Division II student athletes from 11 sports and found that a number of college athletes had one or more risk factors for CVD, including increased waist circumference, elevated blood pressure, high total cholesterol, and low HDL-cholesterol despite participation in sports (33). These factors may predispose the college athletes to cardiac risk later in life when exercise regimens are reduced. Borchers et al reported that of 104 NCAA

TABLE 13.7   Prevalence of Health Problems in College Students (n = 80,121)

Health Problem	Prevalence in Previous Year, %
Allergy problems	47.9
Back pain	46.1
Sinus infection	30.7
Depression	17.0
Strep throat	13.8
Anxiety disorder	13.2
Asthma	11.7
Ear infection	9.5
Bronchitis	8.2
Seasonal affective disorder	8.0
Repetitive stress injury	7.0
Sexually transmitted diseases	5.1
High blood pressure	4.6
High cholesterol	3.8
Substance abuse	3.6
Chronic fatigue syndrome	3.1
Bulimia nervosa	2.1
Anorexia nervosa	1.8
Diabetes	1.0

Source: Data are from reference 22.

Division I football players, 21% were obese (body fat > 25%), 21% had insulin resistance, and 9% had metabolic syndrome (34). Offensive and defensive linemen comprised all of the obese participants in the study and are at a significantly increased risk of insulin resistance and the metabolic syndrome compared with other position players. These data suggest that although Division I collegiate football players participate in high-intensity training, they are at risk of developing metabolic syndrome. Counseling and education on lifestyle modification, exercise, and diet for reduced CVD risk is needed for all athletes, especially as their college sports career is ending.

Diabetes

Athletes with diabetes compete at the highest level in every sport. The sports dietitian should be part of the treatment team providing education and lifestyle strategies to optimize glycemic control (17). The collegiate sports dietitian will more likely encounter type 1 diabetes because of the demographics of the college athlete and should be prepared to address those cases. Refer to Chapter 19 for detailed information on diabetes management in athletes.

Disordered Eating and the Female Athlete Triad

College athletes, especially females, are at increased risk for eating disorders or pathogenic eating and weight-control behaviors. Reasons for this increased risk include the stress of transitioning to college, pressures to be thin, increased academic demands, and participation in college athletics. Eating disorders and disordered eating are associated with serious health problems such as dehydration, electrolyte imbalance, depression, decreased bone density, and cardiac arrhythmia. Greenleaf et al studied 204 NCAA Division I female college athletes from three universities across the United States and found that 25.5% were symptomatic (some symptoms reported but insufficient to warrant a clinical diagnosis) and 2% had eating disorders (anorexia nervosa, bulimia nervosa) (35). These findings are consistent with other research on the prevalence of disordered eating and eating disorders in female college-athletes. There was no relationship between sport type and eating disorder classification, suggesting that eating disorders occur fairly consistently across sports. The NCAA collected information on 1,445 male and female student-athletes from 11 NCAA Division I schools and reported that although rates of clinical eating disorders based on DSM-IV criteria were low (0% for anorexia nervosa for both female and male athletes; 1.1% and 0% for bulimia for female and male athletes, respectively), the number of athletes at risk for disordered eating was significant (25% of female athletes and 9.5% of male athletes) (36). Eating disorders continue to be a problem that predominately affects female athletes, but this study was unique in that it reported on the prevalence of eating disorders and risk of disordered eating in male college student-athletes as well.

Beals and Hill examined the prevalence of the female athlete triad as characterized by disordered eating, menstrual dysfunction, and low bone mineral density (BMD) among 112 female college athletes in seven different sports (37). They found that only one athlete met the criteria for all three disorders of the triad, but 28 athletes met the criteria for disordered eating, 29 athletes met the criteria for menstrual dysfunction, and 2 athletes had low BMD. Although the prevalence of clinical eating disorders is low in female college athletes, many are at risk for disordered eating, which places them at increased risk for menstrual irregularity and bone injuries. The NCAA developed a handbook titled *Managing the Female Athlete Triad,* which is a useful tool for educating athletic department coaches and staff about prevention, detection, and treatment of the female athlete triad (38). Refer to Chapter 18 for more information on eating disorders.

The Athletic Department

Stakeholders

There are many services, operations, and personnel in and around the athletic department that can serve as collaborative and strategic partners for the sports dietitian. The stakeholders are shown in Figure 13.1.

Medical services personnel, coaching staff, athletic administrators, support service staff, and academic faculty can all be important stakeholders in the service the collegiate sports dietitian provides. Team physicians, orthopedic physicians, athletic trainers, and sport psychologists are all important allies in sports nutrition services. The athletic trainer is an especially vital connection to the athletes, given their proximity and level of daily involvement with them. It is crucial to establish positive working relationships with these providers, who will ultimately facilitate the RD's work with the individual athletes and teams. Similarly, student health services often have clinical laboratories and pharmacies on site with staffs who can become valuable colleagues in facilitating nutrition-related biochemical screening protocols and supplement purchasing and distribution.

Coaching staffs, consisting of head and assistant coaches as well as operations staff, and strength and conditioning coaches are obvious partners for the sports dietitian's work. Once these relationships have been established, coaches will be more willing to allocate practice time to nutrition education, offer budgetary support toward nutrition priorities, and help to facilitate a positive nutrition culture within his or her program. Coaching staffs will also often be vocal advocates of nutrition services. In addition, coaches can promote sports nutrition services in the recruiting process in an effort to introduce potential athletes to the comprehensive services offered by the college or university. Parents are often impressed to know that a nutrition program is part of the athletic environment.

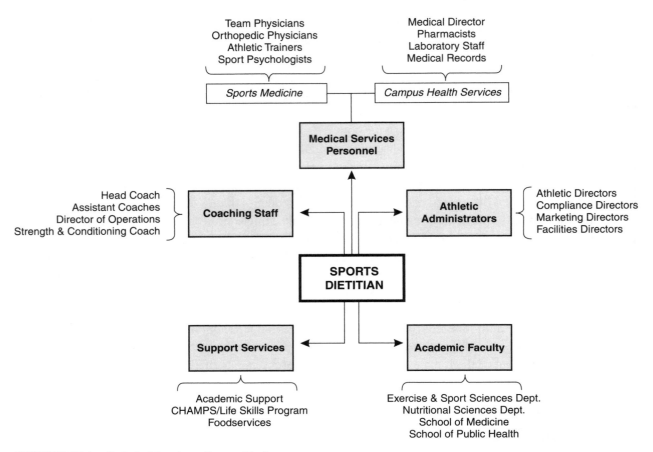

FIGURE 13.1   Stakeholders in college athletics.

Athletic administrators are key stakeholders in establishing nutrition services as well as regulating daily operations. Athletic directors make the decision to invest in nutrition services and to include and offer it as part of the department's plan to carry out its mission. Compliance directors are important in interpreting and overseeing nutrition-related NCAA policies. They can also be helpful in identifying available funding sources for special projects or needs (eg, student-athlete opportunity funds or NCAA grant monies). Marketing administrators can be especially valuable when considering contractual agreements with retail or supplement companies. Elements of these contracts can often be negotiated and structured to provide nutritional products to the athletes, which can provide financial relief for the team's operating budgets, sports medicine supply lines, or nutrition resources. Lastly, some administrators deal with renovating or building athletic facilities. The sports dietitian can suggest the inclusion of nutrition-related spaces, such as meal and training table spaces, an area for cooking demonstrations, nutritional counseling space, and pre- and post-workout recovery space where smoothies or shakes can be made.

Connecting with support services such as academic support, CHAMPS/Life Skills Programs, and campus foodservices also can enhance and assist the sports dietitian in his or her goal of educating and feeding the student-athlete. Nutrition and disordered eating prevention and education are both priorities in the personal development commitment component of the Life Skills Program. Because planning and coordinating meals are major functions of a sports dietitian, the foodservice department is a clear collaborator. The work of creating and implementing training tables, catered meals, and purchase and distribution of other food provisions can be eased with strong relationships with foodservice personnel. The foodservice staff can also benefit from the dietitian's involvement in providing expertise in recipe analysis and management and appropriate menu design.

Lastly, interfacing with academic units on campus can provide cooperative associations with many benefits. For example, the dietitian may be interested in and able to teach a class, lecture, or precept nutrition students in return for the opportunity to create internships or independent study experiences that can help the dietitian research and implement special projects.

Training Table

The NCAA rules allow institutions to provide one training-table meal per day to student-athletes (4). As noted previously, *training table* refers to a meal eaten together as a team in a separate dining facility. The NCAA does not restrict the choice of meal, foods, or cost for the designated training-table meal. This meal can be offered for the breakfast, lunch, or dinner meal and can be specifically designed to meet the needs of the athletes. Often the dinner meal is chosen as the training-table meal so athletes can refuel after practices. Each institution, team, and/or coach in conjunction with the sports dietitian should determine which meal provides the most nutritional benefit to the athletes while considering their academic, practice, and extracurricular schedules. The cost of the training-table meal can exceed the regular on-campus dining hall rate, but the athletic department or the team must pay the difference between the rate and the actual cost of the training-table meal.

Scholarship, recruited nonscholarship, and walk-on athletes who are members of the team are all eligible to participate in the training-table meal. However, any athlete without a room-and-board allowance must pay for their training-table meals. They are required to pay the regular on-campus rate for that specific meal, even though the actual meal cost may exceed the regular student rate. For a scholarship athlete, the established on-campus dining hall rate for the meal is deducted from their room and board allowance (4). For example, if the actual cost of a training-table dinner is $20 and the campus door rate for dinner is $9.50, then the athletic department or team is responsible for paying the $10.50 meal-cost differential.

In addition to subsidizing the meal cost, training tables can require a substantial investment from the athletic department from a facility standpoint. Ideally, the training-table meal would be served in an athletic facility that is convenient and accessible to athletes. However, if a specific athletic dining facility does not exist, the training-table meal can be a catered meal brought on site or to any location. Often individual teams will have the training-table meal delivered to their locker room or team room location. Meals can be provided by on-campus foodservice contractors, outside caterers, local restaurants, or athletic departments can opt to support a self-operation foodservice.

NCAA Compliance

To work in the field of sports nutrition at the collegiate level, sports dietitians need a basic understanding of NCAA rules and regulations. The NCAA, through various committee structures, incorporates legislative actions into adopted operating and administrative bylaws and a constitution. These rules and regulations govern the conduct of intercollegiate member institutions relating to athletic issues such as admissions, financial aid, eligibility, and recruiting. Individual athletic departments are obligated to apply, adhere, and enforce NCAA legislation. Each institution employs a compliance staff that oversees this function to ensure operational integrity.

Training Table and Meal Rules
Most nutrition-related legislation falls within the financial aid, housing and meals, and banned drug list and nutritional supplement bylaws. Box 13.7 outlines the major nutrition-related bylaws. Bylaw 16.5 defines

---

BOX 13.7   Major Nutrition-Related Legislation by the National Collegiate Athletic Association[a]

- **Article 13.3**: Admissions and Graduation Data, Banned Drug List and Initial Eligibility Standards, Bylaw 13.3.2.2: Report Distribution—The NCAA Eligibility Center shall provide the NCAA banned drug list and information about nutritional supplements to a prospective student-athlete and his or her parents or legal guardians after he or she has registered with the Eligibility Center.
- **Article 15.2**: Elements of Financial Aid, Bylaw 15.2.2.1.6: Training Table Meals—The cost of meals provided on the institution's training table shall be deducted from a student-athlete's board allowance, even if the student-athlete is not receiving a full grant-in-aid.
- **Article 16.5**: Housing and Meals, Bylaw 16.5.2: Permissible—Identified housing and meal benefits incidental to a student's participation in intercollegiate athletics that may be financed by the institution are:

    - **16.5.2(c)**: Training Table Meals: An institution may provide only one training table meal per day to a student-athlete during the academic year on those days when regular institutional dining facilities are open.
    - **16.5.2(d)**: Meals Incidental to Participation:

        - 1: Missed Meal Due to Practice Activities: A student-athlete who is not receiving athletically related financial aid (eg, walk-on) may receive the benefit of a training-table meal during the permissible playing and practice season in those instances in which the student-athlete's schedule is affected by involvement in practice activities, provided the student-athlete previously has paid for the same meal (eg, dinner) at an institutional dining facility.
        - 2. Meals in Conjunction with Home Competition: All student-athletes are permitted to receive meals at the institution's discretion beginning with the evening before competition and continuing until they are released by institutional personnel.
        - 3. Meals in Conjunction with Away-from-Home Competition: An institution may provide meals to student-athletes in conjunction with away-from-home competition pursuant to one of the following options, ie regular meals, pre- or post-game meal, or cash in lieu of meals OR meals at the institution's discretion for the duration of travel, in lieu of cash provision.

    - **16.5.2(g)**: Nutritional Supplements—An institution may provide permissible nutritional supplements to a student athlete for the purpose of providing additional calories and electrolytes.
    - **16.5.2(h)**: Fruit, Nuts, and Bagels—An institution may provide fruit, nuts and bagels to a student-athlete at any time.

[a] This information was current at press time but was under review. For the most current information, go to www.ncaa.org.
Source: Data are from reference 4.

---

applications related to training-table meals; nutritional supplements; and fruit, nuts, and bagels. Training-table meals are regulated as discussed previously in this chapter. In addition to training-table meals, an institution is allowed to provide meals incidental to participation in practices or competition. For example, if student-athletes miss a meal due to practice activities or an institutional committee meeting, they can receive a training-table meal from the institution provided they previously paid for the same meal at the institution. Similarly, athletes can be provided meals beginning the evening before a home competition through the time at which they are released at the close of competition. Athletes are also eligible to receive meals or the cash value of the meals in conjunction with away competition and during vacation periods.

Permissible vs Impermissible Ingredients

When considering nutritional supplements, products must be evaluated to ensure that they do not include banned substances. An updated banned substance list is released each year by the NCAA and can be accessed on the NCAA Web site in the drug testing information of the legislative and governance section. Stimulants, anabolic agents, and diuretics are examples of classes of banned substances (39). The published list also provides examples of banned substances in each class, but it is not a complete list.

Sports dietitians must also check whether supplements (or their ingredients) are permissible or impermissible. The NCAA bylaw defines four classes of non–muscle building permissible supplements that an institution can provide to provide additional calories and electrolytes:

- Carbohydrate/electrolyte beverages
- Energy bars
- Carbohydrate boosters
- Vitamins and minerals

Impermissible supplements or ingredients are anything other than these four permissible classes. In 2000 the NCAA published a Legislative Assistance column and an official interpretation for member institutions further explaining the intent and application of the supplement bylaw. For example, a non–muscle building supplement is defined by a protein content limit of ≤ 30% of calories from protein. In addition, a list of common impermissible ingredients identified by the competitive-safeguards committee was published as examples, but this is not to be used as an exhaustive list (40). The following are examples of impermissible ingredients/supplements:

- Amino acids
- Conjugated linoleic acid (CLA)
- Creatine
- Ginseng
- Green tea

The list is updated yearly by the NCAA (www.ncaa.org).

Fruits, Nuts, and Bagels

In 2009 the NCAA Housing and Meal Article 16.5 was amended to include fruit, nuts, and bagels as part of the permissible benefit in the bylaw (4). The amended article simply states that an institution can provide fruit, nuts, and bagels to student-athletes at any time regardless of practice or competition day or time. This recent amendment has been a welcomed opportunity for the sports dietitian to provide additional calories, carbohydrate, and nutrients in whole-food form.

Summary

The role of the sports dietitian at the collegiate level has evolved into a recognized, accepted, and desired component of enhancing performance, assisting in health care needs, and safeguarding the student-athletes' eligibility. The sports dietitian has a unique opportunity to become highly involved in the intercollegiate operation and the institution's academic environment. The skills and experience needed to carry out the responsibilities require an experienced dietitian who is a specialty or advanced practitioner. College sports dietitians do more than provide nutrition services to student-athletes; they also provide administrative and academic duties. Student-athletes have personal and athletic concerns that are often at odds with optimal health. The sports dietitian can improve their nutrition knowledge and help them eliminate nutrition-related barriers to optimal training, performance, and health. The athletic department houses many important stakeholders with whom RDs need to collaborate to support nutrition services. The relationships established in working with college athletes are perhaps the one of most rewarding aspects of the job. The opportunity to contribute to the team and individual successes while becoming part of the team is personally and professionally rewarding.

Future Directions

Nearly 20 year ago, Kristine Clark wrote, "Opportunities for establishing strong sports nutrition positions at major universities are on the horizon" (2). As more positions and opportunities are created across the country, sports dietitians need to be prepared to step into these unique roles and advance the field of sports nutrition. There are many emerging topics of interest that need further research and validation that could lead to key recommendations for the sports dietitian. Some examples are the role of vitamin D in athletic performance, the role of anti-inflammatory foods and supplements in muscle recovery, postsurgical and rehabilitation nutrition interventions, and immune-enhancing nutrition recommendations. The field also needs to focus on using the Nutrition Care Process for documentation of services for potential insurance reimbursement while also demonstrating the cost-effectiveness of nutrition services. In addition, as the group of RDs working in the collegiate setting becomes more focused and expands, organizational efforts should include connecting with the NCAA to provide technical assistance and influence legislative change as well as extending learning and development opportunities for future collegiate sports dietitians.

References

1. National Collegiate Athletic Association. 2008–2009 Membership Report. http://catalog.proemags.com/publication/cc5da338#/cc5da338/1. Accessed January 11, 2010.
2. Clark KL. Working with college athletes, coaches, and trainers at a major university. *Int J Sport Nutr.* 1994;4:135–141.
3. American Dietetic Association standards of practice and standards of professional performance for registered dietitians (generalist, specialty, advanced) in sports dietetics. *J Am Diet Assoc.* 2009;109:544–552.
4. National Collegiate Athletic Association. 2009–2010 NCAA Division 1 Manual: Constitution, Operation Bylaws, Administrative Bylaws. http://www.ncaapublications.com/p-3934-2009-2010-ncaa-division-i-manual.aspx. Accessed January 14, 2010.
5. The World Anti-Doping Code: 2010 Prohibited List International Standard. http://www.wada-ama.org/Documents/World_Anti-Doping_Program/WADP-Prohibited-list/WADA_Prohibited_List_2010_EN.pdf. Accessed March 10, 2010.
6. McNulty KY, Adams CH, Anderson JM, Affenito SG. Development and validation of a screening tool to identify eating disorders in female athletes. *J Am Diet Assoc.* 2001;101:886–892.
7. Morgan JF, Reid F, Lacey JH. The SCOFF questionnaire: assessment of a new screening tool for eating disorders. *BMJ.* 1999;319:1467–1468.
8. Garner DM. *Eating Disorder Inventory 2: Professional Manual.* Odessa, FL: Psychological Assessment Resources; 1991.

9. *Eating Disorder Inventory 3: Professional Manual.* Lutz, FL: Psychological Assessment Resources; 2004.

10. Garner DM, Olmsted MP, Bohr Y, Garfinkel PE. The eating attitudes test: psychometric features and clinical correlates. *Psychol Med.* 1982;12:871–878.

11. Nagel DL, Black DR, Leverenz LJ, Coster DC. Evaluation of a screening test for female college athletes with eating disorders and disordered eating. *J Athl Train.* 2000;35:431–440.

12. Sangenis, P, Drinkwater BL, Loucks A, Sherman RT, Sundgot-Borgen J, Thompson RA. International Olympic Committee Position Stand: The Female Athlete Triad. 2005. http://www.olympic.org/Assets/ImportedNews/Documents/en_report_917.pdf. Accessed March 17, 2010.

13. Smith Rockwell M, Nickols-Richardson SM, Thye F. Nutrition knowledge, opinions, and practices of coaches and athletic trainers at a Division I university. *Int J Sports Nutr Exerc Metab.* 2001;11:174–185.

14. American Diabetes Association position statement: standards of medical care in diabetes 2007. *Diabetes Care.* 2007;30(suppl):S4–S41.

15. Jimenez CC, Corcoran MH, Crawley JT, Hornsby WG, Peer KS, Philbin RD, Riddell MC. National Athletic Trainers' Association position statement: management of the athlete with type 1 diabetes mellitus. *J Athl Train.* 2007;42:536–545.

16. Nattiv A, Loucks AB, Manore MM, Sanborn CF, Sundgot-Borgen J, Warren MP. American College of Sports Medicine position statement: the female athlete triad. *Med Sci Sports Exerc.* 2007;39:1867–1882.

17. Arnett JJ. Emerging adulthood: a theory of development from the late teens to the twenties. *Am Psychol.* 2000; 55:469–480.

18. Jensen, Francis. The Teenage Brain. http://www.npr.org/templates/story/story.php?storyId=124119468. Accessed March 1, 2010.

19. Rosenbloom CA, Jonnalagadda SS, Skinner, R. Nutrition knowledge of collegiate athletes in a Division I National Collegiate Athletic Association institution. *J Am Diet Assoc.* 2002;102:418–420.

20. Ford JA. Substance use among college athletes: a comparison based on sport/team affiliation. *J Am Coll Health.* 2007;55:367–373.

21. National Collegiate Athletic Association. NCAA Study of Substance Use Habits of College Student-Athletes 2005. Presented to: The National Collegiate Athletic Association Committee on Competitive Safeguards and Medical Aspects of Sports by the NCAA Research Staff. http://www.thencaa.biz/wps/wcm/connect/2f0f73004e0b8a4c9a86fa1ad6fc8b25/NCAADrugUseStudy2005.pdf?MOD=AJPERES&CACHEID=2f0f73004e0b8a4c9a86fa1ad6fc8b25. Accessed May 28, 2010.

22. American College Health Association. National College Health Assessment. ACHA-NCHA Reference Group Executive Summary. Alcohol, Tobacco and Other Drug Use. Spring 2008. http://www.achancha.org. Accessed May 28, 2010.

23. American College of Sports position statement on the use of alcohol in sports. *Med Sci Sports Exerc.* 1982;14:ix–xi.

24. Burak LJ. Smokeless tobacco education for college athletes. *J Physical Educ Recreation Dance.* 2001;72:37–45.

25. Rodriguez NR, DiMarco NM, Langley S. Position of the American Dietetic Association, Dietitians of Canada, and the American College of Sports Medicine: nutrition and athletic performance. *J Am Diet Assoc.* 2009;109:509–527.

26. National Collegiate Athletic Association Committee on Competitive Safeguards and Medical Aspects of Sports. NCAA 2009 Survey: Member Institution's Drug-Education and Drug-Testing Programs. http://www.ncaa.org/wps/wcm/connect/86235480437cd009bb24bb6bcdc87ae7/Drug+Education+and+Drug+Testing+Report+2009.pdf?MOD=AJPERES&CACHEID=86235480437cd009bb24bb6bcdc87ae7. Accessed September 22, 2010.

27. Froiland K, Koszewski W, Hingst J, Kopecky L. Nutritional supplement use among college athletes and their sources of information. *Int J Sport Nutr Exerc Metab.* 2004;14:104–120.

28. Cowell BS, Rosenbloom CA, Skinner R, Summers SH. Policies on screening female athletes for iron deficiency in NCAA Division I-A institutions. *Int J Sports Nutr Exerc Metab.* 2003;13:277–285.

29. Eichner R. Anemia and female athletes. *Sports Med Dig.* 2000;22:57

30. Collegiate Athlete Injuries: Trends and Prevention. A Report on the NCAA Injury Surveillance System (ISS). http://www.nata.org/jat/readers/archives/42.2/i1062-6050-42-2-toc.pdf. Accessed March 25, 2010.

31. Assessment of body composition. In: National Collegiate Athletic Association Sports Medicine Handbook 2009–2010. http://www.ncaapublications.com/productdownloads/MD10.pdf. Accessed June 30, 2010.

32. Lloyd-Jones DM, Hong Y, Labarthe D, Mozaffarian D, Appel LJ, Van Horn L, Greenlund K, Daniels S, Nichol G, Tomaselli GF, Arnett DK, Fonarow GC, Ho PM, Lauer MS, Masoudi FA, Robertson RM, Roger V, Schwamm MLH, Sorlie P, Yancy CW, Rosamond WD; American Heart Association Strategic Planning Task Force and Statistics Committee. Defining and setting national goals for cardiovascular health promotion and disease reduction: the American Heart Association's strategic impact goal through 2020 and beyond. *Circulation.* 2010;121:586–613.

33. Muñoz L, Norgan G, Rauschhuber M, Allwein D, Powell BW, Mitchell D, Gilliland I, Beltz S, Mahon M, Milkan V, Cook J, Lowry J, Richardson C, Sethness R, Etnyre A, Jones ME. An exploratory study of cardiac health in college athletes. *Appl Nurs Res.* 2009;22:228–235.

34. Borchers JR, Clem KL, Habash DL, Nagaraja HN, Stokley LM, Best TM. Metabolic syndrome and insulin resistance in Division I collegiate football players. *Med Sci Sports Exerc.* 2009;41:2105–2110.

35. Greenleaf C, Petrie TA, Carter J, Reel JJ. Female collegiate athletes: prevalence of eating disorders and disordered eating behaviors. *J Am Coll Health.* 2009;57:489–495.

36. Johnson C, Powers PS, Dick R. Athletes and eating disorders: the National Collegiate Athletic Association study. *Int J Eat Disord.* 1999;26:179–188.

37. Beals KA, Hill AK. The prevalence of disordered eating, menstrual dysfunction and low bone mineral density among US collegiate athletes. *Int J Sport Nutr Exerc Metab.* 2006;16:1–23

38. Sherman R, Thompson R; National Collegiate Athletic Association. NCAA Coaches Handbook: Managing the Female Athlete Triad. http://www.ncaa.org/wps/wcm/connect/2db7d8004e0db26bac18fc1ad6fc8b25/female_athlete_triad.pdf?MOD=AJPERES&CACHEID=2db7d8004e0db26bac18fc1ad6fc8b25. Accessed March 21, 2010.

39. NCAA Banned Drug List. http://www.ncaa.org/wps/wcm/connect/public/ncaa/student-athlete+experience/ncaa+banned+drugs+list. Accessed June 1, 2010.

40. NCAA issues notice about nutritional supplement provision. NCAA News Archive—2005. May 23, 2005 4:05:10PM. http://fs.ncaa.org/Docs/NCAANewsArchive/2005/Association-wide/index.html. Accessed June 1, 2010.

Chapter 14

MASTERS ATHLETES

Christine A. Rosenbloom, PhD, RD, CSSD

Introduction

What do athletes do when they get older and are no longer competitive in the sport they love? Many of them are taking on a new title: veteran or masters athlete. Events for masters athletes can range from sanctioned events provided through formal governing bodies such as USA Track and Field to events such as the Huntsman World Senior Games held annually in Utah. In 2010 the World Senior Games hosted a record 10,072 athletes competing in 27 sports representing 26 countries, a substantial increase from the 500 athletes who competed in 1985 when the inaugural senior games were held. Almost every city and country in the world—from Auckland, New Zealand, to Vancouver, British Columbia—has an association devoted to masters athlete competitions. It is uncertain how many masters athletes there are worldwide, but almost every country has competitions designed for masters athletes. Table 14.1 provides an overview of some of the major organizations devoted to masters athletics.

Who Are Masters Athletes?

Many sports have masters divisions defined by the rules of the governing body (eg, USA Track and Field, World Masters Athletics, or National Senior Games Association) or a separate organization designed to meet the needs of retired professional athletes (eg, the Champion's Tour in golf, formerly called the Senior Tour, and the Seniors Tennis Tour). The age at which one becomes a "master" ranges from sport to sport and can be as young as 19 years (swimming) or as old as 50 years (golf). The World Masters Athletics (WMA) organization defines the age for masters athletes as beginning at age 35 years for women and men.

Competition is also age-graded, usually in 5-year intervals. The Web site of the International Association of Athletics Federations (IAAF) displays records for masters events in age-graded categories that go as high as 95- to 99-year-olds. The focus of this chapter is on athletes who are 50 years of age or older.

TABLE 14.1   Examples of Masters Athlete Organizations

Organization	Description
National Senior Games (NSG): www.nsga.com	• *History:* Originated as National Senior Olympics in 1985. Held first National Senior Olympics in 1987 with 2,500 competitors. Changed name to US National Senior Organization in 1990. Today known as National Senior Games. Athletes must be 50 years or older and qualify through National Senior Games Association (NSGA) State Games. • *Sponsored activities:* Summer National Senior Games (held in odd-number years). Winter National Games (held even-number years but suspended in 2001; interest in restarting winter games is evident on Web site). First ever Hockey Championships held in 2007.
International Masters Games Association (IMGA): www.imga.ch	• *History:* First World Masters Games held in 1985. Reorganized in 1995 as IMGA from member International Federations to represent masters sports worldwide. • *Sponsored activities:* European Masters Games held every 4 years. World Masters Games held every 4 years. Summer World and Winter Master Games held every other year.
Huntsman World Senior Games: www.seniorgames.net	• *History:* Began as World Senior Games in 1987. Today known as Huntsman World Senior Games. Open to any athletes age 50 years and older. • *Sponsored activities:* Yearly competitions in St George, UT.
World Masters Athletics: www.world-masters-athletics.org	• *History:* Began by middle-aged road runners and first organized event was held in 1975; it has evolved into an international masters organization for track and field for those age ≥ 35 years. • *Sponsored activities:* Sponsors area and world championships in both stadia (events held within a stadium, such as track-and-field and track running events) and nonstadia (events held on the road, such as cross-country and longer distance events).

Increased Aging Population in the United States

The population is aging and it is a global phenomenon. In the United States the number of people aged 65 and older numbered 39.6 million in 2009, an increase of 4.3 million or 12.5% since 1999. In the government-issued report, Profile of Older Americans 2010, the following statistics are presented (1):

- The number of Americans age 45 to 64 years who will reach 65 during the next 20 years increased by 26% during the last 10 years.
- More than one in every eight, or 12.9%, of the population is older than 65 years of age.
- Individuals reaching age 65 have an average life expectancy of an additional 18.6 years (19.9 years for females and 17.2 years for males).

The Baby Boom generation (born between1946 and 1964) is moving into the ranks of older Americans; by 2030 it is estimated that 20% of the population will be 65 years and older. Compare that to 100 years ago, when only 4% of the population was older than 65 years (2).

The number of older people who will be competing at a masters level in athletics is unknown, but growth in masters competitions in recent years suggests increasing numbers in the future. Dychtwald (3) points out that baby boomers are more likely to be active than the generations before them. According to statistics from the health club industry, adults age 55 and older comprise a quarter of the health club memberships in the United States. From 1998 to 2005, the number of age 55-plus fitness participants increased by 33% while the 18- to 34-year-old group showed no growth (4).

Benefits of Exercise in Adults

In 1996 the Surgeon General issued *Physical Activity and Health: A Report of the Surgeon General* (5), the first report of its kind. In the same year, the World Health Organization issued *The Heidelberg Guidelines for Promoting Physical Activity Among Older Persons,* stressing both the individual as well as the societal benefits of physical activity (6). The physical, mental, and societal benefits of a physically active lifestyle are summarized in Box 14.1 (5,6). The reports concluded that regular physical activity induces higher cardiopulmonary fitness, which decreases overall mortality, reduces risk of coronary heart disease and high blood pressure, reduces the risk of colon cancer, protects against the development of type 2 diabetes

---

BOX 14.1   Benefits of a Physically Active Lifestyle

Physiological Responses
- Decreased resting blood pressure
- Increased cardiac output
- Increased blood flow to skeletal muscles and skin
- Increased maximal oxygen uptake (VO_{2max})
- Increased components of immune system such as natural killer cells and circulating T-lymphocytes and B-lymphocytes
- Increased bone mass
- Increased high-density lipoprotein cholesterol
- Increased strength and balance
- Normalized blood glucose levels

Health Benefits
- Decreased overall mortality
- Decreased risk of cardiovascular disease
- Decreased risk of hypertension
- Decreased risk of thrombosis
- Decreased risk of colon cancer
- Decreased risk of type 2 diabetes mellitus
- Decreased risk of obesity
- Decreased risk of falls and fractures in older adults
- Decreased symptoms of depression and anxiety
- Improved sleep
- Enhanced relaxation
- Enhanced mood state
- Increased psychological well-being
- Enhanced social and cultural integration

Societal Benefits
- Reduced health and social care costs
- Enhanced productivity of older adults
- Promoting a positive and active image of older adults

Source: Data are from references 5 and 6.

mellitus, builds bone mass, increases muscle strength and balance, helps control body weight, relieves the symptoms of depression and anxiety, and improves mood (5,6).

The Centers for Disease Control and Prevention recommend that all adult Americans older than 65 years of age get 150 minutes of moderate activity every week and perform muscle-strengthening activities that work the major muscles two or more times per week (7). At every age, exercise induces beneficial physiological adaptations that improve functional abilities.

A report from the Robert Wood Johnson Foundation, *National Blueprint: Increasing Physical Activity Among Adults Age 50 and Older* (8), suggests many strategies for increasing exercise in older adults and calls for more research to identify seniors who are currently active to help develop interventions for all older adults.

Aging and Exercise

It is common to classify aging based on chronological age, but chronological age is a poor predictor of functional age. Someone may be 50 years old (chronological age) but, due to a sedentary lifestyle, may have difficulty performing activities of daily living (functional age). A 75-year-old who has been physically active throughout life may have better functional capacity than a much younger person who has not been active. For example, a masters athlete at 65 years of age may outperform a sedentary 25-year-old on measures of maximum oxygen consumption (VO_{2max}), muscle strength, and flexibility (9).

Astrand (10) reviewed both laboratory data and statistics of world records and noted that personal best performances decreased after the age of 30 to 35 years. At this age range, there is a decrease in maximum aerobic power, even in those athletes who were well conditioned and trained (10).

Peak performance in a sport depends on the key functional element that is required for success. For example, in sports such as gymnastics for which flexibility is crucial, top athletes are usually in their teens (9). In aerobic sports, competitors usually peak in their mid 20s when training improvements and competition experience help athletes before a decrease in VO_{2max} negates those gains. In sports like golf, the best athletes are generally in their 30s or 40s (9).

Maximum oxygen consumption decreases by approximately 5 mL/kg/min each decade beginning at age 25 years. Researchers note that it is hard to determine how much of this loss is due to the normal aging process or to the adoption of a more sedentary lifestyle. Athletes who train regularly experience a rate of decrease as they age that is slightly slower than the general population (9). Early research with masters athletes was done cross-sectionally, but recent longitudinal studies have reported that the decrease in VO_{2max} in masters athletes is more than previously believed (11). In a longitudinal study of 42 athletes, Katzel et al (12) found a 22% decrease in VO_{2max} in older endurance athletes during an 8-year period of follow-up. The greatest decrease in VO_{2max} occurred in those athletes who could not maintain a high volume of training, suggesting that the decrease in VO_{2max} is less related to aging but more related to an inactive lifestyle (12). In this study, only seven athletes (17% of study participants) were still training at high volume at the end of the study. The authors conclude that maintaining a high level of aerobic fitness, even for the highly motivated athlete, becomes more difficult with advancing age (12).

Muscle strength peaks at approximately 25 years of age, plateaus through ages 35 or 40, and then decreases, with 25% loss of peak strength by age 65 (10). The decrease in muscular strength seems to parallel decreases in muscle mass (10). Aging muscle shows an accumulation of fat and connective tissue coupled with protein mass decline that has been called sarcopenia (13). These decreases in muscle mass and strength seem to be due to a combination of alpha motor neuron loss and reduced number and size of muscle fibers (14). The synthesis of both mitochondrial and myofibrillar proteins is reduced in aging and may be related to decreased growth factors, such as IGF-1, as well as an increase in oxidative damage (14). However, Melov and colleagues reported that a 6-month resistance training program can reverse muscle weakness and improve muscle strength in healthy older adults (15).

Research on Masters Athletes

In general, the research on masters athletes shows that participation in competition at the masters level confers physical and psychological benefits (16–22). Shephard et al (16) studied 750 endurance masters athletes during a 7-year period. During the follow-up, 0.6% had a nonfatal heart attack and 0.6% required coronary bypass surgery. Ninety percent said they were very interested in maintaining good health, 76% considered themselves to be less vulnerable to viral infections than their sedentary peers, and 68% reported their quality of life as much better than their sedentary peers. There were some former smokers in the group, most of whom had stopped smoking before they became regular exercisers. Thirty-seven percent of the former smokers reported that exercise helped them with the effects of withdrawal from tobacco. Fifty-nine percent reported getting regular medical checkups, and 88% reported sleeping very well. The authors concluded that participation in masters competition seems to carry real health benefits, but the gains may, in part, reflect an overall healthful lifestyle (16).

Morgan and Costill (17) reported on health behaviors and psychological characteristics of 15 male marathon runners who were first tested in 1969 (N = 8) and again in 1976 (N = 7) with a mean age of 50 years at the time of follow-up. The health behaviors in this sample of men were uniformly positive: all reported moderate use of alcohol, no insomnia, few physical health problems, and good overall mood (17).

Seals et al (18) compared 14 endurance-trained masters athletes with younger endurance athletes and older sedentary men to determine whether the masters athletes had a more favorable lipid profile than did the younger men or sedentary older men. Diet was not assessed, but alcohol intake was recorded and none of the subjects ingested more than 2 oz of alcohol per day. Total cholesterol (TC) and low-density lipo-protein (LDL) cholesterol were higher in the masters athletes than in the young athletes, and high-density lipoprotein (HDL) cholesterol was significantly higher in the masters athletes than in the other groups (66 mg/dL vs 55 mg/dL in young athletes and 45 mg/dL in older untrained men who were lean). The TC:HDL ratios were lower for both the young and the older groups of athletes compared with the older untrained men. The significantly higher HDL cholesterol levels in the older masters athletes compared with their sedentary peers may confer a reduced risk for coronary artery disease (18).

A longitudinal study on coronary heart disease (CHD) risk factors in older track athletes was reported by Mengelkoch et al (19). Twenty-one subjects, ages 60 to 92 years, were assessed at three evaluation points (initial, 10-year, and 20-year). Measurements included smoking history, blood pressure, resting electro-cardiogram, TC, plasma glucose, body weight, percentage body fat, body mass index (BMI), waist-to-hip ratio (WHR), and VO_{2max}. All CHD risk factors remained low, and even after 20 years all values for variables measured were within normal limits. In this study, the prevalence of CHD risk factors remained low into old age in masters athletes (19), indicating that regular activity has a favorable effect on physical measurements that impact chronic disease risk.

Although it is well established that habitual, high levels of physical activity have a positive effect on blood lipid levels, not much is known about coronary artery calcium (CAC) in master athletes. Wilund et al studied a small sample (7 male and 6 female) of masters athletes and 12 sedentary control subjects (ages 60 to 78 years) and found no significant difference in CAC between athletes and control subjects, but when sexes were separated in the analysis, a moderate relationship between CAC and aerobic fitness was found for the men (20).

Giada et al (21) found that a 2-month hiatus from training resulted in a reversal of the favorable lipid profile found in trained cyclists. Like the decreases in VO_{2max} found with decreased training volume, it seems that continued exercise is necessary to maintain a favorable lipid profile in older athletes.

Seals et al (22) compared endurance-trained masters athletes (mean age of 60 years) with young endurance-trained men (mean age of 26 years) to obtain information about glucose tolerance. Each subject had an oral glucose tolerance test. The masters athletes had a significantly blunted insulin response that was similar to the young athletes. These data suggest the deterioration of glucose tolerance is not inevitable in the aging process and that regular vigorous physical activity can prevent the deterioration of glucose tolerance and insulin sensitivity (22).

There is increasing interest in bone health in the older population, and osteoporosis is considered a major public health concern. According to the National Osteoporosis Foundation, approximately 44 million Americans, or 55% of those older than 50 years of age are at risk for fractures associated with low bone density (23). Currently, 10 million individuals have the disease and an estimated 34 million individuals are diagnosed with osteopenia (low bone mass). Eighty percent of those affected by osteoporosis are women (23).

Florindo et al wanted to determine the relationship between habitual physical exercise throughout life and bone mineral density (BMD) in older men (age older than 50 years) (24). More than 300 men in Brazil were recruited for the study, and BMD was measured at four body sites using dual-energy x-ray absorptiometry (DXA). Habitual exercise in the preceding months, as well as lifetime physical activity, was assessed via questionnaires. The authors found significant positive associations between physical activity and BMD at all sites in these older men (24).

In another study on BMD, runners and swimmers recruited from the 2005 National Senior Olympics and nonathlete control subjects, all older than the age of 65 years, were studied by Velez et al (25). BMD was assessed using DXA at four sites (total body, spine, hip, and forearm). Mean age was 73 years for the athletes and 75 years for the control subjects. Age and weight were adjusted and the researchers found that the athletes had greater total body BMD than did control subjects. The difference was most noticeable between runners and control subjects, and less difference was noted between runners and swimmers. However, both athletes and nonathletes had a high percentage of osteopenia at the femoral neck and the distal radius. The female athletes' Z-scores were well above the national average for their age and sex, suggesting that exercise has a positive effect on mediating bone loss in older women (25).

Currently, there is not abundant research on the benefits of physical activity in masters athletes. Most of the studies involve athletes competing in endurance events (predominantly running and cycling), but it is clear from the research reviewed that people who maintain an active lifestyle reap many physical health benefits. Chronic diseases such as cardiovascular disease, hypertension, and diabetes are rare in masters athletes. Changes considered a "normal" consequence of aging, such as reduced muscle mass and strength, reduced aerobic capacity, bone loss, and deterioration of the insulin response to a glucose challenge, seem to be minimized in masters athletes because of their lifelong habit of physical activity. These athletes might very well "use it and not lose it."

Nutrition Concerns

Energy Expenditure and Energy Intake and Exercise

Although there is evidence to suggest that energy needs decrease with age (approximately one third of the decrease is related to a decrease in basal metabolic rate [BMR] and the remainder to decreases in physical activity), these data do not include individuals who vigorously exercise. Adding a layer of complexity to understanding the effect on aging on resting energy metabolic rate (RMR) was the revelation that one of the

TABLE 14.2 Estimated Energy Requirements for Active Older Adults

Age Group, y	Men, kcal/d	Women, kcal/d
50–59	2,757	2,186
60–69	2,657	2,116
70–79	2,557	2,046
80–89	2,457	1,976

Source: Data are from reference 28.

most prolific authors on the topic (Eric T. Poehlman) falsified data and engaged in scientific misconduct (for a good review on Poehlman, see reference 26). However, Van Pelt et al (27) concluded that RMR decreases with age even in highly active older men, but the decrease is related to age-associated decreases in exercise training and intensity.

The Dietary Reference Intakes (DRIs) for energy and macronutrient intakes established Estimated Energy Requirements (EERs) at four levels of energy expenditure (28). But, even the category of "active" physical activity level, as described by the DRI report, may be too low for a masters athlete. Table 14.2 shows EERs for active older adults, which may be used to determine individualized energy needs (28).

Few studies have assessed energy needs of older exercisers. In the studies that have tried to quantify energy needs (29–31), results have shown that energy needs do not differ for masters athletes compared with younger athletes. The main factor predicting energy needs is the volume of exercise, not aging per se. In a review of energy expenditure and aging, Starling (32) concluded that regular participation in physical activity (aerobic activities, primarily running) may attenuate the age-related decrease in RMR.

Even fewer studies have assessed energy needs of masters athletes engaged in strength training. Campbell et al (31) studied the effects of 12 weeks of progressive resistance training on energy balance in sedentary, healthy older adults (eight men and four women, ages 56 to 80 years). At the end of 12 weeks of strength training, muscular strength increased, fat-free mass increased, fat mass decreased, and mean energy intake needed to maintain body weight increased by approximately 15% during the resistance-training program (31).

Studies have reported that exercise training increases the thermic effect of food (TEF) in older subjects. Lundholm et al (33) studied 10 active, well-conditioned men (mean age 70 years) participating in aerobic exercise three to five times per week for at least 1 hour. Case controls were used for comparison. Subjects were fed a liquid formula containing 500 kcal (56% carbohydrate, 24% protein, 20% fat) and BMR was measured. Higher oxygen uptake was found in the well-trained men compared with the sedentary control subjects, and the TEF was significantly increased (~ 56%). The authors concluded that in this study physical activity seemed to have a potentiating effect on TEF in older subjects.

Although scant research exists on energy needs of masters athletes, practitioners can use the same energy equations that they use for younger athletes in assessing energy needs. It is important to quantify activity as much as possible because training tends to decrease in older athletes, and therefore, based on training volume, energy expenditure might not be as high.

Macronutrients

Carbohydrate should provide the major source of energy in any athlete's diet (see Chapter 2). The DRIs suggest a range of carbohydrate of 45% to 65% of total energy (28). Although no ideal level of carbohydrate consumption has been defined for masters athletes, the guidelines used for younger athletes should be recommended: 3 to 5 g/kg/d for very light, low-intensity skill exercise, 5 to 7 g/kg/d for moderate- to high-intensity exercise, and 7 to 12 g/kg/d for the increased needs of endurance athletes. Flexibility is important in establishing carbohydrate goals, recognizing that individual preferences as well as training and competition schedules may necessitate adjustment of carbohydrate intake (34).

To meet fuel needs and general nutrition goals, athletes who exercise less than 1 hour per day with moderate-intensity activity or several hours with low-intensity exercise should aim for 3 to 7 g/kg/d. For recovery after exercise, 1.0 to 1.5 g/kg carbohydrate is recommended within 1 hour of exercise, with the goal of consuming an additional 1 g/kg 2 hours later. This is especially important for those athletes engaged in daily training. Studies suggest that addition of a small amount of protein along with carbohydrate in the recovery period improves the stimulation of protein synthesis by increasing amino acid delivery to the muscle (35).

Many masters athletes may be confused about the role of carbohydrate in sport because they are exposed to media messages that promote protein as "good" and carbohydrate as "bad." Drastically cutting carbohydrate intake while increasing protein foods may diminish the athlete's performance. Aiming for quality carbohydrates (whole grains, fruits, and vegetables) while decreasing refined carbohydrates and sugar-rich foods is one strategy to help athletes to consume adequate carbohydrate to meet the demands of training and competition, maintain energy balance, and reduce risk for some chronic diseases.

The debate about protein needs of exercising individuals is not new, but the context of aging poses the question: What are the dietary protein requirements of masters athletes? Although the question cannot be answered with precision, several researchers have examined protein requirements in active, older people and have concluded that their needs are similar to younger athletes. Both Meredith et al (36) and Campbell et al (37) studied protein requirements of older, active men. Meredith's group conducted a metabolic study of nitrogen balance and found that with adequate energy intake, protein needs were 0.94 ± 0.05 g/kg/d for older subjects (36).

Campbell et al (37) assessed the effect of 12 weeks of strength training in 12 older men and women. The results showed that whole-body protein was significantly increased with strength training, and nitrogen retention was related to the anabolic stimulus of strength training. The efficiency of nitrogen retention was greater when subjects ingested a lower protein intake (0.8 g/kg/d) compared with a higher protein intake (1.62 g/kg/d). This study demonstrates that the anabolic stimulus of strength training enhances nitrogen retention when protein requirements are based on nitrogen balance studies (37). It can be concluded from this study that protein needs seem to be higher in the early phases of strength training, but are not higher when athletes strength train on a regular basis.

It is reasonable to assume that the protein needs of masters athletes are similar to younger athletes. It is important to remember that in research studies, energy intake is usually adequate to support protein utilization. Athletes who ingest low-calorie diets, less-than-recommended carbohydrate intakes, or who are in the beginning stages of endurance- or strength-training programs need more protein than those who get sufficient energy and carbohydrate or who are well trained (38). The current guidelines for daily protein intake for athletes of 1.2 to 1.7 g/kg can be used for the masters athlete. The DRIs suggest a range of protein from 10% to 35% of total energy (28). With such a wide range for protein recommendations, individual assessment of protein needs is imperative.

The recommended daily intake of fat for athletes is approximately 1 g/kg. Fat intake for older active people does not differ from that of younger people. A minimum of 10% of energy from fat ensures adequate intake of essential fatty acids, with 30% to 35% of energy from fat as the upper limit recommended by most professional health organizations (39). The DRIs suggest fat ranges of 20% to 35% of total energy (28).

Micronutrients

Ideal vitamin and mineral requirements for older individuals have yet to be established. The DRIs recognize the increased need for some micronutrients in people older than age 50 years (40). The DRI for vitamins

D, B-6, and B-12, and the mineral calcium are higher for older adults, and the DRI for iron is decreased for older women. Deficiencies in micronutrients can impair exercise tolerance, but little is known about the dietary intakes or requirements of masters athletes.

Only a few studies have assessed nutrient intakes in masters athletes. Nieman et al (41) studied completed 3-day food records from 291 masters men and 56 masters women who participated in the 1987 Los Angeles Marathon. The authors used national survey data from USDA Continuing Survey of Food Intakes by Individuals (CSFII) to compare the masters runners' nutrient intakes. The masters men marathoners averaged 2,526 kcal/d vs 2,426 kcal/d for CSFII data from men; the masters women marathoners averaged 1,868 kcal/d vs 1,602 kcal/d for CSFII data from women. In this study, the marathoners consumed a greater percentage of their energy from carbohydrate and a smaller percentage of energy from fat compared with data for the general population. Nieman et al found that the women runners had low intakes of vitamin D and zinc compared with the RDA (41).

Chatard and colleagues (42) studied 23 French cyclists, runners, swimmers, walkers, and tennis players (mean age = 63 years). Dietary intakes were recorded twice during 3 consecutive weekdays and compared with the French RDA (ie, *Apports Nutritionnels Conseilles*). The athletes consumed a mean of 2,760 kcal/d compared with the RDA of 2,200 kcal/d, 24% more than the recommended energy intake for the general population. Despite the higher energy intakes, the men still had intakes of vitamin D and magnesium that were less than the French RDA.

A 2003 study (43) of 25 female masters cyclists and runners (mean age 50.4 years) compared supplement users with nonusers. Compared to the non-supplementing athletes, those who took dietary supplements consumed significantly more vitamin C (1,042 mg vs 147 mg), vitamin E (268 mg vs 13 mg), calcium (1,000 mg vs 791 mg), and magnesium (601 mg vs 366 mg). When the diets of the athletes who took supplements were analyzed without the supplements, their mean intakes of vitamin D, vitamin E, folic acid, calcium, magnesium, and zinc were less than the DRI.

Although limited studies have shown that masters athletes have increased energy intake, it is often assumed that higher energy intakes will result in improved nutrient intakes. However, that is not always true for all nutrients. Professionals working with masters athletes should pay close attention to vitamins D, E, B-12, folate, riboflavin, pyridoxine, and the minerals calcium, magnesium, and zinc when assessing diet and performance. Masters athletes in age categories older than 60 years may benefit from synthetic forms of vitamins D and B-12 because absorption and utilization of natural forms may be impaired in aging.

Antioxidant supplements are frequently touted to improve performance and help reduce oxidative damage resulting from exercise. If there is a "down" side to exercise it is the production of free radicals during periods of strenuous activity. Although the body increases its natural antioxidant defense systems in the face of activity (44), it is not clear if it is sufficient to fight free radical production without additional antioxidants obtained from supplements (45). Increasing antioxidant-rich foods in the diet is one way to increase these nutrients, but for vitamin E, a fat-soluble vitamin, it is often difficult to get the DRI of 15 mg without including plant oils, seeds, and nuts. Although the evidence for using antioxidant supplements to combat free radical production is equivocal, using the Tolerable Upper Intake Level (UL) established in the DRIs (2,000 mg of vitamin C and 1,000 mg of vitamin E), can provide guidance for a sports dietitian working with masters athletes (40).

Food and Drug Interactions

Food and drug interactions should be monitored in masters athletes who have chronic conditions that require the use of medications. For example, use of thiazide diuretics causes urinary losses of sodium, potassium, and magnesium, and use of salicylates and nonsteroidal anti-inflammatory drugs (NSAIDS) may cause iron losses. Such losses must be considered when determining dietary needs of older athletes. Nutrient and drug interactions should also be investigated for those masters athletes taking cholesterol-lowering medications and hypertension drugs, such as angiotensin-converting enzyme inhibitors.

Some masters athletes' governing bodies have begun testing for banned substances, and this is not without controversy because many of the drugs on the banned substances lists are medications that are commonly used by older adults to treat disease. Box 14.2 highlights this controversy.

Much remains to be learned about the effect of aging and activity on micronutrient intakes. Blumberg and Meydani (46) point out that there is little evidence to support an ergogenic effect of increased intakes of vitamins or minerals; however, optimal intakes of nutrients show promise to reduce tissue injury resulting from exercise.

BOX 14.2   Medication or Doping?

It is estimated that 46% of those older than the age of 65 years have one or more chronic illnesses (2), and most likely a medication is prescribed to treat the condition. Arthritis, osteoporosis, high blood pressure, cardiovascular disease, and breast cancer are not uncommon conditions in older adults, and many of the medications used to treat the disorders—such as diuretics, beta-blockers, glucocortocoids, aromatase inhibitors, and selected estrogen receptor modulators (SERMS)—are all on the banned substance list. Not every organization tests for banned substances, but for those who do (including World Masters Athletics and International Masters Games Association) athletes may find themselves in violation of doping regulations if they do not apply for a therapeutic use exception.

Older athletes are not immune to the pressures of winning, and just like younger athletes may take performance-enhancing drugs. Consider these two headlines from recent masters competitions:

- **Independent Panel Issues Two-Year Suspension to U.S. Track & Field Athlete, Barnwell, For Doping Offense**: "Colorado Springs, Colo. (March 3, 2010)—USADA announced today that Val Barnwell, a Masters track and field athlete, has received a sanction for testing positive for a banned substance at the 2009 Masters World Championships in Lahti, Finland. Barnwell, 52, of Brooklyn, N.Y., tested positive for testosterone prohormones in a sample collected from him on August 3, 2009, after winning a gold medal in the 200 meter event at the Masters World Championships. Testosterone prohormones are prohibited as Anabolic Agents on the World Anti-Doping Agency Prohibited List, which has been adopted by the USADA Protocol for Olympic Movement Testing and the International Association of Athletics Federations ("IAAF") Anti-Doping Rules." (http://masterstrack.com/2010/03/7977)

- **The Irish athlete Geraldine Finegan declared guilty of an anti-doping rule violation and disqualified from the WMA World Indoor Championships in Kamloops, Canada**: "The WMA acknowledges the information recently received from the Irish Sports Council that Ms Geraldine Finegan, a master athlete from Ireland, was found guilty of a doping offence and sanctioned with a 2-month period of ineligibility (from April 27 to June 26, 2010). The analysis of Ms Finegan's urine sample collected on 5 March 2010 at the WMA World Master Indoor Championships in Kamloops (Canada), revealed the presence of a prohibited stimulant (ephedrine). Her results achieved at the World Indoor Championships, 60mH (1st place) and 400m (3rd place), will be disqualified accordingly." (http://www.world-masters-athletics.org/news/172-the-irish-athlete-geraldine-finegan-declared-guilty-of-an-anti-doping-rule-violation-and-disqualified-from-the-wma-world-indoor-championships-in-kamloops-canada).

Fluids

There are several reasons to be concerned about hydration status in masters athletes. First, older adults have less body water. Body water decreases to about 60% to 70% in older adults, from a high of 80% in infancy (47). Second, thirst sensation decreases with age. Body water regulation relies on thirst to control water intake (47). Third, after the age of 40, renal mass declines with a subsequent decrease in renal blood flow. The ability of the older kidney to concentrate urine decreases, meaning more water is needed to remove waste products (47). In addition, sweat glands change as the skin ages, with less sweat produced per gland with aging (48). Normal age-related changes in thirst and fluid requirements, coupled with the increased need for fluids in the exercising individual, make this a topic of paramount concern to masters athletes.

Kenney and Anderson (49) conducted several studies on the effect of exercise and fluid needs in older individuals. They studied 16 women (8 older women, mean age 56 years; and 8 younger women, mean age 25 years) exercising in hot, dry environments and warm, humid environments. Subjects exercised on a motor-driven treadmill for 2 hours at 35% to 40% VO_{2max} and were not allowed to consume fluids during the trials. Four of the older women were unable to complete either the hot-dry or warm-humid exercise trials. In the warm-humid environment, older women sweat at a rate equal to young women, but in the hot-dry environment the older women sweat less. The authors suggest that older women retain the ability to produce high sweat rates, but the sweat rate may be altered if adequate hydration is not available (49).

Zappe et al (50) studied 12 men (6 active older men, 62 to 70 years, and 6 young men, 17 to 34 years) to assess whether older active men showed an expansion of fluid volume after repeated exercise, as has been found in younger men. Subjects exercised with a cycle ergometer at 50% VO_{2max} for 90 minutes on 4 successive days. No fluids were given during exercise, but 3 mL/kg of sport drinks was given at the end of exercise. During the 4 days of exercise, the older subjects were able to maintain body fluid and electrolyte balance similar to the younger subjects. However, the older subjects did not increase their plasma volume compared with the younger men. The older men had a blunted thirst effect in the face of loss of body water (50).

Kenney and Anderson (49) note that older athletes can exercise in hot environments and can tolerate the heat stress as well as younger athletes of similar VO_{2max}, acclimatization state, body size, and composition. However, there are subtle age-related differences in the blood flow to the skin and body fluid balance. Masters athletes who are well conditioned and acclimatized to the heat should not suffer adverse effects associated with normal aging. Kenney and Anderson suggest that the ability to exercise in warm environments is less a function of aging than of physiological health and functional capacity (51,52). Box 14.3 (52) gives tips for older athletes exercising in hot or humid conditions.

The "graying" of the population brings challenges and opportunities to athletes. Today, older people run marathons, climb mountains, skydive, swim competitively, and hike the 2,160-mile Appalachian Trail. Consider these feats by masters athletes:

- Tom Watson finished second at the 2009 British Open, at the age of 59, losing by one stroke in a playoff.
- Dara Torres is the first ever US swimmer to compete in four Olympic Games and she medaled three times in the 2008 Beijing Olympics at the age of 41.
- Morten Anderson kicked in the National Football League until the age of 48 and holds 5 NFL records, including most field goals and most games played.
- Eamonn Coghlan, a dominating indoor runner in the mid 1970s and 1980s, was the first man older than 40 to break the 4-minute mile.
- Randy Johnson, a pitcher for the Arizona Diamondbacks, threw a perfect game at the age of 40—the oldest player to do so. His last pitch was clocked at 98 miles per hour.

BOX 14.3   Fluid Tips for Older Athletes in Hot or Humid Conditions

- **Acclimate.** Perform about half of your usual exercise on the first few days of hot weather. Decrease the duration or slow down the pace, then gradually build it back up.
- **Hydrate.** Drink approximately 16 oz of fluid 30 to 40 minutes before exercise and at least 8 oz every 15 minutes during exercise. Weigh yourself before and after exercise. After exercise, drink enough fluid to get back to, or near, the pre-exercise weight over a 2-hour period. Eat foods with high water content. Use a sport drink to restore lost electrolytes and keep the "drive to drink" alive.
- **Use common sense.** If you are concerned that it is too hot to exercise, it probably is.
- **Learn about exercise in the heat.** Pay attention to warning signs and symptoms of dehydration, heat exhaustion, and heat stroke.

Source: Data are from reference 52.

- Priscilla Welch, a 58-year-old lifelong marathoner, was named the best female masters marathoner in history by *Runner's World*. At age 42 she won the overall women's title at the New York City marathon, the oldest woman to claim that honor.
- Nolan Ryan played major league baseball for 27 seasons and was still hurling his fastball at 95 miles per hour at the age of 45.
- Boxer George Foreman, who is now well known for his low-fat grilling techniques, won the world heavyweight championship 2 months shy of his 46th birthday.

Summary

The evidence is clear that a vigorous lifestyle can be maintained by many older people. Although there is minimal research on the nutritional needs of masters athletes, several conclusions can be drawn. Metabolic rate is driven by lean tissue and physical activity. Older adults who remain physically active have the same needs for energy as active younger athletes. Energy intake should be adjusted when training volume decreases. Fluid may be the most important nutrient for masters athletes—a programmed schedule of drinking can reduce the risk for dehydration. Carbohydrate, protein, and fat recommendations are the same as for younger athletes, but older adults should pay special attention to vitamin and mineral intakes and a "senior" type multivitamin/mineral supplement may be a good addition to supplement dietary intake. Note that "senior"-formulated vitamin/mineral supplements contain less iron but more vitamins B-12, B-6, and D.

References

1. US Department of Health and Human Services. Administration on Aging. Profile of Older Americans: 2010. http://www.aoa.gov/aoaroot/aging_statistics/Profile/2010/docs/2010profile.pdf. Accessed March 7, 2011.
2. Moody HR. *Aging Concepts and Controversies*. 6th ed. Los Angeles, CA: Pine Forge Press; 2010.
3. Dychtwald K. Introduction: healthy aging or Tithonius' revenge? In: Dychtwald K, ed. *Healthy Aging: Challenges and Solutions*. Gaithersburg, MD: Aspen Publishers; 1999:1–16.

4. Health Clubs. http://clubindustry.com/statistics. Accessed July 15, 2010.

5. US Department of Health and Human Services. *Physical Activity and Health: A Report of the Surgeon General.* Atlanta, GA: US Dept Health and Human Services, Centers for Disease Control and Prevention, National Center for Chronic Disease Prevention and Health Promotion; 1996.

6. World Health Organization. *The Heidelberg Guidelines for Promoting Physical Activity Among Older Persons.* Geneva, Switzerland: WHO; 1996.

7. Centers for Disease Control and Prevention. How Much Physical Activity Do Older Adults Need? http://www.cdc.gov/physicalactivity/everyone/guidelines/olderadults.html. Accessed July 18, 2010.

8. Robert Wood Johnson Foundation. *National Blueprint: Increasing Physical Activity Among Adults Age 50 and Older.* Princeton, NJ: Robert Wood Johnson Foundation; 2001. http://www.rwjf.org/publications/publicationsPdfs/Age50_Blueprint_singlepages.pdf. Accessed June 1, 2010.

9. Shephard RJ. Aging and exercise. In: Fahey TD, ed. *Encyclopedia of Sports Medicine and Science.* Internet Society for Sport Science. http://www.sportsci.org/encyc/agingex/agingex.html. Accessed January 10, 2004.

10. Astrand PO. Exercise physiology of the mature athlete. In: Sutton JR, Brock RM, eds. *Sports Medicine for the Mature Athlete.* Indianapolis, IN: Benchmark Press; 1986:3–13.

11. Wiswell RA, Jaque SV, Marcell TJ, Hawkins SA, Tarpenning KM, Constantino N, Hyslop DM. Maximal aerobic power, lactate threshold, and running performance in master athletes. *Med Sci Sports Exerc.* 2000;32:1165–1170.

12. Katzel LI, Sorkin JD, Fleg JL. A comparison of longitudinal changes in aerobic fitness in older endurance athletes and sedentary men. *J Am Geriatr Soc.* 2001;49:1657–1664.

13. Yarasheski KE. Exercise, aging, and muscle protein metabolism. *J Gerontol Med Sci.* 2003;58A:918–922.

14. Tarnopolsky MA. Nutritional considerations in the aging athlete. *Clin J Sport Med.* 2008;18:531–538.

15. Melov S, Tarnopolsky MA, Beckman K, Felkey K, Hubbard A. Resistance exercise reverses aging in human skeletal muscle. *PLoS ONE.* 2007;2:e465. doi:10.1371/journal.pone.0000465.

16. Shephard RJ, Kavanagh T, Mertens DJ, Qureshi S, Clark M. Personal health benefits of Masters athletic competition. *Br J Sports Med.* 1995;29:35–40.

17. Morgan WP, Costill DL. Selected psychological characteristics and health behaviors of aging marathon runners: a longitudinal study. *Int J Sports Med.* 1996;17:305–312.

18. Seals DR, Allen WK, Hurley BF, Dalsky GP, Ehsani AA, Hagberg JM. Elevated high-density lipoprotein cholesterol levels in older endurance athletes. *Am J Cardiol.* 1984;54:390–393.

19. Mengelkoch LJ, Pollock ML, Limacher MC, Graves JE, Shireman RB, Riley WJ, Lowenthal DT, Leon AS. Effects of age, physical training, and physical fitness on coronary heart disease risk factors in older track athletes at twenty-year follow-up. *J Am Geriatr Soc.* 1997;45:1446–1453.

20. Wilund KR, Tomayko EJ, Evans EE, Kim K, Ishaque MR, Fernhall B. Physical activity, coronary artery calcium, and bone mineral density in elderly men and women: a preliminary investigation. *Metab Clin Exp.* 2008;57:584–591.

21. Giada F, Vigna GB, Vitale E, Baldo-Enzi G, Bertaglia M, Crecca R, Fellin R. Effect of age on the response of blood lipids, body composition, and aerobic power to physical conditioning and deconditioning. *Metabolism.* 1995;44:161–165.

22. Seals DR, Hagberg JM, Allen WK, Dalsky GP, Ehsani AA, Holloszy JO. Glucose tolerance in young and older athletes and sedentary men. *J Appl Physiol.* 1984;56:1521–1525.

23. Fast facts on osteoporosis. National Osteoporosis Foundation. http://www.nof.org/osteoporosis/diseasefacts.htm. Accessed July 10, 2010.

24. Florindo AA, Latorre MR, Jaime PC, Tanaka T, Pippa MGB, Zerbini CAF. Past and present habitual physical activity and its relationship with bone mineral density in men aged 50 years and older in Brazil. *J Gerontol Med Sci.* 2002;57A:M654–M657.

25. Velez NF, Zhang A, Stone B, Perera S, Miller M, Greenspan SL. The effect of moderate impact exercise on skeletal integrity in masters athletes. *Osteoporosis Int.* 2008;19:1457–1464.

26. Dunford M. After the storm: body composition, RMR, and aging. *Dietetic Technicians in Practice* (newsletter). 2006;12:1-3–6.

27. Van Pelt RE, Dinneno FA, Seals DR, Jones PP. Age-related decline in RMR in physically active men: relation to exercise volume and energy intake. *Am J Physiol Endocrinol Metab.* 2001;281:E633–E639.

28. Institute of Medicine. *Dietary Reference Intakes for Energy, Carbohydrates, Fiber, Fat, Protein, and Amino Acids (Macronutrients).* Washington, DC: National Academies Press; 2002. http://www.nap.edu/books. Accessed July 26, 2010.

29. Bunyard LB, Katzel LI, Busby-Whitehead MJ, Wu Z, Goldberg AP. Energy requirements of middle-aged men are modifiable by physical activity. *Am J Clin Nutr.* 1998;86:1136–1142.

30. Wilmore JH. Stanforth PR, Hudspeth LA, Gagnon J, Daw EW, Leon AS, Rao DC, Skinner JS, Bouchard C. Alterations in resting metabolic rate as a consequence of 20 wk of endurance training: the HERITAGE Family Study. *Am J Clin Nutr.* 1998;68:66–71.

31. Campbell WW, Crim MC, Young VR, Evan WJ. Increased energy requirements and changes in body composition with resistance training in older adults. *Am J Clin Nutr.* 1994;60:167–175.

32. Starling RD. Energy expenditure and aging: effects of physical activity. *Int J Sport Nutr Exerc Metab.* 2001; 11(suppl):S208–S217.

33. Lundholm K, Holm G, Lindmark L, Larrson B, Sjostrom L, Bjorntop P. Thermogenic effect of food in physically well trained elderly men. *Eur J Appl Physiol.* 1986;55:486–492.

34. Burke LM, Cox GR, Culmmings NK, Desbrow B. Guidelines for daily carbohydrate intake: do athletes need them? *Sports Med.* 2001;31:267–299.

35. Tipton KD, Rasmussen BB, Miller SL, Wolf SE, Owens-Stovall SK, Petrini BE, Wolfe RR. Timing of amino acid-carbohydrate ingestion alters anabolic response of muscle to resistance exercise. *Am J Physiol Endocrinol Metab.* 2001;281:E197–E206.

36. Meredith CN, Zacklin WR, Frontera WR, Evans WJ. Dietary protein requirements and body protein metabolism in endurance-trained men. *J Appl Physiol.* 1989;66:2850–2856.

37. Campbell WW, Crim MC, Young VR, Joseph LJ, Evans WJ. Effects of resistance training and dietary protein intake on protein metabolism in older adults. *Am J Physiol.* 1995;268:E1143–E1153.

38. Lemon PWR. Effects of exercise on dietary protein requirements. *Int J Sport Nutr.* 1998;8:426–447.

39. Krauss RM, Eckel RH, Howard B, Appel LJ, Daniels SR, Dickelbaum RJ, Erdman JW, Kris-Etherton P, Goldberg IJ, Kotchen TA, Lichtenstein AH, Mitch WE, Mullis R, Robinson K, Wylie-Rosett J, St Jeor S, Suttie J, Tribble DL, Bazzarre T. AHA Dietary Guidelines: Revision 2000: a statement for healthcare professionals from the Nutrition Committee of the American Heart Association. *Circulation.* 2000;102:2296–2311.

40. Institute of Medicine. *Dietary Reference Intakes: Recommended Intakes for Individuals.* Washington, DC: National Academies Press; 1998.

41. Nieman DC, Butler JC, Pollett LM, Dietrich SJ, Lutz RD. Nutrient intake of marathon runners. *J Am Diet Assoc.* 1989;89:1273–1278.

42. Chatard JC, Boutet C, Tourny C, Garcia S, Berthouze S, Guezennec CY. Nutritional status and physical fitness in elderly sportsmen. *Eur J Appl Physiol.* 1998;77:157–163.

43. Beshgetoor D, Nichols JF. Dietary intake and supplement use in female master cyclists and runners. *Int J Sport Nutr Exerc Metab.* 2003;13:166–172.

44. Powers SK, Criswell D, Lawler J, Martin D, Lieu F, Ji L, Herb RA. Rigorous exercise training increases superoxide dismutase activity in ventricular myocardium. *Am J Physiol.* 1998;265:H2094–H2098.

45. Clarkson PM, Thompson HS. Antioxidants: what role do they play in physical activity and health? *Am J Clin Nutr.* 2000;72(2 Suppl):637S–646S.

46. Blumberg JB, Meydani M. The relationship between nutrition and exercise in older adults. In: Lamb DR, Gisolfi CV, Nadal E, eds. *Perspectives in Exercise Science and Sports Medicine: Exercise in Older Adults.* Vol 8. Carmel, IN: Cooper Publishing Group; 1995:353–394.

47. Chernoff R. Thirst and fluid requirements. *Nutr Rev.* 1994;52(suppl):S3–S5.

48. Kenney WL, Fowler SR. Methylcholine-activated eccrine sweat gland density and output as a function of age. *J Appl Physiol.* 1988;65:1082–1086.

49. Kenney WL, Anderson RK. Responses of older and younger women to exercise in dry and humid heat without fluid replacement. *Med Sci Sports Exerc.* 1988;20:155–160.

50. Zappe DH, Bell GW, Swartzentruber H, Wideman RF, Kenney WL. Age and regulation of fluid and electrolyte balance during repeated exercise sessions. *Am J Physiol.* 1996;270:R71–R79.

51. Kenney WL. Are there special hydration requirements for older individuals engaged in exercise? *Austral J Nutr Diet.* 1996;53(suppl):S43–S44.

52. Kenney WL. The older athlete: exercise in hot environments. *Sports Sci Exch.* 1993;6(3). http://www.gssiweb.com. Accessed November 11, 2004.

Chapter 15

ELITE ATHLETES

Louise M. Burke, OAM, PhD, APD, FACSM

Introduction

The usual working definition of *elite* is "the best" or "the chosen few." This chapter addresses the nutritional needs of athletes who have reached the professional, world-class, or Olympic rank in their respective sports. These athletes have special nutritional requirements or challenges as a result of their extreme levels of training and competition, as well as the lifestyle that underpins their sporting involvement.

Sports dietitians are drawn to work with top athletes for many reasons, including the following:

- These athletes are often operating at the extremes of human nutrition and physiological capacity. It is fascinating to see what the human body can achieve and how it must be fueled to reach this level of operation.
- Elite athletes represent a motivated group of clients who seek and appreciate the nutrition advice that they are offered and usually adhere to recommendations.
- Sports dietitians have the opportunity to work with famous people and in high-profile situations, which can seem glamorous and publicize a private practice.
- Sports dietitians are surrounded by inspired and inspiring people. They become participants in the excitement and emotion of high-level sports competitions.
- The work can provide opportunities to travel.
- Sports nutrition is a precise discipline with tangible benefits. The athlete and the sports dietitian receive short-term rewards and rapid feedback about the success of their nutrition strategies.
- The work draws on the sports dietitian's creativity and ingenuity to find practical strategies to address the athlete's unique nutritional challenges. Finding individualized solutions to these problems is interesting and challenging.

Of course, these and other ideas about working with elite athletes are usually just perceptions, and some ideas are ill founded. For example, many dietetics students are interested in sports nutrition as an alternative to a career in weight-loss counseling. Yet, the most common reason for athletes to seek the help of a sports dietitian is to reduce weight or body fat. This chapter will provide an overview of some of the nutritional issues that are important to top-level athletes as well as strategies for the sports dietitian to work successfully with such clients.

The Structure of High-Level Sport—Implications for Nutritional Needs and Practice

There are several characteristics of high-level sports that create special nutritional needs or challenges for the athletes involved (1). These include the following:

- Heavy training load
- Demanding competition schedule
- Frequent travel
- Unusual environments for training adaptations or competition preparation (heat, altitude)
- The culture of sport: the price and rewards of fame and publicity
- Influence and power of coaches and other personnel involved with the athlete

Although there are clear differences among sports, the elite or professional athlete typically trains 15 to 30 hours each week. Because this usually involves moderate- to high-intensity exercise, the training program typically results in a high energy cost, targeted carbohydrate needs, and substantial losses of fluids and electrolytes through sweating. Precisely because of the intense training, there is also a new focus on the timing of nutrient intake in relation to exercise, based on the principle that the special nutritional needs of high-level exercise are best met by a strategic intake of carbohydrate and fluid before and during key exercise sessions (2,3) and the intake of carbohydrate (4) and protein (5) during recovery after the workout. To meet such goals, an athlete will need access to a supply of suitable foods or tailor-made sports products providing these nutrients, and will also need an opportunity and appetite to consume them in sufficient amounts. Several factors can challenge these goals, particularly during periods of travel; this will be discussed separately in this chapter

Finally, it is presumed that any increases in nutrient requirements due to sport (see Chapters 2–6) are met within a well-chosen and varied diet that meets the athlete's increased energy needs. However, very few studies have been conducted on the dietary practices of the world's top athletes, and much of the available literature fails to address the potential for biased data due to the limitations of dietary survey methodology (6). Even fewer studies have measured indexes of nutritional status among top athletes. Nevertheless, it seems that most elite male athletes at least have the potential to consume diets that meet the present guidelines for sports nutrition. By contrast, elite female athletes are at greater general risk of suboptimal intakes of a range of nutrients due to their apparent restriction of energy intakes and pursuit of fad diets due to concerns about body mass and body fat (6). Other athletes at risk are those involved in weight-controlled or weight-division sports (eg, boxing, wrestling, weightlifting, lightweight rowing, etc), for which preparation for competition often involves severe energy restriction (7).

The competition schedule of the elite athlete usually presents a different set of nutritional and lifestyle challenges to the training situation. In general, athletes organize their training to "peak" for one to three major competitions each year; however, most will compete in several other events each year. Athletes use these minor competitions to practice and fine-tune their strategies for key events, or to provide themselves with a high-quality "training" session for the more important competitions. In addition, each competition may involve more than one round of events (ie, heats, semifinals, and finals) that ultimately decide the final outcome. Other sports, particularly team sports, can be played in a tournament format with a series of games every 24 to 72 hours. In team sports played seasonally, the traditional weekly game has now developed to have an even more demanding competitive schedule at the elite level. In fact, it is not unusual for professional soccer and basketball players to play a match every 2 or 3 days, especially when the player or the team is entered into more than one association or league (8).

During such competition phases, the athlete is usually focused on acute issues of refueling and rehydration—undertaking special eating strategies before, during, and after an event to meet the needs of the event. Travel and other factors that limit food availability can often challenge the athlete to meet immediate nutritional goals, not to mention the "big picture" issues of energy balance and overall macronutrient and micronutrient needs. The sports dietitian needs to be creative in helping the athlete achieve strategies such as carbohydrate loading, an optimal pre-event meal, food and fluid intake during an event, and proactive recovery eating. However, when competition makes up a substantial proportion of the elite athlete's life and total eating patterns—for example, professional cyclists who compete approximately 100 days each year and ride in stage races lasting up to 3 weeks in duration (9)—there is a need for competition nutrition strategies that also include all dietary goals.

The lifestyle of most top-level athletes is busy and irregular. At the entry point into an elite sport, many younger athletes juggle training and events around the commitments of high school and college. Because many sports are not wholly "professional" or financially rewarding, some top-class athletes must continue to work part- or full-time in addition to their sporting commitments. Meals and snacks eaten during the day must fit into their lifestyles (eg, work, school, and family commitments). A chaotic or displaced eating pattern may challenge some athletes to meet the high energy and nutrient requirements associated with maturational and muscular growth, training, and recovery—in particular, prolonged sessions of high-intensity work or resistance-training programs designed to increase muscle size and strength.

Professional (or otherwise "full-time") athletes generally have the luxury of spreading their training schedule and other commitments, such as medical and testing appointments or team activities, over the day. However, sometimes during periods of multiple daily practices, training camps, or competition travel, athletes are faced with a busy timetable that interferes with a normal eating schedule. At other times, they are left with a considerable amount of free time during the day. In some situations, eating becomes a form of entertainment, which can lead to nutritional problems such as the intake of unnecessary amounts or inappropriate choices of food. In both situations, it is important for athletes to have a clear understanding of their nutritional goals and formulate an eating program that can achieve such goals.

The elite level of sport is a specialized environment, which includes not only the physical aspects of club rooms and training and competition venues, but also the culture of each sport. The pressure to win often means that the athlete is desperate to find dietary shortcuts or "magic bullets," becoming an easy target for the unsupported claims made for fad diets, dietary supplements, and other unusual eating strategies. The athlete is not only susceptible, but also is often specifically targeted by companies and individuals who recognize the benefits of being associated with a high-profile individual or team. Many sports provide an insular world where high-level athletes swap ideas and theories with their peers, trainers, and coaches, or are influenced by material on the Internet and in sports magazines, without necessarily checking the credibility of their information sources. Sports dietitians need to break into these circles to be aware of the latest trends and ideas. They must also contend with a wide array of other, often influential, sources of nutrition advice directed at the athlete. They may also have to fight for the athlete's time, concentration, or resources; these are often limited and must be shared with other sports science and medical professionals, the media, managers, and the coaching and training staff. On the positive side, most top-level athletes take a professional approach to the preparation for their sport and will make effective use of information and practical advice. The structure of many high-level teams and sporting organizations is to surround their athletes with a group of professionals specializing in sports science/medicine and training/conditioning. It is both efficient and rewarding to be part of such a support network.

Nutritional Issues

Meeting Energy and Fuel Needs Across a Range of Extremes

An athlete's energy intake is of interest for several reasons (10):

- It sets the potential for achieving the athlete's requirements for energy-containing macronutrients (especially protein and carbohydrate) and the food needed to provide vitamins, minerals, and other non–energy-containing dietary compounds required for optimal function and health.
- It assists the manipulation of muscle mass and body fat levels to achieve the specific body composition that is ideal for athletic performance.
- It affects the function of hormonal and immune systems.
- It challenges the practical limits to food intake set by issues such as food availability and gastrointestinal comfort.

The total energy expenditure of each athlete is unique, arising from the contribution of basal metabolic rate, the thermic effects of food, and exercise, and, in some cases, growth. Energy expenditure is increased by high levels of lean body mass, growth (including the desired adaptations to a resistance-training program), and a high-volume training program. For some elite athletes these three factors co-exist to create very large energy demands—for example, the male swimmer or rower who faces an increase in training commitment during periods of adolescent growth spurts. Other elite athletes have very large energy requirements due to the extraordinary fuel demands of their competition programs. The energy and fuel costs of very strenuous exercise programs are impressively high. For example, professional cyclists in the Grand Tours have been reported to consume mean daily intakes exceeding 5,500 kcal and 12 g carbohydrate per kg body weight for periods of 3 weeks, albeit during competition (11,12). During the 2008 Beijing Olympic Games, media sources reported that eight-time gold medal–winning swimmer Michael Phelps consumed approximately 12,000 kcal/d. This "fact" created considerable awe among the public, but caused skepticism among sports nutrition experts. Phelps denied this information in his subsequent autobiography (13), claiming his true intake may be up to 8,000 to 10,000 kcal/d. These figures may be estimates of his heaviest days of intake rather than a true average, but nevertheless illustrate the potential for high energy needs among athletes with heavy training loads.

At such extreme levels of energy demand, elite athletes are often advised to consume foods and drinks, particularly in the form of carbohydrate and/or protein, at special times or in greater quantities than would be provided in an everyday diet or dictated by their appetite and hunger. Athletes may also need to consume energy during and after exercise when the availability of foods and fluids, or opportunities to consume them, are limited. Practical issues interfering with the achievement of energy intake goals during postexercise recovery include loss of appetite and fatigue, poor access to suitable foods, and distraction from other activities. In contrast, other elite athletes have low-moderate energy needs—particularly when they are trying to lose body weight or maintain low levels of body fat or are involved in a sport in which training, however prolonged, is based on skill rather than energy expenditure, such as gymnastics, archery, or baseball. Such athletes face many practical challenges in satisfying their nutritional goals and appetite with a smaller energy budget. Specialized advice from a sports dietitian is therefore often useful to assist in the achievement of the energy intake challenges faced by individual athletes. See Box 15.1 for suggestions for increasing energy intake (10) and refer to Chapter 11 for additional information relevant to this topic.

BOX 15.1   Guidelines for Achieving High Energy Intakes by Elite Athletes

Meal Spacing
- Use a food diary to identify *actual* intake rather than perceived intake.
- Consume carbohydrate during prolonged exercises to provide fuel and additional energy.
- Eat a carbohydrate and protein snack after exercise to enhance recovery and increase total daily energy intake.

Food Availability
- Shop for food and prepare meals in advance of hectic periods.
- Overcome postexercise fatigue by preparing meals and snacks in advance.
- When traveling, take snacks that can be easily prepared and eaten (eg, cereal and powdered milk, granola and sport bars, liquid meal supplements, and dried fruit and nuts).
- Have snacks and light meals available at home (eg, fruit, fruit smoothies, yogurt, and sandwiches).
- Consider specialized products such as sport drinks, gels, and bars during exercise and sport bars and liquid meal supplements after exercise. (In most training situations, athletes will need to provide their own products.)

Appetite Management and Gastric Comfort
- Reduce gastric discomfort with small frequent meals.
- Drink liquid meal supplements, flavored milk, fruit smoothies, sport drinks, and juices to provide energy, nutrients, and fluids.
- Choose energy-dense meals and snacks, including sugar-rich foods.
- Avoid excessive intake of high-fiber foods, which may limit total energy intake or lead to gastrointestinal discomfort.
- Appetite suppression may be overcome with small pieces or easy-to-eat foods that do not require considerable cutting and chewing (eg, fruit, sandwiches served as "finger-foods," or a stir-fry).
- Consider postexercise environmental conditions. Heat and dehydration may be matched by cool and liquid-based choices such as fruit smoothies, yogurt, or ice cream. In cold conditions, warm soup, toasted sandwiches, or pizza may be more appetizing.

Source: Data are from reference 10.

The "Ideal" Body Composition for Optimal Performance

Physical characteristics, including height, limb lengths, total body mass (weight), muscle mass, and body fat can all play a role in sports performance. Many elite athletes are subjected to rigid criteria for an "ideal physique," based on the characteristics of other successful competitors. The pressure to conform to such an ideal comes from the athlete's own perfectionism and drive to succeed as well as the influence of coaches, trainers, other athletes, and the media. Although athletes at all levels may battle to achieve their desired weight and body fat level, a disadvantage of being an elite athlete is that this battle may be played out in the public arena, via commentary on Internet sites, in newspapers and magazines, and the discussion of sports reporters. The need to wear skimpy clothing in public has been identified as a risk factor for the development of disordered eating among athletes (14). Imagine how this stress is amplified when the (largely sedentary) audience can be measured in the millions and feels justified in criticizing the athlete for "bulges" made apparent by tight-fitting spandex. Many well-known female swimmers, tennis players, and gymnasts have suffered such humiliation.

Although information about the physique of elite athletes is a source of fascination for the community as well as other athletes, we should be cautious about making rigid prescriptions about the "ideal" physique based on the anthropometrics of successful competitors. The concept of a single "ideal" fails to take into account the considerable variability in the physical characteristics of people, even among individuals in the same sport. Furthermore, athletes sometimes need many years of training and maturation to finally achieve their optimal shape and body composition, and even the best training cannot provide the inherited physical characteristics that predispose some athletes to excel at a sport. Finally, because a wide variety of techniques are used to assess characteristics such as body fat or lean mass, it is impractical to generalize from available data about specific athletes in order to define an "ideal" body type.

A preferable strategy is to use a range of acceptable values for body fat and body weight within each sport, and then monitor the health and performance of individual athletes within this range. Sequential profiling of an athlete can monitor the development of physical characteristics that are associated with good performance for that individual, as well as identify the changes in physique that can be expected over a season or period of specialized training.

A reduction in body mass, particularly through loss of body fat, is a common nutritional goal of elite athletes. There are situations when athletes are clearly carrying excess body fat and will improve their health and performance by reducing body fat levels. This may occur due to heredity or lifestyle factors, or because the athlete has been in a situation in which a sudden change in energy expenditure has occurred without a compensatory change in energy intake—for example, the athlete has failed to reduce energy intake while injured or taking a break from training. Loss of body fat should be achieved through a program based on a sustained and moderate energy deficit, while maintaining adequate energy availability of more than 30 kcal per kg of fat-free mass, where energy availability is defined as the amount of energy made available for general body functions once the energy cost of exercise is subtracted from energy intake (14).

However, in many sports in which a low body mass or body fat level offers distinct advantages to performance, fat loss has become a focus or even obsession. The benefits of leanness can be seen in terms of the energy cost of movement (eg, distance running, cycling), the physics of movement in a tight space or against gravity (eg, gymnastics, diving, cycling uphill), or aesthetics (eg, gymnastics, bodybuilding). In many such "weight-conscious" or "body fat-conscious" sports, elite athletes now strive to achieve minimum body fat levels, with many trying to reduce their body fat to less than the level that seems "natural" or "healthy" for them. In the short term, this may produce an improvement in performance. However, the long-term disadvantages include outcomes related to having very low body-fat stores, as well as the problems associated with unsound weight-loss methods. Excessive training, chronically low intakes of energy and nutrients, and psychological distress are often involved in fat-loss strategies and may cause long-term damage to health, well-being, or performance (14). In recent years, some athletes have died as an apparent result of unsafe weight-loss techniques (15), including training while severely restricting energy, dehydration, and the use of ephedrine-containing fat-loss supplements (16). Weight management is covered in greater detail in Chapter 11.

The Special Challenges of Travel

Travel plays a major role in the lifestyle of the elite athlete, with most world-class athletes traveling within their own state or country as well as internationally for competition or specialized training opportunities. The various challenges imposed by travel are summarized in Box 15.2 (17) and include disruption to the

BOX 15.2 Challenges and Solutions for Traveling Athletes

Challenges of Traveling
- Disruptions to the normal training routine and lifestyle while the athlete is en route
- Changes in climate and environment that create different nutritional needs (especially relevant during training camps at altitude or for heat acclimatization)
- Jet lag
- Changes to food availability, including absence of important and familiar foods
- Reliance on hotels, restaurants, and takeaways instead of home cooking
- Exposure to new foods and eating cultures
- Temptations of an "all you can eat" dining hall in an athletes' village
- Risk of gastrointestinal illnesses due to exposure to food and water with poor hygiene standards
- Excitement and distraction of a new environment

Coping Strategies
- **Planning ahead**: Athletes should investigate food issues on travel routes (eg, airlines) and at the destination before leaving home. Caterers and food organizers should be contacted well ahead of the trip to let them know meal timing and menu needs.
- **Supplies to supplement the local fare**: A supply of portable and nonperishable foods should be taken or sent to the destination to replace important items that may be missing. Useful items include breakfast cereal, cereal bars, crackers, dried fruit, and specialized sport products such as powdered liquid meals and sport drinks. Athletes should be aware that many catering plans only cover meals. Because the athlete's nutrition goals are likely to include well-timed and well-chosen snacks, supplies should be taken to supplement meals en route and at the destination.
- **Eating and drinking well en route**:
  o Many athletes will turn to "boredom eating" when confined. Instead, they should eat according to their real needs, taking into account the forced rest while travelling.
  o When moving to a new time zone, athletes should adopt eating patterns that suit their destination as soon as the trip starts. This will help the body clock adapt.
  o Unseen fluid losses in air conditioned vehicles and pressurized plane cabins should be recognized, and a drinking plan should be organized to keep the athlete well hydrated.
- **Taking care with food/water hygiene**:
  o It is important to find out whether the local water supply is safe to drink. Otherwise, the athlete should stick to drinks from sealed bottles, or hot drinks made from boiled water. Ice added to drinks is often made from tap water and may be a problem.
  o In high-risk environments, the athlete should eat only at reputable hotels or well-known restaurants. Food from local stalls and markets should be avoided, despite the temptation to have an "authentic cultural experience."
  o Food that has been well cooked is the safest; it is best to avoid salads or unpeeled fruit that has been in contact with local water or soil.
- **Adhering to the food plan**:
  o Athletes should choose the best of the local cuisine to meet their nutritional needs, supplementing with their own supplies when needed.
  o Athletes should be assertive in asking for what they need at catering outlets—eg, low-fat cooking styles or an extra carbohydrate choice.
  o The challenges of "all you can eat" dining should be recognized. Athletes should resist the temptation to eat "what is there" or "what everyone else is eating" and instead stick to their own meal plan.

Source: Data are from reference 17.

athlete's normal eating routine and access to his or her preferred foods, as well as exposure to a different standard of food and water hygiene. The process of travel itself is also problematic, exposing the athlete to jet lag, interruption of the normal training program, and "boredom eating" when confined during travel.

Elite athletes need to become organized travelers, identifying the challenges of their intended locations before the trip, and planning to circumvent potential problems (see Box 15.2). During the travel, athletes should adjust their eating to suit a period of inactivity as well as any increases in fluid losses due to a dry atmosphere. They should also switch to a meal routine based on the time zone of their country of destination to assist with the change in "body clock." The travel plan may include organizing catering needs and menus before the trip. In addition, supplies of special foods and drinks may be taken on the trip to complement these catering plans or to make up for the absence of key nutrients or favorite foods.

Of course, these plans must be implemented with understanding of some of the practical constraints involved. For example, quarantine laws in some countries or states may prevent the importation of some food products. In addition, athletes should be aware that heightened security regulations and the increase in oil prices have made travel more challenging. Tighter weight restrictions on checked luggage make it difficult for athletes to include their own specialized sporting equipment let alone food supplies, and large containers of liquids may not be carried onto a flight. Strategies to address these challenges include removing packaging from foodstuffs and taking powdered versions of sports foods to lighten luggage, or organizing supplies to be freighted over or delivered directly to travel destinations rather than transported with the athlete. Elite athletes can sometimes be fortunate in having personal or team-based sponsorships with airlines or other travel agencies that can facilitate the transport of their luggage needs. Being famous can be beneficial when presenting to a check-in with special needs, but a good travel plan should not rely on special last-minute help. If sport foods or supplements are sourced from a local supplier, the athlete should take special caution regarding the potential for contamination with banned substances (see supplements section later in this chapter).

Often, competitions or specialized training protocols occur in physiologically challenging environments, such as a hot climate or moderate altitude. For example, the Summer Olympic Games were held in very hot weather in Atlanta (1996), Athens (2004), and Beijing (2008), and soccer matches during the 2010 World Cup in Johannesburg were played at an altitude of approximately 1,700 meters. In such cases, the athlete usually undertakes a period of acclimatization in a similar environment, or in a chamber that can simulate the same characteristics as the competition site. This is done as a final preparation for the competition. However, on other occasions the athlete may choose to train in hot conditions or at a high altitude (or simulated altitude) to gain physiological adaptations that will be applied to a moderate weather or sea-level environment. Nutritional requirements during these specialized periods will reflect both the type of training, ranging from a precompetition taper to a period of intensified training, as well as the additional needs posed by heat or altitude. In both hot and moderate- to high-altitude environments, the athlete can expect to incur an increase in sweat losses and carbohydrate use compared with exercise in a control condition (18). As a result, the athlete will need to focus on appropriate carbohydrate and fluid replacement strategies before, during, and after each exercise session as well as throughout the day. Iron and micronutrient requirements may increase under these conditions.

Finally, some sporting competitions or environments involve cultural, religious, or practical limitations on the food supply that athletes must plan for. Athletes traveling to Muslim-based countries may find that they are unable to access pork products on menus; in deference to the Hindu population, beef may not be served, as was the case in the athletes' dining hall at the 2010 Commonwealth Games in New Delhi, India. Around the world, many institutions enact a ban on nuts or other high-risk food allergens. When these foods play a large role in the athlete's diet, it can be difficult to find a sufficient range of alternative choices. The 2012 London Olympic Games is of interest because of the overlap between the month of Ramadan (July

20 to August 18) and the competition schedule (July 27 to August 12). Fasting during Ramadan, the ninth month of the lunar calendar, is one of the five pillars of the Islamic faith and involves the abstention from all fluid and food intake during the period from first light to sunset as well as prayer and food rituals involved with the breaking of the fast and throughout the night. Although Ramadan is an annual event that coincides with various sporting competitions each year, the London Olympics will create additional focus on the interaction of fasting on athletic performance because of the potentially large number of Muslim athletes who will participate in these games and the special catering arrangements that will be needed to accommodate this fasting ritual (19).

Do the Results of Studies on Recreational Athletes Apply to Elite Athletes?

Some people think that sport foods and supplements or sports nutrition strategies such as carbohydrate-loading are targeted at the elite athlete. It is true that the pressures and rewards for optimal performance are greater at this level and may justify the expense or effort involved in addressing special nutrition needs. However, the majority of studies on sports nutrition strategies involve subjects throughout the spectrum, from recreationally active to well trained. In fact, few intervention studies have involved world-class or elite athletes. This is understandable, of course, because by definition elite athletes are a scarce resource and it is difficult to arrange a study that does not conflict with their commitments to training and competition (20). However, elite athletes almost certainly have genetic endowment as well as acquired traits gained from their training history and training programs that differ from those of subelite athletes. Because the results of a research study apply with reasonable certainty only to populations that have similar characteristics to the sample involved in the investigation, it is not clear whether elite athletes will respond in the same way to strategies that have been tested on subelite or recreational competitors. An elite athlete may benefit from something that has no detectable effect on recreational athletes. Conversely, strategies that enhance the performance of a recreational performer may not benefit the elite athlete.

Sports dietitians are already familiar with the possibility of individual variability in response to strategies such as caffeine (21) and creatine supplementation (22), although at this stage there is no practical way to distinguish between responders and nonresponders or to suspect that the training status or the genetic characteristics of elite athletes are responsible for differences. Nevertheless, it is possible that certain nutrition strategies "work" by achieving similar benefits to that achieved by a long history or volume of training. Genetics may also play a role in helping an athlete excel in a particular sport. Therefore, working with the elite athlete, a nutrition strategy developed by a food and nutrition professional may have less effect on systems that have already been optimized in the athlete.

With some strategies, variations in actual outcomes in the field may be expected because the real-life practices of elite athletes do not conform to the conditions that were used when the nutrition practice was tested in the laboratory. For example, many studies are done with subjects in a fasted state, with the athlete drinking only water during an exercise session. The results may be different when the same nutrition practice is conducted in real life after a carbohydrate-rich meal (23). At other times, elite athletes may choose or be forced by the circumstances of their event not to follow the existing guidelines. For example, world-class marathon runners typically drink at rates of approximately 200 to 600 mL/h during races, despite hydration guidelines that promote higher rates of intake to better match sweat losses (24). Because these runners are relatively successful (ie, they are the race winners), it is hard to argue that closer adherence to the guidelines is needed.

In summary, at present there is insufficient information to make different recommendations for elite athletes regarding sports nutrition practice other than to recognize that the rules and conditions of their events may provide logistical challenges to fulfilling the existing guidelines. However, sports scientists are encouraged to conduct research with elite athletes and the real-life conditions under which their sport is played so that recommendations can be fine-tuned.

Evaluating the Effects of Supplements When Winning Margins Can Be Measured in Decimals

Most scientific investigations of supplements are biased toward rejecting the hypothesis that the product enhances performance. This bias is due to small sample sizes, performance testing protocols with low reliability, and the use of "statistical significance" to decide whether there was a difference between a treatment and a control or placebo condition. In other words, the framework of most intervention studies is sufficient only to detect large differences in performance outcomes. Yet, most competitions in elite sports are decided by millimeters and fractions of seconds, and many high-level athletes would be happy to consider any supplement or nutrition intervention that could enhance their performance by this tiniest of margins.

Batterham and Hopkins (25) have discussed alternative ways to detect worthwhile performance enhancements in elite sports. This paper considers the challenges in finding middle ground between what scientists and athletes consider "significant." An athlete's required improvement is not the small margin between those individuals who place among the top finishers in a race. Instead, the needed improvement is influenced by a factor related to the day-to-day variability in personal performance in such an event. By modeling the results of various sporting events, Batterham and Hopkins suggest that "worthwhile" changes to the outcome of most events require a performance difference equal to approximately 0.3 to 0.5 times the variability (coefficient of variation [CV]) of performance for that event, and that across a range of events the CV of performance of top athletes is usually within the range of 0.5% to 5%. Such a difference is still outside the realm of detection for many of the studies commonly published in scientific journals. Nevertheless, scientists can interpret their results meaningfully by reporting the outcome as a percentage change in a measure of athletic performance and using 90% to 95% confidence limits to describe the likely range of the true effect of the treatment on the average athlete represented in the study (25).

When weighing pros and cons of using a supplement, elite athletes must consider:

- Expense of the product
- Likelihood of product yielding performance benefits
- Risks of adverse effects
- The risk of a positive drug test

The last item on this list is a recent addition. "Inadvertent doping" through supplement use has emerged as a major concern for athletes who participate in sporting competitions governed by an antidoping code. Some supplements and sport foods contain ingredients, such as prohormones or stimulants, which are included on the Prohibited List of the World Anti-Doping Agency or the international federations governing sports. Taking such a supplement may cause an athlete to have a positive drug test after unintentionally consuming a banned substance found in such products. Because supplements are often regarded as harmless or as alternatives to drugs, some athletes may not carefully read product labels to check the ingredient list for banned substances. In addition, there is convincing evidence that some supplements or sport foods contain these banned substances as undeclared ingredients or contaminants (26,27). Some countries have adopted testing systems for supplements to help to reduce the risk of an inadvertent doping outcome due to contaminated supplements (28). However, this risk can only be reduced rather than eliminated, and sports authorities now warn elite athletes to seek expert advice before using supplements and remind them that strict liability applies in the case of a positive test regardless of the source of the banned substance.

Strategies for Working with Elite Athletes

A successful practice with elite athletes requires certain strategies and personal characteristics of the sports dietitian. The following ideas can help the sports dietitian develop a rewarding career.

Getting Started

Be prepared to start at the bottom to gain experience. Look for opportunities to start with local teams and athletes rather than expecting to start with a job with a national sporting organization or major professional team.

Use your existing contacts and involvement in sports to develop a knowledge base and experience. Your own sporting experiences can earn credibility with athletes and coaches and provide an intimate understanding of what it is like to be an athlete.

Find a mentor. Set a professional development program for yourself that includes regular journal reading and conference attendance—stay up-to-date with both the science and practice of sports nutrition.

Understanding a Sport and Its Special Features

Learn all you can about how a sport influences nutrition needs of competitors, as well as current nutrition practices and beliefs. Get specific information about training practices, competition programs, and lifestyle patterns—including individual differences among players on a team and among different sports (1).

Attend training sessions and events to better understand the culture and experiences of athletes, coaches, and other team members. Let the athletes know that you are interested in their activities.

Stay informed about supplements used or promoted within a sport. Follow the Internet, sports magazines, health food shops, and supplement stores, and the general talk among players to stay abreast of current ideas and practices.

Be a Team Player

Identify all the people who work with an individual athlete or team to provide their nutrition ideas or achieve their nutrition practice. This will include people in the organized support structure and in the personal network that each athlete may develop. Be prepared to listen to the approaches and input of these people, and find a niche in which your services and ideas will be appreciated.

Know when to stand your ground (you are the nutrition expert) and when to be flexible (a compromise of your ideas may be necessary for athletes to accept). Look for middle ground. For example, a coach or trainer may insist that the athlete consume branched-chain amino acids after a training session to promote recovery. Rather than debating whether the present literature provides support for benefits of postexercise supplementation with amino acid supplements, consider setting up recovery snacks for the team including fruit smoothies, flavored yogurt, and cereal/sport bars. Provide educational material showing the coach and athletes that these snacks provide a good source of branched-chain amino acids (similar to amounts found in supplements) as well as carbohydrate and fluid for refueling and rehydration.

Participate (when invited) in all activities of the athlete or team support network, even if these do not directly seem to involve nutrition. Cultivate relationships among other professionals or team support personnel so that they are aware of what you can do and so they will provide early referrals of athletes for your specialty services and support your nutrition plan when you are not present (eg, during team travel).

Be Creative with Nutrition Activities

Create educational resources that target the needs and the interests of your individual athletes and teams. Use innovative ways to provide information rather than relying on standard interview/consultation or lecture formats. Be prepared to put information or activities into "bite-size" chunks or address the issues that are of immediate interest to your athletes rather than following a standard script.

Plan interactive activities, such as cooking classes, supermarket tours, or installation of recovery snacks at training or competition venues. These activities provide tangible outcomes. Many people learn better through practical activities.

Remember, It Isn't All About You

Many people who become involved in the preparation of elite athletes start to identify closely with the success of these athletes. Although it is rewarding to feel that you contributed to a successful outcome or were part of a valued support team, it is important to maintain perspective about your role. High-level sports and high-profile athletes attract an entourage of people, many of whom use a "cult of personality" to make themselves seem indispensable. In some cases, members of this entourage can become as (in)famous as the athlete. Although it is often important to be able to sell your message in a memorable way, this author feels that it is more important to maintain an appropriate and ethical profile.

Stay Ethical

Sport is all about rules and regulations. There is a professional code of conduct that covers your role as nutrition adviser/therapist. Sometimes you may feel pressured to assist an athlete in a dangerous or unethical practice, such as excessive loss of body fat or weight, or use of a prohibited supplement (eg, glycerol, which can be used for hyperhydration and was added to the 2010 WADA Prohibited List [29] but may be undetectable when used in some circumstances). Stay true to professional standards, even when the athlete threatens to undertake the practice without your assistance.

In addition, maintain confidentiality in your work with high-profile athletes. Even when opinions or information about "household names" seem to be discussed as public conversation, guard your knowledge about the athletes with whom you work. This includes the nature of your nutrition work, as well as other information such as inside knowledge of injuries or other problems. At best, breaches of this information are an invasion of the athlete's privacy. At worst, however, they may be considered "insider trading" in a world where betting on sports is a highly lucrative industry.

Tips for Survival in a High-Pressure Environment

Be organized and have definite goals for your activities. Set up a contract with the appropriate person (medical director, head coach, athlete) in which the range of services you can provide is discussed and agreed upon. Provide feedback or summary information on completed services so that your input is documented and appreciated.

Don't forget to build in ways of assessing and rewarding your own progress and achievement of goals. It is easy to overlook your own performance when all the focus is on the athletes.

Finally, make sure you look after your own health and well-being. Sometimes, the service of athletes requires long hours and the elevation of their needs above your own. Be prepared for the politics of high-level sport. Coaches and medical staff are frequently abandoned by their athletes, often for no fault of their own. Expect that this will happen to you. Be prepared to pick yourself up and develop a new plan.

Summary

Working with elite athletes provides an opportunity for the sports dietitian to test his or her sports science knowledge and creativity in solving practical challenges faced by athletes pushing to their extreme limits. The elite environment can be both high pressure and "high return." The sports dietitian will need to remain up-to-date with latest scientific information and adhere to a code of conduct that includes understanding the ethics of sport, respect for confidentiality, and care for their own well-being. It can be rewarding to see that nutrition plays a role in the achievement of the highest levels of success in sport. However, the role is often specific to the needs of a gifted individual and a unique situation.

References

1. Burke LM. Practical and cultural factors. In *Practical Sports Nutrition.* Champaign, IL: Human Kinetics, 2007: 27–39.
2. Burke L. Preparation for competition. In: Burke L, Deakin V, eds. *Clinical Sports Nutrition.* 4th ed. Sydney, Australia: McGraw-Hill; 2010:304–329.
3. Maughan R. Fluid and carbohydrate intake during exercise. In: Burke L, Deakin V, eds. *Clinical Sports Nutrition.* 4th ed. Sydney, Australia: McGraw-Hill; 2010:330–357.
4. Burke L. Nutrition for recovery after training and competition. In: Burke L, Deakin V, eds. *Clinical Sports Nutrition.* 4th ed. Sydney, Australia: McGraw-Hill; 2010:358–392.
5. Burd NA, Tang JE, Moore DR, Phillips SM. Exercise training and protein metabolism: influences of contraction, protein intake, and sex-based differences. *J Appl Physiol.* 2009;106:1692–1701.
6. Burke LM, Cox GR, Cummings NK, Desbrow B. Guidelines for daily carbohydrate intake: do athletes achieve them? *Sports Med.* 2001;31:267–299.
7. Burke L. Weight-making sports. In: *Practical Sports Nutrition.* Champaign, IL: Human Kinetics; 2007:289–312.
8. Reilly T. Football. In: Reilly T, Secher N, Snell P, Williams C, eds. *Physiology of Sports.* London, England: E & FN Spon; 1990:371–426.
9. Mujika I, Padilla S. Physiological and performance characteristics of male professional road cyclists. *Sports Med.* 2001;31:479–487.
10. Burke LM. Energy needs of athletes. *Can J Appl Physiol.* 2001;26(Suppl):S202–S219.
11. Garcia-Roves PM, Terrados N, Fernandez SF, Patterson AM. Macronutrients intake of top level cyclists during continuous competition—change in feeding pattern. *Int J Sports Med.* 1998;19:61–67.
12. Saris WHM, van Erpt-Baart, MA, Brouns F, Westerterp KR, ten Hoor, F. Studies on food intake and energy expenditure during extreme sustained exercise: the Tour de France. *Int J Sports Med.* 1989;10(suppl):S26–S31.
13. Phelps M, Abrahamson A. *No Limits: The Will to Succeed.* Sydney, Australia: Simon and Schuster; 2008.
14. Nattiv A, Loucks AB, Manore MM, Sanborn CF, Sundgot-Borgen J, Warren MP. American College of Sports Medicine position stand. The female athlete triad. *Med Sci Sports Exerc.* 2007;39:1867–1882.
15. Centers for Disease Control and Prevention. Hyperthermia and dehydration-related deaths associated with intentional rapid weight loss in three collegiate wrestlers—North Carolina, Wisconsin, and Michigan, November–December 1998. *JAMA:* 1998;279:824–825.
16. Charatan F. Ephedra supplement may have contributed to sportsman's death. *BMJ.* 2003;326:464.
17. Burke LM. Sports nutrition: practical guidelines for the sports physicians. In: Schwellnus MP, ed. *Olympic Textbook of Medicine in Sport.* Oxford, UK: Blackwell Publishing Ltd; 2008:508–600.

18. Febbraio M, Martin D. Nutritional issues for special environments: training and competing at altitude and in hot climates. In: Burke L, Deakin V, eds. *Clinical Sports Nutrition*. 4th ed. Sydney, Australia: McGraw-Hill; 2010: 659–675.
19. Burke LM. Fasting and recovery from exercise. *Br J Sports Med.* 2010;44:502–508.
20. Hopkins WG, Hawley JA, Burke LM. Design and analysis of research on sport performance enhancement. *Med Sci Sports Exerc.* 1999;31:472–485.
21. Graham TE, Spriet LL. Performance and metabolic responses to a high caffeine dose during prolonged exercise. *J Appl Physiol.* 1991;71:2292–2298.
22. Greenhaff PL, Bodin K, Soderlund K, Hultman E. Effect of oral creatine supplementation on skeletal phospho-creatine resynthesis. *Am J Physiol.* 1994;266:E725–E730.
23. Burke LM, Claassen A, Hawley JA, Noakes TD. Carbohydrate intake during prolonged cycling minimizes effect of glycemic index of preexercise meal. *J Appl Physiol.* 1998;85:2220–2226.
24. Noakes TD. IMMDA advisory statement of guidelines for fluid replacement during marathon running. *New Studies in Athletics.* 2002;17:15–24.
25. Batterham AM, Hopkins WG. Making meaningful inferences about magnitudes. *Int J Sports Physiol Perform.* 2006;1:50–57.
26. Geyer H, Parr MK, Reinhart U, Schrader Y, Mareck U, Schanzer W. Analysis of non-hormonal nutritional supplements for anabolic-androgenic steroids—results of an international study. *Int J Sports Med.* 2004;25: 124–129.
27. Geyer H, Parr MK, Koehler K, Mareck U, Schänzer W, Thevis M. Nutritional supplements cross-contaminated and faked with doping substances. *J Mass Spectrom.* 2008; 43:892–902.
28. Informed Sport Web site. Tested products. http://www.informed-sport.com/about-informed-sport. Accessed October 4, 2011.
29. World Anti-Doping Agency. The 2010 Prohibited List: International Standard. September 19, 2009. http://www.wada-ama.org/rtecontent/document/2010_Prohibited_List_FINAL_EN_Web.pdf. Accessed January 18, 2011.

Chapter 16

VEGETARIAN ATHLETES

D. ENETTE LARSON-MEYER, PhD, RD, CSSD, FACSM

Introduction

Athletes may follow vegetarian diets for many reasons related to health, ethics (animal rights), ecology, the environment, and religious or spiritual beliefs. Well-planned vegetarian diets are nutritionally adequate, appropriate for athletes at all levels—from recreational to elite—and provide health benefits in prevention and treatment of chronic diseases (1–3). Like most athletes, vegetarian athletes will benefit from education about food choices to optimize their health and peak performance.

This chapter reviews the energy, macronutrient, and micronutrient requirements of the vegetarian athlete and provides tips for meeting nutrition needs with a vegetarian diet. The chapter also discusses nutrition recommendations before, during, and after exercise and provides tips for the sports dietitian working with vegetarian athletes.

Sports Nutrition Considerations: Energy and Macronutrients

Energy

The energy needs of athletes and active individuals vary considerably and are dependent on body size, body composition, sex, training regimen, and nontraining physical activity patterns. Using doubly labeled water, energy expenditure is estimated to vary from 2,600 kcal/d in female swimmers to approximately 8,500 kcal/d in male cyclists participating in the Tour de France bicycle race (4). The energy requirements of smaller or less-active individuals may be slightly lower.

In practice, total daily energy expenditure (TDEE) of individual athletes can be estimated using a variety of methods (see Chapter 10). The most straightforward method (5) is to use the predictive equations from the Dietary Reference Intakes (6,7) to estimate resting energy expenditure (REE) *and* then multiply the value by an activity factor of between 1.4 and 2.5, depending on the physical activity category of the athlete. (See Boxes 10.2 and 10.3 and Tables 10.1 and 10.2, in Chapter 10, for equations, activity factors, and examples on using equations.) These equations were developed using the doubly labeled water technique. Another method is to add up the estimates of the components of TDEE, which include REE (8), the energy cost of training or organized physical exercise (ExEE), and the energy cost of occupational and spontaneous

326

physical activity (ie, nonexercise activity thermogenesis; NEAT), as outlined in Box 16.1 (8,9). Although estimation of TDEE from its components may be more cumbersome, it allows for more variation in training and daily activity patterns and can also serve as an educational tool when calculated in the athlete's presence. Estimating TDEE is useful when developing meal plans and when evaluating adequacy of energy intake (along with body weight changes and dietary intake assessments).

Meeting energy needs is a nutrition priority for all athletes (5). Inadequate energy intake relative to energy expenditure negates the benefits of training and compromises performance. Although some athletes who follow vegetarian and vegan diets may have difficulty meeting energy requirements due to the high-fiber content and/or low energy density of plant-based diets (5), sports dietitians are likely to encounter active vegetarians with a variety of energy needs. Some will need to consume six to eight meals and snacks per day and/or avoid excess fiber intake to maintain body weight and meet energy needs. Others may require lower energy intakes to promote weight reduction for health and/or performance. Sports dietitians should work with vegetarian athletes to help them meet their energy needs through consumption of a variety of foods, including whole grains, fruits, vegetables, legumes, nuts, seeds, and, if desired, dairy products and eggs (1). Both the US Department of Agriculture's MyPlate, which has adjustments of energy requirements and tips for vegetarians (10), and the guidelines developed by Larson-Meyer specifically for vegetarian athletes (2) may be useful for educating athletes about healthful eating patterns. Eating plans developed for individuals who consume vegetarian or vegan diets (11,12) may also provide a more useful and better nutritional guideline if the number of servings is increased to meet an athlete's energy needs. Box 16.2 presents sample menus for a 3,000-kcal vegetarian diet and a 4,600-kcal vegan diet. These high energy intakes may be required to meet the needs of individuals who train or exercise regularly. Vegetarian athletes who struggle to consume adequate energy may benefit from consuming only one third to one half of their grains and fruit in the whole, unprocessed form (2). This reduces excessive fiber intake and early onset of satiety as well as promotes increased energy intake.

Carbohydrate

Carbohydrate should make up the bulk of the athlete's diet. Adequate carbohydrate intake maintains muscle and liver glycogen stores (5,13–16) and optimizes mood (17) and performance during prolonged, moderate-intensity exercise (eg, distance running and cycling) (17–21). Carbohydrate also is needed during intermittent and short-duration, high-intensity exercise (22,23), which includes sprinting performance at the end of an endurance event or intermittent bouts of exercise (24,25). For many athletes, maintaining sufficient carbohydrate intake during training results in a longer playing (or exercising) time before fatigue and better sprinting potential at the end of a race or sporting event. The benefits of carbohydrate consumption, however, may not be limited to maintenance of glycogen stores. Dietary carbohydrate may also be important for maintenance of Krebs cycle intermediates (19) and preservation of the bioenergetic state of exercising muscle (23), factors that are also important for optimal muscle function and performance.

The carbohydrate needs of active individuals are easily met on a vegetarian diet. The carbohydrate recommendations for athletes range from 3 to 12 g/kg/d (5). The amount recommended within this range depends on the athlete's TDEE, current training regimen (or phase), and gender. For example, college, elite, or other competitive athletes in heavy training may benefit from a higher carbohydrate intake and should strive for the upper range of close to 7 to 12 g/kg/d. Conversely, smaller female athletes, those participating at a level that demands less training (eg, skill-based, off-season training, or recreational exercise), or those attempting to reduce body weight or fat stores may require only 3 to 5 g/kg/d. Carbohydrate exchanges and label-reading exercises are useful for educating athletes about meeting their carbohydrate needs (2). Knowledge of carbohydrate sources is also useful in planning carbohydrate intake before, during, and after exercise. Carbohydrate needs are discussed in more detail in Chapter 2.

BOX 16.1   Calculation of Total Daily Energy Needs

$$\text{Total Daily Energy Needs} = \text{TDEE} + \text{TEF}$$

$$\text{TDEE} = \text{REE}^a + \text{NEAT} + \text{ExEE}$$

- REE = 22 × Fat-Free Mass (kg)

- NEAT = Physical activity level × REE

  o Light activity = 0.3 × REE
  o Moderate activity = 0.5 × REE
  o Heavy activity = 0.7 × REE

- To determine ExEE, refer to physical activities charts (found in many nutrition or exercise physiology texts).

$$\text{TEF} = 6\% \text{ to } 10\% \text{ of TDEE}$$

- TEF = 0.06 × TDEE

- TEF = 0.10 × TDEE

Example 1
Female college soccer player who practices for 90 minutes and weight trains for 30 minutes.

- Weight = 60 kg with 20% body fat (lean body weight = 48 kg).
- Assume light occupational activity (student).
- A 60-kg female athlete uses ~8.0 kcal/min for soccer practice and 6.8 kcal/min for weight training.

$$\text{REE} = 22 \times 48 = 1{,}056 \text{ kcal}$$

$$\text{NEAT} = 0.3 \times 1{,}056 \text{ kcal} = 317 \text{ kcal}$$

$$\text{ExEE} = (8.0 \text{ kcal/min} \times 90 \text{ min}) + (6.8 \text{ kcal/min} \times 30 \text{ min}) = 720 \text{ kcal} + 204 \text{ kcal} = 924 \text{ kcal}$$

$$\text{TDEE} = 1{,}056 + 317 + 924 = {\sim}2{,}297 \text{ kcal}$$

$$\text{TEF} = 0.06 \times 2{,}297 = {\sim}138 \text{ kcal}$$

$$\text{TEF} = 0.10 \times 2{,}297 = {\sim}230 \text{ kcal}$$

$$\text{Total Daily Energy Needs} = 2{,}297 + 138 = 2{,}435 \text{ kcal}$$

$$\text{Total Daily Energy Needs} = 2{,}297 + 184 = 2{,}527 \text{ kcal}$$

Example 2
Male recreational runner who works as a musician and runs 35 miles/wk (average of 43 min/d at a 7-mph pace).

- Weight = 75 kg.
- Body fat = 16% (lean body weight = 63 kg).
- Assume moderate occupational activity (stands, moves, loads/unloads equipment regularly, some sitting).

continues

BOX 16.1   Calculation of Total Daily Energy Needs (continued)

- A 75-kg male athlete uses ~14.1 kcal/min when running at a steady 7-mph pace.

$$REE = 22 \times 63 = 1{,}386 \text{ kcal}$$

$$NEAT = 0.5 \times 1{,}386 \text{ kcal} = 693 \text{ kcal}$$

$$ExEE = 14.1 \times 43 \text{ min} = 606 \text{ kcal}$$

$$TDEE = 1{,}386 + 693 + 606 = {\sim}2{,}685 \text{ kcal}$$

$$TEF = 0.06 \times 2{,}685 = {\sim}161 \text{ kcal}$$

$$TEF = 0.10 \times 2{,}685 = {\sim}268 \text{ kcal}$$

$$\text{Total Daily Energy Needs} = 2{,}685 + 161 = 2{,}846 \text{ kcal}$$

$$\text{Total Daily Energy Needs} = 2{,}685 + 268 = 2{,}953 \text{ kcal}$$

Abbreviations: TDEE, total daily energy expenditure; REE, resting energy expenditure; NEAT, energy expenditure during nonexercise activity thermogenesis; ExEE, energy expenditure during training; TEF, thermic effect of food.

[a] The Cunningham equation for estimating REE (8) has been shown to more closely estimate the actual REE of endurance-trained men and women (9) than other available equations.

Protein

The protein needs of athletes vary according to the type of activity and level and frequency of training. Protein needs of active vegetarians who engage in light to moderate activity several times per week are likely met by the Recommended Dietary Allowance (RDA) of 0.8 g/kg/d, whereas the protein requirements of those who train more intensely (five or more times a week) are likely to be significantly higher than the RDA. The protein recommendation for athletes is 1.2 to 1.7 g/kg/d (5). The additional protein and essential amino acids during routine endurance and strength training is needed to cover increased protein utilization as an auxiliary fuel during exercise and enhanced protein deposition during muscle development (26). Inadequate intakes of total energy and carbohydrate increase protein needs. During prolonged endurance activity, for example, athletes with low glycogen stores metabolize twice as much protein as those with adequate stores, primarily due to increased gluconeogenesis (27).

There is no research to suggest that protein recommendations are different for athletes following a vegetarian rather than omnivorous diet. Although it has been suggested that vegetarians may need approximately 10% more protein than omnivores to account for the lower digestibility of plant proteins as compared with animal proteins (5,28), the Institute of Medicine currently does not find sufficient evidence to support an additional protein requirement for vegetarians consuming complementary plant proteins (6). A meta-analysis of nitrogen balance studies supported this view and found that the source of dietary protein did not significantly impact the protein needs of healthy individuals (29). However, sports dietitians should be aware that protein needs might be slightly higher in athletes whose dietary protein sources are almost exclusively from less–well-digested plant sources such as legumes and some cereal grains rather than well-digested sources including soy foods (30).

BOX 16.2   Sample 3,000-kcal Vegetarian Menu and 4,600-kcal Vegan Menu

3,000 kcal

Breakfast
  1 cup raisin bran
  1 cup fat-free milk
  2 slices mixed-grain toast
  2 tsp soy margarine
  1 medium banana
  8 oz fruit juice

Lunch
  Whole-wheat pita stuffed with shredded
    spinach, sliced tomato, 2 oz feta cheese,
    2 Tbsp olive oil
  1 large apple
  2 small oatmeal cookies

Snack
  Sesame seed bagel
  1 Tbsp peanut butter
  1 Tbsp jam

Dinner
  Lentil spaghetti sauce (1 cup cooked lentils,
    ½ onion, 1½ cups canned tomatoes,
    1 Tbsp olive oil)
  3 oz dry pasta, cooked
  1 Tbsp parmesan cheese
  2 (1-oz) slices french bread dipped in
    1 Tbsp olive oil
  1 cup steamed broccoli

Snack
  1 cup fruit yogurt

4,600 kcal

Breakfast
  1½ cups raisin bran
  1 cup fortified soy milk
  3 slices mixed-grain toast
  3 tsp soy margarine
  1 medium banana
  8 oz fruit juice

Lunch
  Tofu salad on a 4-oz hoagie roll (1 cup firm
    tofu, 2 tsp mustard, 2 tsp soy
    mayonnaise, lettuce, tomato)
  1 large apple
  3 small oatmeal cookies
  8 oz carrot juice

Snack
  Sesame seed bagel
  1 Tbsp peanut butter
  1 Tbsp jam
  1 cup fortified soy milk

Dinner
  Lentil spaghetti sauce (1½ cup cooked
    lentils, ½ onion, 1½ cups canned
    tomatoes, 1 Tbsp olive oil)
  4 oz dry pasta, cooked
  3 (1-oz) slices french bread dipped in
    2 Tbsp olive oil
  1½ cups steamed collards

Snack
  1 cup fruit sorbet
  1 oz toasted almonds

Vegetarian menu: 3,066 kcal, 106 g protein, 469 g carbohydrate, 85 g fat (14% protein, 25% fat, 61% carbohydrate), 1,600 mg calcium, 29 mg iron, 14 mg zinc. Vegan menu: 4,626 kcal, 146 g protein, 704 g carbohydrate, 136 g fat (13% protein, 26% fat, 61% carbohydrate), 1,133 mg calcium, 60 mg iron, 15 mg zinc.

Note: Both menus assume grain products are made from enriched flour.

Vegetarian athletes can easily achieve adequate protein if their diets are adequate in energy and contain a variety of plant-based protein foods such as legumes (including soy products), nuts, seeds, and grains (see Table 16.1). As reviewed by Young and Pellett (31), vegetarians do not need to be overly concerned with eating specific combinations of plant proteins in the same meal (as was once believed) but should consume an assortment of plant foods during the course of a day. This pattern provides all the essential amino acids

TABLE 16.1 Approximate Protein Content of Selected Vegetarian Food Sources

Food	Portion	Protein, g/portion
Bread, most types	1 oz. (1 slice)	2–3
Rice, pasta, other grains, cooked	⅓–½ cup	2–3
Cheese, medium to hard	1 oz	7
Cheese, cottage	½ cup	13.4
Egg, whole	1 large	6.2
Legumes (most beans, peas, and lentils)	½ cup	7
Milk, all types	1 cup	8
Nuts, most types	2 Tbsp	7
Peanut butter	2 Tbsp	8
Tempeh	½ cup	15
Tofu, firm	1 cup	20
Tofu, soft	1 cup	16
Vegetables, most	½ cup	2–3
Vegetarian "burgers"	1 patty	6–16
Vegetarian "chicken"	1 patty (71 g)	9–12
Vegetarian "dogs"	1 dog	9–12
Yogurt, most types	1 cup	8–10

Source: Data are from the US Department of Agriculture Agricultural Research Service National Nutrient Database (2009) and selected food labels.

and ensures adequate nitrogen retention and utilization in healthy adults (1,31). Emphasizing amino acid balance at each meal is not necessary because "limiting amino acids" in one meal is buffered by the body's free amino acid pools (31) found primarily in skeletal muscle (32). Furthermore, although some plant foods tend to be low in certain amino acids, the usual dietary combinations of protein such as beans and rice tend to be complete (31). However, because cereals tend to be low in the essential amino acid lysine (31), athletes who do not consume dairy and/or eggs should incorporate beans and soy products into their diets to ensure adequate lysine intake and nitrogen balance.

Vegetarian diets generally contain 12.5% of energy from protein, whereas vegan diets typically contain 11% (11). An 80-kg male athlete consuming 3,600 kcal/d would receive 1.41 g protein per kg of body weight from the average vegetarian diet and 1.2 g/kg from the average vegan diet. A 50-kg female gymnast consuming 2,200 kcal/d would receive 1.38 g/kg from a vegetarian diet and 1.21 g/kg from a vegan diet. Most vegetarian athletes meet the requirements for endurance training without special meal planning. However, strength-training athletes (weightlifters, football players, wrestlers) or those with high training volumes or low energy intakes may need to eat more protein-rich foods. This is easily accomplished by encouraging the athlete to incorporate several servings of protein-rich vegetarian foods in regular meals or snacks. Examples include adding soy milk to a fruit snack, lentils to spaghetti sauce, tofu to stir-fry, or garbanzo beans to salad. Furthermore, protein consumption in close proximity to strength or endurance exercise can enhance maintenance of and net gains in skeletal muscle (33,34).

Fat

Dietary fat should make up the remainder of energy intake after carbohydrate and protein needs are met. The American College of Sports Medicine, the Academy of Nutrition and Dietetics (formerly American Dietetic Association), and Dietitians of Canada recommend that fat intake range from 20% to 35% of total energy intake to allow for adequate carbohydrate intake (5). Consumption of less than 20% of energy from fat is not recommended and has the potential to impair endurance performance (35–37), unfavorably alter lipid profile (38–41), and interfere with normal menstrual function in female athletes (42). Fat is particularly important in athletes' diets because it provides energy, essential fatty acids, and other essential elements of cell membranes. Dietary fat is also needed for absorption of fat-soluble vitamins. Recent research also suggests that dietary fat may be necessary for maintaining intramyocellular triglyceride (IMTG) stores (39,43), which serve as an important fuel source during prolonged, moderate-intensity exercise (44,45). Studies to date, however, have not demonstrated that low IMTG stores are responsible for the reduced performance associated with very low–fat diets (40).

The amount and type of fat consumed should be carefully assessed in the vegetarian athlete. Some vegetarian athletes, particularly endurance-trained athletes (runners and triathletes), may consume excessive carbohydrate and inadequate fat, often with the misconception that dietary fat increases body fat and impairs performance. Similarly, recreational athletes with cardiovascular disease or type 2 diabetes may be following the extremely low-fat vegetarian diet plans (< 10% energy from fat) recommended by Ornish et al (46) and Barnard et al (47), which have been shown to promote regression of coronary atherosclerosis (46,48,49) and improve glycemic control (47,50). However, such low-fat diets may be too restrictive for athletes during heavy training. On the other hand, other active vegetarians and vegetarian athletes may be consuming diets that lack carbohydrate and are too rich in saturated fat, mainly from full-fat dairy products, bakery products, or processed foods.

The type of fat included in the diet of vegetarian athletes is important. The proportion of energy from the various fatty acids should be in accord with national guidelines and contain approximately 10% of energy from polyunsaturated fat, at least 10% as monounsaturated fat, less than 7% to 10% from saturated fat, and little to no *trans* fats (51–53) and also meet the Dietary Reference Intake (DRI) of 1.6 and 1.1 g of alpha linolenic acid for men and women, respectively (6). Vegetarian diets are generally rich in sources of n-6 polyunsaturated fatty acids and may be low in n-3 fatty acids. Because n-3 fatty acids may be important for controlling inflammation, vegetarian athletes should focus on incorporating n-3–rich foods (walnuts, flax, canola, hemp, and walnut oils) into the diet and simultaneously decreasing consumption of n-6–rich oils (corn, cotton seed, sunflower, and safflower). Although less than 10% of alpha-linolenic acid is elongated to eicosapentaenoic acid in humans (54), the conversion may be improved when n-6 concentrations in diet or blood are not high (54). Athletes who may benefit from increased n-3 consumption, including pregnant athletes and those with chronic inflammatory injuries or cardiovascular disease, may also benefit from DHA-rich microalgae supplements (55). DHA supplements derived from microalgae are well absorbed and positively influence blood concentrations of both DHA and EPA (56).

Sports Nutrition Considerations: Minerals and Vitamins

Calcium and Vitamin D

Regular exercise has not been shown to increase calcium requirements. Thus, athletes and active individuals should strive to meet the RDA of 1,000 mg for those between 19 and 50 years of age, 1,200 mg for those older than 50 years, and 1,300 mg for those younger than 18 years (57). Limited evidence also suggests that amenorrheic athletes (those not experiencing a menstrual cycle for at least 3 months) may require an additional 500 mg of calcium per day to retain calcium balance (58). Low calcium intake (59) along with reduced vitamin D status (60) have been associated with decreased bone density and increased risk for stress fractures, particularly in amenorrheic athletes (61). One recent study found that 8-week supplementation with 800 IU of vitamin D plus 2,000 mg calcium reduced incidence of stress fracture in female naval recruits by approximately 20% (62).

TABLE 16.2 Vegetarian Sources of Selected Vitamins and Minerals

Nutrient	Good Food Choices
Calcium	Calcium-set tofu, calcium-fortified beverages (orange juice and other fruit juices, soy and rice milks), broccoli, Chinese cabbage, kale, collard, mustard and turnip greens, almonds, tahini, texturized vegetable protein, blackstrap molasses, cow's milk, certain cheeses, and legumes
Iron	Legumes, nuts and seeds, whole/enriched grains, enriched/fortified cereals and pasta, leafy green and root vegetables, and dried fruits
Zinc	Legumes, nuts and seeds, whole-grain products, fortified ready-to-eat cereal, soy products, commercial meat analogues, and hard cheeses
Iodine	Iodized salt and sea vegetables (sea weed, kombu, arame, dulse)
Magnesium	Legumes, nuts and seeds, whole grains, green leafy vegetables, blackstrap molasses
Vitamin D[a]	Fatty fish (salmon, sardines, mackerel), fortified foods (cow's milk, some types/brands of soy and rice milks), orange juice, ready-to-eat breakfast cereals, margarines and yogurt, egg yolks, sun-dried mushrooms
Vitamin B-12	Redstar brand nutritional yeast T6635, fortified foods (ready-to-eat cereal, meat analogues, some types/brands of soy and rice milks, dairy products, and eggs
Riboflavin	Whole-grain and fortified breads and cereals, legumes, tofu, nuts, seeds, tahini, bananas, asparagus, figs, dark-green leafy vegetables, avocado, most sea vegetables (seaweed, kombu, arame, dulse), and dairy products

[a]Sun exposure (~5–30 min on the arms and legs between 10 AM and 2 PM non–Daylight Savings Time, several times a week) is another source of vitamin D.
Source: Data are from the US Department of Agriculture Agricultural Research Service National Nutrient Database (2009) and reference 6.

Eumenorrheic athletes can meet calcium requirements by including several servings of dairy products or eight servings of calcium-containing plant foods daily (Table 16.2) (1). Plant foods that contain calcium that is well absorbed include low-oxalate green leafy vegetables (broccoli, kale, Chinese cabbage, and collard, mustard, and turnip greens), calcium-set tofu, fortified soy and rice milks, textured vegetable protein, tahini, certain legumes, fortified orange juice, and blackstrap molasses (12). Laboratory studies have determined that the calcium bioavailability of most of these foods is as good as or better than cow's milk, which has a fractional absorption of about 32% (63–66). The exceptions include soymilk fortified with tricalcium phosphate, most legumes, nuts, and seeds which have a fractional absorption in the range of 17% to 24% (66). The calcium in spinach, Swiss chard, beet greens, and rhubarb is not well absorbed due to their high oxalate or phytate content. In support of the laboratory studies, a recent clinical study found that young vegetarians maintained positive calcium balance and appropriate bone resorption (measured by urinary deoxypyridinoline) when calcium was provided either from dairy products or exclusively from plant foods, despite a lower calcium intake on the plant-based (843 ± 140 mg) compared to the dairy-containing (1,322 ± 303 mg) diet (67).

Although it is possible to maintain calcium balance on a plant-based diet in a Western diet (1,12,64), some athletes may find it convenient to use fortified foods or calcium supplements to achieve calcium balance, particularly when requirements are elevated due to amenorrhea or menopause. Because vitamin D is also required for adequate calcium absorption and promotion of bone health, a calcium supplement that contains vitamin D is advised. Research, for example, has found that only 10% to 15% dietary calcium is absorbed in the vitamin D–deficient state, whereas 30% to 35% is absorbed when vitamin D status is sufficient (68,69). This effect is due to vitamin D–induced expression of calbindin (an intestinal calcium binding protein) and an epithelial calcium channel protein (70), which increases the efficiency of calcium and phosphorus absorption by active transport across the intestinal mucosa.

Recent research has revealed that vitamin D is involved in many other physiological functions important to the athlete's health (71) and performance (72), including immune function, inflammatory modulation (73,74), and skeletal muscle function (75). Athletes who live at extreme northern or southern latitudes (> 35 to 37 degrees), have dark pigmented skin, or who train primarily indoors or in the early morning or late afternoon throughout the year are at risk for poor vitamin D status (71,76,77). These athletes would benefit from supplementation with enough vitamin D to maintain serum calcium concentrations within the optimal range of 40 to 70 ng/mL (73). Both vitamin D-2 (ergocalciferol) and vitamin D-3 (cholecalciferol) are used in supplements and to fortify foods, including cow's milk as well as some types/brands of soy and rice milks, orange juice, breakfast cereals, margarines, and yogurt. Vitamin D-3 is not vegan because it is obtained through ultraviolet radiation of 7-dehydrocholesterol from lanolin (a product derived from wool), whereas vitamin D-2 is produced from irradiation of ergosterol from yeast (69) and is acceptable to vegans. Recent research has suggested that vitamin D-2 is as effective as vitamin D-3 at lower doses (ie, 1,000 IU) (78) but may be less effective at increasing and maintaining endogenous 25 hydroxy vitamin D (25[OH]D) concentrations when taken in higher doses (> 4,000 IU) (79,80). Natural and fortified sources of vitamin D, listed in Table 16.2, may help meet the RDA of 600 IU (57), but maintaining vitamin D stores in the range thought to promote overall health (> 20 ng/mL) does not seem to be possible through diet alone in the absence of adequate sun exposure (76).

Iron

Iron depletion is one of the most prevalent nutrient deficiencies in athletes—especially in female athletes (81–83). Iron depletion with (stage III) and without (stage II) anemia can impair muscle function and maximal oxygen uptake (84) and decrease endurance (85,86). Whereas iron depletion among athletes is most commonly attributed to insufficient energy and/or low iron intakes (5), other factors that can impact iron status include vegetarian diets, periods of rapid growth, training at high altitude (5), acute inflammation (87), and increased iron losses through gastrointestinal bleeding (88), heavy sweating (89), foot strike or intravascular hemolysis (90), hematuria (91), and/or heavy menstrual blood losses (81).

Most of the iron in a vegetarian diet is nonheme iron, which has a relatively low absorption rate (2% to 20%) compared with heme iron (15% to 35%) (92). Nonheme iron is sensitive to both inhibitors and enhancers of iron absorption. Inhibitors of iron absorption include phytates, calcium, and the polyphenolics (including tannins) in tea, coffee, herb teas, and cocoa (1). Fiber only slightly inhibits iron absorption (93). Vitamin C and other organic acids (citric, malic, lactic, and tartaric acids) can substantially enhance iron absorption and reduce the inhibitory effects of phytates and tannins, thereby improving iron status (6,94). Due to increased iron losses and the lower bioavailabity of iron from a vegetarian diet, the recommended iron requirements of athletes and vegetarians are estimated to be 1.3 to 1.7 and 1.8 times higher than the recommended daily value, respectively (6). Vegetarian athletes should aim for values higher than the RDA.

In most cases, vegetarian athletes can achieve adequate iron status without iron supplementation. Studies in vegetarian athletes (95) and nonathletes (11,96) have found that vegetarians have average iron intakes that are similar to or higher than nonvegetarians but often have lower iron status. Thus, athletes should be educated about plant sources of iron (Table 16.2) and factors that enhance and interfere with iron absorption. For example, an athlete who drinks milk, coffee, or tea when eating legumes at a meal should be advised to replace the beverage with citrus fruit juice to enhance the iron absorbed from that meal. Although supplementation has been shown to improve energy efficiency and endurance performance (97,98) in iron-depleted nonanemic athletes, supplements should be recommended only for those with compromised stores (as indicated by low serum ferritin, elevated total iron binding capacity, or elevated serum transferrin receptor) (83,99). Reduced hemoglobin, hematocrit, and/or red blood cell concentrations in athletes are not good indicators of iron status in endurance athletes (5) because of exercise-induced plasma volume expansion (100). Athletes taking iron supplements should have iron status monitored due to the prevalence of hereditary hemochromatosis and other iron overload abnormalities (6) and the potential association between iron status and chronic disease (101). A recent study in recreational marathon runners found that one in six male runners has signs of iron overload (ferritin concentration > 200 mcg/L) (99).

Zinc

Vegetarian athletes, female athletes, and athletes in heavy training commonly have serum zinc concentrations that are on the low range or less than the recommended level (102,103). In vegetarians, lower zinc status is most likely due to the reduced bioavailability of zinc from plant foods compared to animal foods but may also be related to the selection of zinc-poor foods (1,6). The lower bioavailability in vegetarian diets is mainly due to the higher phytic acid content of many plant foods (104), including phytate-rich unrefined grains and legumes, and may increase the dietary zinc requirement by 50% (6). Although overt zinc deficiency is typically not present in Western vegetarians (1) the significance of marginal deficiency is not known because of the difficulty of evaluating zinc status. Serum zinc concentrations, for example, are often altered with increases in training intensity and may not reflect zinc status (102,105,106). Although more research is needed, zinc supplementation has not been shown to influence serum zinc concentrations during training (105,107) or offer performance benefits (107).

Due to the potential negative effects of zinc status on health and performance, however, sports dietitians should work with vegetarian athletes to ensure that the RDA (or higher) for zinc is met through consumption of zinc-containing plant foods. Consumption of zinc-containing foods with organic acids including citric acid (found in many fruits and vegetables) may enhance zinc absorption (108). In support of this recommendation, a study from the US Department of Agriculture found that nonathletic women consuming a lacto-ovo-vegetarian diet containing legumes and whole grains for 8 weeks maintained zinc status within normal limits, even though the diet was lower in total zinc and higher in phytate and fiber than a control omnivorous diet (109). To maintain adequate zinc status, the authors advised that legumes and whole grains be consumed regularly. Another recent study in women who habitually followed a plant-based diet found that the addition of milk and yogurt to a plant-based diet high in phytates increased zinc bioavailability by more than 70% without altering iron bioavailability (110). The zinc content of selected protein-containing plant foods is shown in Table 16.2.

Iodine

Iodine status has not generally been a concern for athletes living in industrial countries. Evidence is mounting, however, that some vegetarians and vegans may be at increased risk for iodine deficiency (3,111–114). One study that assessed the iodine status of 81 nonathletic adults found that 25% of the vegetarians and 80% of the vegans had iodine deficiency (urinary iodine excretion value less than 100 mcg/L) compared with 9% in nonvegetarians (111). The higher prevalence of iodine deficiency among vegetarians is thought to be a consequence of prevailing (or exclusive) consumption of plant foods grown in soil with low iodine levels (113), limited consumption of cow's milk (112), no intake of fish or sea products (111), and reduced use of iodized salt (111,113). These studies have exposed a need for more research in this area and its possible effect on the health and performance of athletes. Vegetarian athletes can ensure adequate iodine status by consuming ½ t of iodized salt in the diet daily (115). Sea salt, kosher salt, and salty seasonings such as tamari are generally not iodized. Finally, although plant foods such as soybeans, cruciferous vegetables, and sweet potatoes naturally contain goitrogens, these foods have not been associated with thyroid insufficiency if iodine status is adequate (116).

Magnesium

Suboptimal magnesium status is thought to be widespread in the United States (117). Athletes participating in sports requiring weight control (eg, wrestling, ballet, gymnastics) are especially vulnerable to an inadequate magnesium status (5,118). Athletes participating in strenuous exercise may also be at risk due to increased losses in urinary and sweat magnesium that may increase magnesium requirements by 10% to 20% (118). Marginal magnesium deficiency impairs exercise performance and amplifies the negative consequences of strenuous exercise including oxidative stress (118). In athletes with suboptimal magnesium status, increased dietary intake of magnesium, either from food or supplementation, will have beneficial effects on exercise performance (118). Magnesium supplementation for physically active individuals with adequate magnesium status has not been shown to enhance physical performance. Foods rich in magnesium, which are mostly from plant-based sources, are listed in Table 16.2.

B Vitamins

Vegetarian diets can easily meet the requirements for most B vitamins (1,119). However, diets containing little to no eggs or dairy and those low in energy may not supply adequate vitamin B-12 and riboflavin (120).

Vitamin B-12

Because cobalamin, the active form of vitamin B-12, is found exclusively in animal products (121), vegan athletes need to regularly consume vitamin B-12–fortified foods or a vitamin B-12–containing multivitamin. Food sources of vitamin B-12 include Redstar brand nutritional yeast T6635, soymilk, breakfast cereals, and meat analogs that are vitamin B-12–fortified (1). Although there has been some discussion (presented in the lay literature) that fermented soy products and nori and chorella seaweeds can supply bioavailable vitamin B-12, research is not in support of this misconception (which arose because the standard assay for determining vitamin B-12 content does not distinguish between biologically active forms and analogues) (122,123).

Vegetarians who consume dairy products and/or eggs are likely to have adequate intakes of vitamin B-12 (1,121). However, because of the irreversible neurological damage that can occur with vitamin B-12 deficiency, markers of vitamin B-12 status (homocysteine, methylmalonic acid, and holotranscobalamin II) should be measured if there is concern (121). The typical manifestation of vitamin B-12 deficiency as macrocytic anemia can be masked by high folate intake, a likely finding in vegan or vegetarian athletes who consume ample legumes, dark green leafy, and other vegetables rich in folate.

Riboflavin

Riboflavin intake may be low in athletes who avoid dairy products (5), particularly when energy intake is restricted to promote weight loss (119). There is some evidence that riboflavin needs may be increased in individuals who are habitually physically active (6) and in those who begin an exercise program (124,125), particularly if the riboflavin status was marginal prior to exercise initiation. Because dairy products are rich sources of riboflavin, education about plant sources of riboflavin may help ensure adequate intake. Good plant sources of riboflavin are shown in Table 16.2.

Sports Nutrition Considerations: Supplements

Vegetarian athletes, like other athletes, may inquire about nutritional supplements or ergogenic aids to assist their athletic training and performance. Like all athletes, they should first be encouraged to follow a balanced diet before considering supplements. Vegetarian and vegan athletes are also typically concerned about whether the ingredients are animal- or plant-derived (which may vary by manufacturer). An extensive discussion of supplements can be found in Chapter 7, but those of particular interest to vegetarian athletes— protein, creatine, and carnitine—are briefly discussed here.

Protein Supplements

Protein from supplements is not needed if the athlete is consuming adequate energy and making proper food choices (see Table 16.3). For convenience, protein-containing sport beverages and bars can be used occasionally to supplement the diet. However, recent research (126–129) has suggested that supplemental beverages that contain only soy protein are not as effective at promoting muscle protein synthesis and hypertrophy as is milk (see Box 16.3) (33,34,126–132).

Creatine and Carnitine

Creatine and carnitine are supplied by the diet from meat and other animal products. Even though both substances can be endogenously synthesized from amino acid precursors (133), serum concentrations of creatine and carnitine (134,135) and skeletal muscle concentrations of creatine (136–138) are found to be lower in individuals consuming vegetarian diets. Several studies (135,138), but not all (139), have noted that vegetarians who take creatine supplements experience greater increases in skeletal muscle total creatine, phosphocreatine, lean tissue mass, and work performance during weight training (138) and anaerobic

TABLE 16.3 Approximate Leucine, Isoleucine, and Valine Content of Selected Vegetarian Protein Sources

Food	Portion	Protein, g	Leucine, g	Valine, g	Isoleucine, g
Cheese, brie	1 oz	5.9	0.55	0.38	0.29
Cheese, cheddar	1 oz	7.1	0.68	0.47	0.44
Cheese, Swiss	1 oz	7.6	0.84	0.67	0.44
Cottage cheese, 2%	½ cup	13.4	1.34	0.90	0.71
Egg, whole	1 large	6.3	0.54	0.43	0.34
Black beans	½ cup	7.6	0.61	0.40	0.34
Garbanzo beans	½ cup	7.3	0.52	0.31	0.31
Lentils	½ cup	8.9	0.65	0.44	0.39
Pinto beans	½ cup	7.7	0.65	0.45	0.36
Soy beans, mature	½ cup	14.3	1.17	0.72	0.69
Soy beans, green	½ cup	12.4	0.80	0.49	0.49
Tofu, firm	1 cup	19.9	1.51	1.00	0.99
Tofu, soft	½ cup	8.1	0.62	0.40	0.41
Soy protein isolate	1 oz	22.9	1.9	1.2	1.2
Peanut butter	2 Tbsp	8.0	0.49	2.46	0.19
Milk, fat-free (skim)	1 cup	8.3	0.80	0.44	0.37
Milk, reduced-fat (2%)	1 cup	8.1	0.81	0.53	0.45
Yogurt, low-fat vanilla	1 cup	12.1	1.2	1.0	0.66
Whey, sweet fluid	1 cup	2.1	0.19	0.11	0.12
Whey, sweet dry	4 Tbsp	3.9	0.36	0.21	0.22

Source: Data are from the US Department of Agriculture Agricultural Research Service National Nutrient Database (2009).

BOX 16.3   Controversial Topic: Milk as a Postexercise Recovery Beverage?

Who would have thought that milk—particularly chocolate milk—would make a debut as a post-exercise recovery beverage? To the vegetarian athlete, welcoming milk as an acceptable recovery beverage is likely to be dependent on the athlete's philosophy concerning the health benefits of dairy and the animal welfare and environmental impact of dairy production.

Substantial advances over the past several years have found that dietary protein serves as both a substrate and trigger for muscle protein synthesis, thereby promoting adaptation to resistance and aerobic exercise training (see Chapter 3 for review). Although it has been recognized for at least 10 years that protein consumption in the immediate postexercise period promotes a more optimal adaptation to training (33,34) (ie, by stimulating muscle or mitochondrial protein synthesis [130,131]), a handful of recent studies have presented intriguing evidence that milk protein consumption—particularly the whey component—promotes greater muscle protein synthesis than does isonitrogenous and isocaloric amounts of soy protein (126,128,129). The greater "success" of milk protein seems to be due to the quick digestion of whey protein (34), which induces a rapid spike in the branched-chain amino acid (BCAA) leucine along with the other BCAAs isoleucine and valine. The appearance of leucine into systemic circulation is most rapid after whey protein consumption, intermediate with soy protein, and very slow with casein (126). The increase in blood leucine concentration to a "critical threshold" is thought to be necessary to "turn on" muscle protein synthesis (termed the *leucine trigger hypothesis*). Sustaining muscle protein synthesis (MPS) after the initial leucine-mediated activation may be dependent on adequate provision of other essential amino acids, particularly the BCAA, which suggests that supplements of isolated leucine would be of little benefit over consumption of leucine-rich protein foods.

It is important to mention, however, that studies thus far have been done in mostly untrained men. These studies have found that consumption of between 18 and 20 g whey or milk protein immediately after resistance exercise promotes enhanced muscle protein synthesis after a single bout of resistance training (129), and that 12-week consumption of milk (500 mL) in the postexercise period enhanced muscle hypertrophy (particularly in type II fibers) during the early stages of training compared with equal nitrogenous soy protein (127). Thus, studies in women and well-trained men are needed, as are studies looking at mitochondrial and not just MPS.

So, what is the vegetarian athlete to do? For now, vegetarian athletes not opposed to dairy may want to experiment with including milk or other sources of whey protein (including cottage cheese) in the postexercise recovery regimen. Research in men has suggested that consumption of approximately 18 to 20 g protein immediately after exercise along with a source of carbohydrate should offer the most benefit (which is why chocolate milk is often touted over plain, fat-free milk). Higher intake of protein does not seem to offer any more benefit (132). Vegetarian athletes who oppose the typical high-sugar content of chocolate milk can make their own by mixing cocoa powder and table sugar with organic milk or substituting other leucine-rich sources, including cottage cheese with fruit (see Table 16.3). Vegan and vegetarian athletes who consume little to no milk should strive to consume high-quality, leucine-rich protein foods after exercise. As mentioned earlier, soy, particularly fiber-free isolated protein, is a rich source of leucine as are most legumes. The leucine in these products is not as rapidly absorbed as the leucine in whey. Nuts, seeds, and grains, on the other hand, are not leucine-rich and may be better as source of protein at other times of the day. Vegetarian athletes should stay tuned as additional research unfolds.

bicycle performance (135) than do nonvegetarians taking the same dose. There is no evidence, however, that vegetarians benefit from carnitine supplementation.

Nutrition Before, During, and After Exercise

Pre-exercise Nutrition

Eating before exercise has been shown to improve performance (5). The meal or snack before a competition or exercise session should be high in carbohydrate (to maintain blood glucose and top off glycogen stores), provide adequate hydration, and prevent both hunger and gastrointestinal distress. Studies have shown that consumption of between 1 and 4 g carbohydrate per kg of body weight 1 to 4 hours before endurance exercise has the potential to improve endurance performance by as much as 14% (140–142) and is also thought to be beneficial in high-intensity activity lasting several hours. Vegetarian athletes should be encouraged to consume familiar, well-tolerated, high-carbohydrate meals that are low in fiber (5). Smaller meals should be consumed in close proximity (1 to 2 hours) to exercise or a sport event to allow for gastric emptying, whereas larger meals may be consumed when more time is available before the activity (3 to 4 hours) (5). Guidelines for carbohydrate intake before exercise are found in Chapter 2. Vegetarian athletes who are accustomed to eating gas-producing foods such as legumes, which are not typically recommended in the pre-event meal, may tolerate these foods without complications. Athletes who experience gastrointestinal distress may find liquid meals such as fruit smoothies more tolerable before exercise. Although some research suggests that emphasizing low– rather than high–glycemic index (GI) foods (eg, lentils vs mashed potatoes) may offer a performance advantage—particularly during prolonged submaximal exercise (143), other research has found no performance advantages (144). Athletes interested in trying new pre-event regimens should experiment with new foods and beverages during practice sessions. Strategies for overcoming gastrointestinal distress are discussed in Chapter 2.

In addition, vegetarian athletes should follow the recommended guidelines for fluid consumption to avoid initiating exercise in a dehydrated state. This includes maintaining adequate hydration in the 12- to 24-hour period before exercise. Chapter 6 provides detailed information on hydration and fluid guidelines.

Carbohydrate During Exercise

Carbohydrate ingestion at levels between 30 and 60 g/h has been shown to benefit both prolonged, moderate-intensity exercise lasting 2 hours or more (18) and variable-intensity exercise of shorter duration (145–147), such as playing soccer (148) or other team sports. This performance benefit is presumed to result from maintenance of blood glucose concentrations and preservation of carbohydrate oxidation, which decreases as glycogen stores become depleted (149). Ingestion of fluid-replacement beverages, at the recommended carbohydrate concentration of 6% to 8% (5,150), provides carbohydrate while simultaneously meeting fluid needs and may be beneficial to performance in events lasting 1 hour or less (particularly when exercise is initiated in the fasting or near-fasting state) (5). Recent work has suggested that ingestion of up to 136 g carbohydrate per hour in the form of mixed sugars that use different intestinal transporters for absorption, may provide additional benefits for events lasting longer than 2 to 3 hours (151,152).

Adequate fluid intake is also essential for maintaining endurance performance and has a cumulative effect (as does carbohydrate on performance (147). Intake of carbohydrate and fluid should be initiated shortly after the start of exercise to maximize time for sugar and other nutrients to reach the bloodstream.

Fluid-replacement goals depend on the athletes' sweat rate, exercise intensity and duration, and environmental temperatures. In general, enough fluid should be consumed during the exercise to avert a fluid deficit in excess of 2% of body weight (5,150).

Although commercial sport drinks and gels consumed with water work well for delivering easily absorbed carbohydrate (153), some vegetarian athletes may prefer natural sources of carbohydrate. Diluted fruit juices (4 oz juice in 4 oz water = 6% solution), low-sodium vegetable juices such as carrot juice (7% solution), and honey or solid foods ingested with water may be appropriate. Research has shown that solid food (154–156) and honey (157) consumed with water are as effective as liquids in increasing blood glucose and enhancing performance and are easily digested. The guideline is to drink approximately 240 mL (8 oz) of water with every 15 g carbohydrate ingested to create a 6% solution. A pinch of table salt can also be added to juices or low-sodium solids as necessary for events lasting longer than 3 to 4 hours (158). Although many vegetarians are interested in honey because it is perceived as a "natural" sugar, vegans typically do not consume honey because it is an animal product. Although there is some evidence that the addition of protein to fluid replacement beverages may have an additional benefit to performance or postexercise recovery (159,160), more research is needed (161–163).

Postexercise Nutrition

Athletes should consume a mixed meal or snack providing carbohydrates, protein, and fat soon after a strenuous competition or training session. Vegetarian athletes who have performed prolonged or strenuous exercise should make an effort to consume carbohydrate and possibly protein immediately after exercise to promote recovery, particularly if exercise training is to be resumed the following day.

Carbohydrate intake of between 1 and 1.5 g/kg within 30 minutes of exercise and again every 2 hours for the subsequent 4 to 6 hours is recommended to replace muscle glycogen and ensure rapid recovery (5). Foods with a high GI (144,164,165) or those containing both carbohydrate and protein (166) may increase the rate of muscle glycogen storage after exercise by stimulating greater insulin secretion. Evidence suggests that consuming protein along with carbohydrate after endurance or resistance training may provide needed amino acids for building and repair of muscle tissue to maximize nitrogen retention and stimulate muscle protein synthesis (33,167–171).

Current recommendations for postexercise fluid requirements are to consume up to 150% of the weight lost during the exercise session (5,150), which may be better retained if consumed at several settings rather than as a bolus (172). Athletes participating in heavy, prolonged workouts should also include sodium and potassium in the recovery meals (150,173). Although vegetarians are likely to choose potassium-containing foods (eg, fruits, vegetables), many may avoid sodium-containing foods. Sodium intake can be of concern during periods of heavy training in athletes who avoid salt or processed foods (ie, the typical sweat loss is approximately 50 mEq/L or 1 g sodium per hour) (5,150). Thus, more liberal intakes of sodium are often appropriate in the athletic population.

Special Concerns for Female Athletes

Low energy availability, with or without eating disorders, amenorrhea, and reduced bone density, alone or in combination, provide substantial health risk for female athletes (174). Although there is some evidence that several components of the female athlete triad, including low energy availability (174) and menstrual cycle disturbances, may be more common in vegetarians (175) and vegetarian athletes, the findings are not consistent (175,176). In some cases, the increased prevalence may be explained by study design or recruitment bias (175). For example, studies may define *vegetarian* differently (ie, those who eat a small amount of meat are not truly vegetarians), which may tend to recruit a biased sample of "vegetarians" (175). Furthermore, for some people proclaiming to be vegetarian may be perceived as a socially acceptable way to mask an eating disorder (177–180).

The mechanism mediating the disruption of normal hypothalamic reproductive function is unknown, but evidence points to a negative energy availability (ie, the energy drain hypothesis, in which athletes consistently eat less than they expend), rather than stress or an overly lean body composition (181). (See Box 18.2 in Chapter 18 for discussion of Female Athlete Triad and energy drain.) Other factors, however, have been linked to amenorrhea in individuals consuming a plant-based diet. In nonathletic females, Goldin et al (182) found that vegetarians, compared with nonvegetarians, had lower circulating estrogen concentrations, which was associated with higher fiber and lower fat intakes, higher fecal outputs, and two to three times more estrogen in feces. Among athletes, retrospective recall studies have generally documented lower intakes of energy (183,184), protein (183,184), fat (183,185), and zinc (185), and higher intakes of fiber (185,186) and vitamin A (185) in amenorrheic compared with eumenorrheic athletes. Collectively, these findings suggest that the energy and/or nutrient composition of some vegetarian diets could predispose vegetarian athletes to amenorrhea and reduced bone density.

Because available research suggests that reproductive disruption typically occurs when energy availability (dietary energy intake minus exercise energy expenditure) is less than a threshold of 30 kcal per kg of lean body mass (174,181), amenorrheic vegetarian athletes should be counseled on how to meet energy needs on a vegetarian diet, which may include reducing fiber intake. For athletes in heavy training, a diet with excessive fiber may lower energy intake and potentially reduce enterohepatic circulation of sex steroid hormones (182,187).

Nutrition Assessment of Vegetarian Athletes

The body sizes and shapes of vegetarian athletes vary, as do their dietary practices, food choices, and reasons for being vegetarian. It is important that the sports dietitian initially obtain and evaluate anthropometric measures, biochemical (laboratory) values, pertinent clinical information, and dietary and environmental factors as discussed in Chapter 8. Although laboratory and clinical data collected will vary, evaluation of mean corpuscular volume (MCV), hemoglobin, hematocrit, and 25(OH)D (71) concentrations may be helpful, along with information on training regimen, fatigue, injury history, and exercise performance. Menstrual cycle function and other components of the female athlete triad should also be assessed in female athletes (174). Unintended weight or muscle loss, fatigue, reduced strength gains, reduced performance, and/or loss of menstrual cycle function are signs that the diet may be lacking in total energy and possibly in certain macronutrients or micronutrients.

The dietary component of the assessment should begin by determining which foods the athlete normally eliminates from the diet and which foods are included. This will help assess nutrient adequacy and ensure that nutrients in omitted foods (such as dairy products) can be met with acceptable vegetarian foods. Although terms such as *lacto-ovo-vegetarian, lacto-vegetarian, vegan,* or *strict vegetarian* are commonly used to describe vegetarians, recent evidence-based analysis suggests that these very broad categories mask important variations within vegetarian diets and dietary practices (1). For example, two lacto-ovo-vegetarian athletes may have different philosophies about dairy products that would require different intervention plans. One of these athletes may consume several servings of dairy products per day, whereas the other may eat only cheese and small amounts of dairy found in processed foods. Similarly, some vegans may be extremely strict, eliminating all commercially available foods that contain any ingredient that is animal-derived or processed with an animal derivative (eg, commercial bread), while another will avoid foods of obvious animal origin. Also, some individuals claim to follow vegetarian diets when they mean that they avoid red meat but occasionally eat fish or poultry.

A thorough diet history followed by an analysis of energy and key nutrients (such as carbohydrate, protein, fat, fiber, calcium, vitamin D, iron, zinc, iodine, riboflavin, and vitamin B-12) is the best way to reliably assess the vegetarian athlete's diet. Computer nutrient databases may be helpful, but many do not contain an adequate selection of commercial vegetarian foods. In many cases, it is useful to have the athlete keep food records and bring in food labels from vegetarian products that he or she consumes.

Collection of environmental and behavioral information should include discussion on the athlete's belief system (ie, why he or she has chosen to follow a vegetarian diet) and barriers to healthful eating. Although health, ecology, animal welfare, and religion are admirable reasons for following a vegetarian diet, the desire to lose weight, a lack of time, or the desire to create a certain social image may warrant further investigation. Individuals who "don't eat meat" because they perceive vegetarianism to be a socially acceptable way to lose weight or because they have limited time or restricted food budgets have been labeled "new wave" vegetarians (188). These individuals may be at health and nutritional risk due to their haphazard eating patterns and lack of a solid philosophy that drives many nutritionally successful vegetarians in their desire to eat well. The focus when working with "new wave" vegetarians should be on improving the diet with more healthful plant-based (but not necessarily vegetarian) foods. A final concern is that vegetarianism may be used as a convenient and socially acceptable way for individuals with disordered eating tendencies to reduce energy and fat intake and thus mask their disordered eating behaviors (177–180), Occasionally, vegetarianism may be a sign of disordered eating and increased risk for the female athlete triad (5,174).

Counseling and Nutrition Treatment

The role of the sports dietitian during counseling, nutrition education, and treatment is to work with athletes to ensure adequate nutritional status within their vegetarian beliefs, budget, and lifestyle. Guidelines initially developed for counseling pregnant vegetarians (189) are useful when working with the vegetarian population in general (190). These guidelines include establishing rapport, reinforcing positive nutrition practices, prioritizing nutrition concerns, and providing individualized counseling (189). It is also important to remember that DRIs and other comparable nutritional requirements are recommended for essential nutrients (including protein, calcium, and iron) rather than for specific foods or food groups. As stated in the position of the Academy of Nutrition and Dietetics on vegetarian diets, vegetarian athletes should never be advised that they need to consume meat or dairy to be healthy. Box 16.4 contains tips for helping vegetarian athletes select a well-balanced vegetarian diet. Some male athletes, vegetarian or not, often ask about soy consumption and the risk of eating soy. Box 16.5 discusses the controversy of soy and feminization (190–194).

Resources for Improving the Diet

Some athletes or active individuals—vegetarian or omnivorous—may find it difficult to select a healthful, well-balanced diet with adequate variety (195). Factors such as lack of knowledge about food preparation,

---

BOX 16.4   Tips for Vegetarian Athletes

- Choose a variety of foods including whole and enriched grains, fruits, vegetables, legumes, nuts, seeds, and, if desired, dairy products and eggs.
- Consume adequate energy to optimize performance and help meet other nutrient needs, including protein, iron, zinc, magnesium, and riboflavin. Decrease fiber and possibly increase energy intake by consuming one third to one half of cereal/grain servings from refined rather than whole-grain sources and by replacing some high-fiber fruit or vegetable servings with juice servings.
- To help meet energy needs, consume small, frequent meals and snacks and strive to obtain one third to one half of grains, fruits, and vegetables from more refined rather than whole-food sources including enriched pasta, white rice, and fruit juice.
- Strive to consume a variety of protein-rich foods over the course of the day. Consumption of protein-rich foods along with carbohydrate foods in the 30 minutes after strenuous exercise may enhance recovery.
- Incorporate healthful fats in cooking and in dressing up foods, and limit foods that are high in saturated and *trans* fats.
- Include foods rich in n-3 fatty acids such as flax seeds; walnuts; and canola, flaxseed, hemp, and walnut oils.
- If dairy products are not consumed, chose eight or more servings per day of calcium-rich foods (see Table 16.2).
- Obtain adequate vitamin D from regular sun exposure or through fortified foods or supplements. In the absence of adequate sun exposure, intake of between 1,000 and 7,000 IU vitamin D is needed daily to maintain optimal vitamin D status.
- To meet iron needs, consume a variety of iron-rich grains and legumes daily. Aim to consume a fruit or vegetable that contains vitamin C along with most meals to boost absorption.
- Incorporate legumes and a serving or two of nuts into the diet almost daily. These foods provide protein and an abundance of other nutrients, including iron, zinc, magnesium, and some calcium. Nuts also provide additional energy and healthful fats.
- Use iodized salt when cooking and in salting foods, particularly in areas where the concentration of iodine in the soil is low. Remember the sodium needs of athletes are often increased due to sodium losses in sweat.
- Incorporate sources of vitamin B-12 in the diet each day. Vegan sources include one Tbsp of Red StarT6635 nutritional yeast, 1 cup (8 oz) of fortified soy milk, 1 oz (28 g) of fortified cereal, and 1.5 oz (42 g) of fortified meat analogue. Servings for vegetarians include ½ cup (4 oz) of cow's milk, 6 oz (172 g) yogurt, and one egg.
- Limit consumption of overly processed foods, which typically contain added sugars and unhealthful fats.

---

lack of time, and economic constraints may lead to a monotonous diet. Vegetarian cookbooks (particularly with pictures) and videos can be used to provide ideas for both increasing dietary variety and preparing simple meals. A tour of a supermarket or natural foods store may help identify products that are suitable for a vegetarian diet. Vegetarian cooking classes for teams or individual athletes are also a great way to provide hands-on education and introduce new vegetarian foods and recipes. (See Box 16.6 for recommended resources.)

BOX 16.5   Does Soy Consumption Lead to Feminization in Male Athletes?

In addition to being a source of quality protein, iron, calcium, magnesium, and other minerals, soy foods may offer health benefits beyond nutrient content. These benefits—which include reduced risk of cardiovascular disease, osteoporosis, and certain cancers—are linked to the high isoflavone content of soy (190). The isoflavone content is also the cause of the controversy because the chemical structure is close to that of estrogen (191) and it functions as selective estrogen receptor modulators (mixed estrogen agonists/antagonists) (192). For males, the concern is that xenoestrogen exposure, which includes phytoestrogens, has been hypothesized to produce a variety of undesirable side effects, including gynecomastia, erectile dysfunction, low sperm count, and reduced fertility. Such concerns have been referred to as "feminizing" effects of soy, and fueled by sensationalized media stories.

There are a few reports in the literature—mainly from isolated case reports or animal studies—that have linked excess isoflavone exposure to gynecomastia, erectile dysfunction, and reduced fertility (191). According to a recent critical analysis by Messina, however, the majority of clinical studies overwhelmingly indicate that isoflavone exposure at levels close to or in slight excess of typical Japanese intakes does not alter estrogen or testosterone concentrations (in men), sperm parameters, erectile dysfunction, or reproductive status (191). In contrast, one case study suggested a possible therapeutic role of soy isoflavones for infertility due to low sperm count (193).

One serving of traditional soy foods contains approximately 25 mg of isoflavones (3.5 mg per gram of protein) (194) whereas some isolated soy proteins contain little isoflavones due to processing. By comparison the estimated average daily intake of Asian adults is 25 to 50 mg of isoflavones, with about 10% consuming as much as 100 mg/day (194).

Male athletes can therefore rest assured that incorporating soy foods into the well-balanced vegetarian diet will not compromise virility or reproductive health. The interested reader is referred to a critical review by Messina (191) for additional information on soy exposure in men.

Summary

Athletes at all levels of performance can meet their energy and nutrient needs on a vegetarian diet that contains a variety of plant foods. Depending on their food patterns, some athletes may experience challenges in meeting their dietary needs for energy and key nutrients, including carbohydrate, protein, fat, calcium, vitamin D, iron, zinc, iodine, riboflavin, and vitamin B-12. Therefore, vegetarian athletes, like most athletes, may benefit from education about food choices that provide adequate nutrients and promote optimal training, optimal performance, and good health.

Sports dietitians who work with vegetarian athletes and their coaches and trainers need to be sensitive to and knowledgeable about vegetarianism and exercise training. Athletes should be encouraged to eat a wide variety of plant foods; they should not be told that they need poultry, fish, or dairy products to obtain adequate nutrition. It is the position of the Academy of Nutrition and Dietetics that "appropriately planned vegetarian diets are healthful, nutritionally adequate, and provide health benefits in the prevention and treatment of certain diseases" and can also "meet the needs of competitive athletes" (1).

BOX 16.6   Vegetarian Resources

Consumer Publications
- Davis B, Melina V. *Becoming Vegan.* Summertown, TN: Book Publishing Co; 2000.
- Larson-Meyer E. *Vegetarian Sports Nutrition: Food Choices and Eating Plans for Fitness and Performance.* Champaign, IL: Human Kinetics; 2007.
- Melina V, Davis B. *The New Becoming Vegetarian.* Summertown, TN: Healthy Living Publications; 2003.
- *Vegetarian Journal.* Bimonthly publication by the Vegetarian Resource Group, PO Box 1463, Baltimore, MD 21203. http://www.vrg.org.
- *Vegetarian Journal's Guide to Natural Food Restaurants in the US & Canada.* 4th ed. Baltimore, MD: Vegetarian Resource Group; 2005. Updates available at: http://www.vrg.org/restaurant/index.php.
- Wassernan D, Stahler C. *Meatless Meals for Working People: Quick and Easy Vegetarian Recipes.* 5th ed. Baltimore, MD: Vegetarian Resource Group; 2009.
- Wasserman D, Mangels R. *Simply Vegan.* 4th ed. Baltimore, MD: Vegetarian Resource Group; 2006.

Professional Publications
- Position of the American Dietetic Association: vegetarian diets. *J Am Diet Assoc.* 2009;109: 1266–1282.
- Carlson P, ed. *The Complete Vegetarian: The Essential Guide to Good Health.* Champaign, IL: University of Illinois Press; 2009.
- Messing V, Mangels R, Messina M. *A Dietitian's Guide to Vegetarian Diets: Issues and Applications.* 2nd ed. Sudbury, MA: Jones and Bartlett Publishers; 2004.
- Sabate J. *Vegetarian Nutrition.* Boca Raton, FL: CRC Press; 2001.

Quantity Recipes
- Berkoff N. *Vegan in Volume: Vegan Quantity Recipes for Every Occasion.* Revised ed. Baltimore, MD: Vegetarian Resource Group; 2007.
- *Vegetarian Journal's Foodservice Update.* Periodic publication by the Vegetarian Resource Group, PO Box 1463, Baltimore, MD 21203. http://www.vrg.org.

Resource Groups
- **Vegetarian Nutrition Dietetic Practice Group** of the Academy of Nutrition and Dietetics. http://www.vegetariannutrition.net.
- **The Vegetarian Resource Group**. http://www.vrg.org.

References

1. Craig WJ, Mangels AR. Position of the American Dietetic Association: vegetarian diets. *J Am Diet Assoc.* 2009; 109:1266–1282.
2. Larson-Meyer D. *Vegetarian Sports Nutrition. Food Choices and Eating Plans for Fitness and Performance.* Champaign, IL: Human Kinetics; 2007.
3. Leitzmann C. Vegetarian diets: what are the advantages? *Forum Nutr.* 2005;56:147–156.

4. Goran M. Variation in total energy expenditure in humans. *Obes Res.* 1995;3:59–66.

5. Rodriguez NR, DiMarco NM, Langley S. Position of the American Dietetic Association, Dietitians of Canada, and the American College of Sports Medicine: nutrition and athletic performance. *J Am Diet Assoc.* 2009;109:509–527.

6. Otten JJ, Hellwig JP, Meyers LD; Institute of Medicine. *The Dietary Reference Intakes: The Essential Guide to Nutrient Requirements.* Washington, DC: National Academy Press; 2006.

7. Institute of Medicine. *Dietary Reference Intakes for Energy, Carbohydrate, Fiber, Fat, Fatty Acids, Cholesterol, Protein, and Amino Acids.* Washington, DC: National Academies Press; 2005.

8. Cunningham J. A reanalysis of the factors influencing basal metabolic rate in normal adults. *Am J Clin Nutr.* 1980;33:2372–2374.

9. Thompson J, Manore M. Predicted and measured resting metabolic rate of male and female endurance athletes. *J Am Diet Assoc.* 1996;96:30–34.

10. US Department of Agriculture. MyPlate. http://www.choosemyplate.gov/tipsresources/vegetarian_diets.html. Accessed July 19, 2011.

11. Messina V, Mangels AR, Messina M. *A Dietitian's Guide to Vegetarian Diets: Issues and Applications.* 2nd ed. Boston, MA: Jones and Bartlett Publishers; 2004.

12. Messina V, Melina V, Mangels AR. A new food guide for North American vegetarians. *J Am Diet Assoc.* 2003;103: 771–775.

13. Casey A, Mann R, Banister K, Fox J, Morris PG, Macdonald IA, Greenhaff PL. Effect of carbohydrate ingestion on glycogen resynthesis in human liver and skeletal muscle, measured by (13)C MRS. *Am J Physiol Endocrinol Metab.* 2000;278:E65–E75.

14. Bergstrom J, Hermansen L, Hultman E, Saltin B. Diet, muscle glycogen and physical performance. *Acta Physiol Scand.* 1967;71:140–150.

15. Goforth HW, Laurent D, Prusaczyk WK, Schneider KE, Petersen KF, Shulman GI. Effects of depletion exercise and light training on muscle glycogen supercompensation in men. *Am J Physiol.* 2003;285:E1304–E1311.

16. Nilsson L, Hultman E. Liver glycogen in man—the effect of total starvation or a carbohydrate-poor diet followed by carbohydrate refeeding. *Scand J Clin Lab Invest.* 1973;32:325–330.

17. Achten J, Halson SL, Moseley L, Rayson MP, Casey A, Jeukendrup AE. Higher dietary carbohydrate content during intensified running training results in better maintenance of performance and mood state. *J Appl Physiol.* 2004;96:1331–1340.

18. Coggan AR, Swanson SC. Nutritional manipulations before and during endurance exercise: effects on performance. *Med Sci Sports Exerc.* 1992;24(suppl):S331–S335.

19. Spencer MK, Yan Z, Katz A. Carbohydrate supplementation attenuates IMP accumulation in human muscle during prolonged exercise. *Am J Physiol.* 1991;261:C71–C76.

20. O'Keeffe K, Keith R, Wilson G, Blessing D. Dietary carbohydrate intake and endurance exercise performance of trained female cyclists. *Nutr Res.* 1989;9:819–830.

21. Brewer J, Williams C, Patton A. The influence of high carbohydrate diets on endurance running performance. *Eur J Appl Physiol.* 1988;57:698–706.

22. Pizza F, Flynn M, Duscha B, Holden J, Kubitz E. A carbohydrate loading regimen improves high intensity, short duration exercise performance. *Int J Sport Nutr.* 1995;5:110–116.

23. Larson DE, Hesslink RL, Hrovat MI, Fishman RS, Systrom DM. Dietary effects on exercising muscle metabolism and performance by 31P-MRS. *J Appl Physiol.* 1994;77:1108–1115.

24. Sugiura K, Kobayashi K. Effect of carbohydrate ingestion on sprint performance following continuous and intermittent exercise. *Med Sci Sports Exerc.* 1998;30:1624–1630.

25. Hargreaves M, Costill D, Coggan A, Fink W, Nishibata I. Effect of carbohydrate feedings on muscle glycogen utilization and exercise performance. *Med Sci Sports Exerc.* 1984;16:219–222.

26. Tipton KD, Witard OC. Protein requirements and recommendations for athletes: relevance of ivory tower arguments for practical recommendations. *Clin Sports Med.* 2007;26:17–36.

27. Lemon P, Mullin J. Effect of initial muscle glycogen levels on protein catabolism during exercise. *J Appl Physiol.* 1980;48:624–629.

28. Institute of Medicine. *Recommended Dietary Allowances*. 10th ed. Washington, DC: National Academies Press; 1989.

29. Rand WM, Pellett PL, Young VR. Meta-analysis of nitrogen balance studies for estimating protein requirements in healthy adults. *Am J Clin Nutr*. 2003;77:109–127.

30. *FAO/WHO/UNU Expert Consultation on Protein and Amino Acid Requirements in Human Nutrition*. Report of a Joint FAO/WHO/UNU Expert Consultation. Geneva, Switzerland: World Health Organization; 2002.

31. Young VR, Pellett PL. Plant proteins in relation to human protein and amino acid nutrition. *Am J Clin Nutr*. 1994;59(5 Suppl):1203S–1212S.

32. Bergstrom J, Furst P, Vinnars E. Effect of a test meal, without and with protein, on muscle and plasma free amino acids. *Clin Sci (Lond)*. 1990;79:331–337.

33. Tipton KD, Rasmussen BB, Miller SL, Wolf SE, Owens-Stovall SK, Petrini BE, Wolfe RR. Timing of amino acid-carbohydrate ingestion alters anabolic response of muscle to resistance exercise. *Am J Physiol Endocrinol Metab*. 2001;281:E197–E206.

34. Tipton KD, Elliott TA, Cree MG, Aarsland AA, Sanford AP, Wolfe RR. Stimulation of net muscle protein synthesis by whey protein ingestion before and after exercise. *Am J Physiol Endocrinol Metab*. 2007;292:E71–E76.

35. Horvath PJ, Eagen CK, Fisher NM, Leddy JJ, Pendergast DR. The effects of varying dietary fat on performance and metabolism in trained male and female runners. *J Am Coll Nutr*. 2000;19:52–60.

36. Muoio DM, Leddy JJ, Horvath PJ, Awad AB, Pendergast DR. Effect of dietary fat on metabolic adjustments to maximal VO2 and endurance in runners. *Med Sci Sports Exerc*. 1994;26:81–88.

37. Hoppeler H, Billeter R, Horvath PJ, Leddy JJ, Pendergast DR. Muscle structure with low- and high-fat diets in well trained male runners. *Int J Sports Med*. 1999;20:522–526.

38. Brown RC, Cox CM. Effects of high fat versus high carbohydrate diets on plasma lipids and lipoproteins in endurance athletes. *Med Sci Sports Exerc*. 1998;30:1677–1683.

39. Larson-Meyer DE, Hunter GR, Newcomer BR. Influence of endurance running and recovery diet on intramyocellular lipid content in women: A 1H-NMR study. *Am J Physiol*. 2002;282:E95–E106.

40. Larson-Meyer DE, Borkhsenious ON, Gullett JC, Russell RR, Devries MC, Smith SR, Ravussin E. Effect of dietary fat on serum and intramyocellular lipids and running performance. *Med Sci Sports Exerc*. 2008;40:892–902.

41. Thompson PD, Cullinane EM, Eshleman R, Kantor MA, Herbert PN. The effects of high-carbohydrate and high-fat diets on the serum lipid and lipoprotein concentrations of endurance athletes. *Metabolism*. 1984;33:1003–1010.

42. Laughlin GA, Yen SS. Nutritional and endocrine-metabolic aberrations in amenorrheic athletes. *J Clin Endocrinol Metab*. 1996;81:4301–4309.

43. Decombaz J, Schmitt B, Ith M, Decarli B, Diem P, Kreis R, Hoppeler H, Boesch C. Postexercise fat intake repletes intramyocellular lipids but no faster in trained than in sedentary subjects. *Am J Physiol Regul Integr Comp Physiol*. 2001;281:R760–769.

44. Romijn J, Coyle EF, Sidossis LS, Gastaldelli A, Horowitz JF, Endert E, Wolfe RR. Regulation of endogenous fat and carbohydrate metabolism in relation to exercise intensity and duration. *Am J Physiol Endocrinol Metab*. 1993;265:E380–E391.

45. Romijn JA, Coyle EF, Sidossis LS, Rosenblatt J, Wolfe RR. Substrate metabolism during different exercise intensities in endurance-trained women. *J Appl Physiol*. 2000;88:1707–1714.

46. Ornish D, Brown S, Scherwitz L, Billings J, Armstrong W, Ports T, McLanahan S, Kirkeeide R, Brand R, Gould K. Can lifestyle changes reverse coronary heart disease? The Lifestyle Heart Trial. *Lancet*. 1990;336:129–133.

47. Barnard ND, Katcher HI, Jenkins DJ, Cohen J, Turner-McGrievy G. Vegetarian and vegan diets in type 2 diabetes management. *Nutr Rev*. 2009;67:255–263.

48. Gould KL, Ornish D, Kirkeeide R, Brown S, Stuart Y, Buchi M, Billings J, Armstrong W, Ports T, Scherwitz L. Improved stenosis geometry by quantitative coronary arteriography after vigorous risk factor modification. *Am J Cardiol*. 1992;69:845–853.

49. Gould KL, Ornish D, Scherwitz L, Brown S, Edens RP, Hess MJ, Mullani N, Bolomey L, Dobbs F, Armstrong WT, Merritt T, Ports T, Sparler S, Billings J. Changes in myocardial perfusion abnormalities by positron emission tomography after long-term, intense risk factor modification. *JAMA*. 1995;274:894–901.

50. Barnard ND, Cohen J, Jenkins DJ, Turner-McGrievy G, Gloede L, Green A, Ferdowsian H. A low-fat vegan diet and a conventional diabetes diet in the treatment of type 2 diabetes: a randomized, controlled, 74-wk clinical trial. *Am J Clin Nutr.* 2009;89(suppl);1588S–1596S.

51. Lichtenstein AH, Appel LJ, Brands M, Carnethon M, Daniels S, Franch HA, Franklin B, Kris-Etherton P, Harris WS, Howard B, Karanja N, Lefevre M, Rudel L, Sacks F, Van Horn L, Winston M, Wylie-Rosett J. Diet and lifestyle recommendations revision 2006: a scientific statement from the American Heart Association Nutrition Committee. *Circulation.* 2006;114:82–96.

52. Executive Summary of the Third Report of the National Cholesterol Education Program (NCEP) Expert Panel on Detection, Evaluation, and Treatment of High Blood Cholesterol in Adults (Adult Treatment Panel III). *JAMA.* 2001;285:2486–2497.

53. US Department of Health and Human Services; US Department of Agriculture. Dietary Guidelines for Americans, 2010. 7th ed. http://www.health.gov/dietaryguidelines/2010.asp. Accessed October 12, 2011.

54. Williams CM, Burdge G. Long-chain n-3 PUFA: plant v. marine sources. *Proc Nutr Soc.* 2006;65:42–50.

55. Geppert J, Kraft V, Demmelmair H, Koletzko B. Docosahexaenoic acid supplementation in vegetarians effectively increases omega-3 index: a randomized trial. *Lipids.* 2005;40:807–814.

56. Conquer JA, Holub BJ. Supplementation with an algae source of docosahexaenoic acid increases (n-3) fatty acid status and alters selected risk factors for heart disease in vegetarian subjects. *J Nutr.* 1996;126:3032–3039.

57. Institute of Medicine. *Dietary Reference Intakes for Calcium and Vitamin D.* Washington, DC: National Academies Press; 2010.

58. Heaney R, Recker R, Saville P. Menopausal changes in calcium balance performance. *J Lab Clin Med.* 1978;92:953–962.

59. Myburgh K, Hutchins J, Fataar A, Hough S, Noakes T. Low bone density is an etiologic factor for stress fractures in athletes. *Ann Intern Med.* 1990;113:754–759.

60. Ruohola JP, Laaksi I, Ylikomi T, Haataja R, Mattila VM, Sahi T, Tuohimaa P, Pihlajamaki H. Association between serum 25(OH)D concentrations and bone stress fractures in Finnish young men. *J Bone Miner Res.* 2006;21:1483–1488.

61. Wolman R, Clark P, McNally E, Harries M, Reeve J. Dietary calcium as a statistical determinant of trabecular bone density in amenorrhoeic and oestrogen-replete athletes. *Bone Miner.* 1992;17:415–423.

62. Lappe J, Cullen D, Haynatzki G, Recker R, Ahlf R, Thompson K. Calcium and vitamin D supplementation decreases incidence of stress fractures in female navy recruits. *J Bone Miner Res.* 2008;23:741–749.

63. Weaver C, Plawecki K. Dietary calcium: adequacy of a vegetarian diet. *Am J Clin Nutr.* 1994;59(5 Suppl):1238S–1241S.

64. Weaver CM, Proulx WR, Heaney R. Choices for achieving adequate dietary calcium with a vegetarian diet. *Am J Clin Nutr.* 1999;70(3 Suppl):543S–548S.

65. Heaney RP, Dowell MS, Rafferty K, Bierman J. Bioavailability of the calcium in fortified soy imitation milk, with some observations on method. *Am J Clin Nutr.* 2000;71:1166–1169.

66. Zhao Y, Martin BR, Weaver CM. Calcium bioavailability of calcium carbonate fortified soymilk is equivalent to cow's milk in young women. *J Nutr.* 2005;135:2379–2382.

67. Kohlenberg-Mueller K, Raschka L. Calcium balance in young adults on a vegan and lactovegetarian diet. *J Bone Miner Metab.* 2003;21:28–33.

68. Heaney RP, Dowell MS, Hale CA, Bendich A. Calcium absorption varies within the reference range for serum 25-hydroxyvitamin D. *J Am Coll Nutr.* 2003;22:142–146.

69. Holick MF. Sunlight and vitamin D for bone health and prevention of autoimmune diseases, cancers, and cardiovascular disease. *Am J Clin Nutr.* 2004;80(6 Suppl):1678S–1688S.

70. Holick MF. The vitamin D epidemic and its health consequences. *J Nutr.* 2005;135(suppl):2739S–2748S.

71. Larson-Meyer DE, Willis KS. Vitamin D and athletes. *Curr Sports Med Rep.* 2010;9:220–226.

72. Cannell JJ, Hollis BW, Sorenson MB, Taft TN, Anderson JJ. Athletic performance and vitamin D. *Med Sci Sports Exerc.* 2009;41:1102–1110.

73. Cannell JJ, Hollis BW. Use of vitamin D in clinical practice. *Altern Med Rev.* 2008;13:6–20.

74. Cannell JJ, Zasloff M, Garland CF, Scragg R, Giovannucci E. On the epidemiology of influenza. *Virol J*. 2008; 5:29.

75. Hamilton B. Vitamin D and human skeletal muscle. *Scand J Med Sci Sports*. 2009;20:182–190.

76. Halliday T, Peterson N, Thomas J, Kleppinger K, Hollis B, Larson-Meyer D. Vitamin D status relative to diet, lifestyle, injury and illness in college athletes. *Med Sci Sports Exerc*. 2011;43:335–343.

77. Hamilton B, Grantham J, Racinais S, Chalabi H. Vitamin D deficiency is endemic in Middle Eastern sportsmen. *Public Health Nutr*. 2010;13:1528–1534.

78. Holick MF, Biancuzzo RM, Chen TC, Klein EK, Young A, Bibuld D, Reitz R, Salameh W, Ameri A, Tannenbaum AD. Vitamin D2 is as effective as vitamin D3 in maintaining circulating concentrations of 25-hydroxyvitamin D. *J Clin Endocrinol Metab*. 2008;93:677–681.

79. Trang HM, Cole DE, Rubin LA, Pierratos A, Siu S, Vieth R. Evidence that vitamin D3 increases serum 25-hydroxyvitamin D more efficiently than does vitamin D2. *Am J Clin Nutr*. 1998;68:854–858.

80. Armas LA, Hollis BW, Heaney RP. Vitamin D2 is much less effective than vitamin D3 in humans. *J Clin Endocrinol Metab*. 2004;89:5387–5391.

81. Malczewska J, Raczynski G, Stupnicki R. Iron status in female endurance athletes and in non-athletes. *Int J Sport Nutr*. 2000;10:260–276.

82. Malczewska J, Szczepanska B, Stupnicki R, Sendecki W. The assessment of frequency of iron deficiency in athletes from the transferrin receptor-ferritin index. *Int J Sport Nutr Exerc Metab*. 2001;11:42–52.

83. Woolf K, St Thomas MM, Hahn N, Vaughan LA, Carlson AG, Hinton P. Iron status in highly active and sedentary young women. *Int J Sport Nutr Exerc Metab*. 2009;19:519–535.

84. Zhu Y, Haas J. Iron depletion without anemia and physical performance. *Am J Clin Nutr*. 1997;66:334–341.

85. Brownlie T, Utermohlen V, Hinton PS, Haas JD. Tissue iron deficiency without anemia impairs adaptation in endurance capacity after aerobic training in previously untrained women. *Am J Clin Nutr*. 2004;79:437–443.

86. Lamanca J, Haymes E. Effects of low ferritin concentrations on endurance performance. *Int J Sports Med*. 1992; 2:376–385.

87. Peeling P, Dawson B, Goodman C, Landers G, Trinder D. Athletic induced iron deficiency: new insights into the role of inflammation, cytokines and hormones. *Eur J Appl Physiol*. 2008;103:381–391.

88. Robertson J, Maughan R, Davidson R. Faecal blood loss in response to exercise. *BMJ*. 1987;295:303–305.

89. Waller M, Haymes E. The effects of heat and exercise on sweat iron loss. *Med Sci Sports Exerc*. 1996;28:197–203.

90. Eichner E. Runner's macrocytosis: a clue to footstrike hemolysis. *Am J Med*. 1985;78:321–325.

91. Jones GR, Newhouse I. Sport-related hematuria: a review. *Clin J Sport Med*. 1997;7:119–125.

92. Craig W. Iron status of vegetarians. *Am J Clin Nutr*. 1994;59(5 Suppl):1233S–1237S.

93. Coudray C, Bellanger J, Castiglia-Delavaud C, Remesy C, Vermorel M, Rayssignuier Y. Effect of soluble or partly soluble dietary fibres supplementation on absorption and balance of calcium, magnesium, iron and zinc in healthy young men. *Eur J Clin Nutr*. 1997;51:375–380.

94. Hallberg L, Hulthen L. Prediction of dietary iron absorption: an algorithm for calculating absorption and bioavailability of dietary iron. *Am J Clin Nutr*. 2000;71:1147–1160.

95. Snyder A, Dvorak L, Roepke J. Influence of dietary iron source on measures of iron status among female runners. *Med Sci Sports Exerc*. 1989;21:7–10.

96. Ball MJ, Bartlett MA. Dietary intake and iron status of Australian vegetarian women. *Am J Clin Nutr*. 1999;70: 353–358.

97. Hinton PS, Giordano C, Brownlie T, Haas JD. Iron supplementation improves endurance after training in iron-depleted, nonanemic women. *J Appl Physiol*. 2000;88:1103–1111.

98. Hinton PS, Sinclair LM. Iron supplementation maintains ventilatory threshold and improves energetic efficiency in iron-deficient nonanemic athletes. *Eur J Clin Nutr*. 2007;61:30–39.

99. Mettler S, Zimmermann MB. Iron excess in recreational marathon runners. *Eur J Clin Nutr*. 2010;64:490–494.

100. Schumacher YO, Schmid A, Grathwohl D, Bultermann D, Berg A. Hematological indices and iron status in athletes of various sports and performances. *Med Sci Sports Exerc*. 2002;34:869–875.

101. Herbert V. Everyone should be tested for iron disorders. *J Am Diet Assoc*. 1992;92:1502–1509.

102. Micheletti A, Rossi R, Rufini S. Zinc status in athletes: relation to diet and exercise. *Sports Med.* 2001;31:577–582.

103. Lukaski HC. Micronutrients (magnesium, zinc, and copper): are mineral supplements needed for athletes? *Int J Sport Nutr.* 1995;5(Suppl):S74–S83.

104. Hunt JR. Bioavailability of iron, zinc, and other trace minerals from vegetarian diets. *Am J Clin Nutr.* 2003;78 (3 Suppl):633S–639S.

105. Manore MM, Helleksen JM, Merkel J, Skinner JS. Longitudinal changes in zinc status in untrained men: effects of two different 12-week exercise training programs and zinc supplementation. *J Am Diet Assoc.* 1993;93: 1165–1168.

106. Lukaski HC. Vitamin and mineral status: effects on physical performance. *Nutrition.* 2004;20:632–644.

107. Singh A, Moses FM, Deuster PA. Vitamin and mineral status in physically active men: effects of a high-potency supplement. *Am J Clin Nutr.* 1992;55:1–7.

108. Lonnerdal B. Dietary factors influencing zinc absorption. *J Nutr.* 2000;130(5S Suppl):1378S–1383S.

109. Hunt JR, Matthys LA, Johnson LK. Zinc absorption, mineral balance, and blood lipids in women consuming controlled lactoovovegetarian and omnivorous diets for 8 wk. *Am J Clin Nutr.* 1998;67:421–430.

110. Rosado JL, Diaz M, Gonzalez K, Griffin I, Abrams SA, Preciado R. The addition of milk or yogurt to a plant-based diet increases zinc bioavailability but does not affect iron bioavailability in women. *J Nutr.* 2005;135:465–468.

111. Krajcovicova-Kudlackova M, Buckova K, Klimes I, Sebokova E. Iodine deficiency in vegetarians and vegans. *Ann Nutr Metab.* 2003;47:183–185.

112. Lightowler HJ, Davies GJ. Iodine intake and iodine deficiency in vegans as assessed by the duplicate-portion technique and urinary iodine excretion. *Br J Nutr.* 1998;80:529–535.

113. Remer T, Neubert A, Manz F. Increased risk of iodine deficiency with vegetarian nutrition. *Br J Nutr.* 1999;81: 45–49.

114. Waldmann A, Koschizke JW, Leitzmann C, Hahn A. Dietary intakes and lifestyle factors of a vegan population in Germany: results from the German Vegan Study. *Eur J Clin Nutr.* 2003;57:947–955.

115. Mangels AR, Messina V, Melina V. Position of the American Dietetic Association and Dietitians of Canada: vegetarian diets. *J Am Diet Assoc.* 2003;103:748–765.

116. Messina M, Redmond G. Effects of soy protein and soybean isoflavones on thyroid function in healthy adults and hypothyroid patients: a review of the relevant literature. *Thyroid.* 2006;16:249–258.

117. Rude RK, Singer FR, Gruber HE. Skeletal and hormonal effects of magnesium deficiency. *J Am Coll Nutr.* 2009; 28:131–141.

118. Nielsen FH, Lukaski HC. Update on the relationship between magnesium and exercise. *Magnes Res.* 2006;19: 180–189.

119. Woolf K, Manore MM. B-vitamins and exercise: does exercise alter requirements? *Int J Sport Nutr Exerc Metab.* 2006;16:453–484.

120. Herrmann W, Schorr H, Obeid R, Geisel J. Vitamin B-12 status, particularly holotranscobalamin II and methyl-malonic acid concentrations, and hyperhomocysteinemia in vegetarians. *Am J Clin Nutr.* 2003;78:131–136.

121. Herrmann W, Geisel J. Vegetarian lifestyle and monitoring of vitamin B-12 status. *Clin Chim Acta.* 2002;326: 47–59.

122. Rauma A, Torronen R, Hanninen O, Mykkanen H. Vitamin B-12 status of long-term adherents of a strict uncooked vegan diet ("living food diet") is compromised. *J Nutr.* 1995;125:2511–2515.

123. Donaldson MS. Metabolic vitamin B12 status on a mostly raw vegan diet with follow-up using tablets, nutritional yeast, or probiotic supplements. *Ann Nutr Metab.* 2000;44:229–234.

124. Belko A, Obarzanek E, Kalkwarf H, Rotter M, Bogusz S, Miller D, Haas J, Daphne D. Effects of exercise on riboflavin requirements of young women. *Am J Clin Nutr.* 1983;37:509–517.

125. Soares M, Satyanarayana K, Bamji M, Jacob C, Ramana Y, Rao S. The effect of exercise on the riboflavin status of adult men. *Br J Nutr.* 1993;69:541–551.

126. Tang JE, Moore DR, Kujbida GW, Tarnopolsky MA, Phillips SM. Ingestion of whey hydrolysate, casein, or soy protein isolate: effects on mixed muscle protein synthesis at rest and following resistance exercise in young men. *J Appl Physiol.* 2009;107:987–992.

127. Hartman JW, Tang JE, Wilkinson SB, Tarnopolsky MA, Lawrence RL, Fullerton AV, Phillips SM. Consumption of fat-free fluid milk after resistance exercise promotes greater lean mass accretion than does consumption of soy or carbohydrate in young, novice, male weightlifters. *Am J Clin Nutr.* 2007;86:373–381.

128. Phillips SM, Hartman JW, Wilkinson SB. Dietary protein to support anabolism with resistance exercise in young men. *J Am Coll Nutr.* 2005;24(suppl):134S–139S.

129. Wilkinson SB, Tarnopolsky MA, Macdonald MJ, Macdonald JR, Armstrong D, Phillips SM. Consumption of fluid skim milk promotes greater muscle protein accretion after resistance exercise than does consumption of an isonitrogenous and isoenergetic soy-protein beverage. *Am J Clin Nutr.* 2007;85:1031–1040.

130. Wilkinson SB, Phillips SM, Atherton PJ, Patel R, Yarasheski KE, Tarnopolsky MA, Rennie MJ. Differential effects of resistance and endurance exercise in the fed state on signaling molecule phosphorylation and protein synthesis in human muscle. *J Physiol.* 2008;586:3701–3717.

131. Howarth KR, Moreau NA, Phillips SM, Gibala MJ. Coingestion of protein with carbohydrate during recovery from endurance exercise stimulates skeletal muscle protein synthesis in humans. *J Appl Physiol.* 2009;106:1394–1402.

132. Moore DR, Robinson MJ, Fry JL, Tang JE, Glover EI, Wilkinson SB, Prior T, Tarnopolsky MA, Phillips SM. Ingested protein dose response of muscle and albumin protein synthesis after resistance exercise in young men. *Am J Clin Nutr.* 2009;89:161–168.

133. Balsom PD, Ekblom B, Soderlund K, Sjodin B, Hultman E. Creatine supplementation and dynamic high-intensity intermittent exercise. *Scand J Med Sci Sports.* 1993;3:143–149.

134. Delanghe J, De Slypere J-P, De Buyzere M, Robbrecht J, Wieme R, Vermeulen A. Normal reference values for creatine, creatinine, and carnitine are lower in vegetarians. *Clin Chem.* 1989;35:1802–1803.

135. Shomrat A, Weinstein Y, Katz A. Effect of creatine feeding on maximal exercise performance in vegetarians. *Eur J Appl Physiol.* 2000;82:321–325.

136. Harris RC, Soderlund K, Hultman E. Elevation of creatine in resting and exercised muscle of normal subjects by creatine supplementation. *Clin Sci.* 1992;83:367–374.

137. Lukaszuk JM, Robertson RJ, Arch JE, Moore GE, Yaw KM, Kelley DE, Rubin JT, Moyna NM. Effect of creatine supplementation and a lacto-ovo-vegetarian diet on muscle creatine concentration. *Int J Sport Nutr.* 2002;12:336–348.

138. Burke DG, Chilibeck PD, Parise G, Candow DG, Mahoney D, Tarnopolsky M. Effect of creatine and weight training on muscle creatine and performance in vegetarians. *Med Sci Sports Exerc.* 2003;35:1946–1955.

139. Clarys P, Zinzen E, Hebbelinck M. The effect of oral creatine supplementation on torque production in a vegetarian and non-vegetarian population: a double blind study. *Veg Nutr.* 1997;1:100–105.

140. Coyle E, Coggan A, Davis J, Sherman W. Current thoughts and practical considerations concerning substrate utilization during exercise. *Sports Sci Exch.* 1992;7:1–4.

141. Sherman W, Brodowicz G, Wright D, Allen W, Somonsen J, Dernbach A. Effects of 4 h preexercise carbohydrate feedings on cycling performance. *Med Sci Sports Exerc.* 1989;21:598–604.

142. Wright D, Sherman W, Dernbach A. Carbohydrate feedings before, during, or in combination improve cycling endurance performance. *J Appl Physiol.* 1991;71:1082–1088.

143. Wu CL, Williams C. A low glycemic index meal before exercise improves endurance running capacity in men. *Int J Sport Nutr Exerc Metab.* 2006;16:510–527.

144. Mondazzi L, Arcelli E. Glycemic index in sports nutrition. *J Am Coll Nutr.* 2009;28(Suppl):455S–463S.

145. Below P, Mora-Rodriguez R, Gonzalez-Alonso J, Coyle E. Fluid and carbohydrate ingestion independently improve performance during 1 h of intense exercise. *Med Sci Sports Exerc.* 1995;27:200–210.

146. Ball TC, Headley SA, Vanderburgh PM, Smith JC. Periodic carbohydrate replacement during 50 min of high-intensity cycling improves subsequent sprint performance. *Int J Sport Nutr.* 1995;5:151–158.

147. Nicholas C, Williams C, Phillips G, Nowitz A. Influence of ingesting a carbohydrate-electrolyte solution on endurance capacity during intermittent, high intensity shuttle running. *J Sports Sci.* 1995;13:283–290.

148. Currell K, Conway S, Jeukendrup AE. Carbohydrate ingestion improves performance of a new reliable test of soccer performance. *Int J Sport Nutr Exerc Metab.* 2009;19:34–46.

149. Hulston CJ, Jeukendrup AE. No placebo effect from carbohydrate intake during prolonged exercise. *Int J Sport Nutr Exerc Metab.* 2009;19:275–284.

150. Sawka MN, Burke LM, Eichner ER, Maughan RJ, Montain SJ, Stachenfeld NS. American College of Sports Medicine position stand. Exercise and fluid replacement. *Med Sci Sports Exerc.* 2007;39:377–390.

151. Jeukendrup AE. Carbohydrate intake during exercise and performance. *Nutrition.* 2004;20:669–677.

152. Currell K, Jeukendrup AE. Superior endurance performance with ingestion of multiple transportable carbohydrates. *Med Sci Sports Exerc.* 2008;40:275–281.

153. Pfeiffer B, Cotterill A, Grathwohl D, Stellingwerff T, Jeukendrup AE. The effect of carbohydrate gels on gastrointestinal tolerance during a 16-km run. *Int J Sport Nutr Exerc Metab.* 2009;19:485–503.

154. Neufer P, Costill D, Flynn M, Kirwan J, Mitchell J, Houmard J. Improvements in exercise performance: effects of carbohydrate feedings and diet. *J Appl Physiol.* 1987;62:983–988.

155. van der Brug GE, Peters HP, Hardeman MR, Schep G, Mosterd WL. Hemorheological response to prolonged exercise—no effects of different kinds of feedings. *Int J Sports Med.* 1995;16:231–237.

156. Lugo M, Sherman WM, Wimer GS, Garleb K. Metabolic responses when different forms of carbohydrate energy are consumed during cycling. *Int J Sport Nutr.* 1993;3:398–407.

157. Lancaster S, Kreider RB, Rasmussen C, Kerksick C, Greenwood M, Milnor P, Almada AL, Earnest CP. Effects of honey supplementation on glucose, insulin, and endurance cycling performance. *FASEB J.* 2001;15(supplement): LB315.

158. Gisolfi C, Duchman S. Guidelines for optimal replacement beverages for different athletic events. *Med Sci Sports Exerc.* 1992;24:679–687.

159. Saunders MJ, Kane MD, Todd MK. Effects of a carbohydrate-protein beverage on cycling endurance and muscle damage. *Med Sci Sports Exerc.* 2004;36:1233–1238.

160. Saunders MJ, Moore RW, Kies AK, Luden ND, Pratt CA. Carbohydrate and protein hydrolysate coingestions improvement of late-exercise time-trial performance. *Int J Sport Nutr Exerc Metab.* 2009;19:136–149.

161. Breen L, Tipton KD, Jeukendrup AE. No effect of carbohydrate-protein on cycling performance and indices of recovery. *Med Sci Sports Exerc.* 2010;42:1140–1148.

162. Jeukendrup AE, Tipton KD, Gibala MJ. Protein plus carbohydrate does not enhance 60-km time-trial performance. *Int J Sport Nutr Exerc Metab.* 2009;19:335–337.

163. van Essen M, Gibala MJ. Failure of protein to improve time trial performance when added to a sports drink. *Med Sci Sports Exerc.* 2006;38:1476–1483.

164. Burke L, Collier G, Hargreaves M. Muscle glycogen storage after prolonged exercise: effect of the glycemic index of carbohydrate feedings. *J Appl Physiol.* 1993;75:1019–1023.

165. Jozsi AC, Trappe TA, Starling RD, Goodpaster B, Trappe SW, Fink WJ, Costill DL. The influence of starch structure on glycogen resynthesis and subsequent cycling performance. *Int J Sports Med.* 1996;17:373–378.

166. Ivy JL, Goforth HW Jr, Damon BM, McCauley TR, Parsons EC, Price TB. Early postexercise muscle glycogen recovery is enhanced with a carbohydrate-protein supplement. *J Appl Physiol.* 2002;93:1337–1344.

167. Rodriguez NR, Vislocky LM, Gaine PC. Dietary protein, endurance exercise, and human skeletal-muscle protein turnover. *Curr Opin Clin Nutr Metab Care.* 2007;10:40–45.

168. Roy BD, Tarnopolsky MA, MacDougall JD, Fowles J, Yarasheski KE. Effect of glucose supplement on protein metabolism after resistance training. *J Appl Physiol.* 1997;82:1882–1888.

169. Roy BD, Luttmer K, Bosman MJ, Tarnopolsky MA. The influence of post-exercise macronutrient intake on energy balance and protein metabolism in active females participating in endurance training. *Int J Sport Nutr.* 2002;12:172–188.

170. Levenhagen DK, Gresham JD, Carlson MG, Maron DJ, Borel MJ, Flakoll PJ. Postexercise nutrient intake timing in humans is critical to recovery of leg glucose and protein homeostasis. *Am J Physiol Endocrinol Metab.* 2001;280:E982–E993.

171. Miller SL, Tipton KD, Chinkes DL, Wolf SE, Wolfe RR. Independent and combined effects of amino acids and glucose after resistance exercise. *Med Sci Sports Exerc.* 2003;35:449–455.

172. Jones EJ, Bishop PA, Green JM, Richardson MT. Effects of metered versus bolus water consumption on urine production and rehydration. *Int J Sport Nutr Exerc Metab.* 2010;20:139–144.

173. Maughan R, Leiper J, Shirreffs S. Restoration of fluid balance after exercise-induced dehydration: effects of food and fluid intake. *Eur J Appl Physiol*. 1996;73:317–325.

174. Nattiv A, Loucks AB, Manore MM, Sanborn CF, Sundgot-Borgen J, Warren MP. American College of Sports Medicine position stand. The female athlete triad. *Med Sci Sports Exerc*. 2007;39:1867–1882.

175. Barr SI. Vegetarianism and menstrual cycle disturbances: is there an association? *Am J Clin Nutr*. 1999;70(3 Suppl):549S–554S.

176. Slavin J, Lutter J, Cushman S. Amenorrhea in vegetarian athletes [letter]. *Lancet*. 1984;1:1474–1475.

177. O'Connor MA, Touyz SW, Dunn SM, Beumont JV. Vegetarianism in anorexia nervosa? A review of 116 consecutive cases. *Med J Aust*. 1987;147:540–542.

178. Huse DM, Lucas AR. Dietary patterns in anorexia nervosa. *Am J Clin Nutr*. 1984;40:251–254.

179. Robinson-O'Brien R, Perry CL, Wall MM, Story M, Neumark-Sztainer D. Adolescent and young adult vegetarianism: better dietary intake and weight outcomes but increased risk of disordered eating behaviors. *J Am Diet Assoc*. 2009;109:648–655.

180. Neumark-Sztainer D, Story M, Resnick MD, Blum RW. Adolescent vegetarians. A behavioral profile of a school-based population in Minnesota. *Arch Pediatr Adolesc Med*. 1997;151:833–838.

181. Loucks AB. Energy availability, not body fatness, regulates reproductive function in women. *Exerc Sport Sci Rev*. 2003;31:144–148.

182. Goldin B, Adlercreutz H, Gorbach S, Warram J, Dwyer J, Swenson L, Woods M. Estrogen excretion patterns and plasma levels in vegetarian and omnivorous women. *N Engl J Med*. 1982;307:1542–1547.

183. Kaiserauer S, Snyder A, Sleeper M, Zierath J. Nutritional, physiological, and menstrual status of distance runners. *Med Sci Sports Exerc*. 1989;21:120–125.

184. Nelson M, Fisher E, Catsos P, Meredith C, Turksoy R, Evans W. Diet and bone status in amenorrheic runners. *Am J Clin Nutr*. 1986;43:910–916.

185. Deuster PA, Kyle SB, Moser PB, Vigersky RA, Singh A, Schoomaker EB. Nutritional intakes and status of highly trained amenorrheic and eumenorrheic women runners. *Fertil Steril*. 1986;46:636–643.

186. Lloyd T, Buchanen J, Bitzer S, Waldman C, Myers C, Ford B. Interrelationship of diet, athletic activity, menstrual status, and bone density in collegiate women. *Am J Clin Nutr*. 1987;46:681–684.

187. Raben A, Kiens B, Richter EA, Rasmussen LB, Svenstrup B, Micic S, Bennett P. Serum sex hormones and endurance performance after a lacto-ovo vegetarian and a mixed diet. *Med Sci Sports Exerc*. 1992;24:1290–1297.

188. Szabo L. The health risks of new-wave vegetarianism. *Can Med Assoc J*. 1997;156:1454–1455.

189. Johnston P. Counseling the pregnant vegetarian. *Am J Clin Nutr*. 1988;48(3 Suppl):S901–S905.

190. Messina M, Watanabe S, Setchell KD. Report on the 8th International Symposium on the Role of Soy in Health Promotion and Chronic Disease Prevention and Treatment. *J Nutr*. 2009;139(suppl):796S–802S.

191. Messina M. Soybean isoflavone exposure does not have feminizing effects on men: a critical examination of the clinical evidence. *Fertil Steril*. 2010;93:2095–2104.

192. Setchell KD. Soy isoflavones—benefits and risks from nature's selective estrogen receptor modulators (SERMs). *J Am Coll Nutr*. 2001;20(5 Suppl):354S–362S; discussion 381S–383S.

193. Casini ML, Gerli S, Unfer V. An infertile couple suffering from oligospermia by partial sperm maturation arrest: can phytoestrogens play a therapeutic role? A case report study. *Gynecol Endocrinol*. 2006;22:399–401.

194. Messina M, Nagata C, Wu AH. Estimated Asian adult soy protein and isoflavone intakes. *Nutr Cancer*. 2006;55:1–12.

195. Mangels A. Working with vegetarian clients. *Issues in Vegetarian Dietetics*. 1995;5(1):1,4,5.

Chapter 17

PREGNANCY AND EXERCISE

MICHELLE F. MOTTOLA, PhD, FACSM

Introduction

Pregnancy is a special time during which many women change to a healthier lifestyle because of concern for the developing fetus. Many women eat more nutritious foods, stop smoking, stop drinking alcohol, moderate caffeine consumption, and think about active living. This is a unique opportunity for health care professionals to educate pregnant women on the benefits of healthful eating and being physically active.

There are many physiological alterations that occur during pregnancy that make meeting the nutritional needs of the mother and growing fetus a potential challenge. These physiological alterations must also be considered to prescribe safe exercise guidelines. Pregnant women must be medically prescreened before they start or continue an exercise program. They should be counseled on appropriate food choices and portion sizes. Pregnant women should not "eat for two," but rather eat "twice as healthy."

This chapter will begin with the major physiological changes that occur during pregnancy that have implications for an exercise prescription. Metabolic adaptations during pregnancy are important for the growth and development of the fetus because the major energy source is maternal blood glucose. An unhealthy diet and a sedentary lifestyle can tip the balance of these normal metabolic changes and lead to high and uncontrolled maternal blood glucose, which places the woman at risk for excessive weight gain and gestational diabetes mellitus (GDM).

An unhealthy lifestyle may lead to potential chronic disease risk factors for both mother and child. The environment of the developing fetus has an important impact on the future health of the child, adolescent, and adult. Prevention of excessive weight gain during pregnancy by adopting a healthful lifestyle approach is vital for the health of the pregnant woman. This can be accomplished by ensuring that her nutrient intake is adequate to meet the needs of pregnancy and using a medical prescreening tool (PARmed-X for Pregnancy) to screen for contraindications to exercise. An exercise prescription for aerobic and muscle conditioning exercise for the expectant woman is recommended for a healthy pregnancy as is the use of an intervention program to prevent excessive weight gain in overweight and obese pregnant women. The importance of emphasizing active living during pregnancy is paramount.

Physiological Adaptations During Pregnancy

Physiological adaptations that occur during pregnancy affect nutritional needs and exercise performance. The following descriptions of maternal physiological adaptations at rest represent complicated examples of the many changes occurring to support the growth and development of the fetus. Further readings that summarize these pregnancy-induced alterations are suggested (1–6). This section will focus on the physiological changes that impact exercise capacity and performance, namely the cardiorespiratory system, thermoregulation, and metabolism.

Cardiorespiratory System

The cardiorespiratory system adapts early in pregnancy, mediated by ovarian and placental hormones. Resting cardiac output increases significantly in the first trimester (typically 4 to 5 L/min) (2), reflecting a 50% increase from nonpregnant values (7), with smaller gradual increases until midway through the second trimester, after which cardiac output will plateau (3,8). These changes are observed in association with increases in aortic capacitance (9), a reduction in peripheral vascular resistance (10), and ventricular cavity dilation without an increase in wall thickness of the heart (11). The maternal cardiovascular system is remodeled in early gestation (12) to accommodate the increasing blood volume.

The early pregnancy-induced changes in cardiac output are thought to occur in response to increases in resting heart rate, as most of the 15- to 20-beat increase in heart rate from nonpregnant values also occurs during the first trimester (6). Stroke volume has been shown to increase by approximately 10% at the end of the first trimester (7). The stroke volume increase occurs before substantial enhancement of maternal blood volume (10), which may increase up to 50% above nonpregnant values by late pregnancy (13). The gradual increase in maternal plasma volume may be caused by pregnancy-induced hormones that reduce peripheral vascular resistance (10), leading to fluid retention so that blood pressure is maintained or slightly reduced from nonpregnant values (10).

Pregnancy-induced hormones also cause a remodeling of the thoracic cage so that the diaphragm is in a higher midthoracic position (4). In addition, during early pregnancy there is an increase in respiratory sensitivity to carbon dioxide (4), with little or no change in respiratory frequency (14). Although pregnant women with no history of cardiorespiratory disease complain of respiratory discomfort or shortness of breath (dyspnea), especially in late pregnancy, one potential cause both at rest and upon exertion (15) may be an increased respiratory effort due to mechanical alterations of the respiratory system (16).

Thermoregulation During Pregnancy

Thermoregulation steadily improves during pregnancy, reflected by a continuous decrease in rectal temperature (17,18). This is related to the downward shift in the temperature set point for the initiation of sweating that allows evaporative heat loss to occur at a lower body temperature as pregnancy advances (17). Maternal heat regulation and dissipation are important because fetal metabolism generates heat and fetal temperature is dependent upon maternal temperature, fetal metabolism, and uterine blood flow (18).

Metabolic Adaptations to Pregnancy

Maternal blood glucose is the primary energy source for growth of the fetus and placenta, and maternal metabolic adaptations ensure an adequate supply (19). A cascade of hormonal events results in an increase in maternal blood glucose production from the liver (20), an increase in pancreatic insulin production (21), an increase in insulin resistance at the skeletal muscle level (22), and a decrease in the use of blood glucose by maternal skeletal muscles (23). This normal insulin resistance at the muscle level ensures more maternal blood glucose for fetal use, which can be as high as 30% to 50% in late gestation (24). Maternal body fat is stored early in pregnancy (perhaps due to the action of the increased insulin concentrations) (25), to ensure that these fat stores can be used for lipolysis in late pregnancy as an alternate fuel source for the mother to conserve maternal glucose for fetal needs (26).

If a woman has risk factors for type 2 diabetes, such as being overweight, a family history of diabetes, from a certain ethnic/ancestry (Native American, Hispanic, South Asian, Asian, or African descent) or is age 35 years or older at the time of pregnancy (27), pregnancy may tip the balance and abnormally high maternal blood glucose and insulin concentrations may result (27). These abnormally high concentrations result in GDM, which is defined as a form of diabetes first diagnosed during pregnancy (28). The high concentration of blood glucose in women diagnosed with GDM is used by the fetus for growth and development, increasing baby size and weight and leading to a difficult labor and birth, especially if the baby weighs more than 9 lb (macrosomia) (28).

Energy Balance and Maternal Weight Gain

Although the normal metabolic adaptations mentioned earlier are necessary for fetal growth and development, the energy balance equation still applies during pregnancy. Excessive energy input without corresponding energy output will cause excessive pregnancy weight gain. Excessive pregnancy weight gain and weight retention after delivery have been linked to type 2 diabetes and the increasing epidemic of obesity (29). The prevalence of maternal obesity and being overweight ranges from 34% to 39% (30,31) worldwide, with an increasing prevalence of 69% over 10 years (1993 to 2003) in nine US states (32), which may be an underestimation of the current situation.

Overweight women who retained previous pregnancy weight start their next pregnancy with a higher early rate of weight gain (33), which has been strongly associated with weight retention at 6 and 12 months' postpartum. This growing epidemic of maternal obesity and excessive gestational weight gain and retention after delivery prompted the Institute of Medicine (IOM) to publish new pregnancy weight-gain guidelines (Table 17.1), which are now based on prepregnancy body mass index (BMI) as suggested by the World Health Organization and have a specific recommendation for women who are obese (34). Table 17.2 represents the total body weight gain distribution necessary for a normal-weight pregnant woman, assuming the

TABLE 17.1 Institute of Medicine Recommendations for Weight Gain in Pregnancy

Prepregnancy Weight Classification Classification	Prepregnancy Body Mass Index	Recommended Total Pregnancy Weight Gain, lb	Recommended Rates of Weight Gain for 2nd and 3rd Trimesters, lb/wk (Mean Range, lb/wk)
Underweight	< 18.5	28–40	1 (1–1.3)
Normal weight	18.5–24.9	25–35	1 (0.8–1)
Overweight	25.0–29.9	15–25	0.6 (0.5–0.7)
Obese (including all classes)	≥ 30.0	11–20	0.5 (0.4–0.6)

Source: Data are from reference 34.

TABLE 17.2 Approximate Body Weight Gain Distribution Necessary for Normal-Weight Pregnant Women[a]

Body Tissue	Weight Gain, kg (lb)
Breasts	0.5 (1.1)
Placenta	0.6 (1.3)
Baby	3.4 (7.5)
Uterus	1.0 (2.2)
Blood	1.5 (3.3)
Amniotic fluid	1.0 (2.2)
Maternal fluids	1.5 (3.3)
Body reserves (fat stores)[b]	3.0 (6.6)

[a]Estimates assume a baby who weighs 7.5 lb.
[b]Excessive body weight gain more than the recommended range for normal-weight women will be stored as fat reserves.
Source: Data are from reference 35.

baby weighs approximately 7.5 lb (35). The weight gain guidelines are presented as a range because every pregnant woman should be treated as an individual, with stature and race/ethnicity as important considerations for weight gain (34). Excessive weight gain more than the recommended range may be added to fat reserves (Table 17.2) (35), and may contribute to the problem of weight retention after delivery. Gaining excessive weight adds increased risk to being diagnosed with GDM (36), pregnancy-induced hypertension (37), and a difficult labor and birth. Women who gain excessive weight are also more likely to have adverse fetal outcomes such as large-for-gestational age babies, and, in turn, these babies are at risk for obesity and the resultant comorbidities (38).

Macronutrient and Micronutrient Considerations During Pregnancy

Adequate maternal weight gain supports the products of conception (fetus, placenta, and amniotic fluid) and the maternal tissues needed to support the pregnancy (extra blood volume, fluids, uterus, mammary glands, and fat stores) as shown in Table 17.2 (35). Many physiological adaptations occur early in pregnancy; however, compared to the needs of a nonpregnant woman of childbearing age, the total amount of extra energy required does not markedly increase until the second and third trimesters (39), as long as the woman is consuming a healthful, well-balanced diet required for adult women. Table 17.3 lists the macronutrients and micronutrients necessary for adult women, pregnant women, and breastfeeding women up to 6 months after delivery (39–41). The extra energy requirement beyond the usual energy requirement of an adult woman is approximately 340 kcal in the second trimester and 452 kcal in the third (39). (See Table 17.3.) Many pregnant women do not realize that meeting their extra daily energy requirements does not mean doubling the amount of food. The extra daily energy requirement in the second trimester may be met by consuming, for example, a medium apple (85 kcal), a cup of fat-free milk (90 kcal), ½ cup of fruit yogurt (128 kcal), and ½ cup of baby carrots (40 kcal). In the third trimester, a woman could add the equivalent of a large apple (115 kcal) to the second-trimester sample food list and meet her extra daily energy needs. In addition to Table 17.3, specific estimated energy requirements (EER) can be calculated for pregnant women by using the equations provided in the IOM 2009 full report (42).

TABLE 17.3   Dietary Reference Intakes for Women[a]

Nutrient	Women (Not Pregnant, Not Lactating)	Pregnant Women	Lactating Women, 0–6 mo Postdelivery
Energy, kcal	2,403	2,743 (2nd trimester); 2,855 (3rd trimester)	2,698
Protein, g/kg	0.8	1.1	1.1
Carbohydrate, g	130	175	210
Total fiber, g	25	28	29
Linoleic acid, g	12	13	13
Alpha-Linolenic acid, g	1.1	1.4	1.3
Vitamin A, mcg retinol activity equivalents	700	770	1,300
Vitamin D, mcg	15	15	15
Vitamin E, mg alpha-tocopherol	15	15	19
Vitamin K, mcg	90	90	90
Vitamin C, mg	75	85	120
Thiamin, mg	1.1	1.4	1.4
Riboflavin, mg	1.1	1.4	1.6
Vitamin B-6, mg	1.3	1.9	2.0
Niacin, mg niacin equivalents	14	18	17
Folate, mcg dietary folate equivalents	400	600	500
Vitamin B-12, mcg	2.4	2.6	2.8
Pantothenic acid, mg	5	6	7
Biotin, mcg	30	30	35
Choline, mg	425	450	550
Calcium, mg	1,000	1,000	1,000
Phosphorus, mg	700	700	700
Magnesium, mg	320	350	310
Iron, mg	8	27	9
Zinc, mg	8	11	12
Iodine, mcg	150	220	290
Selenium, mcg	55	60	70
Fluoride, mg	3	3	3
Manganese, mg	1.8	2.0	2.6
Molybdenum, mcg	45	50	50
Chromium, mcg	25	30	45
Copper, mcg	900	1,000	1,300
Sodium, mg	2,300	2,300	2,300
Potassium, mg	4,700	4,700	5,100

[a]Dietary Reference Intakes (DRIs) are for women ages 19 to 50 y. Energy DRI is the Estimated Energy Requirement. DRIs for total fiber, linoleic acid, alpha-linolenic acid, vitamin K, pantothenic acid, biotin, choline, chromium, manganese, potassium, and sodium are Adequate Intakes. All other DRIs are Recommended Dietary Allowances.
Source: Data are from references 39, 40, and 41.

It is particularly important to assess pregnant women's intake of folic acid and iron because many women do not meet the daily requirements. The US Department of Agriculture's MyPlate Web site includes pregnancy-specific nutrition information that can be used to make healthful food choices to ensure that appropriate requirements are met (43). Eating foods with dietary fiber, such as whole grain products, vegetables, fruit, and legumes, is important for pregnant women (39). In addition to a well-balanced diet, pregnant women should consume approximately 8 to 10 cups of fluid per day for adequate hydration. Fluids include milk and water in fruits and vegetables; sugary drinks and soda should be minimized (39).

Maternal-Fetal Link to Chronic Disease

Eating well and maintaining a healthful lifestyle is extremely important because there is an increasing body of scientific literature suggesting a robust link between the fetal environment and the profound influence on lifelong health and the future disease risk of the offspring (44,45). Maternal ingestion of heavily processed, high-calorie "junk food" during pregnancy and lactation may increase her offspring's preference for junk food and the propensity for offspring obesity (46). In addition, if the metabolic state of the mother is altered by an increasing hyperglycemia during pregnancy (GDM and impaired glucose tolerance), her child is at increased risk of obesity and type 2 diabetes at 5 to 7 years of age (47). However, this increased risk is modifiable if the GDM is treated or prevented (47), which strongly suggests that the influence of the intrauterine milieu can be passed on to the next generation nongenetically, and that by maintaining a healthy fetal environment, undesirable influences affecting the offspring can be reversed and prevented (48).

Achievement and maintenance of a healthy weight must be encouraged, and support must be provided to assist women in reaching and maintaining this goal during and after pregnancy (49). In addition to overeating, a sedentary lifestyle is a common link between excessive weight gain and obesity and GDM (49). The prevention of excessive weight gain during pregnancy through healthful eating and increased physical activity is highly recommended as an intervention to reduce the occurrence of chronic disease risk for both the mother and her future child.

Exercise During Pregnancy

The benefits of being active during pregnancy include an increase in maternal metabolic and cardiopulmonary reserve, promotion of normal glucose tolerance, and improved psychological well-being (50). In addition, there are beneficial fetal and placental adaptations in a low-risk pregnancy (1). However, the absence of adequate and habitual physical activity, in which these beneficial adaptive benefits occur, may ultimately lead to future obesity, type 2 diabetes, and cardiovascular disease (49). The American College of Obstetricians and Gynecologists (ACOG) suggests that all pregnant women with low-risk pregnancies should exercise on most if not all days of the week (51). The Physical Activity Guidelines for Americans recommends at least 150 minutes (2 hours and 30 minutes) of moderate-intensity aerobic activity per week for pregnant women, with this activity spread throughout the week (52). These guidelines also suggest that pregnant women who begin an exercise program should increase the amount gradually over time (52). Before prescribing exercise, the medical provider should thoroughly evaluate a pregnant patient to ensure low obstetric risk. The Physical Activity Readiness Medical Examination (PARmed-X) for Pregnancy (53) is a tool that can be used by health care providers for medical prescreening in a simple checklist format. This document also provides more specific guidelines that use the FITT principle (frequency, intensity, time [duration], and type of exercise) after medical prescreening (53,54).

The PARmed-X for Pregnancy document is based on scientific evidence that suggests that pregnant women who are medically prescreened and have no contraindications to exercise can safely exercise at 60% to 80% of their aerobic capacity (50,54,55). This document contains a brief medical history questionnaire for the pregnant woman to complete, a list of contraindications to exercise (both absolute and relative), guidelines for aerobic and muscular conditioning exercise, a list of safety considerations, and reasons to stop exercise and seek medical advice (53). The PARmed-X for Pregnancy has been endorsed by various professional organizations in the United States (56) and Canada (54,57,58).

Aerobic Exercise Prescription

Exercise prescriptions should be based on the FITT principle (59), which should be individualized to each pregnant woman. With medical approval, women with low-risk pregnancies can begin an exercise program; they may prefer to start in the second trimester after the fatigue and other pregnancy-induced discomforts of first trimester have diminished.

Frequency

ACOG (51) recommends exercise on most if not all days of the week for pregnant women, and the latest Physical Activity Guidelines for Americans suggest that this activity be spread throughout the week (52). A recent study suggests caution, however, because frequency of structured exercise, especially during late pregnancy, was a determinant of birth weight (60). In this case-control study of 526 women, the odds of giving birth to a small-for-gestational age baby was 4.6 times more likely for women who engaged in structured exercise more than five times per week (which may be too much) and also 2.6 times more likely for those women who engaged in structured exercise two or fewer times per week (which may be too little) (60). Because small-for-gestational age babies are at risk for obesity and cardiovascular disease later in life (45), structured exercise three to four times per week would seem ideal. Starting an exercise program at three times per week with a day of rest between each exercise day may also help eliminate fatigue (50).

Intensity

The PARmed-X for Pregnancy document presents target heart rate zones based on age that is related to approximately 60% to 80% of aerobic capacity (moderate-intensity exercise) for pregnant women (55). These heart rate zones were modified from the zones suggested for nonpregnant individuals for two reasons. First, heart rate reserve during pregnancy is decreased because heart rate during maximal exercise is attenuated (61). Second, resting heart rate during pregnancy increases by about 15 to 20 beats per minute above nonpregnant values (55). Although it has been suggested that target heart rate zones should not be used to monitor exercise intensity in pregnant women, the safety and efficacy of the target heart rate zones presented in the PARmed-X for Pregnancy have been verified in controlled studies (14,50,62) and are appropriate for pregnant women with a normal BMI (62).

Women on either end of the exercise continuum, either unfit and slightly overweight, or very fit, may find that the target heart rate zones listed in the PARmed-X for Pregnancy are not appropriate. New target heart rate zones for pregnant women were developed and validated in a population of 156 pregnant women and are now based on maternal age and fitness level, reflecting 60% to 80% of aerobic capacity (62). These modified target heart rate zones based on age and fitness levels are presented in Table 17.4 (53,62).

For overweight and obese pregnant women (prepregnancy BMI ≥ 25), an exercise program of moderate-intensity exercise (60% to 80% aerobic capacity) may be too much. The American College of Sports Medicine (ACSM) suggested that previously sedentary overweight and obese pregnant women should initiate an aerobic exercise program at a milder intensity equivalent to 20% to 39% aerobic capacity, which indicates the lowest level of physical activity to provide health benefits (63). Target heart rate zones were developed and validated on 106 overweight and obese low-risk pregnant women using the equivalent of 20% to 39% of aerobic capacity (64). These exercise target heart rate zones are also based on maternal age and are between 102 and 124 beats per minute for women 20 to 29 years of age and between 101 and 120 beats per minute for women 30 to 39 years of age (64). Overweight and obese pregnant women who use these lower intensities may be more compliant, especially if walking is the mode of activity (65).

TABLE 17.4 Target Heart Rate Zones for Aerobic Exercise Prescription in Pregnancy

Fitness Level	Target Heart Rate, beats/min	
	Age 20–29 y	*Age 30–39 y*
Low	129–144	128–144
Active	140–155	130–145
Fit	145–160	140–156

Source: Data are from references 53 and 62.

A pregnant woman starting an exercise program should begin at the lower end of the target heart rate range for her age, whereas women continuing an existing exercise program can exercise at the upper end of the target heart rate range (53). Additional checks on the appropriate intensity during exercise include using the rating of perceived exertion scale (66), in which a range of "somewhat hard" is appropriate for most pregnant women (53). The final check is called the "talk test," in which a pregnant woman carries on a conversation during exercise without being out of breath to avoid overexertion (55).

Time (Duration of Exercise Session)
The Physical Activity Guidelines for Americans (52) suggest that pregnant women who begin an exercise program should increase the amount gradually over time. The PARmed-X for Pregnancy document recommends that it is safe for healthy pregnant women who are just beginning an exercise program to start with 15 minutes at the appropriate target heart rate, with a 10- to 15-minute warm-up and a 10- to 15-minute cooldown at a lower intensity before and after the exercise session (53). The best time to progress to a longer duration is during the second trimester, when many of the pregnancy-induced discomforts are minimal, by adding 2 minutes per week to the exercise session until 30 minutes is reached (54). Overweight and obese pregnant women should initially attempt 15 minutes at the appropriate target heart rate, building slowly to a maximum of 30 minutes of aerobic activity, even if it means reducing the intensity and using rest intervals (53,65). The Physical Activity Guidelines for Americans (52) recommendation of 150 minutes (2 hours and 30 minutes) of moderate-intensity exercise per week for healthy pregnant women may be too difficult for women who are unfit or overweight or obese. If these women were to exercise three to four times per week, they would have to engage in exercise of 50 minutes per session three times per week or 38 minutes per session four times per week.

Type (Mode of Activity)
Aerobic exercise should include the movement of large muscle groups, such as walking, stationary cycling, aquatic exercise, or low-impact aerobics (53). Water aerobics has also been shown to be safe for the mother and fetus (67,68). Exercises that are contraindicated are those activities that increase the risk of falling, abdominal trauma and collision, and contact sports, including gymnastics, horseback riding, downhill skiing, soccer, and basketball (54). Scuba diving should also be avoided, and pregnant women should be cautious if they exercise at high altitude (51).

Rate of Progression
The best time to progress is during the second trimester because risks and discomforts of pregnancy are lowest at that time (54). Aerobic exercise should be increased gradually during the second trimester from a minimum of 15 minutes per session, three times per week (at the appropriate target heart rate or perceived rating

of exertion) to a maximum of approximately 30 minutes per session, four times per week (at the appropriate target heart rate or rating of exertion), preceded by a warm-up and followed by a cool-down (53).

Muscle Strength and Conditioning Exercise

The PARmed-X for Pregnancy document includes precautions for muscle-conditioning activity as well as examples of appropriate exercises (53). A prescription for muscular conditioning includes full range of motion for all major muscle groups to increase strength and endurance. One to two types of exercises should be used for each major muscle group for each side of the body. These areas should include: back and shoulders; chest and arms; legs and buttocks; abdominal and lower back muscles (body core support); and pelvic floor muscles. Resistance exercise (moving a specific muscle group continuously with a weight added for resistance as a tool) should include high repetitions (eg, 12 to 15 repetitions without fatigue) with a low comfortable mass, emphasizing continuous breathing while exhaling on exertion and inhaling on relaxation (53,69). During pregnancy, technique and proper breathing are extremely important to prevent injury. The Valsalva maneuver (holding one's breath while exercising) should be avoided during pregnancy as this may cause a change in blood pressure (53). In addition, pregnant women should take the following precautions:

- Avoid exercise in the supine (lying on the back) position past 16 weeks of gestation due to potential pressing of the pregnant uterus on the inferior vena cava (diminishing blood flow back to the heart) and/or the abdominal aorta (main blood supply to the uterine arteries) (53,70).
- Avoid exercise with rapid changes of direction and jarring of joints because of a potential relaxation of ligaments and joint instability (53). Caution should be used for stretching activities to avoid ligament and joint injury.
- As pregnancy progresses, avoid abdominal exercise if diastasis recti (tearing of the connective tissue line or linea alba) occurs (53). Diastasis recti presents as a rippling or bulging along the abdominal midline. If abdominal exercise continues, this condition may get worse, and thus further strengthening of these abdominal muscles is not recommended once diagnosed (71).
- Focus on correct posture, which includes a neutral pelvic alignment (53). Incorrect posture may lead to back and pelvic pain. To find a neutral pelvic alignment, the pregnant woman should stand with feet shoulder-width apart, knees slightly bent, with pelvic placement halfway between an accentuated lordosis (one extreme) and posterior pelvic tilt position (pushing the pelvis as far forward as possible, other extreme). These extreme positions should be avoided during pregnancy, with the neutral pelvic alignment maintained midway between these two extreme positions.

Safety Precautions and Reasons to Stop Exercise and Seek Medical Advice

Although regular physical activity should be part of the routine of healthy pregnant women, and the adverse consequences of the sedentary lifestyle are well established, one must proceed with some caution when the health and well-being of the fetus are potentially at risk. Safety considerations are outlined in Box 17.1 (53,54). Pregnant women should avoid exercise in hot, humid environments, and this would include monitoring the temperature of heated pools because a warm environment may augment the exercise-induced increase in maternal body core temperature and thermoregulation (50,62). It is also recommended that athletic competition be avoided while pregnant (53). This is related to the stress of competition, the risk of fatigue and athletic injury, and unknown risks to the fetus.

Throughout pregnancy, but particularly when regularly exercising, it is important to maintain proper nutrition and hydration (72). In a pilot study examining the dietary intakes of 11 active women who exercised

---

BOX 17.1   Safety Considerations for Exercising Pregnant Women

- Avoid exercising in warm or humid environments, especially in the first trimester.
- Avoid isometric exercise or straining while holding your breath.
- Maintain adequate nutrition and hydration; drink liquids before and after exercise.
- Avoid exercise while lying on your back after the 4th month (16 weeks) of pregnancy.
- Avoid activities that involve physical contact or danger of falling.
- **Know your limits**—pregnancy is not a good time to train for athletic competition.
- Know the reasons to stop exercise (Box 17.2) and consult a qualified health care provider immediately if they occur.

Source: Data are from references 53 and 54.

---

for 40 minutes at 70% of peak aerobic capacity three to four times per week, results showed on average a lower energy intake than recommended for second and third trimesters. This was partially due to a lower consumption of dairy products in some of the women. However, on average the daily protein intake was higher than recommended levels, whereas the overall micronutrient intake was low in iron, folate, potassium, calcium, and vitamin D. With a nutrient supplement, these women were within the guidelines (72). Although this was a small convenience sample, the study illustrates the importance of ensuring proper nutrition in very fit, active women. Exercising pregnant women should sip water before, during, and after the activity to maintain hydration.

Reasons to stop exercise and seek medical advice are listed in Box 17.2 (51,53,54). These are medical issues and should be dealt with as soon as possible.

BOX 17.2   Reasons to Stop Exercise and Seek Medical Advice

- Persistent and painful uterine contractions (> 6 to 8 per hour)
- Bloody vaginal discharge
- Gush of fluid from vagina (suggesting ruptured membranes)
- Unexplained abdominal pain
- Sudden swelling of extremities (ankles, hands, or face)
- Swelling, pain, and redness in the calf of one leg (suggesting phlebitis)
- Persistent headaches or blurring of vision
- Dizziness or faintness
- Marked fatigue, chest pain, or heart palpitations
- Excessive shortness of breath
- Absence of usual fetal movement (once detected)

Source: Data are from references 51, 53, and 54.

Prevention of Excessive Weight Gain for Overweight and Obese Pregnant Women

Although the healthful eating and lifestyle approach is intuitive to prevent excessive weight gain (65), several studies were not successful in achieving this goal for overweight and obese pregnant women (73–75) when behavior-based education alone was used as the intervention. Interventions that use dietary control in combination with exercise as part of a lifestyle change were the most successful (65). A recent study using a Nutrition and Exercise Lifestyle Intervention Program (NELIP) starting at 16 to 20 weeks' gestation was successful in preventing excessive gestational weight gain in 65 overweight and obese pregnant women (76). Specific goals of the nutrition component were to individualize the total energy intake to approximately 2,000 kcal/d. Total carbohydrate intake was 40% to 55% of total energy intake, distributed throughout the day with three balanced meals, plus three to four snacks per day, with the entire meal plan emphasizing complex carbohydrates and low–glycemic index foods. Total fat intake was 30% of total energy intake (substituting monounsaturated fatty acids for saturated and *trans* fatty acids), with the remaining 20% to 30% of energy dedicated to protein intake, while also meeting the micronutrient and fluid needs recommended during pregnancy (40).

The exercise component of the NELIP used mild walking (30% peak heart rate reserve) to facilitate compliance (64). The exercise session started at 25 minutes of walking per session, three to four times per week, thereafter increasing the exercise time by 2 minutes per week, until a maximum of 40 minutes was reached and maintained until delivery (76). Pedometers were used to count steps, and daily step counts increased from approximately 5,600 steps to more than 10,000 steps on the days the women exercised (76). Taking 10,000 steps has been shown to improve health outcomes of several population groups (77). A similar walking program has been used in women with GDM, resulting in a decrease in insulin use per kg body mass in the walking group compared with matched control subjects (78). Previous research has also shown that walking is the most popular activity of pregnant women (79).

Exercise in the Prevention and Treatment of Gestational Diabetes

Conventional management for women with gestational diabetes includes controlling energy intake or medical nutrition therapy (MNT) (80). MNT consists of a dietary intervention to achieve normal glycemia through good food choices, eating smaller meals more often, and controlling carbohydrate intake, while meeting the needs of pregnancy (the nutrition component of NELIP discussed previously is based on these components as a tool for preventing excessive weight gain and GDM in overweight and obese women). After 2 weeks of MNT, if capillary glucose concentrations are not controlled, women may progress to insulin injections to manage their blood glucose (28).

Exercise has been used as an adjunctive therapy, even though women who were the most active during pregnancy had the lowest prevalence of GDM (81), and the addition of exercise to MNT in obese GDM women limited weight gain and decreased macrosomia (82). Exercise continues to be an adjunctive therapy, with advice to be more active (28), or a recommendation of planned physical activity of 30 minutes per day (83), without suggesting a cost-effective, easily accessible evidence-based program with guidelines based on the FITT principle (frequency, intensity, time, and type of activity) that would produce the best possible outcomes for women with GDM (80). Although preliminary results are encouraging with a NELIP walking program (as described previously), the true effectiveness of a structured exercise program in controlling glucose and reducing the incidence of insulin therapy remains untapped (80). Continuing research is necessary in this important area.

Active Living During Pregnancy

With guidelines in place for medical prescreening and an exercise prescription appropriate for pregnant women (including overweight and obese women and those women with low or high fitness levels), it is imperative that all pregnant women with low-risk pregnancies remain active or start being active during pregnancy. Promoting active living during pregnancy will have many benefits to both mother and fetus, such as healthful living habits that will last a lifetime. Pregnant women, and women with young children, have a strong influence on family life, and healthful eating habits and active lifestyle may be transferred to the children, hopefully diminishing potential health risks for the next generation. Prevention of excessive weight gain during pregnancy, through active living and prevention of weight retention after the baby is born, may be important strategies in helping to stem the obesity and diabetes epidemics. Although postpartum exercise and guidelines are not mentioned in this chapter, further reading is suggested on practical applications, breastfeeding, and postpartum exercise (84).

Summary

It is clear that unhealthy eating habits and physical inactivity during pregnancy may cause increased risk for obesity, diabetes, and cardiovascular disease later in life for both the mother and her offspring (49,85). Armed with a medical prescreening tool with safe guidelines for aerobic and muscle conditioning exercises, health care professionals with interest in special populations, such as pregnant women, can work closely with low-risk women, educating them about healthful food choices, ensuring adequate nutrient requirements for pregnancy, and prescribing safe physical activity that will benefit the lifestyle of prenatal women and their families.

References

1. Clapp JF. Influence of endurance exercise and diet on human placental development and fetal growth. *Placenta.* 2006;27:527–534.
2. Pivarnik JM. Cardiovascular responses to aerobic exercise during pregnancy and postpartum. *Semin Perinat.* 1996;20:242–249.
3. Weissgerber TL, Wolfe LA. Physiological adaptation in early pregnancy: adaptation to balance maternal-fetal demands. *Appl Physiol Nutr Metabol.* 2006;31:1–11.
4. Wolfe LA, Weissgerber TL. Clinical physiology of exercise in pregnancy: a literature review. *J Obstet Gynecol Can.* 2003;25:451–453.
5. Wolfe LA, Brenner IK, Mottola MF. Maternal exercise, fetal well-being and pregnancy outcome. *Exerc Sports Sci Rev.* 1994;22:145–194.
6. Wolfe LA, Ohtake PJ, Mottola MF, McGrath MJ. Physiological interactions between pregnancy and aerobic exercise. *Exerc Sports Sci Rev.* 1989;17:295–351.
7. Pivarnik JM, Lee W, Clark S, Cotton D, Spillman M, Miller JF. Cardiac output responses of primigravid women during exercise determined by the direct Fick technique. *Obst Gynecol.* 1990;75:954–959.
8. Wolfe LA, Hall P, Webb K, Goodman L, Monga M, McGrath M. Prescription of aerobic exercise in pregnancy. *Sports Med.* 1989;8:273–301.
9. Hart MV, Morton MJ, Hosenpud J, Metcalfe J. Aortic function during normal human pregnancy. *Am J Obstet Gynecol.* 1996;154:887–891.

10. Duvekot J, Cheriex E, Pieters F, Menheere P, Peeters L. Early pregnancy changes in hemodynamics and volume homeostasis are consecutive adjustments triggered by a primary fall in systemic vascular tone. *Am J Obstet Gynecol.* 1993;169:1382–1392.

11. Rubler S, Damani P, Pinto E. Cardiac size and performance during pregnancy estimated with echocardiography. *Am J Cardiol.* 1997;40:534–540.

12. Wolfe LA, Preston R, Burggraf G, McGrath M. Effects of pregnancy and chronic exercise on maternal cardiac structure and function. *Can J Physiol Pharmacol.* 1999;77:909–917.

13. Pivarnik JM, Mauer MB, Ayers N, Kirshon B, Dildy G, Cotton DB. Effect of chronic exercise on blood volume expansion and hematologic indices during pregnancy. *Obstet Gynecol.* 1994;83:265–269.

14. Ohtake PJ, Wolfe LA. Physical conditioning attenuates respiratory responses to steady-state exercise in late gestation. *Med Sci Sports Exerc.* 1998;30:17–27.

15. Milne J, Howie A, Pack A. Dyspnea during normal pregnancy. *Br J Obstet Gynaecol.* 1978;85:260–263.

16. Bader RA, Bader ME, Rosse DJ. The oxygen cost of breathing in dyspnoeic subjects as studied in normal pregnant women. *Clin Sci (Lond).* 1959;18:223–235.

17. Clapp JF. The changing thermal response to endurance exercise during pregnancy. *Am J Obstet Gynecol.* 1991;165:1684–1689.

18. Lindqvist PG, Marsal K, Merlo J, Pirhonen JP. Thermal response to submaximal exercise before, during and after pregnancy: a longitudinal study. *J Matern Fetal Neonatal Med.* 2003;13:152–156.

19. Bauer MK, Harding JE, Bassett NS, Breier BH, Oliver MH, Gallaher BH, Evans PC, Woodall SM, Gluckman PD. Foetal growth and placental function. *Mol Cell Endocrin.* 1998;140:115–120.

20. Mottola MF, Christopher PD. Effects of maternal exercise on liver and skeletal muscle glycogen storage in pregnant rats. *J Appl Physiol.* 1991;71:1015–1019.

21. Catalano PM, Tyzbir E, Roman N. Longitudinal changes in insulin release and insulin resistance in non-obese pregnant women. *Am J Obstet Gynecol.* 1991;165:1667–1672.

22. Buchanan TA, Metzer B, Freinkel N. Insulin sensitivity and B-cell responsiveness to glucose during late pregnancy in lean and moderately obese women with normal glucose tolerance or gestational diabetes. *Am J Obstet Gynaecol.* 1990;162:1008–1014.

23. Lesser KB, Carpenter M. Metabolic changes associated with normal pregnancy and pregnancy complicated by diabetes mellitus. *Semin Perinatol.* 1994;18:399–406.

24. Clapp JF. Maternal carbohydrate intake and pregnancy outcome. *Proc Nutr Soc.* 2002;61:45–50.

25. Boden G. Fuel metabolism in pregnancy and in gestational diabetes mellitus. *Obstet Gynecol Clin North Am.* 1996;23:1–10.

26. Bessinger R, McMurray R. Substrate utilization and hormonal responses to exercise in pregnancy. *Clin Obstet Gynecol.* 2003;46: 467–478.

27. Dornhorst A, Rossi M. Risk and prevention of type 2 diabetes in women with gestational diabetes. *Diabetes Care.* 1998;21:B43–B49.

28. Canadian Diabetes Association. Diabetes in pregnancy. *Can J Diabetes.* 2008;22(suppl):S168–S180.

29. Rooney B, Schauberger C, Mathiason M. Impact of perinatal weight change on long-term obesity and obesity-related illnesses. *Obstet Gynecol.* 2005;106:1349–1356.

30. Callaway L, Prins JB, Chang AM, McIntyre HD. The prevalence and impact of overweight and obesity in an Australian obstetric population. *Med J Austr.* 2006;184:56–59.

31. LaCoursiere D, Bloebaum Y, Duncan L, Varner MW. Population-based trends and correlates of maternal overweight and obesity, Utah 1991–2001. *Am J Obstet Gynecol.* 2005;192:832–839.

32. Kim S, Dietz P, England L, Morrow B, Callaghan WM. Trends in pre-pregnancy obesity in nine states, 1993–2003. *Obesity.* 2007;15:986–993.

33. Muscati SK, Gray-Donald K, Koski KG. Timing of weight gain during pregnancy: promoting fetal growth and minimizing maternal weight retention. *Int J Obes Relat Metab Disord.* 1996;20:526–532.

34. Institute of Medicine. Weight gain during pregnancy: reexamining the guidelines. *Report Brief.* 2009(May);1–4.

35. Hytten FE, Leitch I. *The Physiology of Human Pregnancy.* 2nd ed. Oxford, UK: Blackwell Scientific Publications; 1971.

36. Artenisio A, Corrado F, Sobbrio G, Bruno L, Todisco L, Galletta MG, Galletta MR, Campisi R, Mancuso A. Glucose tolerance and insulin secretion in pregnancy. *Diabetes Nutr Metab.* 1999;12:264–270.

37. Pole JD, Dodds LA. Maternal outcomes associated with weight change between pregnancies. *Can J Public Health.* 1999;90:233–236.

38. Rooney B, Schauberger C. Excess pregnancy weight gain and long-term obesity: one decade later. *Obstet Gynecol.* 2002;100:245–252.

39. American Dietetic Association. Position of the American Dietetic Association: nutrition and lifestyle for a healthy pregnancy outcome. *J Am Diet Assoc.* 2008;108:553–561.

40. Institute of Medicine. *Dietary Reference Intakes: The Essential Guide to Nutrient Requirements.* Washington, DC: National Academies Press; 2006.

41. Institute of Medicine. Dietary Reference Intakes Tables and Applications. http://iom.edu/Activities/Nutrition/SummaryDRIs/DRI-Tables.aspx. Accessed July 25, 2011.

42. Institute of Medicine. *Weight Gain During Pregnancy: Reexamining the Guidelines.* Washington, DC: National Academies Press; 2009:316. http://www.nap.edu/catalog.php?record_id=12584. Accessed November 11, 2010.

43. US Department of Agriculture. MyPlate Web site. www.choosemyplate.gov. Accessed October 12, 2011.

44. Catalano PM, Ehrenberg HM. The short- and long-term implications of maternal obesity on the mother and her offspring. *Br J Obstet Gynecol.* 2006;113:1126–1133.

45. Oken E, Gillman MW. Fetal origins of obesity. *Obes Res.* 2003;11:496–506.

46. Bayol S, Farrington S, Stickland N. A maternal "junk food" diet in pregnancy and lactation promotes an exacerbated taste for "junk food" and a greater propensity for obesity in rat offspring. *Br J Nutr.* 2007;98:843–851.

47. Hillier T, Mullen J, Pedula K, Mullen JA, Charles MA, Pettitt DJ. Childhood obesity and metabolic imprinting: the ongoing effects of maternal hyperglycemia. *Diabetes Care.* 2007;30:2287–2292.

48. Miles J, Huber K, Thompson N, Davison M, Breier BH. Moderate daily exercise activates metabolic flexibility to prevent prenatally induced obesity. *Endocrinology.* 2009;150:179–186.

49. Pivarnik JM, Chambliss H, Clapp JF, Dugan SA, Hatch M, Lovelady CA, Mottola MF, Williams MA. Impact of physical activity during pregnancy and postpartum on chronic disease risk: an ACSM roundtable consensus statement. *Med Sci Sports Exerc.* 2006;38:989–1005.

50. Mottola MF, Wolfe LA. The pregnant athlete. In: Drinkwater B, ed. *Encyclopaedia of Sports Medicine: Women in Sport.* Oxford, U.K: Blackwell Science; 2000:194–207.

51. American College of Obstetricians and Gynecologists. Opinion no. 267: exercise during pregnancy and the postpartum period. *Obst Gynecol.* 2002;99:171–173.

52. US Department of Health and Human Services. Physical Activity Guidelines for Americans. Chapter 7. 2008. http://www.health.gov/paguidelines/guidelines/chapter7.aspx. Accessed November 11, 2010.

53. Wolfe LA, Mottola MF. PARmed-X for Pregnancy: Physical Activity Readiness Medical Examination. Ottawa, ON: Canadian Society for Exercise Physiology and Health Canada; 2002:1–4. http://www.csep.ca/cmfiles/publications/parq/parmed-xpreg.pdf. Accessed November 11, 2010.

54. Davies G, Wolfe LA, Mottola MF, MacKinnon C. Joint SOGC/CSEP clinical practice guideline: exercise in pregnancy and the postpartum period. *J Obstet Gynecol Can.* 2003;25:516–522.

55. Wolfe LA, Davies G. Canadian guidelines for exercise in pregnancy. *Clin Obstet Gynecol.* 2003;46:488–495.

56. American College of Sports Medicine. Endorsements. *Sports Med Bull.* 2004;39(5).

57. Davies G, Wolfe LA, Mottola MF, MacKinnon C. Joint SOGC/CSEP clinical practice guideline: exercise in pregnancy and the postpartum period. *Can J Appl Physiol.* 2003;28:329–341.

58. Canadian Academy of Sport and Exercise Medicine; Alleyne J, Peticca P. Exercise and Pregnancy. Discussion Paper. Rev ed. 2008. http://www.casm-acms.org/Media/Content/files/Discussion%20Paper%20Pregnancy.pdf. Accessed September 30, 2011.

59. Thompson W, Gordon N, Pescatello L, eds. *ACSM's Guidelines for Exercise Testing and Prescription.* 8th ed. Philadelphia, PA: Lippincott Williams & Wilkins; 2009.

60. Campbell MK, Mottola MF. Recreational exercise and occupational activity during pregnancy and birth weight: a case-control study. *Am J Obstet Gynecol.* 2001;184:403–408.

61. Wolfe LA, Mottola MF. Aerobic exercise in pregnancy: an update. *Can J Appl Physiol.* 1993;18:119–147.

62. Mottola MF, Davenport M, Brun CR, Inglis SD, Charlesworth S, Sopper MM. VO2peak prediction and exercise prescription for pregnant women. *Med Sci Sports Exerc*. 2006;38:1389–1395.

63. American College of Sports Medicine. *Guidelines for Exercise Testing and Exercise Prescription*. 7th ed. Philadelphia, PA: Lippincott, Williams & Wilkins; 2005.

64. Davenport M, Sopper MM, Charlesworth S, Vanderspank D, Mottola MF. Development and validation of exercise target heart rate zones for overweight and obese pregnant women. *Appl Physiol Nutr Metabol*. 2008;33:984–989.

65. Mottola MF. Exercise prescription for overweight and obese women: pregnant and postpartum. *Obstet Gynecol Clinics NA*. 2009;36:301–316.

66. Borg GAV. Psychophysical bases of perceived exertion. *Med Sci Sports Exerc*. 1982;14:377–381.

67. Baciuk E, Pereira R, Cecatti J, Braga A, Cavalcante S. Water aerobics in pregnancy: cardiovascular response, labor and neonatal outcomes. *Reprod Health*. 2008;5:10–22.

68. Cavalcante S, Cecatti J, Pereira R, Baciuk E, Bernardo A, Silveira C. Water aerobics II: maternal body composition and perinatal outcomes after a program for low risk pregnant women. *Reprod Health*. 2009;6:1–7.

69. Brankston G, Mitchell B, Ryan E, Okun N. Resistance exercise decreases the need for insulin in overweight women with gestational diabetes mellitus. *Am J Obstet Gynecol*. 2004;190:188–193.

70. Ueland K, Novy MJ, Peterson EN, Metcalfe J. Maternal cardiovascular dynamics. IV. The influence of gestational age on the maternal cardiovascular response to posture and exercise. *Am J Obstet Gynecol*. 1969;104:856–864.

71. Bursch SG. Interrater reliability of diastasis recti abdominis measurement. *Phys Ther*. 1987;67:1077–1079.

72. Giroux I, Inglis S, Lander S, Gerrie S, Mottola MF. Dietary intake, weight gain and birth outcomes of physically active pregnant women: a pilot study. *Appl Physiol Nutr Metab*. 2006;31:483–489.

73. Polley BA, Wing RR, Sims CJ. Randomized controlled trial to prevent excessive weight gain in pregnant women. *Int J Obes Relat Metab Disord*. 2002;26:1494–1502.

74. Gray-Donald K, Robinson E, Collier A. Intervening to reduce weight gain in pregnancy and gestational diabetes mellitus in Cree communities: an evaluation. *CMAJ*. 2000;163;1247–1251.

75. Olsen CM, Strawderman MS, Reed RG. Efficacy of an intervention to prevent excessive gestational weight gain. *Am J Obstet Gynecol*. 2004;191:530–536.

76. Mottola MF, Giroux I, Gratton R, Hammond J, Hanley A, Harris S, McManus R, Davenport M, Sopper MM. Nutrition and exercise prevents excess weight gain in pregnant overweight women. *Med Sci Sports Exerc*. 2010;42: 265–272.

77. Tudor-Locke C, Bassett D. How many steps/day are enough? Preliminary pedometer indices for public health. *Sports Med*. 2004;43:1–8.

78. Davenport MH, McManus R, Gratton R, Mottola MF. A walking intervention improves capillary glucose control in women with gestational diabetes mellitus: a pilot study. *Appl Physiol Nutr Metabol*. 2008;33:511–517.

79. Mottola MF, Campbell MK. Activity patterns during pregnancy. *Can J Appl Physiol*. 2003;28:642–653.

80. Mottola MF. The role of exercise in the prevention and treatment of gestational diabetes mellitus. *Curr Diab Rep*. 2008;8:299–304.

81. Dyck R, Klomp H, Tan L, Turnell RW, Boctor MA. A comparison of rates, risk factors and outcomes of gestational diabetes between aboriginal and non-aboriginal women in the Saskatoon health district. *Diabetes Care*. 2002;25:487–493.

82. Artal R, Catanzaro RB, Gavard JA, Mostello DJ, Friganza JC. A lifestyle intervention of weight-gain restriction: diet and exercise in obese women with gestational diabetes mellitus. *Appl Physiol Nutr Metab*. 2007;32:596–601.

83. Metzger BE, Buchanan TA, Coustan DR, de Leiva A, Dunger DB, Hadden DR, Hod M, Kitzmiller JL, Kjos SL, Oats JN, Pettitt DJ, Sacks DA, Zoupas C. Summary and recommendations of the Fifth International Workshop-Conference on Gestational Diabetes Mellitus. *Diabetes Care*. 2007;30(Suppl):S251–S260.

84. Mottola MF. Exercise in the postpartum period: practical applications. *Curr Sports Med Rep*. 2002;1:362–368.

85. Weissgerber T, Wolfe LA, Davies G, Mottola MF. Exercise in the prevention and treatment of maternal-fetal disease: A review of the literature. *Appl Physiol Nutr Metab*. 2006;31:661–674.

Acknowledgment: This work is supported by the Canadian Institute of Health Research, the Lawson Foundation, Rx & D Health Research Foundation of Canada, and the Molly Towell Perinatal Research Foundation.

Chapter 18

DISORDERED EATING IN ATHLETES

Katherine A. Beals, PhD, RD, FACSM, CSSD

Introduction

Since the early 1980s, a growing body of literature has documented eating disturbances and body-weight issues in athletes. Despite the interest of the scientific community, disordered eating in athletes did not garner mainstream attention until Christy Henrich's much-publicized battle with, and eventual death from, anorexia nervosa in 1994. The death of this 22-year-old gymnast seemed to open the door to the eating disorder closet, as several other well-recognized athletes (eg, Nadia Comaneci, Dara Torres, and Zina Garrison) as well as collegiate and even recreational athletes began to reveal their own personal struggles with disordered eating.

With the increasing visibility of eating disorders in athletes has come the need to create programs and recruit personnel to identify, prevent, and treat them. The sports dietitian is often one of the first individuals to come into contact with an athlete with an eating disorder and is almost always an integral member of the treatment team. Thus, it is essential that he or she has a firm understanding of eating disorders and is prepared to provide appropriate nutrition care. This chapter provides sports nutrition professionals with background information as well as the tools needed to successfully manage disordered eating in athletes.

Eating Disorder Categories and Classification

The terms *eating disorder* and *disordered eating* are frequently, yet erroneously, used interchangeably, both in the literature and in general practice. Strictly speaking, the term *eating disorder* refers to one of the three clinically diagnosable conditions—anorexia nervosa, bulimia nervosa, or eating disorders not otherwise specified (EDNOS)—recognized in the 4th edition of the American Psychiatric Association's *Diagnostic and Statistical Manual of Mental Disorders* (DSM-IV) (1). (Note: A draft of the fifth edition of the DSM has been released, with the final release scheduled for May 2013. For more information, go to: www.dsm5.org.) To be diagnosed with a clinical eating disorder, an individual must meet a standard set of criteria as outlined in the DSM (1). (See Appendix A.) *Disordered eating,* on the other hand, is a general term used to describe the spectrum of abnormal and harmful eating behaviors that are used in a misguided attempt to lose weight or maintain a lower than normal body weight (2). The two categories are described in detail in this chapter.

The Clinical Conditions

According to the current (4th) edition of the DSM, the clinical eating disorders—anorexia nervosa, bulimia nervosa, and EDNOS—are characterized by severe disturbances in eating behavior and body image (1). It must be emphasized that the clinical eating disorders are psychiatric conditions and, as such, they go beyond body weight/shape dissatisfaction and involve more than just abnormal eating patterns and pathogenic weight-control behaviors. For individuals with clinical eating disorders, body weight concerns and eating pathology are symptoms of the underlying psychiatric disturbance; they are the means to an end, not the end itself. Not surprisingly then, individuals with clinical eating disorders often experience comorbid psychological conditions, such as obsessive-compulsive disorders, depression, and anxiety disorders (3). In addition, they often display severe feelings of insecurity and worthlessness, have trouble identifying and displaying emotions, and experience difficulty in forming close relationships with others.

Athletes with clinical eating disorders resemble their nonathletic counterparts in many ways; however, there are some subtle but important differences. Athletes with anorexia nervosa, like nonathletes, are driven by the need for control, including controlling their body weight, which translates into an obsession with thinness. However, unlike nonathletes with anorexia, who generally view thinness as the only goal, athletes with anorexia strive for thinness *and* the improvement in performance that they believe will accompany it. This is particularly (although not exclusively) true for female athletes, especially those participating in sports that emphasize leanness (eg, gymnastics, figure skating, diving, distance running, and triathlon). Although starving in the name of improved performance may seem counterproductive, the athlete with anorexia, like her nonathletic counterpart, is not logical regarding the topic of body weight and often has come to embrace (and embody) the notion that thinner is better (ie, faster, stronger, more pleasing to the judges, etc) (4).

Athletes with anorexia are often more difficult to identify and may be more resistant to treatment than nonathletes with the condition. To be competitive, athletes must engage in intense, and what might be considered excessive, physical training. They often follow rigid and obscure dietary practices, thus making it difficult to distinguish the committed athlete from the diet- and exercise-obsessed individual with anorexia (4).

Athletes with bulimia nervosa, like nonathletes with the clinical condition, engage in regular binge-purge cycles; however, both the binge and purge may be somewhat less clear when it comes to athletes. According to the DSM-IV (1), a binge is defined as eating "a large amount of food in a discrete period of time." As might be expected, there are challenges in interpreting the phrases "large amount of food" (larger than most individuals under similar circumstances) and "discrete period of time," particularly as they apply to athletes. It could be argued that because of increased energy expenditure and therefore increased energy requirements, athletes generally consume more food than most individuals. Moreover, the varied energy needs of athletes make it difficult to characterize or compare "similar circumstances." The context of eating must also be considered. For example, what may be thought of as excessive consumption at a typical meal might be considered normal under certain circumstances, such as carbohydrate loading for a competitive event or refueling after a particularly prolonged or intense training session or competition.

The factors precipitating binge-purge cycles and the rationalizations accompanying them also serve to differentiate athletes with bulimia nervosa from nonathletes (4). For example, the nonathlete with bulimia generally restricts food intake for weight loss alone, whereas food restriction for the athlete with the same condition often serves a dual purpose: weight loss and performance enhancement (or at least the athlete uses the guise of performance to justify food restriction). Although typically triggered by periods of food restriction or dieting, the bingeing and purging cycles of the athlete with bulimia nervosa may be caused by other factors unique to the sport setting, including athletic identity crises and performance dynamics. As is true for athletes with anorexia, athletes with bulimia tend to connect self-esteem and self-worth to athletic performance. Anything that threatens these athletes' fragile sense of self-esteem (eg, a poor performance, negative comment from a coach or teammates) can serve to elicit a binge-and-purge cycle.

Finally, the athletic environment provides unique situations for bingeing as well as purging that are generally not available to the nonathlete with bulimia. The common practice of carbohydrate loading before an endurance event is a key example of a situation in which the athlete with bulimia is actually encouraged to engage in the very behavior that epitomizes the disease. Team meals may further complicate matters because the social situation and peer pressure may increase food consumption. These environmental cues, individually or collectively, can increase the likelihood of a binge and a subsequent purge.

It has also been suggested that athletes with bulimia nervosa are more likely to engage in excessive exercise after a binge than nonathletes, who are more apt to purge using vomiting or laxatives (5). This difference in purging behaviors is again largely explained by the nature of the sport setting. That is, because exercise is a behavior that athletes already engage in, it is easier for athletes with bulimia, like those with anorexia, to disguise their condition with excessive physical activity or at least to rationalize increased exercise in the name of improved performance. Conversely, concealing vomiting or the use of laxatives and diuretics is much more difficult for the athlete, particularly during road trips or other team functions (5).

Subclinical Variants

In some cases, athletes may exhibit many of the overt behaviors of a clinical eating disorder but do not harbor the severe psychological disturbances that underlie the clinical eating disorders (5–9). These partial or subclinical eating disorder syndromes have been classified and characterized in a variety of ways by several researchers and practitioners.

A prominent researcher in the area of eating disorders in athletes, Sundgot-Borgen (10) has developed a set of criteria to describe a variant of anorexia nervosa in athletes, which she refers to as *anorexia athletica*. The following is a list of essential features of anorexia athletica. Features marked with + are absolute criteria; (+) are relative criteria.

- Weight loss of more than 5% of expected body weight: +
- Delayed menarche (ie, no menstrual bleeding by 16 years of age):   (+)
- Menstrual dysfunction (amenorrhea or oligomenorrhea):   (+)
- Gastrointestinal complaints: (+)
- Absence of medical illness or affective disorder to explain the weight loss: +
- Body image distortion: (+)
- Excessive fear of weight gain or becoming obese: +
- Restriction of energy intake (less than 1,200 kcal/d):   +
- Use of purging methods (eg, self-induced vomiting, laxatives, diuretics):   (+)
- Binge eating: (+)
- Compulsive exercise: (+)

It should be noted that the criteria for anorexia athletica were derived largely from a set criteria used to describe a disorder referred to as "fear of obesity" observed in a small sample of nonathletic adolescents (11).

More broadly, the term *subclinical eating disorder* has frequently been used by researchers to describe individuals, both athletes and nonathletes, who have considerable eating pathology and body weight concerns but do not demonstrate significant psychopathology and/or fail to meet all of the DSM-IV (1) criteria for anorexia nervosa, bulimia nervosa, or EDNOS (6–8,12,13). Indeed, many athletes who report using pathogenic weight-control methods (eg, laxatives, diet pills, and excessive exercise) do not technically meet the criteria for a clinical eating disorder as outlined in the DSM-IV; nonetheless, their behaviors place them at considerable health risk.

For example, one female collegiate distance runner reported routinely eating approximately 1,000 kcal/d while running an average of 60 miles/wk (and "working out" at the gym in addition to her regular training regimen). She ate similar foods every day and severely limited her fat intake (no more than 20 g/d). Occasionally (less than once a week) she would "binge" by eating a forbidden food (eg, a piece of cake or french fries) and she would train longer or harder at her next workout to make up for what she had eaten. Although she was openly dissatisfied with her body weight and shape (despite the fact her body weight was on the low end of normal for her height), she did not display any substantial emotional distress or psychological disturbance pertaining to these constructs.

This athlete definitely displays disordered eating behaviors; however, she does not meet the diagnostic criteria for either anorexia nervosa or bulimia nervosa. In fact, depending on the context of the evaluation, she might not even meet the criteria necessary for a diagnosis of EDNOS. This example serves to emphasize that it should not be the precise eating disorder diagnosis that is of primary concern, but rather the extent to which the disordered eating *behaviors* compromise the athlete's physical and mental health.

Prevalence

Current estimates of the prevalence of disordered eating among athletes are highly variable, ranging from less than 1% to as high as 62% in female athletes (2,14–18), and between 0% and 57% in male athletes (19–21). This wide range of estimates is due to differences in screening instruments/assessment tools used (eg, self-report questionnaires vs in-depth interviews), definitions of eating disorders applied (few have used the DSM-IV criteria), and the athletic populations studied (eg, collegiate vs high school athletes; elite athletes vs recreational athletes vs those who are physically active but noncompetitive). Only a few studies have used large (n > 100) heterogeneous samples of athletes and validated measures of disordered eating (see Table 18.1) (10,16–18,20–24).

Despite differences in methodology and the seemingly wide-ranging estimates derived from the available research, the current data are consistent in indicating the following four points: (*a*) the prevalence of clinical eating disorders among athletes is similar to that of nonathletes; (*b*) the prevalence of subclinical eating disorders exceeds that of the clinical eating disorders among athletes; (*c*) female athletes are at greater risk for disordered eating behaviors than their male counterparts; and (*d*) there is a higher incidence of disordered eating (including both clinical and subclinical eating disorders) in athletes participating in sports or activities in which a lean physique is considered advantageous or the norm (5,6,14,15,20,25,26).

Etiology

Not unlike many other health conditions (eg, obesity, cancer, heart disease), there has been much speculation about whether the cause of eating disorders is due to genetic (nature) or environmental (nurture) factors. Although some eating disorder experts might gravitate toward one side or another, most would agree that the etiology of disordered eating is multifactorial and encompasses a complex interaction between environmental (eg, sociocultural, demographic, psychological, behavioral) and genetic factors (27,28). There are a few sport-specific risk factors, but research suggests that athletes are susceptible to the same risk factors as their nonathletic counterparts (29). The etiological factors for disordered eating are described in the following sections.

TABLE 18.1   Summary of Prevalence Studies Including Large, Heterogeneous Samples of Athletes and Validated Assessments of Disordered Eating

Study (Reference)	Subjects	Instruments	Findings
Beals and Hill, 2006 (16)	112 female collegiate athletes	Questionnaire developed by the authors including the EDE-Q and Eating Disorder Symptom Checklist	3% of athletes self-reported a clinical eating disorder; 23% of athletes met the criteria for disordered eating.
Beals and Manore, 2002 (22)	425 female collegiate athletes	EAT-26 and EDI-BD	3.3% and 2.4% of the athletes self-reported a diagnosis of clinical anorexia and bulimia nervosa, respectively; 15% and 31.5% of the athletes scored more than the designated cutoff scores on the EAT-26 and EDI-BD, respectively.
Johnson et al, 1999 (24)	1,445 collegiate athletes (883 men and 562 women) from 11 NCAA Division I Schools	EDI-2 and questionnaire developed by the authors using DSM-IV criteria	None of the men met the criteria for anorexia or bulimia nervosa; 1.1% of the women met the criteria for bulimia nervosa. 9.2% of the women and 0.01% of the men met the criteria for subclinical bulimia; 2.8% met the criteria for subclinical anorexia. 5.5% of the women and 2% of the men reported purging (vomiting, using laxatives or diuretics) on a weekly basis.
Nichols et al, 2007 (17)	423 female high school athletes	EDE-Q	20% of athletes met the EDE-Q criteria for disordered eating.
Nichols et al, 2006 (18)	170 female high school athletes	In-depth interview developed by the author using the EDE.	18.2% met the criteria for disordered eating.
Sundgot-Borgen, 1993 (10)	522 Norwegian elite female athletes	EDI and in-depth interview developed by the author based on DSM-III criteria	1.3%, 8.0%, and 8.2% were diagnosed with anorexia nervosa, bulimia nervosa, and anorexia athletica, respectively.
Sundgot-Borgen and Torstveit, 2004 (20)	1,620 Norwegian elite male and female athletes	EDI-2 and in-depth interview developed by the author based on DSM-IV criteria	13.5% of athletes met the criteria for clinical and subclinical eating disorders; more female athletes than male athletes met the criteria for disordered eating.
Sundgot-Borgen et al, 1999 (23)	The total population of Norwegian elite athletes (960 men and 660 women) representing 60 different sporting events.	A questionnaire developed by the authors, including subscales of the EDI, weight history, and self-reported history of eating disorders	20% (n = 156) of the female athletes and 8% (n = 27) of the male athletes met the DSM-IV criteria for a clinical eating disorders (ie, anorexia nervosa, bulimia nervosa, or EDNOS).
Toro et al, 2005 (21)	283 elite female athletes competing in 20 different sports.	EAT and the Eating Disorder Assessment Questionnaire (CETCA; based on DSM-III-R criteria)	11% of the athletes exceeded the EAT cutoff score. 2.5% and 20.1% of the athletes met the CETCA criteria for anorexia nervosa and bulimia nervosa, respectively.

Abbreviations: EDE-Q, Eating Disorder Examination Questionnaire; DSM, *Diagnostic and Statistical Manual of Mental Disorders;* EAT-26, Eating Attitudes Test; EDI-BD, Eating Disorder Inventory Body Dissatisfaction Subscale; EDI-2, Eating Disorder Inventory 2; EDNOS, eating disorder not otherwise specified; NCAA, National Collegiate Athletic Association.

Environmental Factors

Environmental risk factors for disordered eating include those circumstances and events external to the individual that increase the likelihood that he or she may develop an eating disorder. The most frequently studied environmental risk factors include sociocultural (including the athletic subculture) and familial factors (27).

Sociocultural Factors

Sociocultural models of eating disorders highlight the Western culture's objectification of the female body and the overemphasis of extreme thinness as the epitome of the beauty ideal as key risk factors for the development of eating disorders. According to the sociocultural model, disordered eating develops over time and through a sequential series of steps, including: (*a*) exposure to the thin ideal, (*b*) internalization of the ideal, and (*c*) realization of a considerable discrepancy between the ideal and the actual "self," which results in body dissatisfaction and disordered eating (27).

Support for this sociocultural model come from data indicating that eating disorders are more prevalent in Westernized cultures (eg, Australia, Canada, England, France, and the United States) where thinness is highly valued and not only equates to physical beauty but is also believed to be associated with several other positive attributes, including intelligence, kindness, success, and power (27). Despite some methodological limitations, cross-cultural studies have confirmed that where Westernized beauty ideals (particularly those related to body weight and the cult of thinness) have infiltrated, the incidence of disordered eating has and will likely continue to increase (27).

An additional line of evidence supporting the sociocultural model comes from the discrepancy in eating disorder prevalence between males and females. Indeed, leading eating disorder researchers assert that the single best predictor of risk for developing an eating disorder is being female (27). Their contention is supported by research indicating that worldwide the number of females suffering from eating disorders outnumbers that of males by a significant margin (30–32). This is particularly true for those disorders in which body weight (and, more specifically striving for a lower body weight) are paramount, such as anorexia nervosa and bulimia nervosa. Interestingly, sex differences in eating disorder prevalence are far less pronounced in binge-eating disorder (33,34), in which body weight/shape obsession is not a key factor.

Research also suggests that homosexual men experience higher levels of disordered eating than heterosexuals, not because of their sexual orientation, but because of the social and psychological factors that are present among the gay culture—that is, the emphasis on a lean and muscular body shape/size (32). Nonetheless, it should be noted that over the last three decades there has been increasing objectification of the male body and an emphasis on a hypermuscular lean physique. With this societal shift has come an increase in body dissatisfaction and disordered eating among men, although it more often takes the form of an obsession with muscularity (vs thinness) and has been referred to as *muscle dysmorphia* (see Box 18.1) (35–37).

The Athletic Subculture

It has been hypothesized that the athletic "subculture" (ie, the inherent pressures and demands of the sport setting) puts additional pressure on athletes and may serve to "trigger" the development of an eating disorder in those who are psychologically susceptible (5,13,29). This pressure may be particularly high for athletes in thin-build sports or activities that require a low body weight or lean physique, such as dance (especially ballet), gymnastics, distance running, triathlon, swimming, diving, figure skating, cheerleading, wrestling, and lightweight rowing. Moreover, the pressure can be particularly strong (rendering the development of an eating disorder much more likely) when there is a discrepancy between the athlete's actual body weight and the perceived ideal body weight for the athlete's particular sport (14). For example, a naturally larger athlete

---

BOX 18.1   Muscle Dysmorphia

In 1997 a group of researchers, led by Harrison G. Pope, described a form of body image disturbance seen in male weightlifters, which they referred to as *muscle dysmorphia* (36). According to
the researchers, muscle dysmorphia is a subtype of body dysmorphic disorder (BDD), which has
been defined as an intense and excessive preoccupation/dissatisfaction with a perceived defect
in appearance. Once referred to as *reverse anorexia*, muscle dysmorphia is characterized by inor-
dinate preoccupation and dissatisfaction with body size and muscularity. Individuals with muscle
dysmorphia perceive themselves as small and frail even though they are actually quite large and
muscular. Muscle dysmorphia shares some similarities with eating disorders—body image dis-
turbance/distortion, preoccupation with body weight and size, excessive exercise, preoccupation
with food and dieting, and use of pathogenic weight-control behaviors. Another common feature
among individuals with muscle dysmorphia is the abuse of performance-enhancing drugs and
supplements. In their initial report, Pope and his colleagues noted that 13% (n = 9) of the weightlifters with muscle dysmorphia also reported a history of disordered eating and all reported a
history of anabolic steroid abuse (36). In a follow-up study by the same authors, one third of the
weightlifters with muscle dysmorphia reported coexistent eating disorders and more than half
reported currently using anabolic steroids.

Source: Data are from references 35, 36, and 37.

---

who wants to compete in gymnastics or a naturally heavier wrestler who is trying to compete in a lower
weight class may feel especially strong pressure to alter his or her body weight. Indeed, research clearly
shows that the prevalence of disordered eating among athletes—both males and females—is substantially
higher among those involved in aesthetic or thin-build sports and when a lower body weight is thought to
confer a competitive advantage (4,5,20,38,39).

In a study investigating risk and trigger factors for the development of eating disorders among female
athletes, Sundgot-Borgen et al (23) found that those with disordered eating reported engaging in sport-
specific training and dieting at considerably earlier ages than athletes without eating disorders. In addition,
prolonged periods of dieting, frequent weight fluctuations, sudden increases in training volume, or traumatic
life events such as an injury or a change of coach tended to trigger the development of eating disorders (29).

Conversely, some researchers have proposed that specific sports or physical activities (ie, those that
emphasize leanness or muscularity or require large training volumes) may attract individuals with eating
disorders, particularly anorexia nervosa, because these activities provide a setting in which individuals can
use or abuse exercise to expend extra energy and hide or justify their excessive exercise and abnormal eating and dieting behaviors (25,39). Moreover, the stereotypical standards of body shape in women's sports
and physical activities that emphasize leanness make it difficult for observers to notice when an individual
has lost too much weight. These common and accepted low weight standards may help active women with
disordered eating deny their problem and delay intervention (29). Similarly, the muscular physique characteristic of weightlifting and bodybuilding may attract males with body image and eating disturbances (eg,
muscle dysmorphia) (32,38).

Familial Factors

Individuals with eating disorders often have dysfunctional families, particularly those with overbearing or
controlling parents, victims of physical or sexual abuse, or those whose parents have a history of alcoholism

or substance abuse (27,40). Such family environments can cause severe psychological and emotional distress, undermine the development of self-esteem, and lead to inadequate coping skills, all of which may increase the risk that an eating disorder might develop. Although family dysfunction may not be a common causative factor in athletes, it should always be considered a possibility. For example, an athlete may feel overwhelmed or out of control as a result of an injury, a particularly poor performance, or the excessive demands of a coach. Because of a dysfunctional family environment, the athlete may have never developed the coping skills necessary to handle these problems, and thus the athlete concentrates on something that can be managed, such as body weight (4).

Genetic Factors

Although environmental factors undoubtedly contribute to the development of an eating disorder, they are unlikely to be the sole cause. Not all individuals exposed to the same environmental stimuli will develop disordered eating; thus, there must be some other underlying or mediating factor. Most eating disorder experts contend that the mediating factor is genetics.

Over the past 10 years, there has been an accumulating body of evidence indicating that an individual's genetic makeup determines his or her susceptibility to developing an eating disorder (41). Evidence from familial and twin studies suggests that as much as 50% of the variance in anorexia and up to 83% of the variance in bulimia nervosa can be accounted for by genetic factors (27,41). Molecular genetic studies have identified several candidate genes; however, the most promising results have been from genes encoding for the proteins that clear serotonin from the synapse (42,43).

To date there have been no genetic studies of eating disorders specific to an athletic population, but it can be assumed that the genetic models previously described could be generalized to athletes. A biological-behavioral model of activity-based anorexia nervosa was proposed in a series of studies by Epling and colleagues (44,45). They theorized that dieting and exercising initiate the anorexic cycle and claimed that as many as 75% of the cases of anorexia nervosa are exercise-induced. The theory is that strenuous exercise suppresses appetite, which leads to a decrease in food intake and subsequent reduction in body weight. It should be noted that this research was conducted with rats and has not been replicated in humans (46).

Effects on Health and Performance

The effects of disordered eating on health and performance of the athlete can be surprisingly variable, but they are generally dependent on the severity and duration of the disorder. Some athletes may be able to engage in disordered eating behaviors for extended periods of time with few long-term negative effects (5). For most, however, it is simply a matter of time before the pathogenic weight-control behaviors and chronic energy restriction negatively affect their physical performance and, more importantly, their physical and emotional health.

Health

The morbidity associated with disordered eating can be explained by (a) the restriction of calories and the resulting state of starvation or semistarvation, and (b) the purging techniques used to rid the body of ingested energy. Athletes who chronically or severely restrict energy intake will likely have macro- and micronutrient deficiencies, anemia, chronic fatigue, and an increased risk of infections, injury, and illnesses (2,47,48). Additional health effects associated with chronic or severe energy restriction and the resulting weight loss (or maintenance of a dangerously low body weight) include decreased basal metabolic rate, cardiovascular and gastrointestinal disorders, depression, reductions in bone mineral density, menstrual dysfunction in female athletes, and possibly reduced testosterone levels in male athletes (see Table 18.2 and Box 18.2) (2,4,48–52).

Athletes who engage in bingeing and purging have many of the same health complications as those with anorexia nervosa (eg, nutrient deficiencies, chronic fatigue, endocrine abnormalities, and bone mineral density reductions); however, the gastrointestinal and cardiovascular complications are somewhat distinct. Bingeing frequently causes gastric distention that, in rare cases, can result in gastric necrosis and even rupture (2,51). Esophageal reflux and subsequent chronic throat irritation are also common and may increase the risk for esophageal cancer (53). The gastrointestinal complications associated with purging depend on the purging methods used and can include throat and mouth ulcers, dental caries, abdominal cramping, diarrhea, and hemorrhoids (see Table 18.2) (51).

TABLE 18.2   Health Consequences of Disordered Eating Behaviors

Weight Control Behavior	Physiological Effects and Health Consequences
Fasting or starvation	Promotes loss of lean body mass, a decrease in metabolic rate, and a reduction in bone mineral density. Increases the risk of nutrient deficiencies. Promotes glycogen depletion, resulting in poor exercise performance. May cause cardiovascular abnormalities.
Diet pills	Typically function by suppressing appetite and may cause a slight increase in metabolic rate (if they contain ephedrine or caffeine). May induce rapid heart rate, anxiety, inability to concentrate, nervousness, inability to sleep, and dehydration. Any weight lost is quickly regained once use is discontinued.
Diuretics	Weight loss is primarily water, and any weight lost is quickly regained once use is discontinued. Dehydration and electrolyte imbalances are common and may disrupt thermoregulatory function and induce cardiac arrhythmia.
Laxatives or enemas	Weight loss is primarily water, and any weight lost is quickly regained once use is discontinued. Dehydration and electrolyte imbalances, constipation, cathartic colon (a condition in which the colon becomes unable to function properly on its own), and steatorrhea (excessive fat in the feces) are common. May be addictive, and athlete can develop resistance, thus requiring larger and larger doses to produce the same effect (or even to induce a normal bowel movement).
Self-induced vomiting	Largely ineffective in promoting weight (body fat) loss. Large body water losses can lead to dehydration and electrolyte imbalances. Gastrointestinal problems, including esophagitis, esophageal perforation, and esophageal and stomach ulcers, are common. May promote erosion of tooth enamel and increase the risk for dental caries. Finger calluses and abrasions are often present.
Fat-free diets	May be lacking in essential nutrients, especially fat-soluble vitamins and essential fatty acids. Total energy intake must still be reduced to produce weight loss. Many fat-free convenience foods are highly processed, with high sugar contents and few micronutrients unless the foods are fortified. The diet is often difficult to follow and may promote binge eating.
Saunas	Weight loss is primarily water, and any weight lost is quickly regained once fluids are replaced. Dehydration and electrolyte imbalances are common and may disrupt thermoregulatory function and induce cardiac arrhythmia.
Excessive exercise	Increases risk of staleness, chronic fatigue, illness, overuse injuries, and menstrual dysfunction.

Source: Reprinted from Beals KA. *Disordered Eating Among Athletes: A Comprehensive Guide for Health Professionals.* Champaign, IL: Human Kinetics; 2004:84–85, by permission of the author.

BOX 18.2   The Female Athlete Triad

The female athlete triad (triad) was officially described in 1997 in a position stand published by the American College of Sports Medicine (ACSM) as a collection of three distinct yet interrelated disorders including disordered eating, amenorrhea, and osteoporosis. Ten years later (2007), a second position stand by the ACSM was released in which the triad categories were substantially altered to better reflect the "spectrum" of disorders that can afflict female athletes. Specifically, the term *disordered eating* was replaced by *energy availability*, *amenorrhea* was replaced by *menstrual function*, and *osteoporosis* by *bone health*. In addition, the newly revised position stand asserts that *low energy availabilty* is the cornerstone of the metabolic and health consequences associated with the triad. *Energy availability* is defined as the amount of energy available for the metabolic processes of the body after energy is used for exercise, normalized for fat-free mass (Energy availability = Energy intake – Energy expenditure per kilogram of fat-free mass [FFM]). Although low energy availability can (and often does) result from disordered eating, it may also result from the athlete inadvertently failing to meet exercise energy requirements due to time constraints, food availability issues, or lack of appropriate nutrition knowledge. In female athletes, disordered eating is associated with menstrual dysfunction as well as low bone mineral density (even in the absence of menstrual dysfunction). In addition, research on amenorrheic female athletes and amenorrheic patients suffering from anorexia nervosa point to low energy availability as the mechanism leading to compromised bone and reproductive health.

Source: Data are from reference 2.

Electrolyte imbalances, particularly hypokalemia (ie, low blood potassium levels), are also common in individuals who engage in purging behaviors and can have debilitating effects on health. The cardiovascular complications associated with bingeing and purging are usually secondary to the electrolyte imbalances induced by purging. As described earlier, hypokalemia can result in life-threatening cardiac arrhythmia. In addition, individuals who abuse ipecac may have myocarditis (inflammation of the middle layer of the heart muscle) and various cardiomyopathies (54). Alterations in electrolytes as a result of purging can lead to dangerous disruptions in the body's acid-base balance and life-threatening alterations in the body's pH. Self-induced vomiting typically results in an increase in serum bicarbonate levels and thus leads to metabolic alkalosis (increase in blood pH). On the other hand, individuals who abuse laxatives are most likely to develop metabolic acidosis (decrease in blood pH) due to loss of bicarbonate in the stool (54).

Performance

Surprisingly, anecdotal evidence (ie, reports from coaches and personal accounts by athletes with disordered eating) suggests that athletes practicing disordered eating behaviors often experience an initial, albeit transient, increase in performance. The reasons for this temporary increase in performance are not completely understood, but are thought to be related to the initial physiological and psychological effects of starvation and purging (55). Starvation and purging are physiological stressors and, as such, produce an up-regulation of the hypothalamic-pituitary-adrenal axis, (ie, "the fight-or-flight response") and an increase in the adrenal hormones (cortisol, epinephrine, and norepinephrine). These hormones have a stimulatory effect on the central nervous system that can mask fatigue and evoke feelings of euphoria in the eating disordered athlete. In addition, the initial decrease in body weight (particularly before there is a substantial decrease in muscle mass) may induce a transient increase in relative maximal oxygen uptake per kilogram of body weight (VO_{2max}) (56). Moreover, with weight loss athletes may feel lighter, which may afford them a psychological boost, particularly if they believe that lighter is always better in terms of performance.

It should be emphasized that the increase in performance sometimes noted with disordered eating is only temporary. Eventually, the body will break down and performance will suffer. The decrement in performance with chronic or severe energy restriction is likely due to one or more of the following factors: nutrient deficiencies, anemia, fatigue, reduced cardiovascular function, frequent infection, illness, and/or injuries (4). As previously described, individuals with bulimia nervosa may purge or attempt to compensate for their bingeing episodes by using diuretics, laxatives, or enemas; self-induced vomiting; or exercising excessively. If the purging or compensatory behaviors place the athlete in a state of negative energy balance, then the potential effects on performance are similar to those that occur with chronic or severe energy restriction. Also, the gastrointestinal blood losses that often result from chronic vomiting can contribute to iron losses and increase the risk of iron-deficiency anemia. Excessive exercise, especially given inadequate energy and nutrient intakes, invariably leads to overuse injuries. In addition to the resulting energy and nutrient deficiencies, purging poses some unique problems regarding athletic performance, most notably dehydration and electrolyte abnormalities (57).

The effects of disordered eating on athletic performance are a function of the severity and duration of the disordered eating behaviors as well as the physiological demands of the sport (4). Thus, an individual who engages in severe energy restriction or who has been bingeing and purging for a long time will likely experience a greater decrement in performance than one who has engaged in milder weight-control behaviors for a shorter period of time. Likewise, endurance sports and other physical activities with high energy demands (eg, distance running, swimming, cycling, basketball, field hockey, and ice hockey) are likely to be more negatively affected than sports with lower energy demands (eg, diving, gymnastics, weightlifting). Finally, athletes who train at a high intensity (eg, elite athletes) are apt to have greater performance decrements than those who engage in lower-intensity exercise (eg, recreational athletes).

Prevention

Eating disorder prevention efforts and strategies should focus on the environmental risk factors that have been shown to predispose athletes to developing disordered eating, including the sociocultural emphasis on thinness, unrealistic body weight ideals, and unhealthful eating and weight-control practices that continue to permeate the athletic environment.

Educational programming for the prevention of disordered eating in athletes should be provided by an appropriate health professional, such as an exercise physiologist, psychiatrist/psychologist, registered dietitian (RD), or physician, and should target coaches, trainers, athletic support staff and administration, and the athletes themselves. For the younger athlete with disordered eating, education should also be directed toward the athlete's parents because they maintain a considerable influence over the athlete and may facilitate, albeit unknowingly, the athlete's disordered eating behaviors. The focus of education should be on dispelling the myths and misconceptions about nutrition, body weight and composition, weight loss, and the impact of these factors on athletic performance. Equally important is providing accurate and appropriate nutrition information and dietary guidelines to promote optimal health and athletic performance. An RD with expertise in sports nutrition as well as eating disorders is the most qualified individual to provide such nutrition education (4).

Nonetheless, education is unlikely to be effective unless it is accompanied by preventive efforts designed to change the beliefs and behaviors of athletes and athletic staff. Prevention strategies should build on the educational information supplied and thus should de-emphasize body weight and body composition, promote healthful eating behaviors, destigmatize disordered eating, and recognize and encourage the athlete's individuality while fostering a team environment (4). Examples of these strategies follow.

De-emphasizing Weight and Body Composition

There are several ways that coaches, trainers, and athletic staff can help de-emphasize body weight and composition among their athletes. As mentioned in the previous section, simply educating the athletes and athletic staff about the limitations of anthropometric measurements can help to reduce the emphasis on body weight and composition (or at least put it into proper perspective). Of course, the most obvious way to de-emphasize body weight or composition is to simply eliminate anthropometric assessments altogether (58).

Promoting Healthful Eating Behaviors

To successfully promote healthful eating behaviors among athletes, nutrition education and information must be reinforced by practice. All those involved in the management of athletes must therefore practice what they preach. Coaches are probably in the best position to reinforce nutrition education messages by bringing healthful foods to practice, choosing healthful restaurants before and after competitions, and, of course, eating healthfully themselves.

Destigmatizing Eating Disorders

Coaches, trainers, and other athletic personnel can help reduce the stigma of disordered eating by creating an atmosphere in which athletes feel comfortable discussing their concerns about body image, eating, and weight control. Athletic personnel should strive to promote understanding and foster trust with their athletes. The goal is to create an atmosphere in which athletes feel comfortable confiding an eating problem. In short, coaches, trainers, and athletic administrators must make it clear that they place the athletes' health and well-being ahead of athletic performance.

Fostering Individuality Within a Team Environment

Most coaches, trainers, and athletes have come to realize the importance of individualizing physical training regimens. Thus, it is surprising that they still have difficulty accepting that each athlete has a unique body size, shape, and composition with distinct nutritional requirements. Individualization of each athlete's body weight or composition goals and dietary practices, taking into account weight and nutritional history, current training and dietary practices, and weight, diet, and performance goals, is not only key to optimal performance but also to the prevention of disordered eating.

Although it is important to recognize and respect the athlete's individuality, it is also important to foster a team environment, one in which all athletes work together toward the common goal of optimal health and performance. This may be somewhat challenging because athletes, by their very nature, are competitive. The environment dictates that athletes be competitive not only with their opponents, but also often within their own team to secure playing time or their position on the team. Unfortunately, this competitive drive sometimes goes beyond the playing field and affects other aspects of the athlete's life, such as eating behaviors, body weight, and/or body composition.

Comparing oneself physically to another individual is certainly not a practice limited to athletes, but it may be more prevalent in the athletic setting simply because athletes have more opportunities for comparison (eg, athletes frequently change clothes and shower in the same locker room; athletic apparel or uniforms are becoming increasingly revealing; group weigh-ins and body composition assessments remain prevalent in many sports) (5). Coaches, trainers, and athletic administrators can help reduce this "competitive thinness" by not comparing athletes' body weights or body compositions and by not using the bodies of certain athletes on the team as the gold standard by which all others are measured. Instead, coaches and trainers should try to downplay body weight and encourage healthful eating behaviors among all of their athletes.

Peer-Led Approaches to Reducing Eating Disorder Risk

A novel approach to the prevention of disordered eating among female athletes has recently been described (59). Created by Carolyn Black Becker, PhD, and based on cognitive dissonance theory, this theory states that the possession of inconsistent cognitions creates psychological discomfort that motivates people to alter their cognitions to produce greater consistency. It has been argued that dissonance approaches are more effective than educational approaches to prevention because attitudinal changes in the former are achieved by challenging a person's self-concept, which is more enduring than change motivated by an external source (ie, providing information).

The Female Athlete Body Project used a peer-led eating disorder prevention program for athletes at Trinity University (59,60). A peer leader was selected from each of the Trinity varsity athletic teams. The peer leaders completed an intensive training session with the researcher and then conducted three, 75-minute education/intervention sessions over a 6-week period. The sessions were athlete-centered, interactive, and included discussions of the sport-specific ideal of thinness; the pressure to conform to the sport-specific thin ideal; the athlete-specific, healthy ideal; factors that can inhibit and enhance performance; and the female athlete triad. The results showed that athletes who participated in the peer-led prevention program had a decrease in several of the constructs measured at baseline, including thin-ideal internalization, negative affect, dietary restraint, bulimic pathology, and body dissatisfaction. Moreover, 1-year follow-up assessment indicated that all constructs except for thin-ideal internalization remained below baseline.

Identification, Approach, and Referral

Athletes with disordered eating often either deny that the problem exists or do not realize that they have a problem. In either case, they are unlikely to come forward and admit to disordered eating. Thus, it is up to others to recognize the signs and symptoms of disordered eating and initiate intervention. A variety of eating disorder questionnaires and screening instruments are available (see Table 18.3) (61–70). However, many researchers and practitioners contend that the best method for identifying athletes with disordered eating is probably direct observation (4,71). Table 18.4 lists common signs and symptoms of disordered eating (4). For direct observation to be effective, every individual who works closely with athletes needs to be familiar with the warning signs and symptoms of disordered eating.

Once disordered eating has been identified, the next steps are approaching and referring the athlete to a treatment program. Approaching an athlete with disordered eating and convincing him or her to seek treatment can be extremely difficult. Although the athlete with disordered eating may seem to be the most compliant individual on the team, when threatened with exposure and the potential consequences (eg, embarrassment, disapproval by coaches and teammates, being withheld from competition or removed from the team, having to relinquish the pathogenic weight-control behaviors and possibly gain weight), denial and defiance often take over (5). Thus, it is crucial to be sensitive yet firm when approaching an athlete who is suspected of having an eating disorder and attempting to convince him or her to seek treatment.

TABLE 18.3 Self-Report Surveys and Questionnaires for Identifying Disordered Eating in Athletes

Instrument (Reference)	Description
General Questionnaires	
Bulimia Test-Revised (BULIT-R) (61)	28-item multiple-choice questionnaire designed to assess the severity of symptoms and behaviors associated with bulimia nervosa (eg, weight preoccupation and bingeing and purging frequency). Respondents rate each item on a 5-point Likert scale in which higher scores are more indicative of bulimia nervosa.
Eating Attitudes Test, 26 items (EAT-26) (62)	Shortened (26-item) version of the EAT-40 that also identifies thoughts, feelings, and behaviors associated with anorexia nervosa. Uses a 6-point Likert scale ranging from *rarely* to *always*. A score of ≥ 20 indicates risk of anorexia nervosa.
Eating Disorder Examination Questionnaire (EDE-Q) (63)	Self-report version of the Eating Disorder Examination interview. It assesses the features of eating disorders via the following four subscales: (*a*) dietary restraint, (*b*) eating concern, (*c*) body shape concern, (*d*) weight concern along with a global (total) score.
Eating Disorder Inventory (EDI) (64)	64-item questionnaire with eight subscales. The first three subscales (drive for thinness; bulimia; and body dissatisfaction) assess behaviors regarding body image, eating, and weight-control practices. The remaining five subscales (interpersonal distrust; perfectionism; interoceptive awareness; maturity fears; and ineffectiveness) assess the various psychological disturbances characteristic of those with clinical eating disorders. Items are answered using a 6-point Likert scale ranging from *always* to *never.*
Eating Disorder Inventory-2 (EDI-2) (65)	91-item multidimensional inventory designed to assess the symptoms of anorexia nervosa and bulimia nervosa. The EDI-2 contains the same eight subscales as the EDI and adds three additional subscales (27 more items), including asceticism; impulse regulation; and social insecurity. Items are answered using a 6-point Likert scale ranging from *always* to *never.*
Eating Disorder Inventory-3 (EDI-3) (66)	91-item questionnaire organized into 12 primary scales that yield six composite scores: eating disorder, risk ineffectiveness, interpersonal problems, affective problems, overcontrol, and general psychological maladjustment.
Three-Factor Eating Questionnaire (TFEQ) (67)	58-item true/false and multiple-choice questionnaire that measures the tendency toward voluntary and excessive restriction of food intake as a means of controlling body weight. The questionnaire contains 3 subscales: restrained eating (eg, "I often stop eating when I am not full as a conscious means of controlling my weight"); tendency toward disinhibition (eg, "When I feel lonely, I console myself by eating"); and perceived hunger (eg, "I am always hungry enough to eat at any time").
Athlete-Specific Questionnaires	
Athletic Milieu Direct Questionnaire (AMDQ) (68)	19-item questionnaire. Assesses behaviors associated with anorexia nervosa and bulimia nervosa (eg, body image, dieting practices, body weight changes). A variety of response categories are used.
Female Athlete Screening Tool (FAST) (69)	33-item multiple-choice questionnaire. Assesses the unique issues of disordered eating and excessive exercise as they pertain to athletes (eg, "I think that being thin is associated with winning).
Physiologic Screening Test (70)	18-item questionnaire consisting of four physiological measures: (*a*) body fat percentage, (*b*) waist-to-hip ratio, (*c*) standing diastolic blood pressure, (*d*) parotid gland enlargement; and 14 self-report items including physical symptoms (dizziness, abdominal bloating /cramping, bowel movements, menstrual dysfunction) and behaviors and cognitions (excessive exercise, body dissatisfaction, weight loss attempts, highest, lowest, and ideal body weight).

TABLE 18.4   Signs and Symptoms of Disordered Eating

Behavioral	Physical
• Excessive criticism of one's body weight or shape • Preoccupation with food, calories, or weight • Compulsive, excessive exercise • Mood swings, irritability • Depression • Social withdrawal • Secretly eating or stealing food • Bathroom visits after eating • Avoiding food-related social activities • Excessive use of laxatives, diuretics, or diet pills • Consumption of large amounts of food inconsistent with the athlete's weight • Excessive fear of being overweight or becoming fat that does not diminish as weight loss continues • Preoccupation with the dietary patterns and eating behaviors of other people • Lack of concern for excessive weight loss or extremely low body weight	• Chronic fatigue • Noticeable weight loss or gain • Anemia • Frequent gastrointestinal problems or complaints (eg, excessive gas, abdominal bloating, constipation, ulcers) • Cold intolerance • Lanugo (fine hair on the face and body) • Tooth erosion, excessive dental caries • Callused fingers • Frequent musculoskeletal injuries (particularly stress fractures) • Delayed or prolonged healing of wounds or injuries • Frequent or prolonged illnesses • Dry skin and hair • Brittle nails • Alopecia (hair loss) • In women, irregular or absent menstrual cycles • Cardiovascular abnormalities (eg, palpitations, bradycardia, prolonged QT intervals) • Orthostatic hypotension

Source: Adapted from Beals KA. *Disordered Eating Among Athletes: A Comprehensive Guide for Health Professionals.* Champaign, IL: Human Kinetics; 2004:129, by permission of the author.

The potential for a successful intervention increases if the following three conditions are met: (*a*) the athlete is approached in a timely fashion; (*b*) there is an established rapport between the athlete and the individual attempting the intervention; and (*c*) the athlete is approached with caring and concern. The Ohio State University athletic department's eating disorders policy (72), which is presented in Box 18.3, is a good model for approaching and referring athletes identified with disordered eating.

Treatment

Treatment of disordered eating involves the application of specific therapeutic modalities—psychological, nutritional, and medical—by qualified health professionals, such as psychiatrists, psychologists, RDs, and physicians. Because eating disorders are psychological disorders, psychological counseling is considered the cornerstone of treatment. Because medical complications often accompany disordered eating, a physician should also be included in the overall treatment plan. Finally, nutrition counseling, provided by an RD specializing in eating disorders, is a vital component of the total treatment regimen for disordered eating.

Psychological Treatment

A variety of psychological approaches have been used successfully to treat eating disorders, including psychodynamic, cognitive-behavioral, and behavioral methods. Additional variables to consider when selecting a treatment approach include the treatment setting (eg, inpatient vs outpatient) and format (eg, individual

---

BOX 18.3   Strategies for Approaching an Athlete Suspected of Having an Eating Disorder

- The individual (eg, coach, staff member) who has the best rapport with the student athlete should be the one to approach the athlete, and it should be done in a private setting (eg, a private meeting).
- In a respectful tone, indicate specific observations that led to the concern, being sure to give the athlete time to respond.
- Choose "I" statements over "you" statements to avoid placing the athlete on the defensive. For example, "I've noticed that you've been fatigued lately, and I'm concerned about you" is preferable to "You need to eat and everything will be fine."
- Avoid giving simple solutions (eg, "Just eat something") to a complex problem. This will only encourage the student athlete to hide the behavior from you in the future.
- Avoid discussing implications for team participation and instead affirm that the student athlete's role on the team will not be jeopardized by an admission to a problem. The team may be the athlete's only diversion from his or her disordered eating. By eliminating this opportunity for social support and the supervision of a coach or trainer, the athlete may dive into further pathology.
- Regardless of whether the student athlete responds with denial or hostility, it is important to encourage him or her to meet with a professional for an assessment. Acknowledge that seeking outside help is often beneficial and is not a sign of weakness.

Source: Data are from reference 72.

---

vs group, with or without family). For additional information about psychological treatment, refer to the *Handbook of Treatment for Eating Disorders* (73).

Nutrition Counseling

Psychological counseling aims to uncover and correct the underlying mental and emotional issues fueling the eating disorder, whereas nutrition counseling focuses on eliminating the disordered eating behaviors (ie, the energy restriction, bingeing, and/or purging), treating any nutritional deficiencies, addressing nutrition beliefs and thoughts about food, improving body image, and reeducating the athlete about sound sport nutrition practices (4).

It is beyond the scope of this chapter to provide an in-depth discussion of nutrition counseling for individuals with disordered eating. There are several books and review articles that cover this topic, and the reader is encouraged to examine those for more detailed information (74–77). A brief summary of the general components of nutrition interventions for disordered eating in athletes is presented here.

As a result of their high energy expenditures combined with inadequate energy intake, athletes with disordered eating often suffer from low energy availability and nutrient deficiencies that can range from mild to severe. Thus, one of the first steps in treatment should be to identify and rectify existing nutritional deficiencies. Dietary intake assessments and nutritional status measures can be used to determine nutritional deficiencies and even to verify the presence of disordered eating (see Table 18.5) (4,57). Negative energy balance (ie, energy intake less than energy expenditure) and/or low energy availability (energy expenditure in exercise that is not adequately covered by energy intake—see Box 18.2) can be corrected by

TABLE 18.5 Laboratory and Biochemical Findings Associated with Eating Disorders

Anorexia Nervosa	Bulimia Nervosa
• Decreased iron status measures (anemia is common) • Elevation of liver enzymes • Hypoglycemia • Decreased serum creatinine • Decreased blood urea nitrogen (BUN) • Low thyroid function (decreased T4) • Hypophosphatemia • Hyponatremia • Dyslipidemia	• Decreased iron status measures (anemia is common) • Hyponatremia • Hypokalemia • Metabolic alkalosis (associated with self-induced vomiting) • Metabolic acidosis (associated with laxative abuse; may mask a potassium deficiency) • Hypomagnesemia • Hypoglycemia (due to purging) • Hyperglycemia (due to bingeing) • Dehydration

Source: Adapted from Beals KA. *Disordered Eating Among Athletes: A Comprehensive Guide for Health Professionals.* Champaign, IL: Human Kinetics; 2004:185–188, by permission of the author.

increasing the athlete's energy intake and/or decreasing his/her training load (47). As simple as this sounds, it is actually one of the most difficult aspects of nutrition treatment for the athlete with disordered eating. Specific meal plans providing a gradual increase in energy intake and/or energy density may be helpful at first, with the idea of eventually moving toward more of an intuitive eating plan (75,76). Micronutrient deficiencies are common, particularly deficiencies of the B vitamins and the minerals, iron, calcium, zinc, and magnesium. Efforts to supply these nutrients via whole foods should be made first (47). However, because the disordered eating athlete will likely be resistant to substantial changes/increases in food intake, supplementation may be necessary during the early stages of treatment. Supplementation of iron should not ensue without status measures indicative of poor iron status.

Individuals with disordered eating are obsessed with nutrition and often seem to be experts on the topic; however, the knowledge that they possess is frequently wrought with myths and misconceptions (4). Moreover, they have often been engaged in abnormal eating patterns for so long that they do not recognize what constitutes normal or healthful eating. Thus, the primary goals of nutrition management for eating disorders are to dispel the myths and misconceptions regarding food and diet and to reestablish healthful eating patterns. To help extinguish disordered eating beliefs and behaviors, RDs should provide accurate information about such topics as energy balance, vitamin and mineral functions and requirements, and fluid needs.

Individuals with disordered eating have often lost touch with internal (physiological) feelings of hunger and satiety, instead relying on external cues and rigid rules for eating. Thus, nutrition counseling must focus on helping them recognize and respond appropriately to body signals of hunger and satiety (74). Meal management (ie, creating meal plans and strategies to deal with irrational food thoughts and behaviors) can aid in the reestablishment of "normal eating" and may also help empower the individual with an eating disorder to take control of mealtimes and food intake.

Summary

In the world of athletics, a fraction of a second or one tenth of a point can mean the difference between winning and losing. These high stakes can place enormous pressure on athletes. Under such pressure, many athletes develop a "win at any cost" attitude and some may resort to disordered eating behaviors in an attempt to lose weight and therefore improve performance. Unfortunately, these weight-loss behaviors are often self-defeating. Any initial improvement in performance (as a result of weight loss) is transient. The pathogenic weight-control practices will eventually take their toll on the athlete's health and performance.

Prevention of disordered eating in athletes involves the development of educational programs and strategies designed to dispel the myths and misconceptions surrounding nutrition, dieting, body weight, and body composition, and their impact on performance, as well as stressing the role of nutrition in promoting health and optimal physical performance. Early identification is paramount to limiting progression and shortening the duration of the disordered eating. Thus, all those individuals working with athletes must be familiar with the warning signs and symptoms of disordered eating in athletes.

The primary treatment goals for eating disorders in athletes are to normalize eating behaviors and body weight and identify and correct the underlying psychological issues that initiated and perpetuate the eating disorder. As the individual who is most knowledgeable in the area of nutrition as it relates to athletes, the sports dietitian plays an integral role in the treatment of disordered eating in athletes.

References

1. *Diagnostic and Statistical Manual of Mental Disorders*. 4th ed. Washington, DC: American Psychiatric Association; 1994.
2. Nattiv A, Loucks AB, Manore MM, Sanborn CF, Sundgot-Borgen J, Warren MP. American College of Sports Medicine position stand. The female athlete triad. *Med Sci Sports Exerc*. 2007;39:1867–1882.
3. Fairburn CG, Brownell KD, eds. *Eating Disorders and Obesity: A Comprehensive Handbook*. 2nd ed. New York, NY: Guilford Press; 2001.
4. Beals KA. *Disordered Eating Among Athletes: A Comprehensive Guide for Health Professionals*. Champaign, IL: Human Kinetics; 2004.
5. Thompson RA, Sherman RT. *Disordered Eating in Sport*. London, England: Routledge UK; 2010.
6. Beals KA, Manore MM. The prevalence and consequences of subclinical eating disorders in female athletes. *Int J Sport Nutr*. 1994;4:175–195.
7. Beals KA, Manore MM. Subclinical eating disorders in active women. *Topics Clin Nutr*. 1999;14:14–24.
8. Beals KA, Manore MM. Behavioral, psychological and physical characteristics of female athletes with subclinical eating disorders. *Int J Sport Nutr Exerc Metab*. 2000;10:128–143.
9. Smith NJ. Excessive weight loss and food aversion in athletes simulating anorexia nervosa. *Pediatrics*. 1980; 66:139–142.
10. Sundgot-Borgen J. Prevalence of eating disorders in elite female athletes. *Int J Sport Nutr*. 1993;3:29–40.
11. Pugliese MT, Liftshitz F, Grad G, Fort P, Marks-Katz M. Fear of obesity: a cause for short stature and delayed puberty. *N Engl J Med*. 1983;309:513–518.
12. Bunnell DW, Shenker IR, Nussbaum MP, Jacobson MS, Cooper P. Subclinical versus formal eating disorders: differentiating psychological features. *Int J Eat Disord*. 1990;9:357–362.
13. Williamson DA, Netemeyer RG, Jackman LP, Anderson DA, Funsch CL, Rabalais JY. Structural equation modeling for risks for the development of eating disorder symptoms in female athletes. *Int J Eat Disord*. 1995;4:387–393.
14. Brownell KD, Rodin J. Prevalence of eating disorders in athletes. In: Brownell KD, Rodin J, Wilmore JH, eds. *Eating, Body Weight and Performance in Athletes: Disorders of Modern Society*. Philadelphia, PA: Lea and Febiger; 1992:128–145.
15. Byrne S, McLean N. Eating disorders in athletes: a review of the literature. *J Sci Med Sport*. 2001;4:145–159.
16. Beals KA, Hill AK. The prevalence of disordered eating, menstrual dysfunction and low bone mineral density among US collegiate athletes. *Int J Sport Nutr Exerc Metab*. 2006;16:1–23.
17. Nichols JF, Raugh MJ, Barrack MT, Barkai HS, Pernick Y. Disordered eating and menstrual irregularity in high school athletes in lean-build and non-lean build sports. *Int J Sport Nutr Exerc Metab*. 2007;17:364–377.
18. Nichols JF, Raugh MJ, Lawson MJ, Ji M, Barkai HS. Prevalence of the female athlete triad syndrome among high school athletes. *Arch Pediatr Adolesc Med*. 2006;160:137–142.

19. Andersen AE, Holman JE. Males with eating disorders: challenges for treatment and research. *Psychopharmacol Bull.* 1997;33:391–397.

20. Sundgot-Borgen J, Torstveit MK. Prevalence of eating disorders in elite athletes is higher than in the general population. *Clin J Sport Med.* 2004;14:25–32.

21. Toro J, Galilea B, Martinez-Mallen E, Salamero M, Capdevila l, Mari J, Mayolas J, Toro E. Eating disorders in Spanish female athletes. *Int J Sports Med.* 2005;26:696–700.

22. Beals KA, Manore MM. Disorders of the female athlete triad among collegiate athletes. *Int J Sport Nutr Exerc Metab.* 2002;12:281–293.

23. Sundgot-Borgen J, Dlungland M, Torstveit G, Rolland C. Prevalence of eating disorders in male and female elite athletes. *Med Sci Sports Exerc.* 1999;31(suppl):S297.

24. Johnson C, Powers PS, Dick R. Athletes and eating disorders: the National Collegiate Athletic Association study. *Int J Eat Disord.* 1999;26:179–188.

25. Sundgot-Borgen J. Eating disorders. In: Berning JR, Steen SN, eds. *Nutrition for Exercise and Sport.* Gaithersburg, MD: Aspen Publishers; 1998:187–204.

26. Wilmore JH. Eating and weight disorders in the female athlete. *Int J Sport Nutr.* 1991;1:104–107.

27. Striegel-Moore RH, Bulik CM. Risk factors for eating disorders. *Am Psychol.* 2007;62:181–198.

28. Polivy J, Herman P. Causes of eating disorders. *Ann Rev Psychol.* 2002;53:187–213.

29. Sundgot-Borgen J. Risk and trigger factors for the development of eating disorders in female athletes. *Med Sci Sports Exerc.* 1994;26:414–419.

30. Hoek HW. Incidence, prevalence, and mortality of anorexia nervosa and other eating disorders. *Curr Opin Psychiatry.* 2006;19:389–394.

31. Witchen HU, Jacobi F. Size and burden of mental disorders in Europe. A critical review and appraisal of 27 studies. *Eur Neuropsychopharmacol.* 2005;15:357–376.

32. Petrie TA, McFarland MB. Men and muscles: the increasing objectification of the male body. In: *The Hidden Faces of Eating Disorders and Body Image.* Reel JJ, Beals KA, eds. Reston, VA: National Association for Girls and Women in Sports; 2009:39–61.

33. Woodside DB, Garfinkel PE, Lin E, Goeing P, Kaplan AS, Goldbloom DS, Kennedy SH. Comparisons of men with full or partial eating disorders, men without eating disorders and women with eating disorders in the community. *Am J Psychiatry.* 2001;158:570–574.

34. Hudson J, Hiripi E, Pope HG Jr, Kessler RC. The prevalence and correlates of eating disorders in the National Comorbidity Survey Replication. *Biol Psychiatry.* 2007;61:348–358.

35. Pope HG Jr, Phillips KA, Olivardia R. *The Adonis Complex: The Secret Crisis of Male Body Obsession.* New York, NY: Free Press; 2000.

36. Pope HG, Gruber AJ, Choi P. Muscle dysmorphia: an unrecognized form of body dysmorphic disorder. *Psychosomatics.* 1997;38:548–557.

37. Beals KA. Mirror, mirror on the wall, who is the most muscular of them all? Disordered eating and body image disturbances in male athletes. *ACSM Health Fit J.* 2003;7:6–11.

38. Glazer JL. Eating disorders among male athletes. *Curr Sports Med Rep.* 2008;7:332–337.

39. Baum A. Eating disorders in the male athlete. *Sports Med.* 2006;36:1–6.

40. Fairburn CG, Welch SL, Doll HA, Davies BA, O'Connor ME. Risk factors for bulimia nervosa: a community-based, case-control study. *Arch Gen Psychiatry.* 1997;54:509–517.

41. Bulik CM, Slof-Opt Landt MCT, van Furth EF, Sullivan PF. The genetics of anorexia nervosa. *Annu Rev Nutr.* 2007;27:263–275.

42. Gorwood P, Kipman A, Foulon C. The human genetics of anorexia nervosa. *Eur J Pharmacol.* 2003;480:163–170.

43. Matsushita S, Suzuki K, Murayama M, Nishiguchi N, Hishimoto A, Takeda A, Shirakawa O, Higuchi S. Serotonin transporter regulatory region polymorphism is associated with anorexia nervosa. *Am J Med Genet B Neuropsychiatr Genet.* 2004;128:114–117.

44. Epling WF, Pierce WD. Activity-based anorexia nervosa. *Int J Eat Disord.* 1988;7:475–485.

45. Epling WF, Pierce WD, Stefan L. A theory of activity-based anorexia nervosa. *Int J Eat Disord.* 1983;3:27–46.

46. O'Connor PJ, Smith JC. Physical activity and eating disorders. In: Rippe JM, ed. *Lifestyle Medicine*. Oxford, England: Blackwell Science; 1999:1005–1015.

47. Beals KA, Manore MM. Nutritional status of female athletes with subclinical eating disorders. *J Am Diet Assoc.* 1998;98:419–425.

48. Manore MM, Kam LC, Loucks AB. The female athlete triad: components, nutrition issues, and health consequences. *J Sports Sci.* 2007;25(Suppl 1):S61–S71.

49. Loucks AB, Verdun M, Heath EM. Low energy availability, not stress of exercise, alters LH pulsatility in exercising women. *J Appl Physiol.* 1998;84:37–46.

50. Keen AD, Drinkwater BL. Irreversible bone loss in former amenorrheic athletes. *Osteoporosis Int.* 1997;7: 311–315.

51. Pomeroy C, Mitchell JE. Medical issues in the eating disorders. In: Brownell KD, Rodin J, Wilmore JH, eds. *Eating, Body Weight and Performance in Athletes: Disorders of Modern Society*. Philadelphia, PA: Lea and Febiger; 1992:202–221.

52. Misra M, Katzman DK, Cord J, Manning SJ, Mendes N, Herzog DB, Miller KK, Kibanski A. Bone metabolism in adolescent boys with anorexia nervosa. *J Clin Endocrinol Metab.* 2008;93:3029–3036.

53. Carney CP, Andersen AE. Eating disorders: guide to medical evaluation and complications. *Psychiatr Clin North Am.* 1996;19:657–679.

54. Bo-Linn GW. Understanding medical complications in eating disorders. In: Larocca F. *Eating Disorders*. San Francisco, CA: Jossey-Bass; 1986:5–12.

55. Johnson MD. Disordered eating in active and athletic women. *Clin Sports Med.* 1994;13:355–369.

56. Ingjer F, Sundgot-Borgen J. Influence of body weight reduction on maximal oxygen uptake in female elite athletes. *Scand J Med Sci Sport.* 1991;1:141–146.

57. Otis CL, Goldingay R. *The Athletic Woman's Survival Guide: How to Win the Battle Against Eating Disorders, Amenorrhea, and Osteoporosis*. Champaign, IL: Human Kinetics; 2000.

58. Carson JD, Bridges E. Abandoning routine body composition assessment: a strategy to reduce disordered eating among female athletes and dancers. Canadian Academy of Sport Medicine Position Statement. *Clin J Sports Med.* 2001;11:280.

59. Black Becker C. Peer-led approaches to reducing eating disorder risk factors and increasing awareness of the female athlete triad. Presented at the 26th SCAN Symposium. San Diego, CA. Mar 27–30, 2010.

60. Stice E, Shaw H, Black Becker C, Rohde P. Dissonance-based interventions for the prevention of eating disorders: using persuasion principles to promote health. *Prev Sci.* 2008;9:114–128.

61. Thelen MH, Farmer J, Wonderlich S, Smith M. A revision of the bulimia test: the BULIT-R. *J Consult Clin Psychol.* 1991;3:119–124.

62. Garner DM, Olmstead MP, Bohr Y, Garfinkel PE. The Eating Attitudes Test: psychometric features and clinical correlates. *Psychol Med.* 1982;12:871–878.

63. Fairburn CG, Cooper Z, Doll HA, Davies BA. Identifying dieters who will develop an eating disorder: a prospective, population-based study. *Am J Psychiatry.* 2005;162:2249–2255.

64. Garner DM, Olmsted MP, Polivy J. Development and validation of a multidimensional eating disorder inventory for anorexia nervosa and bulimia. *Int J Eat Disord.* 1983;2:15–34.

65. Garner DM. *Eating Disorder Inventory-2 Manual*. Odessa, FL: Psychological Assessment Resources; 1991.

66. Garner DM. *Eating Disorder Inventory-3 (EDI-3)*. Lutz, FL: Psychological Assessment Resources; 2004.

67. Stunkard AJ. "Restrained eating": what it is and a new scale to measure it. In: Cioffi LA, ed. *The Body Weight Regulatory System: Normal and Disturbed Mechanisms*. New York, NY: Raven Press; 1981:243–251.

68. Nagel DL, Black DR, Leverenz LJ, Coster DC. Evaluation of a screening test for female college athletes with eating disorders and disordered eating. *J Athl Train.* 2000;35:431–440.

69. McNulty KY, Adams CH, Anderson JM, Affenito SG. Development and validation of a screening tool to identify eating disorders in female athletes. *J Am Diet Assoc.* 2001;101:886–892.

70. Black DR, Larkin LJ, Coster DC, Leverenz LJ, Abood DA. Physiologic screening test for eating disorders/ disordered eating among female collegiate athletes. *J Athl Train.* 2003;3:286–297.

71. Ryan R. Management of eating problems in the athletic setting. In: Brownell KD, Rodin J, Wilmore JH, eds. *Eating, Body Weight and Performance in Athletes: Disorders of Modern Society.* Philadelphia, PA: Lea and Febiger; 1992:344–362.

72. Hill L. The Ohio State University Department of Athletics Eating Disorder Policy 2001. http://ehe.osu.edu/sports nut/policy/ED.pdf. Accessed October 15, 2011.

73. Garner DM, Garfinkel PE. *Handbook of Treatment for Eating Disorders.* New York, NY: Guilford Press; 1997.

74. Kahm A. Recovery through nutritional counseling. In: Kinovy BP. *Eating Disorders: New Directions in Treatment and Recovery.* 2nd ed. New York, NY: Columbia University Press; 2001:15–47.

75. Reiter CS, Graves L. Nutrition therapy for eating disorders. *Nutr Clin Pract.* 2010;25:122–136.

76. Tribole E, Resch E. *Intuitive Eating: A Revolutionary Program That Works.* New York, NY: St Martin's Griffin; 2003.

77. Herrin M. *Nutrition Counseling in the Treatment of Eating Disorders.* 2nd ed. New York, NY: Brunner-Routledge; 2003.

Chapter 19

DIABETES AND EXERCISE

CHARLOTTE HAYES, MMSc, MS, RD, CDE, ACSM-CES

Introduction

Physical activity is a cornerstone in diabetes management and prevention (1). The important health benefits of activity for people with diabetes and for those at risk of diabetes include a reduction in cardiovascular risk factors, improved success with weight loss and maintenance, lower percentage of body fat, and a heightened sense of well-being (1–4). Exercise also affects glucose metabolism (3,5). It increases muscle and liver insulin sensitivity, enhances muscle glucose uptake and utilization, and improves overall glycemic control (3,5). Unfortunately, although metabolic adaptations to exercise generally improve blood glucose control for individuals with type 2 diabetes and normalize glucose homeostasis in those with pre-diabetes (4–6), these same adaptations can lead to glucose variability and considerable management challenges for individuals with type 1 diabetes (5,7,8).

The health-focused exerciser, as well as the elite athlete with diabetes, often faces the need to adjust diabetes management to achieve and maintain euglycemia with activity. Adjustments may be necessary in medications, meal planning, and in the exercise routine itself. The need for multiple, complex adjustments may require input from a specialized diabetes team. Registered dietitians (RDs) play a central role in integrating diabetes nutrition management and activity. The desired outcome of nutrition intervention is the achievement of optimal glycemic control with exercise so that the individual with diabetes can realize the many health benefits of an active lifestyle and the athlete with diabetes can achieve optimal competitive performance.

The Role of Exercise in Diabetes Prevention

Type 2 diabetes is a progressive condition that is closely linked to obesity. The prevalence of both disease states has dramatically increased during the past decade (9,10). Furthermore, the prevalence of type 2 diabetes in youth has increased at an alarming rate (11). In part, the dual epidemics of obesity and diabetes are attributed to the built environment, which supports physical inactivity and easy access to foods that are often calorie-dense yet nutrient-poor. The dramatic increases in obesity and type 2 diabetes are important public health concerns (10).

Prior to the onset of type 2 diabetes, metabolic syndrome and associated cardiovascular risk factors often become apparent. Unless lifestyle changes are made, metabolic syndrome typically progresses to pre-diabetes, defined as fasting plasma glucose (FPG) of 100 to 120 mg/dL, impaired glucose tolerance (IGT; 2-hour blood glucose value of 140 to 199 mg/dL in an oral glucose tolerance test), or hemoglobin A1C of 5.7% to 6.4% (7). Within 3 to 10 years of onset, pre-diabetes can progress to overt type 2 diabetes (12). Recognition of the link between the metabolic disorders associated with pre-diabetes/type 2 diabetes and cardiovascular diseases is essential because adults with diabetes have a two to four times greater risk of cardiovascular disease than those without diabetes (13). The Look AHEAD Trial (Action for Health in Diabetes) is an 11-year trial investigating the effectiveness of intensive lifestyle interventions aimed at weight loss through calorie restriction, increased physical activity, and behavior modification on cardiovascular outcomes in people with diabetes. One-year results of the trial showed clinically significant weight loss as well as improved diabetes control and CVD risk factors (14). At end point, this trial should elucidate the effects of long-term weight loss and lifestyle modification on cardiovascular disease outcomes.

The role of exercise in diabetes prevention cannot be overlooked. Exercise reduces insulin resistance, improves insulin action, and increases glucose tolerance. Furthermore, exercise improves cardiovascular risk factors and aids with weight loss and maintenance (2,15). Because exercise improves the constellation of metabolic abnormalities that lead to type 2 diabetes (see Box 19.1) and its complications, physical activity is considered an essential modality for its prevention (7,15,16).

Landmark clinical trials investigating the feasibility and effectiveness of preventing type 2 diabetes through lifestyle interventions have provided strong evidence that early lifestyle intervention can lead to prevention (17–20). In these trials, modest lifestyle modifications aimed at increasing physical activity to an average of 150 minutes per week, reducing dietary fat and energy intake, and moderately reducing weight by 5% to 7% of starting weight were shown to decrease progression of pre-diabetes to overt diabetes by 31% to 63% in individuals with impaired fasting glucose. Intensive lifestyle interventions resulted in a 58% reduction in risk of developing type 2 diabetes both in the Diabetes Prevention Program (17) and Finnish Diabetes Prevention Program (18), two large randomized controlled trials.

BOX 19.1   Risk Factors for Development of Type 2 Diabetes

- Physical inactivity
- Other conditions associated with insulin resistance such as overweight and obesity
- Age ≥ 45 years
- A1C > 5.7%, impaired fasting glucose or impaired glucose tolerance on previous testing
- Hypertension (blood pressure ≥ 140/90) or being treated for hypertension
- Dyslipidemia (high-density lipoprotein cholesterol ≤ 35 mg/dL or triglycerides ≥ 250 mg/dL)
- History of cardiovascular disease
- Having a parent or sibling with diabetes
- Diagnosis of gestational diabetes or giving birth to a baby weighing > 9 lb
- Polycystic ovary syndrome
- Racial/ethnic group (African American, Alaska Native, American Indian, Asian American, Hispanic/Latino, Pacific Islander)

Source: Data are from references 7, 15, and 16.

Physical activity recommendations for prevention of diabetes are similar to those recommended for the general population by the US Department of Health and Human Services' Physical Activity Guidelines for Americans. These evidence-based guidelines advise adults to accrue at least 150 minutes of moderate-intensity or 75 minutes of vigorous activity per week (21).

Type 2 Diabetes

Type 2 diabetes is the predominant form of diabetes. It is characterized by reduced insulin-mediated glucose uptake due to insulin resistance, defects in insulin secretion, and, over time, insulin deficiency (7). Risk factors for developing type 2 diabetes are multiple (see Box 19.1) (7,15,16). Lack of physical activity is a considerable risk factor, and potential benefits of exercise to the individual with type 2 diabetes are numerous (see Box 19.2) (1–3,22). The benefit of exercise in improving the metabolic abnormalities associated with type 2 diabetes seems to be greatest early in the progression of the disease (1,3).

Medical nutrition therapy (MNT) is an integral part of type 2 diabetes management. Desired goals of MNT include achievement and maintenance of glucose, lipid, and blood pressure levels as close to normal ranges as safely possible and prevention or delay of chronic diabetes complications (23). Weight loss is often an important aspect of management as well. A moderate loss of 5% to 7% of initial body weight (approximately 10 to 20 lb) is sufficient to considerably improve glycemic control, blood lipids, and blood pressure (10,15,24). Lifestyle modification that includes diet and exercise has been shown to optimize weight loss (10,15,24), decrease the reductions in lean body mass and resting metabolic rate that often accompany weight loss (24), and improve cardiovascular risk factors (13,15). Diet and exercise should be considered adjunctive therapies in type 2 diabetes management.

Diabetes MNT and Exercise for Optimal Glycemic Control

When advising individuals with type 2 diabetes, it is important to emphasize that the combined therapies of meal planning plus exercise can lead to optimal blood glucose control and provide other health benefits. In contrast, the consumption of unnecessary extra calories when exercising can easily counter the energy deficit and blood glucose–lowering effect of activity, especially if an individual's physical capacity is limited and the energy deficit created is small.

Individuals who control their diabetes by diet and exercise alone are not at increased risk of hypoglycemia when active (5). Extra food for exercise is often unnecessary and should certainly be avoided if weight

---

BOX 19.2   Potential Health Benefits of Exercise in Type 2 Diabetes

- Improved glycemic control
- Improved insulin sensitivity
- Reduced cardiovascular risk factors:
  - Improved lipid profile; decrease in triglyceride-rich, very low–density lipoproteins
  - Lower blood pressure
  - Increased fibrinolytic activity
  - Greater success with weight loss and maintenance
  - Possible delay or prevention of onset of type 2 diabetes complications

Source: Data are from references 1–3 and 22.

TABLE 19.1 Oral Glucose-Lowering Medications and Associated Hypoglycemia Risk

Medications	Potential for Hypoglycemia
Insulin Secretagogues	
Second-generation sulfonylureas: glyburide (Micronase, Diabeta); micronized glyburide (Glynase PresTab); glipizide (Glucotrol); glipizide extended release (Glucotrol XL); glimepiride (Amaryl)	Moderate
Meglitinides: repaglinide (Prandin)	Low-moderate
D-Phenylalanine derivative: nateglinide (Starlix)	Low-moderate
Starch Blockers	
Alpha-glucosidase inhibitors: acarbose (Precose); miglitol (Glycet)[a,b]	Low
Biguanides	
metformin (Glucophage)[a]; metformin sustained-release (Glucophage XR); metformin extended release (Fortamet, Glumetza)	Low
Insulin Sensitizers	
pioglitazone (Actos)[a]; rosiglitazone (Avandia)	Low
DPP-4 Inhibitors	
sitagliptin phosphate (Januvia); saxagliptin (Onglyza); linagliptin (Tradjenta)	Low

[a]Can contribute to hypoglycemia if used as combination therapy with insulin or sulfonylureas.
[b]Glucose must be used as treatment for hypoglycemia; alpha-glucosidase inhibitors prevent the conversion of sucrose to metabolically available sugars.
Source: Data are from references 25, 26, and 27.

management is a goal. An exception is during periods of prolonged, vigorous exercise, when the intake of extra calories is typically necessary to support sustained, increased energy expenditure.

For those on oral antidiabetes medication(s), moderate exercise typically leads to a gradual reduction in blood glucose that is unlikely to result in hypoglycemia. However, with certain medications, hypoglycemia is still possible (25,26) (see Tables 19.1 and 19.2) (25–27), and prolonged activity increases the possibility of blood glucose levels falling too low (3,5). If the blood glucose decreases to less than a desirable range, a reduction in the dosage of medication(s) should be discussed with the diabetes team. Extra food to maintain adequate blood glucose values should be used conservatively.

Individuals treated with insulin are at risk of experiencing exercise-related blood glucose fluctuations and hypoglycemia. To maintain euglycemia with activity, the principles of adjusting insulin, carbohydrates, and exercise that guide individuals with type 1 diabetes should be applied to type 2 diabetes management (5).

Postmeal exercise may reduce blood glucose response to food consumed. Individuals who experience postprandial hyperglycemia may benefit from exercising 1 to 2 hours after eating. Exercise at this time may reduce postmeal blood glucose increases and certainly will reduce risk of exercise-related hypoglycemia.

Exercise Recommendations for Type 2 Diabetes

The 2008 Physical Activity Guidelines for Americans recommend that all adults older than 18 years accumulate at least 150 minutes of moderate physical activity per week (21). Individuals are encouraged to begin by taking small steps each day to informally increase activity levels. These general recommendations

TABLE 19.2 Injected Glucose-Lowering Medications and Associated Hypoglycemia Risk

Medications	*Potential for Hypoglycemia*
Incretin Mimetics	
exenatide (Byetta)	Low-moderate (risk increases when used in combination with insulin secretagogues)
pramlintide (Symlin)	Low-moderate (premeal insulin dose may need to be reduced by 30%–50%)
Glucagon-like Peptide-1(GLP-1)Analog	
Victoza (liraglutide)	Moderate-high (when used in combination with an insulin secretagogue)
Insulin	
Rapid-acting: aspart (Novalog); glulisine (Apidra); lispro (Humalog)	High (peak time 30 min–2 h postinjection)
Short-acting: regular (Humulin R, ReliOn/Novolin R)	High (peak time 2–3 h postinjection)
Intermediate-acting: NPH (Humulin N, Novolin N)	High (peak time 4–12 h postinjection)
Long-acting: glargine (Lantus); detemir (Levemir)	Moderate-high (glargine: flat, no pronounced peak; detemir: relatively flat peak)
Combination drugs	
Various	Varies

Source: Data are from references 25, 26, and 27.

are safe and effective for most people with type 2 diabetes and are consistent with recommendations that successfully guided increases in physical activity in the diabetes prevention trials (4). The beneficial effects of exercise on insulin sensitivity last for only 24 to 72 hours (depending on intensity and duration of exercise); therefore, clinicians should emphasize the importance of routine activity for optimal blood glucose control. Planned exercise at least 5 days per week, with no more than two consecutive days without aerobic activity, is recommended (3). Resistance exercise has been shown to improve insulin sensitivity and hemoglobin A1C and offers additional health benefits, including increased muscle mass, strength, and endurance, and improved body composition. For these reasons, individuals with type 2 diabetes should be encouraged to do resistance exercises that include all major muscle groups three times per week (3,7).

In the past decade, the optimal level of exercise to support weight loss and maintenance has been debated and clarified. Based on recent review of scientific literature, the American College of Sports Medicine (ACSM) recommends that overweight and obese individuals participate in at least 150 to 250 minutes of moderate-intensity physical activity per week to prevent further weight gain. Accrual of 250 to 300 minutes of weekly moderate activity, or an approximate 2,000-kcal energy expenditure, is likely to result in greater success with weight loss and prevention of weight regain (28). When advising individuals with type 2 diabetes, the majority of whom are overweight, it is important to encourage stepwise increases in physical activity and apply strategies that will encourage adoption and maintenance of lifelong activity (29). Physical activity goals that seem beyond reach will only dissuade the most sedentary, who have the most to gain from moderate increases in physical activity.

BOX 19.3   Macrovascular and Microvascular Complications of Diabetes

Macrovascular
- Coronary artery disease
- Peripheral vascular disease
- Cerebrovascular disease

Microvascular
- Retinopathy
- Neuropathy
  - Peripheral
  - Autonomic
- Nephropathy

Source: Data are from reference 7.

Prior to beginning exercise, a thorough medical evaluation to screen for macrovascular and microvascular complications of diabetes may be indicated (see Box 19.3) (1,3,7). This will minimize exercise risk and assure the appropriateness of an exercise prescription.

Type 1 Diabetes

Type 1 diabetes accounts for 5% to 10% of all diabetes cases. However, most athletes with diabetes have type 1, which is characterized by pancreatic beta cell destruction and absolute insulin deficiency (30,31). Athletes with type 1 diabetes must overcome considerable obstacles during exercise because for them metabolic adjustments to maintain fuel homeostasis (see Table 19.3) are lacking (3,5). The result can be a mismatch between hepatic glucose production and muscle glucose utilization, and substantial deviation from euglycemia. Exercise must be carefully integrated into the diabetes management regimen so that optimal blood glucose levels are maintained and training and performance goals are achieved.

Many variables influence the glycemic response to exercise (see Box 19.4) (1,3,5). Those that can most readily be modified are circulating insulin levels and nutrition intake. Insulin adjustments and carbohydrate supplementation can be used independently or together to maintain optimal blood glucose levels during and after exercise. The individual with type 1 diabetes must monitor glucose regularly to understand glycemic

TABLE 19.3   Hormonal Adjustments to Maintain Fuel Homeostasis

Hormone	Response to Exercise	Metabolic Effect
Insulin	Decreases	Restricts use of glucose by nonexercising skeletal muscle; increases hepatic glycogenolysis; facilitates lipolysis
Glucagon	Increases	Stimulates hepatic glycogenolysis and gluconeogenesis
Epinephrine	Increases	Stimulates glucose production during prolonged exercise; increases muscle glycogenolysis; increases adipose tissue lypolysis
Norepinephrine	Increases	Modulates initial hepatic glucose release
Cortisol	Increases	Increases hepatic glucose production

Source: Data are from references 3 and 5.

BOX 19.4   Variables That Influence the Effect of Exercise on Blood Glucose Levels in Type 1 Diabetes

- Level of training and fitness
- Intensity of exercise
- Duration of exercise
- Time of exercise

- Type of exercise
- Metabolic control
- Nutritional status and glycogen stores
- Circulating insulin levels

Source: Data are from references 1, 3, and 5.

---

response to exercise, learn to make appropriate exercise-related management decisions, and evaluate the effectiveness of these decisions.

Self-Monitoring of Blood Glucose and Pattern Management

Self-monitoring of blood glucose (SMBG), careful record-keeping, and recognition of blood-glucose patterns with exercise are important skills for the individual with type 1 diabetes. These skills enhance the ability to make sound self-adjustment decisions that improve exercise safety and optimize competitive performance (1,7). SMBG should be done regularly before exercise, after exercise, during prolonged events, or when the type, duration, or intensity of exercise is not routine. Frequent monitoring helps predict potential for hypoglycemia or hyperglycemia occurring during or after exercise and thus reduces risk for these acute complications. Data from monitoring, when carefully recorded and analyzed, become the basis for decision-making about adjustments in management for subsequent exercise sessions (see Figure 19.1) (5). Pattern management, the methodical process of data collection, analysis, and decision-making, is the foundation of successful blood-glucose control with exercise (see Box 19.5) (32).

Continuous glucose monitoring (CGM) systems have recently emerged as an important adjunct to SMBG for athletes and active individuals with type 1 diabetes. CGM measurement devices continually (every few minutes) measure "real time" glucose values and glucose trends data. These systems use small sensors inserted under the skin to measure interstitial glucose, which correlates with plasma glucose levels (7). Each sensor stays in place from 3 to 7 days after insertion (depending on system), and information is transmitted wirelessly from a transmitter to a monitor that stores and displays data for viewing. CGM systems contain alarm features that warn of predicted hypo- or hyperglycemia (based on an individual's preset target glucose range) and indicate the direction and rate of change of the glucose level during the prior 20- to 60-minute period. Additionally, sensor data can be downloaded to a computer for in-depth review and identification of glucose patterns and trends (33,34). For more information on CGM systems, see reference 35 as well as Web sites for specific products.

For athletes with diabetes, CGM has considerable utility before, during, and after exercise, when glucose levels can be highly variable. Awareness of direction and rate of change of glucose and pending hypo- or hyperglycemia allows preemptive adjustments in carbohydrate intake or insulin doses. Such "on-time" adjustments can help athletes with diabetes to maintain optimal competitive performance and avoid exercise-related hypoglycemia, which is a serious concern for all individuals who require insulin (36,37).

Current CGM devices still do not have the level of accuracy of standard blood glucose meters (see Box 19.6) (34,38). They tend to be least accurate for 12 to 24 hours after insertion of a new sensor, during periods of hypoglycemia, and during periods of rapid blood glucose change. Because interstitial glucose readings lag 5 to 10 minutes behind capillary glucose readings (measured by SMBG by finger stick), a

Name: _____   For: Month _____   Year _____

Address: _____   Home Phone: _____   Work: _____

City: _____   State: _____   Zip: _____

<u>Blood Glucose Target Range: 70–140 mg/dL</u>
<u>Blood Glucose Target Range at Bedtime: 90–150 mg/dL</u>

TIME	2–4 AM	PRE-BREAKFAST			PC	NOON			PC	PRE-SUPPER			PC	BEDTIME			REMARKS
DATE	BG	BG	RA	Sup		BG	RA	Sup		BG	RA	Sup		BG	L	Sup	*Reaction # Exercise
6/14	98	126	7	0	(57)	(61)	7	-1 / 0		77	7	-1 / 0		106	17	0	*#Work in yard 2 hrs. 9:30–11:30a
6/15	—	121	5	0		[178]	7	2	2:30 (59)	[157]	7	1		120	17	0	*#Aerobics class 1:00–2:00p ↑ 30 g CHO
6/16	133	132	5	0		136	5	0		125	7	0		97	17	0	
6/17	97	104	5	0		[141]	5	1	3:00 (63)	97	7	0		112	17	0	*#Brisk walk 1:30–12:25p ↑ 20 g CHO
6/18	—	110	5	0		137	4	0		129	7	0		141	17	0	
6/19	141	97	5	0		115	4	0	2:30 108	134	7	0		138	17	0	#Aerobics class 1:00–2:00p 0 ↑ CHO
6/20	104	[152]	5	1		75	4	-1 / 0	3:00 92	86	7	0		126	17	0	*#Brisk walk 2:00–3:00p 0 ↑ CHO
6/21	—	128	5	0		[148]	4	1		112	7	0		1	17	0	

◯ = BG < target range
▢ = BG > target range

FIGURE 19.1 Sample blood glucose flow sheet. Abbreviations: BG, blood glucose; L, long-acting insulin; RA, rapid-acting insulin; Sup, supplement/compensatory insulin. Copyright © Atlanta Diabetes Associates.

BOX 19.5   Exercise Pattern Management: A Seven-Step Process

Step 1: Record blood glucose values surrounding exercise.
Step 2: Study the recorded information.
Step 3: Find and interpret exercise-related blood glucose patterns.
Step 4: Make adjustments in carbohydrate intake or insulin based on identified patterns.
Step 5: Try adjustment strategies.
Step 6: Evaluate blood glucose responses and effectiveness of adjustments.
Step 7: Continue to modify and fine-tune strategies as needed.

Source: Data are from reference 32.

CGM reading can be significantly higher than the capillary value when the blood glucose level is rapidly decreasing and can be significantly lower than the capillary value when the blood glucose level is rapidly increasing (34,38,39). Thus, routine SMBG is necessary for individuals who use CGM, and adjustments in diabetes management should be based on blood glucose meter readings rather than sensor readings alone (7,37).

BOX 19.6   Continuous Glucose Monitoring (CGM) Accuracy Considerations Related to Lag Time

- Interstitial glucose levels equilibrate more slowly than blood glucose levels.
  - When glucose levels are increasing, sensor readings will be lower than simultaneous meter readings.
  - When glucose levels are decreasing, sensor readings will be higher than simultaneous meter readings.
- CGM systems take multiple glucose readings over 5 minutes and average these values to generate a single glucose number that is displayed on the monitor screen. This data that appear on the screen are, on average, 2½ minutes old.
- Duration of processing glucose values may cause CGM to underestimate rate of decline when glucose is decreasing, as during exercise.

Source: Data are from references 34 and 38.

Carbohydrate Supplements

Carbohydrate supplements, though necessary in many exercise situations, should be used conservatively in some circumstances. When deciding about the need for additional carbohydrate during exercise, several factors should be considered (see Box 19.7) (1,5). Unnecessary or immoderate carbohydrate intake can quickly offset the beneficial blood glucose–lowering effects of exercise and can supply excessive energy.

Carbohydrate supplements are useful when activity is spontaneous or unplanned and is typically necessary during long-duration training or competitive events when energy expenditure is high. Carbohydrate can be consumed before, during, or after such exercise. As a general rule, intake of supplemental carbohydrate is indicated pre-exercise when the blood glucose is less than 100 mg/dL prior to the start of activity (1,7). Individuals who participate in long-duration or competitive events that last longer than 60 minutes will likely need to consume carbohydrate during exercise to maintain optimal blood glucose control and to delay fatigue. Muscle efficiency and performance seem to be best when blood glucose values are maintained between 80 and 180 mg/dL, or as near normal as possible, during exercise (40). However, as more

---

BOX 19.7   Factors That Influence Carbohydrate Supplement and Insulin Adjustment Decisions

- Blood glucose level before exercise
- Planned exercise intensity
- Planned exercise duration
- Level of training
- Time of day for planned exercise

- Time of last meal
- Insulin therapy
- Previously measured metabolic response to exercise

Source: Data are from references 1 and 5.

athletes use CGM technology, refinement of current understanding of optimal glucose levels for competitive performance is possible.

Enough carbohydrate should be consumed during exercise to keep the blood glucose in this optimal range. Intake of 15 to 30 g carbohydrate every 30 to 60 minutes of exercise is a general, safe starting guideline for supplementing carbohydrate (39,40). Sport drinks and diluted juices (< 8% carbohydrate) replace fluid as well as carbohydrate and are certainly appropriate for individuals with diabetes. Energy gels or sport bars are easy to carry, portion-controlled, carbohydrate-controlled supplement options and are convenient to use during training and competition. Taking additional insulin to cover carbohydrate consumed for the purpose of maintaining target range blood glucose levels during exercise is generally not advised. Because numerous variables can influence blood glucose response to exercise, strategies for supplementing carbohydrate must be highly individualized (1,5). Glucose monitoring and pattern management allow the individual to draw on prior exercise experience, fine-tune carbohydrate supplementation strategies, and achieve optimal blood glucose levels for peak performance.

Endurance athletes with diabetes may use strategies for manipulating carbohydrate intake to optimize muscle and liver glycogen stores prior to long events. Frequent SMBG and insulin adjustment is necessary to maintain glycemic control when carbohydrate intake and training are altered before an event. Carbohydrate loading can be used with caution and meticulous care by athletes with diabetes (41). Extra carbohydrate is often necessary after exercise when insulin sensitivity is increased and glycogen synthesis is enhanced (5,41,42). Intake of additional carbohydrate at this time both promotes glycogen storage and reduces the likelihood of hypoglycemia. SMBG should be done every 1 to 2 hours after exercise to assess the blood glucose response and make necessary adjustments in food intake and insulin doses (41).

Insulin Adjustment

Because insulin sensitivity and responsiveness change with exercise, substantial blood glucose fluctuations can occur if circulating insulin levels are too high or too low (see Table 19.4) (3,5). Pre-exercise insulin adjustment to reduce the usual dose and thus reduce circulating insulin levels is often necessary, especially before long-duration exercise or sports competition. Insulin adjustment to reduce insulin can also be used by those who are concerned about weight management and wish to limit the need for extra carbohydrate

TABLE 19.4   Metabolic Response to Exercise Based on Insulin Status

Insulin Level	Liver Glucose Output	Muscle Glucose Uptake	Metabolic Effect
High	↑	↑↑	↓ BG ↑ Hypoglycemia risk ↓ FFA mobilization
Desirable	↑↑	↑↑	Stable BG Efficient fuel flux
Low	↑↑	↑	↑ BG ↑ Potential for hyperglycemia ↑ Lipolysis ↑ Ketones

Key: ↑ = moderate increase; ↑↑= large increase; ↓ = decrease.
Abbreviations: BG, blood glucose level; FFA, free fatty acid.
Source: Data are from references 3 and 5.

(and calories) to maintain optimal blood glucose levels. Elevated pre-exercise blood glucose can indicate insulin deficiency. Supplemental insulin may be necessary to correct low insulin levels and improve metabolic control before beginning exercise. Adjustment decisions should always be made with consideration of several important variables (refer to Box 19.6). SMBG, careful record-keeping, and evaluation of blood glucose patterns are crucial for determining successful adjustment strategies.

Several guidelines for reducing insulin doses prior to planned exercise have been suggested (5,40,41,43). A 30% to 50% reduction in the dose of insulin acting during the time of exercise is generally accepted as a safe starting guideline. Greater reductions are often needed for prolonged training or during competition (5,40,43). Because adjustment decisions require recognition of the insulin acting during the time of exercise, familiarity with the time course of insulin action is important (see Table 19.2).

Intensive insulin therapy, either multiple daily injections (MDI) or continuous subcutaneous insulin infusion (CSII), is considered standard treatment for type 1 diabetes (43). The advantage of intensive therapy is that it offers multiple opportunities to adjust insulin doses throughout the day; thus, adjustments for exercise can be made with great precision. Conventional (or twice-daily insulin therapy) offers fewer opportunities to manipulate doses to reflect changes in insulin requirements. Therefore, adjustments for exercise tend to be less precise. Conventional therapy depends on intermediate-acting insulin (NPH), which has a pronounced and extended peak. Intensive therapy depends on use of rapid- or short-acting insulin in combination with a long-acting insulin analog, glargine or detemir, which has little or no peak. For these reasons, intensive therapy is more likely to allow safe and optimal exercise performance and is certainly the therapy of choice for athletes with type 1 diabetes.

Doses of insulin may need to be modified for an extended time after extreme or prolonged activity, when insulin sensitivity and muscle glycogen repletion are increased. The period of heightened sensitivity to insulin can last for up to 36 hours after extreme or unusual exercise. Reduction in insulin doses during this period may be necessary to prevent postexercise hypoglycemia, which can be quite severe. Frequent SMBG, including monitoring during the night (eg, at 3:00 AM), is an advisable precautionary measure. In contrast, high-intensity, short-duration activity can result in postexercise hyperglycemia due to release of the counter-regulatory hormones norepinephrine and epinephrine and excessive hepatic glucose production (3,43).

Blood glucose elevation in this situation is usually transient, and use of supplemental insulin as a corrective measure is typically not indicated. Extra insulin could contribute to hypoglycemia if its action coincides with an increase in insulin sensitivity after exercise (43,44).

Interpretation of Blood Glucose Patterns and Appropriate Corrective Actions

Pre-exercise blood glucose levels and changes that occur during and after exercise reflect circulating insulin levels (36). When diabetes medications are properly adjusted and carbohydrate intake is appropriate, blood glucose levels are more likely to remain within a desired target range during and after exercise.

If circulating insulin levels are too high, glucose will enter the exercising muscle cell rapidly, resulting in a substantial decrease in blood glucose (34). Too much circulating insulin also restricts glucose production by the liver and reduces free fatty acid mobilization from fat cells, thus making other important fuels for exercise unavailable (3,5). The result can be hypoglycemia, which is a risk to all intensively treated individuals with type 1 diabetes but is especially a concern during extreme or competitive sports events. Both antecedent exercise and antecedent hypoglycemia have been shown to reduce the ability to defend against subsequent hypoglycemia; thus, preventing hypoglycemia is vitally important (45–47).

The appropriate corrective action is to reduce the dose of insulin or oral antidiabetes medication and supplement carbohydrate in controlled amounts at the next exercise session. Whenever hypoglycemia is suspected, exercise must be delayed until the blood glucose level is verified by SMBG. A blood glucose value less than 70 mg/dL indicates hypoglycemia (7). This must be treated appropriately before exercise is resumed (see Figure 19.2) (41,48).

If circulating insulin levels are too low, glucose has difficulty entering exercising muscle cells. Glucose production and release from the liver and fatty acid mobilization are increased. The result can be hyperglycemia and ketosis (3,5). If the fasting blood glucose is elevated prior to exercise, blood or urine ketones should be tested. The combination of elevated fasting blood glucose and positive ketones indicates insulinopenia and poor metabolic control (1). Supplemental insulin should be administered and exercise should be delayed until improved metabolic control is achieved (5). Intake of noncaloric fluids should be encouraged to prevent dehydration associated with hyperglycemia and to help clear ketones. Hyperglycemia in the absence of ketones is often due to factors such as prior dietary indiscretion or psychological stress, including anticipation of sports competition. If this is the case, exercise will usually result in a reduction in blood glucose and improved control. If an individual feels well, there is no reason to postpone exercise based solely on hyperglycemia (3,7).

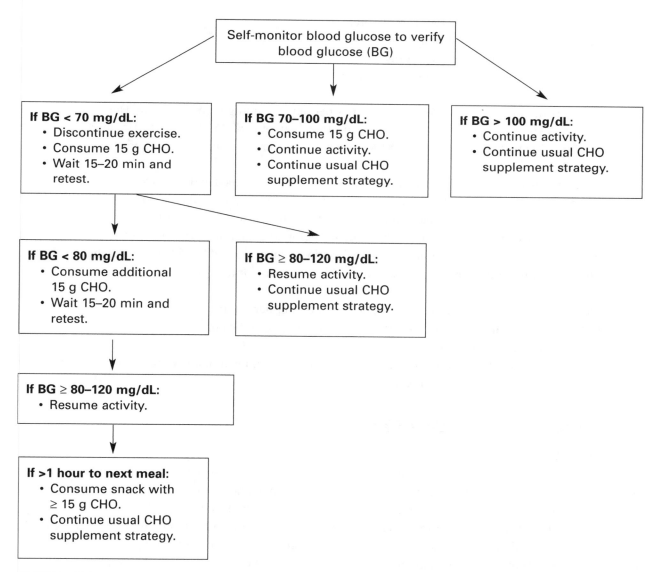

FIGURE 19.2 Carbohydrate supplement use during exercise. Data are from references 41 and 48.

Diabetes and Exercise Case Study

Client History

SJ is a 22-year-old female student who has been running 3 miles three to four times per week. Three weeks ago, she began training for a half-marathon, which will be held 3 months from now. She has had challenges with her blood glucose control during and after her training runs, and a week ago she experienced severe nighttime hypoglycemia after running 5 miles in the late afternoon. SJ has had type 1 diabetes for 9 years. Her height is 5 feet, 5 inches and she weighs 122 pounds.

SJ is on a basal-bolus insulin program of evening glargine (Lantus) and premeal lispro (Humalog). Her usual insulin doses are 14 units of glargine at 9:00 PM and premeal lispro based on an insulin-to-carbohydrate ratio (ICR) of 1 unit of insulin to 10 g carbohydrate (1:10 ratio) at breakfast and 1 unit to 15 g carbohydrate (1:15 ratio) at lunch and dinner. SJ estimates that she consumes 1,700 kcal/d and her usual premeal insulin doses are:

- **Breakfast**: 4 units per 40–45 g carbohydrate
- **Lunch**: 4 units per 60 g carbohydrate
- **Dinner**: 5 units per 75 g carbohydrate
- **Snack(s)**: 1–3 units per 15–45 g carbohydrate

SJ monitors her blood glucose four or five times per day, including before running. Her premeal blood glucose target is 70 to 140 mg/dL and her 2-hour postmeal target is 60 to 160 mg/dL. Having been trained in insulin correction by her diabetes team, SJ adjusts her rapid-acting insulin using a correction dose calculated by her diabetes care provider.

SJ is training with two friends, and their program includes both speed and distance workouts. SJ scheduled an appointment with her RD for assistance with adjusting her food intake and insulin regimen to accommodate the longer distances that she is beginning to run. A priority is to avoid reoccurrence of hypoglycemia. SJ was asked to monitor her blood glucose before, during, and after her workouts for the past week, and to bring her training and glucose log to the appointment. SJ and her RD reviewed the log (Figure 19.3) at the beginning of the appointment and used this as a basis for the following:

- Identifying SJ's blood glucose patterns during and after her training runs.
- Determining the amount of extra carbohydrate and unplanned calories SJ has needed to consume to maintain her glucose level in a safe range.
- Considering options for adjusting SJ's carbohydrate intake, insulin, and training schedule to reduce blood glucose fluctuations during and after her workouts and reduce hypoglycemia risk.

SJ's Diabetes Nutrition Care Plan

Assessment

Although SJ had excellent comprehension and skills regarding her diabetes self-management including SMBG, carbohydrate counting, use of her ICR and insulin adjustment, she is experiencing considerable glucose variability during and after exercise. Her blood glucose patterns during her distance runs are target-range blood glucose levels before exercise; low glucose levels 20 to 30 minutes into her runs; glucose elevations immediately postexercise; and below target-range glucose levels, including hypoglycemia, 4 to 6 hours later. SJ has had to consume 30 to 50 additional g carbohydrate and 100 to 200 unplanned calories

Day, Time of Exercise	Pre-Run BG	Run BG	Post-Run BG	4–6 hour Post-Run BG	Notes
Mon, 5:00 PM	132	N/A	97	115 (9:15 PM)	Walk 2 mile
Tues, 5:30 PM	119	(72) (20 min) / (75) (35 min)	[196]	(56) (10:30 PM)	5-mile run 15 g carb @ 20 min 25 g carb @ 35 min
Wed, 5:00 PM	122	(85) (20 min)	[166]	(82) (11:00 PM)	3-mile run 25 g carb @ 20 min
Thurs, 4:30 PM	155	[187] (30 min)	[201]	112 (10:00 PM)	Fast-slow intervals (30 min)
Fri, 8:30 AM	142	102 (30 min)	140	(77) (11:45 AM)	Run 3 miles/ walk 1 mile 15 g carb @ 30 min
Sat, 9:30 AM	149	(62) (25 min) / (70) (40 min)	[193]	(62) (12:30 PM)	6-mile run 15 g carb @ 25 min 15 g carb @ 40 min 15 g carb @ 55 min
Sun, 4:00 PM	122	[175] (18 min)	[179]	130 (6:00 PM) 158 (10:00 PM)	Fast-slow intervals (35 min)

FIGURE 19.3   SJ's 1-week activity and blood glucose (BG) log. Circled numbers note BG < target range. Boxed numbers are BG > target range.

to treat or prevent hypoglycemia during these runs. SJ's glucose patterns during and after speed workouts show transient hyperglycemia during and immediately postexercise with normalization of glucose levels 4 to 6 hours later.

Management

SJ and her RD decided to focus first on improving SJ's glucose patterns during and after her distance runs. They discussed the following strategies:

- Pre-exercise:
  - Reducing the prelunch insulin dose by 25%, or by 1 unit, on days of SJ's late-afternoon training runs and reducing her prebreakfast insulin dose by 25%, or by 1 unit, on days of her morning distance runs.
  - Blood glucose monitoring 30 minutes before the start of each training run. Consuming a 15- to 20-g carbohydrate snack that includes some protein (eg, Greek yogurt) 15 to 20 minutes before starting exercise *if* SJ's glucose level is ≤ 100mg/dL.
  - Using combined insulin adjustment and carbohydrate supplementation strategies to achieve a pre-exercise glucose level ≥ 120 mg/dL.

- During exercise:
  - Monitoring glucose every 30 to 45 minutes.
  - Consuming approximately 15 g carbohydrate every 30 to 60 minutes, as needed, to maintain her glucose levels above 100 mg/dL. This carbohydrate also provides fuel for working muscles and supports optimal training and race performance.
  - Focusing on hydration by drinking 1 to 1½ cups of fluid per 15 to 20 minutes of exercise. Carbohydrate-containing sport beverages provide both carbohydrate and fluid.
- Postexercise: Continuing to monitor glucose immediately after exercise to verify glucose patterns. The trend toward hyperglycemia at this time may be corrected by the insulin adjustment and planned carbohydrate supplementation strategies applied during exercise.

If the pattern persists, SJ will consider the following strategies:
- After late-afternoon exercise, consider taking premeal lispro 20 to 25 minutes (rather than 15 minutes) before dinner to allow additional time for the insulin to lower her glucose level before she consumes the meal.
- After morning exercise, consider taking a small amount of supplemental insulin to correct the glucose elevation. However, be aware of heightened insulin sensitivity at this time and the potential for hypoglycemia, especially if lunch is delayed.
- Continuing to monitor blood glucose 4 to 6 hours postexercise and make adjustments to reduce hypoglycemia risk at this time and during the night. Possible adjustments include the following:
  - Routinely consuming an evening snack with 15 to 30 g carbohydrate (ideally with some protein).
  - Reducing dosage of glargine insulin, initially by 2 units, to correct a pattern of nighttime hypoglycemia. With physiologic adaptations to training, overall insulin requirements will likely decrease.
  - For morning exercise, considering timing of lunch meal in relation to the end of exercise and incorporating an additional carbohydrate choice in that meal.
  - Changing time of day of training runs from late afternoon to morning may reduce risk of nighttime hypoglycemia.

SJ's RD explained that some "trial and error" with careful record-keeping will enable SJ to find strategies that work best for her. SJ will follow up with her RD and diabetes care provider in 2 weeks to review and fine-tune her revised management strategies. By working with her RD and diabetes team, SJ can expect to successfully train and complete her half-marathon in her goal of less than 2½ hours.

Summary

For individuals with type 2 diabetes and those with pre-diabetes, regular physical activity can improve blood glucose control and may even alleviate symptoms of the disease. However, for individuals with type 1 diabetes, exercise does not have the same tendency to improve glycemic control. Rather, it has the potential to contribute to substantial blood glucose variability and considerable management challenges (5). Even so, all individuals with diabetes should be encouraged to follow active lifestyles to achieve the many health benefits of physical activity. The athlete with diabetes who is striving for competitive performance should be offered the support and self-management training needed to achieve optimal performance.

This chapter provides general guidelines and strategies for adapting diabetes medications and MNT to accommodate exercise. The information presented should be considered a starting point (see Box 19.8 and reference list for additional resources). Strategies must be modified and individualized based on the

---

BOX 19.8   Selected Online Resources on Diabetes and Exercise

- **Insulindependence.** *http://www.insulindependence.org.* This nonprofit service organization helps people with diabetes (including youths) set personal fitness goals and provides education on managing diabetes and exercise. Individuals can join communities to learn more about various activities and glucose management.
- **National Diabetes Education Program.** *http://ndep.nih.gov/partners-community-organization/campaigns/SmallStepsBigRewards.aspx.* This is a valuable resource; publishes *Small Steps, Big Rewards* materials on the prevention of type 2 diabetes.
- **Team Type 1.** *http://www.teamtype1.org.* Team type 1 "strives to instill hope and inspiration for people around the world affected by diabetes. With appropriate diet, exercise, treatment, and technology, we believe anyone with diabetes can achieve their dreams."

---

uniqueness of each client and each exercise situation. SMBG and pattern management allow successful strategies to be developed and fine-tuned to minimize exercise risk while maximizing performance.

References

1. American Diabetes Association. Position statement: physical activity/exercise and diabetes. *Diabetes Care.* 2004; 27(Suppl 1):S58–S62.
2. American College of Sports Medicine, American Diabetes Association. Joint position statement: exercise and type 2 diabetes. *Med Sci Sports Exerc.* 2010;42:2282–2303.
3. Sigal R, Kenny GP, Wasserman D, Casteneda-Sceppa C. Physical activity/exercise and type 2 diabetes. *Diabetes Care.* 2004;27:2518–2539.
4. Kriska A. Can a physically active lifestyle prevent type 2 diabetes? *Exerc Sports Sci Rev.* 2003;31:132–137.
5. Wasserman D, Davis S, Zinman B. Fuel metabolism during exercise in health and diabetes. In: Ruderman N, Devlin J, Schneider S, eds. *Handbook of Exercise in Diabetes.* Alexandria, VA: American Diabetes Association; 2002:63–99.
6. Sherwin RS, Anderson RM, Buse JB, Chin MH, Eddy D, Fradkin J, Ganiats TG, Ginsberg HN, Kahn R, Nwankwo R, Rewers M, Schlessinger L, Stern M, Vinicor F, Zinman B; American Diabetes Association; National Institute of Diabetes and Digestive and Kidney Diseases. The prevention or delay of type 2 diabetes. *Diabetes Care.* 2004;27 (Suppl 1):S47–S54.
7. American Diabetes Association. Standards of medical care in diabetes, 2010. *Diabetes Care.* 2011;34(Suppl 1): S11–S61.
8. Raguso CA, Coggan AR, Gastadelli A, Sidossis LS, Bastyr EJ III, Wolfe RR. Lipid and carbohydrate metabolism in IDDM during moderate and intense exercise. *Diabetes.* 1995;44:1066–1074.
9. Fonseca V. Defining and characterizing the progression of type 2 diabetes. *Diabetes Care.* 2009; 32 (Suppl 2): S151–S156.
10. Position of the American Dietetic Association: weight management. *J Am Diet Assoc.* 2009;109:330–346.
11. Diabetes in Children and Adolescents Work Group of the National Diabetes Education Program. An update on type 2 diabetes in youth from the National Diabetes Education Program. *Pediatrics.* 2004; 114:259–263.
12. Nichols GA, Hiller TA, Brown JB. Progression from newly acquired impaired fasting glucose to type 2 diabetes. *Diabetes Care.* 2007;30:228–233.

13. Eckel RH, Kahn R, Robertson RM, Rizza RA. Preventing cardiovascular disease and diabetes: a call to action from the American Diabetes Association and the American Heart Association. *Circulation*. 2006;113: 2943–2946.

14. The Look AHEAD Research Group. Reduction in weight and cardiovascular disease risk factors in individuals with type 2 diabetes. *Diabetes Care*. 2007;30:1374–1383.

15. Klein S, Sheard NF, Pi-Sunyer X, Daly A, Wylie-Rosett J, Kulkarni K, Clark NG. Weight management through lifestyle modification for the prevention and management of type 2 diabetes: rationale and strategies. *Diabetes Care*. 2004;27:2067–2073.

16. National Institute of Diabetes and Digestive and Kidney Diseases. National Diabetes Information Clearinghouse. Insulin Resistance and Pre-diabetes. http://diabetes.niddk.nih.gov/dm/pubs/insulinresistance/index.htm# prediabetes. Accessed March 14, 2010.

17. Diabetes Prevention Research Group. Reduction in the incidence of type 2 diabetes with lifestyle intervention or metformin. *N Engl J Med*. 2002;346:393–403.

18. Tuomilehto J, Lindstrom J, Eriksson T, Valle T, Hamalainen H, Ilanne-Paprikka P, Keinanen-Kiukaanniemi S, Laasko M, Louheranta A, Rastas M, Salminen V, Uusitupa M. Prevention of type 2 diabetes mellitus by changes in lifestyle among subjects with impaired glucose tolerance. *N Engl J Med*. 2001;344:1343–1350.

19. Eriksson K, Lindgarde F. Prevention of type 2 (non-insulin dependent) diabetes by diet and physical exercise. *Diabetologia*. 1991;34:891–898.

20. Pan X, Li G, Hu Y, Wang J, Yang W, An Z, Hu Z, Lin J, Xiao J, Cao H, Liu P, Jiang X, Jiang Y, Wang J, Zheng H, Zhang H, Bennett P, Howard B. Effects of diet and exercise in preventing NIDDM in people with impaired glucose tolerance: the Da Quin IGT and Diabetes Study. *Diabetes Care*. 1997;20:537–544.

21. US Department of Health and Human Services. *2008 Physical Activity Guidelines for Americans*. Atlanta, GA: Centers for Disease Control and Prevention; 2008.

22. Marwick TH, Hordern MD, Miller T, Chyun DA, Bertoni AG, Blumenthal RS, Philippides G, Rocchini A. Exercise training for type 2 diabetes mellitus; impact on cardiovascular risk: a scientific statement from the American Heart Association. *Circulation*. 2009;119:3244–3262.

23. American Diabetes Association. Nutrition recommendations and interventions for diabetes. *Diabetes Care*. 2008; 31(Suppl 1):S61–S78.

24. Wing RR. Exercise and weight control. In: Ruderman N, Devlin J, Schneider S, eds. *Handbook of Exercise in Diabetes*. Alexandria, VA: American Diabetes Association; 2002:355–364.

25. Meece J. Oral agent use in type 2 diabetes. *On the Cutting Edge*. 2004;25:23–27.

26. Joslin Diabetes Center. Oral Diabetes Medications Summary Chart. http://www.joslin.org/info/oral_diabetes_medications_summary_chart.html. Accessed March 14, 2010.

27. National Institute of Diabetes and Digestive and Kidney Diseases. National Diabetes Information Clearinghouse. Types of Insulin. http://diabetes.niddk.nih.gov/dm/pubs/medicines_ez/insert_C.htm. Accessed March 14, 2010.

28. Donnelly J, Blair SN, Jakicic JM, Manore M, Rankin JW, Smith BK. Appropriate physical activity intervention strategies for weight loss and prevention of weight regain for adults. *Med Sci Sports Exerc*. 2009;41:459–471.

29. Jakicic JM, Gallagher KI. Exercise considerations for the sedentary overweight adult. *Exerc Sport Sci Rev*. 2003; 31:91–95.

30. American Diabetes Association. Diagnosis and classification of diabetes mellitus. *Diabetes Care*. 2011;34 (Suppl 1): S62–S69.

31. Hornsby GW, Chetlin RD. Management of competitive athletes with diabetes. *Diabetes Spectrum*. 2005;18: 102–107.

32. Hayes C. Physical activity and exercise. In: Ross T, Boucher J, O'Connell B, eds. *American Dietetic Association Guide to Diabetes Medical Nutrition Therapy and Education*. Chicago, IL: American Dietetic Association; 2005: 71–80.

33. National Institute of Diabetes and Digestive and Kidney Diseases. National Diabetes Information Clearinghouse. Continuous Glucose Monitoring. http://diabetes.niddk.nih.gov/dm/pubs/glucosemonitor/index.htm. Accessed March 23, 2010.

34. Diabetes Self-Management Blog. Continuous Glucose Monitoring: Making Sense of Your Numbers. http://www .diabetesselfmanagement.com/blood-glucose-monitoring/continuous_glucose_monitoring_making_sense_of_ your_numbers. Accessed March 25, 2010.

35. Burge MR, Mitchell S, Sawyer A, Schade DS. Continuous glucose monitoring: the future of diabetes management. *Diabetes Spectrum.* 2008;21:112–119.

36. Iscoe KE, Campbell JE, Jamnik V, Perkins BA, Ridell MC. Efficacy of continuous real-time blood glucose monitoring during and after prolonged high-intensity cycling exercise: spinning with a continuous glucose monitoring system. *Diabetes Technol Ther.* 2006;8:627–635.

37. Demma L, Hayes C, Bode B. The utility of a continuous glucose monitoring system for elite cyclists during the Race Across America. *Infusystems USA.* 2007;4:4–8.

38. Bloomgarden Z. Type 1 diabetes and glucose monitoring. *Diabetes Care.* 2007;30:2965–2971.

39. Klonoff DC. Continuous glucose monitoring: roadmap for 21st century diabetes therapy. *Diabetes Care.* 2005; 28:1231–1239.

40. Colberg SR. Working with athletes with diabetes. *On the Cutting Edge.* 2006;26:19–23.

41. Franz M. Nutrition, physical activity, and diabetes. In: Ruderman N, Devlin J, Schneider S, eds. *Handbook of Exercise in Diabetes.* Alexandria, VA: American Diabetes Association; 2002:321–337.

42. Sherman W, Jacobs K, Ferrara C. Nutritional strategies to optimize athletic performance. In: Ruderman N, Devlin J, Schneider S, eds. *Handbook of Exercise in Diabetes.* Alexandria, VA: American Diabetes Association; 2002: 339–354.

43. Berger M. Adjustment of insulin and oral agent therapy. In: Ruderman N, Devlin J, Schneider S, eds. *Handbook of Exercise in Diabetes.* Alexandria, VA: American Diabetes Association; 2002:365–376.

44. Bennett J. Trends in insulin therapy: an update. *On the Cutting Edge.* 2004;25(2):29–31,36.

45. Ertl AC, Davis SN. The evidence for a vicious cycle of exercise and hypoglycemia in type 1 diabetes mellitus. *Diabetes Metab Res Rev.* 2004;20:124–130.

46. Sandoval D, Guy D, Richardson M, Ertl A, Davis S. Effects of low and moderate antecedent exercise on counter-regulatory responses to subsequent hypoglycemia in type 1 diabetes. *Diabetes.* 2004;53:1798–1804.

47. Cryer PE. The barrier of hypoglycemia in diabetes. *Diabetes.* 2008;57:3169–3176.

48. National Institute of Diabetes and Digestive and Kidney Diseases. National Diabetes Information Clearinghouse. Hypoglycemia. http://diabetes.niddk.gov/dm/pubs/hypoglycemia. Accessed March 28, 2010.

Section 4

Sports-Specific Nutrition Guidelines

The practice of sports nutrition has come a long way. The chapters in this section synthesize the science of sports nutrition and exercise to provide guidelines for athletes participating in sports ranging from the very high–intensity but short all-out effort (like the 100-meter sprint that crowns the "fastest" athlete in the world) to the ultra-endurance events (like the Run Around Australia, which covers 9,053 miles in 191 days of competition). Athletes have very different nutritional needs depending on exercise intensity and duration. These chapters pinpoint the nutritional requirements for training as well as competition for athletes competing in very high–intensity, high-intensity short-duration, high-intensity intermittent exercise, endurance, and ultra-endurance events. The science, as well as practical tips for fueling athletes, is provided to help sports dietitians establish food and fluid tips to help athletes achieve their dreams.

Chapter 20

NUTRITION FOR VERY HIGH– AND HIGH-INTENSITY, SHORT-DURATION SPORTS

Janet Walberg Rankin, PhD, FACSM

Introduction

Most sports nutrition research has centered on endurance activities, such as distance running and cycling, or "stop-and-go" sports like soccer. Although fewer studies have been done with athletes in high-intensity, shorter events, athletes participating in these events need science-informed advice regarding their diets to avoid being vulnerable to dietary myths or the mistaken belief that what they eat does not matter because their activity is of short duration. This chapter reviews the evidence that the diet of athletes performing in high- or very high–intensity sports of short duration does affect athletic success. For the purposes of this chapter, very high–intensity sports will be those requiring maximal, all-out effort of less than 30 seconds, and high-intensity refers to maximal efforts up to several minutes. Table 20.1 lists examples of sports and events that would be categorized in these groupings. The recommendations will have implications for athletes involved in single sprints of various modes (eg, swim, run, cycle, skate); jumping and throwing events; sports with episodic, intense but brief muscle power efforts during the course of a game or match (eg, football, volleyball, or baseball); and in middle-distance events (eg, rowing, running) that take several minutes to complete.

Most athletes are involved in intensive workouts, often daily and sometimes even several times per day, which influence their dietary needs. Although a high school–level athlete may work out approximately 3 or 4 days per week for 1 to 2 hours per session, a college or elite athlete may be involved in as many as 14 sessions per week or more. On the day of competition, although the actual event might be brief, the athlete may compete in multiple events in one day (eg, relay, sprint, and jump). This chapter reviews the energy systems used to fuel very high–intensity activity, diets typically consumed, and evidence-based dietary recommendations for athletes doing high- and very high–intensity exercise.

TABLE 20.1   Events and Sports That Involve Very High–Intensity or High-Intensity Exercise

Mode	Event (Approximate Duration)
Very high–intensity	
Running sprint	50-m dash (6 sec), 100 m (10 sec), 200 m (20 sec)
Jumping or hurdles	100-/110-m hurdle, high jump, long jump, triple jump, pole vault
Cycle sprint	200 m (10 sec)
Swimming sprint	50 m (22 sec)
Throwing	Shot, javelin, discus, hammer (several seconds)
Olympic weightlifting	Snatch, clean and jerk ($\leq$ 1 sec)
Power lifting	Bench press, squat, dead lift (seconds)
Gymnastics	Multiple events
Team sports with sprints	Multiple, including football, baseball
High-intensity	
Running	400 m (50 s); 600 m (1:30); 800 m (2:00)
Swimming	100 m (1:00); 200 m (2:00)
Skating	1,000 m (1:15); 1,500 m (2:00)

Energy System and Fuel Use

The performance of high- and very high–intensity efforts in sport depends on many factors, including reaction time, muscle power, skill, muscle fiber type, and psychological issues. From a metabolic standpoint, adenosine triphosphate (ATP) availability, rate of breakdown, and rate of ATP resynthesis are critical. The rate of ATP production needed to perform these events is high. For example, the power output during a 30-second sprint is approximately twice that achieved at maximum oxygen consumption (VO_{2max}) and the energy need for a 1,500-meter running race may be approximately 115% of maximal oxygen consumption (1). A substantial amount of the ATP to fuel these events is produced anaerobically. The shorter the maximal effort, the higher the percentage of ATP from anaerobic sources used. For example, the ATP used in a 30-second sprint is approximately 80% anaerobically generated, whereas a 10-second sprint is approximately 97% anaerobically fueled (2). Although the specific crossover point varies by individual, in general, events of effort longer than 2 minutes obtain a majority of ATP from the aerobic system and the contribution from anaerobic pathways diminishes.

The briefest, highest intensity efforts are fueled by ATP produced anaerobically by the breakdown of creatine phosphate (PCr) within the muscle. Estimates are that the maximal rate of ATP production (μmol/sec/kg) is 6.0 for PCr but only 1.5 for anaerobic glycolysis, and 0.24 and 0.5 for aerobic generation via fat and carbohydrate, respectively (3). This means that efforts that require very rapid ATP use will rely heavily on PCr breakdown. Because creatine phosphate stores are limited and the use of these stores is rapid with high-intensity work, it is possible to substantially reduce them during a brief exercise bout. For example, research shows that a 30-second sprint decreased PCr by 75%, a 20-second sprint (eg, 200-meter run, 50-meter swim) decreased it by about half, while even a 10-second maximal effort (eg, 100-meter run, 200-meter cycle) decreased PCr by 40% (2,3). So, a limiting factor for performance of these very high–intensity efforts could be initial muscle PCr stores. It is logical to begin the event, game, or match with high muscle PCr. Sprint training can increase PCr stores. Another way to boost muscle creatine stores is through a

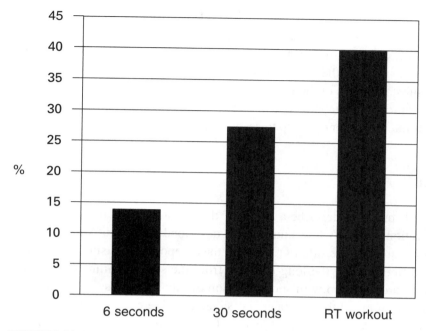

FIGURE 20.1 Percentage muscle glycogen reduction for sprints and resistance exercise workout. RT = multiple-set resistance training. Data are from references 4, 5, and 6.

supplementation strategy with oral creatine (discussed later in this chapter). Although PCr is resynthesized rapidly, replenishment may not be complete if a second very high–intensity bout occurs close to the first. The rate of recovery for muscular PCr depends on many factors, including the magnitude of reduction, oxygen availability, pH, and substrate levels, but it can take up to a minute to regain the initial levels.

In addition to PCr, the other fuel that provides ATP anaerobically for high- and very high–intensity efforts is carbohydrate through glycolysis. The use of glycolysis for ATP generation rather than PCr increases with the duration of a sprint. A 10-second sprint depends on glycolysis for approximately 44% of the ATP used, whereas a 30-second sprint will likely get more than 50% of the ATP from this system (2). Even so, because muscles have much more glycogen than PCr, these brief, very high–intensity efforts do not substantially reduce muscle glycogen. The magnitude of reduction in muscle glycogen depends on the intensity and duration of an exercise bout as well as the type of activity (see Figure 20.1) (4–6). The magnitude of glycogen depletion during resistance exercise will be related to the intensity of the lift and to the amount of work performed. Most of the studies used a high-volume resistance exercise workout; little research has been done on glycogen use with low-volume, high-intensity workouts.

Although the reductions described earlier are meaningful, glycogen is not reduced to a level shown to actually be detrimental to performance of aerobic events. Although it is unlikely that modestly reduced glycogen stores will influence performance of a single very high–intensity effort, it could impair high-intensity efforts interspersed within a game that involves substantial aerobic exercise (eg, basketball or soccer) or if it is concurrent with a low-carbohydrate diet (eg, less than 3 to 4 g per kg body weight).

A limiting factor for the performance of high-intensity events of several minutes is acidosis that occurs secondary to lactate production during anaerobic glycolysis. Some research suggests that acidosis directly impairs muscle force development, whereas others suggest it may have an indirect effect via impairment of enzyme activity critical for ATP generation. Other metabolic factors such as the accumulation of intracellular phosphate with the subsequent disruption of calcium release from the sarcoplasmic reticulum could play a role in fatigue for middle-distance events (7).

In summary, brief, very high–intensity efforts rely primarily on PCr stores, with increasing reliance on glycogen stores occurring with the longer sprints or middle-distance events such as the 800-meter sprint. This can result in substantial use of the PCr stores, but typically less than one third of the muscle glycogen stores. The accumulation of metabolites such as hydrogen ion and inorganic phosphate can contribute to fatigue during high-intensity events for up to several minutes.

Typical Diets

There are no unified studies to describe a "typical" diet for athletes participating in very high– and high-intensity short-duration sports. A few studies have described the diet of very high–intensity athletes, but the manner in which athletes are often grouped in these reports (eg, using the category "swimmers," for instance, without differentiating the long-distance from the sprint swimmer) can make it difficult to differentiate those who are involved with short-duration events from those who participate in long-duration events (8). In addition, some of these data are collected on athletes from different countries, adding variation due to different cultures and different levels of competition (8–13). Some of the studies that evaluated the diet of high- or very high–intensity athletes using dietary records are shown in Tables 20.2 and 20.3 (7–13).

The study of Japanese track and field athletes separated the athletes by event (9). The diets of male sprinters and jumpers were similar in energy content, whereas throwers and long-distance runners similarly consumed approximately 30% more energy than the sprinters or jumpers. The proportion of macronutrients in the diet was remarkably consistent among all types of athletes, although the absolute amount of all macronutrients was higher for athletes with the greatest energy consumption. The dietary habits of elite male and female Flemish adolescent sprint athletes were studied using 7-day weighed food records (13). Total carbohydrate intake was moderate—5.1 and 6.0 g/kg for girls and boys, respectively—whereas both genders consumed 1.5 g protein per kg body weight. Mineral intake (eg, calcium and iron) as well as some

TABLE 20.2 Reported Diet Quality and Quantity for Female Athletes Involved in Brief High-Intensity Exercise

Type of Athlete (Reference)	Energy, kcal/d (kcal/kg)	Energy from Carbohydrate, %	Carbohydrate, (g/kg)	Energy from Protein, %	Energy from Fat, %
Gymnasts (8)	2,298 (51.0)	42	5.4	16	42
Gymnasts (12)	1,838 (42.5)	49	5.1	15	36
Gymnasts (11)	1,678 (34.4)	66	5.8	17	18
Field athletes (10)	2,215 (26.2)	46	3.0	17	38
Throwers (8)	4,446 (53.0)	35	4.6	19	47
Throwers (9)	2,617 (40.0)	54	5.1	14	32
Sprinters (9)	2,393 (45.7)	53	5.8	15	33
Sprinters (13)	2,007 (54.7)	55	5.1	15.7	29.9
Jumpers (9)	1,982 (36.5)	51	4.5	16	33
Swimmers (8)	4,595 (71)	35	6.2	26	49

TABLE 20.3 Reported Diet Quality and Quantity for Male Athletes Involved in Brief High-Intensity Exercise

Type of Athlete (Reference)	Energy, kcal/d (kcal/kg)	Energy from Carbohydrate, %	Carbohydrate, (g/kg)	Energy from Protein, %	Energy from Fat, %
Gymnasts (8)	3,310 (56.0)	43	6.1	18	38
Throwers (8)	5,353 (49.0)	34	4.1	20	47
Throwers (9)	3,591 (34.6)	55	4.1	15	30
Field athletes (10)	3,485 (36.0)	41	3.7	19	40
Sprinters (7)	2,653 (40.0)	54	5.1	15	30
Sprinters (13)	3,117 (50.9)	55.7	6.0	14.1	30.3
Jumpers (7)	2,863 (41.6)	54	5.2	15	31
Swimmers (8)	5,938(80)	33	6.5	22	48
Weightlifters (8)	4,597 (57)	38	5.4	22	40

of the fat-soluble vitamins (ie, vitamins E and A) were less than the Belgian Recommended Dietary Intake for most of the athletes. Although it is difficult to find consistent patterns, the sprinters and jumpers tended to consume lower-energy diets than throwers and weightlifters.

Nutrition Issues

The effect of nutritional quality or quantity on performance of high- or very high–intensity efforts is not as well researched as nutrition's impact on performance in endurance events. The nutrition recommendations that follow are based on the theoretical limitations to performance discussed earlier as well as the limited research that has been done.

Energy, Body Weight, and Body Composition

Track and field coaches encourage athletes to increase lean mass while minimizing body fat for most events (except throwers). Increased muscle mass has the advantage of enhanced force generation, but any extra body fat can be a disadvantage for performance. Wilmore (14) evaluated body fat for a cross section of athletes and reported that male sprinters and discus throwers had approximately 16% body fat, whereas shot-putters ranged from 16% to 20% body fat. The female athletes in these events had more body fat than the men did, with female sprinters and jumpers at approximately 19% to 20% fat and the female throwers from 25% to 28% body fat. Although these averages are helpful to provide some context, there are too many other important factors that determine performance and, as discussed later in this chapter, potential unintended consequences of weight loss to encourage rigid minimum body-fat standards.

Sprinters tend to have much higher muscularity and somewhat higher body fat than do distance runners. The higher muscularity obviously helps produce more power for rapid acceleration and maximal speed. However, because more energy is required to perform events at a heavier body weight when the body is moved through space, overemphasis on muscle growth is detrimental to some speed events.

There is evidence that weight loss is common in high-power athletes. Folgelholm and Hiilloskorpi (15) reported that approximately 50% of men and women in speed sports were trying to lose weight. Almost half of the elite gymnasts studied by Jonnalagadda et al (11) were on a "self-prescribed diet."

Weight loss and negative energy balance may impair physical performance. Some studies report no effect of short-term weight loss on performance of high-intensity exercise, whereas others report decrements. In general, rapid or substantial weight loss is more likely to impair performance than gradual or modest loss (16). A study from Virginia Tech showed that short-term weight loss through energy restriction reduced dynamic muscle strength approximately 8% in athletes who lost 3.3 kg in 10 days (17). So, a substantial weight loss that is done quickly (eg, 5% within several days) is more likely to be detrimental to high-intensity performance than a more gradual weight loss.

The macronutrient mix, especially the amount of carbohydrate in a weight-loss diet, may influence performance. For example, resistance trainers who consumed a low-energy diet with 50% of energy from carbohydrate had decreased muscle endurance after 7 days of the diet, whereas those who consumed the same amount of energy, but with 70% of the energy derived from carbohydrate, maintained their rates of isometric fatigue at baseline levels (18). For sprinters, there is evidence for a reduction in sprint performance and muscle strength or endurance in some, but not all, studies examining acute weight loss in athletes. Very high–intensity efforts are likely less affected by negative energy balance than more prolonged exercise bouts.

Because there could be the negative impact of energy restriction on sports performance, body composition recommendations should be flexible and individualized for athletes with different body types and weight histories. There is no guarantee that any individual athlete will improve performance as a result of weight loss. In fact, as discussed, performance may be impaired during the weight loss. Other potential consequences of rapid weight loss include decreases in muscle mass and possible effects on linear growth, hormonal changes, and nutrient deficiencies (16). Female athletes dieting for weight loss are particularly susceptible to the female athlete triad: disruption of reproductive hormones, reduced bone strength concurrent with disordered eating, and poor diet (see Chapter 18). Athletes who need to lose weight should be encouraged to lose weight gradually and during the off-season to minimize any detrimental effect on performance.

Athletes interested in muscle mass gain need to boost their energy intake above the amount required for maintenance, ensure that they are ingesting adequate protein, and participate in strenuous resistance training (19). Protein for lean mass gain is discussed in Chapter 3.

Hydration

Strenuous activity in a hot and humid environment makes it challenging to maintain hydration. Football players, for example, have been shown to come to practice dehydrated, as shown by reduced body weight and increased urine-specific gravity (20). Judelson et al (21) reviewed the research evidence for an effect of dehydration on performance of muscle strength, power, and high-intensity endurance. They determined that dehydration of 3% to 4% causes a reduction in muscle strength of approximately 2%, muscle power of approximately 3%, and muscle high-intensity endurance of approximately 10%.

The value of hydration on maximal power output during prolonged endurance exercise was illustrated in a study by Fritzsche et al (22). Eight endurance-trained cyclists exercised 122 minutes at 62% VO_{2max} in a hot and humid environment on four separate occasions. Volume of fluid ingested was either low (~0.4 liters) or high (~3.3 liters), and with either 204 g or no carbohydrate. Maximal power production over 4 seconds was measured four times during each 2-hour cycling bout. Although there was no difference in maximum power production sprints during the treatments at the first power test, the decrease in power near the end of the bout was the least for the treatment with the highest fluid volume with carbohydrate (Figure 20.2) (22). The subjects could produce more power with this treatment than when they had the same volume of water alone. Both of these treatments were superior to both treatments with the small volume of water (whether

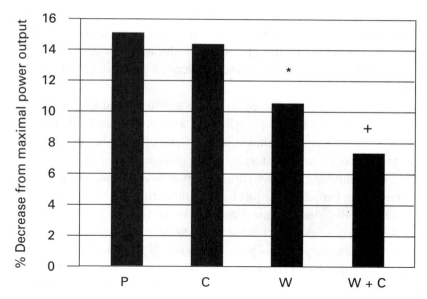

FIGURE 20.2   Decrease in power output for 4-sec maximal power test during 2-h endurance exercise bout for treatments varying in hydration and carbohydrate. **Key:** P, placebo consumed (0.4 L water); C, carbohydrate consumed (204 g carbohydrate in 0.5 L water); W, water consumed (3.3 L water); W + C, water with carbohydrate consumed (3.4 L water with 204 g carbohydrate). * indicates significantly different from P or C; + indicates significantly different from all other groups. Data are from reference 22.

containing carbohydrate or not). The researchers concluded that maximal power is best maintained by consuming high volumes of fluid with carbohydrate. This illustrates the importance of hydration to athletes involved in games that include substantial aerobic activity with sporadic sprints or high muscle-power generation.

In summary, acute dehydration is modestly harmful to sport performance involving maximal muscle strength and power but becomes more detrimental if the high-intensity effort in a sport or exercise is longer, or if sprints are interspersed within prolonged aerobic exercise, as in the case of runners. As with weight loss through energy restriction, the magnitude of dehydration will influence performance. Because some evidence suggests that even modest amounts of dehydration can impair performance in some athletes, weight loss through dehydration should not exceed 2% of body weight.

Carbohydrate

Dietary carbohydrate can ensure that glycogen stores are adequate and that blood glucose is maintained. As discussed earlier, very high–intensity exercise drains some muscle glycogen, but not to the extent that it causes impaired performance as may occur in longer events or events involving repeated sprints. Therefore, the value of high initial muscle glycogen on short, maximal efforts is debatable.

Muscle Strength and Power

Some studies suggest that a low initial muscle glycogen concentration will adversely affect muscle strength and power (23), but a careful subsequent study suggested that some of this impairment was due to the exhaustive exercise performed, rather than the glycogen reduction itself (24). It was discerned that a reduction of more than half of the muscle glycogen through diet and exercise resulted in a decrease in muscle strength and endurance, but repletion of muscle glycogen through diet did not allow recovery of muscle force. Thus, there is not good evidence that muscle glycogen has any effect on maximal, single-effort muscle strength or power.

The effect of muscle glycogen on muscle endurance is not supported in a study of 11 resistance-trained athletes who completed a resistance training workout in a carbohydrate-loaded or carbohydrate-depleted condition (25). There was no difference in total volume lifted between the two dietary conditions, suggesting that muscle glycogen was not a limiting factor for the resistance exercises.

The effect of acute consumption of carbohydrate on muscle endurance is controversial. Several studies support the value of consuming carbohydrate just before and during a resistance exercise bout on total work performed during a workout. Resistance-trained males who consumed a glucose polymer solution before and during a repeated-set leg-extension bout tended to have better muscle endurance, as reflected by number of repetitions (149 vs 129 for carbohydrate vs placebo) and sets (17.1 vs 14.4 for carbohydrate vs placebo), but the differences were not significant (26). Haff et al (27) reported that resistance-trained males could do approximately 8% more total work during an exercise test of 16 sets of 10 repetitions. However, another study from the same laboratory (28) using a similar design found no positive results from acute carbohydrate ingestion before and between sets of a 39-minute isotonic exercise bout. This was in spite of the fact that the carbohydrate ingestion lessened the amount of total muscle glycogen reduction during the exercise workout.

Another study did not support the value of a single high-carbohydrate feeding (1 g/kg) on the performance of multiple-set resistance exercise when 14 subjects were losing weight on a low-energy diet for 3 days (29). The number of repetitions performed until exhaustion in the last set of leg extensions and the weight supported in a bench press portion of a four-exercise resistance workout were not different if the subjects consumed a high-carbohydrate beverage as compared to a placebo beverage.

In summary, most studies do not support the value of high muscle glycogen or acute carbohydrate ingestion on muscle strength or endurance. The majority of the studies done in a weight-room setting with multiple sets and exercise workouts have not demonstrated a benefit of a continuously high-carbohydrate diet or acute carbohydrate ingestion on performance. Some of the variation among studies may relate to the performance tests used (eg, large-muscle vs small-muscle exercises, number of repetitions, and intensity) as well as the subjects (athletes trained in that event compared with those less familiar and thus less reliable in their performance of the test).

Sprint Performance

Few studies have examined the effect of muscle glycogen on single sprint performance. However, one study (30) reported a detrimental effect of a low-carbohydrate diet over 3 days on high-intensity exercise. Eight subjects produced a higher mean power output (but the same peak power) in a 30-second maximal cycling test when they consumed a 50% carbohydrate diet with approximately 3.9 g/kg compared with an isocaloric diet of only 5% carbohydrate (~0.4 g/kg) for 3 days (Figure 20.3) (30). It should be pointed out that few athletes are likely consuming such a low-carbohydrate diet, so the practical value of this study is limited.

Even if sprint performance is impaired by a very low–carbohydrate diet, most studies do not observe a benefit of moving from a moderate-carbohydrate diet to a high-carbohydrate diet for sprint performance. Lamb et al (31) found no benefit of a high-carbohydrate diet (80% of energy; 12.1 g/kg) compared with a moderate-carbohydrate diet (43% of energy; 6.5 g/kg) consumed for 9 days on 50-meter swim sprint performance in collegiate male swimmers. Vandenberghe et al (32) found no difference in cycling time to exhaustion (~125% VO_{2max}) for a moderate- compared with a high-carbohydrate diet (70% of energy and ~7.7 g/kg vs 50% of energy and ~ 4.6 g/kg).

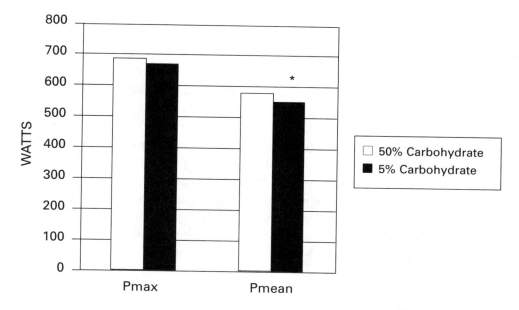

FIGURE 20.3   Effect of 3 days of low-carbohydrate diet on 30-sec cycle sprint maximum and mean power. Pmax = maximum power; Pmean = mean power. * indicates significant difference between dietary treatment groups. Data are from reference 30.

Limited research suggests that sprint performance may be reduced with very low–carbohydrate diets, but few athletes are likely to actually consume diets too low in carbohydrate. The exception could be athletes attempting to lose weight on the low-carbohydrate diets that recommend severe limits on carbohydrate intake, a practice that should be discouraged. Conversely, there is little evidence for the value of increasing dietary carbohydrate to higher than moderate levels (5–7 g/kg).

Recovery

Some athletes perform repeated events or games during a single day, so they need to recover as quickly as possible. Consumption of carbohydrate after exercise will accelerate glycogen replenishment. For example, Pascoe et al (33) showed that muscle glycogen decreased to approximately 70% of resting values after a multiset resistance exercise bout, but consumption of a carbohydrate beverage (1.5 g/kg) after exercise increased muscle glycogen to 75% of baseline after 2 hours and to 91% of baseline after 6 hours. On the other hand, there was no restoration of muscle glycogen after 6 hours when a water placebo was ingested after exercise.

The evidence is not conclusive that a high-carbohydrate diet between two high-intensity exercise bouts enhances subsequent performance. Two studies using similar methodology but different subject populations yielded completely different conclusions regarding the importance of high carbohydrate intake between bouts. Haub et al (34) reported that six moderately trained men were able to maintain their maximal exercise performance of a 100-KJ cycle ergometer test to that of an initial test when they had consumed carbohydrate (0.7 g/kg) during the 60 minutes between the two tests; time to complete the 100-KJ test was longer if subjects consumed a placebo during the recovery period. Although this suggests a benefit of high carbohydrate ingestion on recovery from high-intensity performance, a subsequent study with the same protocol (35) using seven competitive cyclists found no benefit on performance after high carbohydrate consumption between bouts. Because training, especially sport-specific training, is such an important variable, it is difficult to compare the two studies. The differences between these studies emphasize the importance of using athletes specific to the event in these dietary intervention studies.

To summarize, the information from research on dietary carbohydrate for sprinting or muscle strength translates into more flexibility for the diet of athletes involved in very high–intensity events than for those participating in prolonged endurance exercise (36). Several studies show superior performance of single sprints when athletes have consumed high-carbohydrate diets (> 65% of energy from carbohydrate; > 7 g/kg) compared with low-carbohydrate diets (< 10% of energy; < 1.5 g/kg), but this is not consistent among studies. There is no consensus that a high-carbohydrate diet is superior to a moderate-carbohydrate diet for the performance of single sprints or maximum muscle power. Therefore, although glycogen stores can be supercompensated using glycogen loading, there is no evidence that this could help performance, and, in fact, it may be counterproductive, owing to weight gain that coincides with the additional carbohydrate stores. The carbohydrate content of the diet may come into play for athletes competing in multiple events over a day or for those doing substantial amounts of aerobic activity in addition to the sprints (eg, basketball). In addition, athletes who do high-volume aerobic training but compete in very high–intensity, brief events (eg, swimmers) will need to consume substantial amounts of carbohydrate to replenish the glycogen used during training. In most cases, it is recommended that athletes involved in very high–intensity sports or events consume approximately 5 to 7 g of carbohydrate per kg body weight, with the lower end of the range recommended for athletes with lower energy needs and little aerobic training, and the higher end recommended for those participating in modest amounts of aerobic training in addition to the high-intensity work. The consumption of carbohydrate foods shortly after an event will enhance the rate of glycogen replacement.

Protein

Because most athletes performing brief, maximal efforts depend on high muscularity and function, they want nutritional strategies that enhance lean body mass. Although most research does not support consuming a chronically high protein intake (> 1.8 g/kg) in the daily diet (37), research is accumulating that consumption of at least 1.2 to 1.7 g/kg protein throughout the day with emphasis on timing of protein-containing food just before or after a resistance exercise bout can improve muscle protein balance (19,38,39). The consumption of food containing protein moves muscle protein balance from negative when fasting to positive, allowing muscle growth.

Recent research has expanded our knowledge regarding the effect of dietary protein on muscle protein balance or lean mass gain (19,38). Most of this research tested a single exercise bout and used untrained subjects. Resistance exercise is a strong anabolic stimulus, but nutrient intake is important to cause a positive muscle protein balance. Ideal muscle protein synthesis depends on the provision of substrate (amino acids) as well as the appropriate hormonal environment (eg, insulin) to enhance protein synthesis. Most studies are consistent in the conclusion that the consumption of protein before or after a resistance exercise bout is beneficial for protein retention and superior to the same energy as carbohydrate alone (19,38). The areas of continued research include optimal dose and type of amino acid or protein. The type of protein that is best for muscle protein gains is controversial; studies have reported either no difference in muscle protein synthesis response to ingestion of different protein types (40,41) or that one is superior to the others (42,43). A dose-response study of the acute muscle protein synthesis response to consumption of four doses of egg albumin (between 5 and 40 g) demonstrated that the synthesis increased until a plateau at 20 g (44). However, the study design does not allow determination of the optimal protein intake because no doses were tested between 10 and 20 g. This suggests that somewhere between 10 and 20 g protein after a resistance exercise workout will allow optimal muscle protein synthesis, but that ingestion of more than 20 g of protein at one time is superfluous; the extra protein will be oxidized rather than used for protein synthesis. Coingestion of carbohydrate with the protein makes practical sense for glycogen replacement, but it is not likely to amplify muscle protein synthesis if the protein ingestion is ideal.

The verification that the results of these acute studies translate to greater lean mass gain with ongoing training is difficult because of problems of individual variability in muscle hypertrophy response as well as maintaining tight control on exercise and diet over a long enough period to measure muscle hypertrophy. Two studies (45,46) reported similar results that show there was a statistical trend for improved lean gain when subjects consumed a protein-containing postexercise beverage compared to an isoenergetic carbo-hydrate drink after each workout during 10 weeks of training. Two studies of training for 12 to 14 weeks (47,48) reported significantly greater muscle hypertrophy for a protein-containing supplement compared to a carbohydrate supplement. The timing of ingestion of the protein-containing food or beverage has been reported to have no effect in some studies (49), or to have a critical role to enhance muscle hypertrophy in others (50).

Because there is no disadvantage and some evidence of benefit to consuming foods with protein just before or after a workout, consuming foods with protein is recommended to athletes desiring lean mass gain. This could be accomplished, for example, by consuming a dairy product, a lean meat sandwich, or nuts before or after a resistance workout. It should be emphasized that the most important dietary factor for weight gain is energy. An athlete will not gain lean tissue without a positive energy balance.

Supplements and Ergogenic Aids

Dietary supplements that are attractive to athletes involved in very high–intensity events or sports are those that may increase the availability of PCr, increase lean body mass, or improve reaction time; enhancement of buffering capacity may be helpful for high-intensity events lasting up to several minutes.

Improving PCr Availability

Research shows that daily consumption of creatine monohydrate increases muscle stores of PCr up to 20%. Apparently, some individuals are responders whereas others are nonresponders, and athletes cannot predict to which group they belong (51). A meta-analysis showed that supplemental creatine was effec-tive in improving performance for the majority of the studies and was most likely to improve performance of repeated exercise bouts of less than 30 seconds (eg, resistance exercise, cycle sprints) and upper-body exercise (52). Predictably, the benefits diminished as the bouts lengthened in duration because PCr is the primary fuel source for brief efforts. For example, Tipton et al (39) infer that creatine is more likely to be ergogenic for 60- to 100-meter sprints rather than 200- to 400-meter events. There have been claims that creatine supplementation will enhance muscle hypertrophy. Some research suggests that this may be more through an anticatabolic effect rather than stimulation of protein synthesis (53). Fortunately, there is not much evidence of harm from creatine supplementation for healthy adult athletes. However, it should not be recommended for anyone younger than 18 years (there is not enough research to support its safety in this population), and it is potentially dangerous for those with abnormal kidney function (54). More information on creatine is found in Chapter 7.

Enhancing Muscle Gain

A variety of supplements have been sold with claims that they promote muscle gain. There is inadequate research on most of these supplements to make unequivocal statements of efficacy, but the majority of studies do not support a benefit of chromium, boron, vanadyl sulfate, androstenedione, or dehydroepian-drosterone (DHEA) (55–57). There is limited evidence that beta-hydroxy beta-methylbuterate (HMB) may improve lean mass gain for untrained individuals beginning a resistance exercise program, but it does not seem to benefit trained individuals (45,58). See Chapter 7 for more information.

Stimulants

Stimulants can improve reaction time and are tempting for those who must react with quick acceleration from a start signal. However, these chemicals can also reduce perception of effort and influence fuel utilization. Caffeine is an example of a commonly used stimulant that is not currently banned by the World Anti-Doping Agency (WADA) for use by athletes. Caffeine is a central nervous system stimulant that antagonizes adenosine receptors in the brain to reduce perception of pain or fatigue (59). Although studies of maximal strength or very brief single sprints do not typically observe a benefit of caffeine on performance, there is evidence that caffeine has potential to improve performance of maximal efforts lasting 60 to 180 seconds (60). Two (61,62) of three studies that examined the effect of caffeine ingestion (6 or 9 mg/kg) on 2,000-meter rowing performance (~7 minute maximal effort) reported an ergogenic effect whereas the other study did not (63). Thus, the balance of research supports a potential value of caffeine on performance of high-intensity but not very high–intensity exercise. Caffeine can have adverse effects, including nervousness, sleeplessness, and cardiac arrhythmia.

Buffers

Events longer than a sprint and up to several minutes depend highly on the anaerobic glycolysis system for ATP regeneration. The consequent accumulation of hydrogen ions leads to acidosis within the muscle and some leakage into the bloodstream. The blood contains some endogenous buffers to reduce the hydrogen ion load, and supplements have been studied to determine their ability to further buffer these ions and reduce fatigue. Bicarbonate is the most studied buffer supplement. Although not fully consistent, the balance of research suggests that bicarbonate ingestion before high-intensity exercise can improve performance (64). The optimal dose is estimated to be 0.3 g/kg as either bicarbonate or citrate from approximately 1 to 2 hours before the event (1), but up to 10% of athletes will experience gastrointestinal distress with this strategy. Therefore, it is critical that athletes experiment with bicarbonate ingestion prior to a competition.

Creating a Nutrition Plan

Based on evidence from current research, the overall goals of nutrition planning for athletes in very high–intensity sports/events should be to maintain:

- Energy balance (or positive if muscle growth is a goal)
- Hydration
- Blood glucose
- Adequate muscle glycogen
- Muscle mass
- Comfort before competition
- A healthful diet (eg, adequate intake of micronutrients)

These objectives can be accomplished by recommending a balanced, varied diet that maintains body weight, with 5 to 7 g/kg or approximately 55% of energy from carbohydrate and at least 1.2 g protein per kg. Fluids should be consumed at each meal, between meals, and during workouts to maintain hydration. Measurement of body weight before and after a workout can be used as an index of dehydration, and effort should be made to rehydrate before the next workout or competition. To avoid gastrointestinal distress during the event, a pre-event meal should be consumed at least 1½ hours prior, with only liquids closer to the event. A low-fiber, low-fat meal is recommended because it will leave the stomach and intestine more quickly. Inclusion of protein with carbohydrate in the meal will make it more likely that blood glucose will be at a normal concentration before the event.

During a high volume of training, initiation of training, or when an increase in lean mass gain is desired, athletes may require a higher energy intake (~ 500 additional kcal/d), with special efforts made to consume food with protein and carbohydrate just before or after (as tolerated) each resistance training workout to maximize muscle glycogen replacement and protein synthesis. During recovery, consumption of between 10 and 20 g of protein with 1.2 g carbohydrate per kg per hour is ideal for muscle protein and glycogen synthesis.

Many athletes are tempted by various claims from supplement companies, so the sports dietitian should find out what supplements the athletes may be taking (see Chapter 7). Supplements that have no evidence of benefit, have evidence that they could be harmful, or are banned by sports governing bodies should be strongly discouraged. Ongoing education should be provided because new supplements continually become popular. See Box 20.1 for a discussion of beta-alanine, a new supplement that is being touted for very high–intensity exercise (65–69).

BOX 20.1   Beta-Alanine as an Ergogenic Aid in High-Intensity Exercise

A number of studies have been published related to the potential benefits of supplementation with beta-alanine on performance of high-intensity exercise, in which accumulation of lactate can contribute to fatigue. The theoretical basis for this supplement is that muscle carnosine, a dipeptide, can serve as an intracellular buffer and may affect calcium release from the sarcoplasmic reticulum (65). Carnosine is synthesized in the muscle cell from histidine and beta-alanine, the latter being the limiting substrate. High-intensity training can increase muscle carnosine but provision of additional beta-alanine through a supplement can also increase muscle carnosine up to 80% (65). This requires daily, chronic ingestion of 4-6 g/d supplemental beta-alanine for 4 to 10 weeks. Doses higher than this have been associated with flushing and paraesthesia, nerve-related pain. Although no other side effects have been reported, long-term studies have not been completed.

A handful of studies report an ergogenic effect of chronic beta-alanine ingestion. For example, one study (66) observed an 11% increase in peak power and 5% increase in mean power during a 30-second cycle sprint that was performed after a prolonged endurance cycle bout in subjects who consumed beta-alanine. The supplement did not influence performance of a longer 10-minute time trial in that study, however. Although one study suggested that consumption of this supplement reduced perception of fatigue and improved training volumes of football players during a training camp (67), there is insufficient evidence that this will result in superior lean tissue and strength gains resulting from a training program. Two training studies observed different outcomes. Although both studies, one using 4 weeks (68) and another 10 weeks of supplementation (69), demonstrated that daily beta-alanine ingestion increased muscle carnosine content, only one study (68) noted an enhancement of muscle function with no effect on performance of a 400-meter sprint. The other study (69) did not observe any effect of the supplement on body composition or muscle function. Thus, some of the research suggests potential value of this supplement, but the lack of consistency in results suggests that this is an area of research to watch for future developments.

Athletes competing in several events or matches during one day have a special challenge in deciding what they can tolerate that will also help their performance. A light snack such as yogurt with fruit, small sandwich (without high-fat sauces or cheeses), cereal with milk, regular or dried fruit, a commercial liquid meal, fruit cookies, or muffins along with sport drinks or water are appropriate between events. Because the food provided at the concession stands at most sporting events do not fit this profile, it is best if athletes or the trainers pack their own snacks for the day.

All athletes, including those who compete in very high–intensity sports, should be discouraged from consuming a very low–carbohydrate diet. This diet may impair performance and is often less healthful due to low vitamin, mineral, and fiber content.

Some athletes may know that there is less evidence for an effect of diet on performance in very high–intensity events, and therefore believe they can eat whatever they want. Any dietary recommendations for these athletes must consider the same health issues as for any other individual. Therefore, it is important that the sports dietitian assess the overall diet and provide education about making changes to improve the quality and healthfulness of the diet as well to improve performance.

Summary

For most very high–intensity, brief exercise events, a balanced diet will have less of an impact than genetics, training, and motivational factors. The benefits of nutrition for high-intensity exercise performance are most often observed when high-intensity efforts are interspersed with substantial amounts of other aerobic exercise. Only very low–carbohydrate diets or moderately low–carbohydrate diets paired with low energy intake had a detrimental effect on performance of single, maximal efforts. Dehydration in the range of 3% to 4% can reduce muscle strength and power slightly but can substantially reduce muscle high-intensity endurance. Nutrition can be a valuable adjunct to resistance training in maximizing gain in lean mass. Consuming more total energy as well as protein before or after each resistance exercise bout can improve muscle protein balance and long-term gain. Although not without controversy, most evidence suggests that supplements such as creatine, caffeine, and bicarbonate may benefit those athletes performing high-intensity exercise. Ethical, health, and legal issues should always be considered before using supplements.

References

1. Stellingwerff T, Boit MK, Res PT. Nutritional strategies to optimize training and racing in middle-distance athletes. *J Sports Sci.* 2007;25(suppl):S17–S28.
2. Spriet LL. Anaerobic metabolism during high-intensity exercise. In: Hargreaves EM. *Exercise Metabolism.* Champaign, IL: Human Kinetics; 1995:10–20.
3. Lamb DR. *Physiology of Exercise.* 2nd ed. New York, NY: Macmillan; 1984.
4. Gaitanos GC, Williams C, Boobis LH, Brooks S. Human muscle metabolism during intermittent maximal exercise. *J Appl Physiol.* 1993;75:712–719.
5. Esbjornsson-Liljedahl M, Sundberg CJ, Norman B, Jansson E. Metabolic response in type I and type II muscle fibers during a 30-s cycle sprint in men and women. *J Appl Physiol.* 1999;87:1326–1332.
6. Haff GG, Lehmkuhl MJ, McCoy LB, Stone MH. Carbohydrate supplementation and resistance training. *J Stength Cond Res.* 2003;17:187–196.
7. Ament W, Verkerke GJ. Exercise and fatigue. *Sports Med.* 2009: 39: 389–422.
8. Chen JD, Wang JF, Li KJ, Zhao YW, Wang SW, Jiao Y, Hou XY. Nutritional problems and measures in elite and amateur athletes. *Am J Clin Nutr.* 1989;49:1084–1089.

9. Sugiura K, Suzuki I, Kobayashi K. Nutritional intake of elite Japanese track-and-field athletes. *Int J Sport Nutr.* 1999;9:202–212.

10. Faber M, Benade AJ. Mineral and vitamin intake in field athletes (discus-, hammer-, and javelin-throwers and shotputters). *Int J Sports Med.* 1991;12:324–327.

11. Jonnalagadda SS, Bernadot D, Nelson M. Energy and nutrient intakes of the United States National Women's Artistic Gymnastics Team. *Int J Sport Nutr.* 1998;8:331–344.

12. Loosli AR, Benson J, Gillien DM, Bourdet K. Nutrition habits and knowledge in competitive adolescent female gymnasts. *Phys Sportsmed.* 1986;14:118–130.

13. Aerenhouts D, Hebbelinck, Poortmans JR, Clarys P. Nutritional habits of Flemish adolescent sprint athletes. *Int J Sport Nutr Exerc Metab.* 2008;18:509–523.

14. Wilmore JH. Body composition in sports medicine: directions for future research. *Med Sci Sports Exerc.* 1983;15:21–31.

15. Fogelholm M, Hiilloskorpi H. Weight and diet concerns in Finnish female and male athletes. *Med Sci Sports Exerc.* 1999;31:229–235.

16. Rankin JW. Weight loss and gain in athletes. *Curr Sports Med Rep.* 2002;1:208–213.

17. Walberg-Rankin J, Hawkins CE, Fild DS, Sebolt DR. The effect of oral arginine during energy restriction in male weight trainers. *J Strength Cond Res.* 1994;8:170–177.

18. Walberg J, Leidy M, Sturgill D, Hinkle D, Ritchey S, Sebolt D. Macronutrient content of a hypoenergy diet affects nitrogen retention and muscle function in weight lifters. *Int J Sports Med.* 1988;4:261–266.

19. Koopman R, Saris WHM, Wagenmakers AJM, van Loon LJC. Nutritional interventions to promote post-exercise muscle protein synthesis. *Sports Med.* 2007;37:895–906.

20. Godek SF, Godek JJ, Bartolozzi AR. Hydration status in college football players during consecutive days of twice-a-day preseason practices. *Am J Sports Med.* 2005;33:843–851.

21. Judelson DA, Maresh CM, Anderson JM, Armstrong LE, Casa DJ, Kraemer WJ, Volek JS. Hydration and muscle performance: does fluid balance affect strength, power and high-intensity endurance? *Sports Med.* 2007;37: 907–921.

22. Fritzsche RG, Switzer TW, Hodgkinson BJ, Lee SH, Martin JC, Coyle EF. Water and carbohydrate ingestion during prolonged exercise increase maximal neuromuscular power. *J Appl Physiol.* 2000;88:730–737.

23. Jacobs I, Kaiser P, Tesch P. Muscle strength and fatigue after selective glycogen depletion in human skeletal muscle fibers. *Eur J Appl Physiol.* 1981;46:47–53.

24. Grisdale RK, Jabobs I, Cafarelli E. Relative effects of glycogen depletion and previous exercise on muscle force and endurance capacity. *J Appl Physiol.* 1990;69:1276–1282.

25. Mitchell JB, DiLauro PC, Pizza FX, Cavender DL. The effect of preexercise carbohydrate status on resistance exercise performance. *Int J Sport Nutr.* 1997;7:185–196.

26. Lambert CP, Flynn MG, Boone JB, Michaud T, Rodriguez-Zayas J. Effects of carbohydrate feeding on multiple-bout resistance exercise. *J Appl Sport Sci Res.* 1991;5:192–197.

27. Haff GG, Schroeder CA, Koch AJ, Kuphal KE, Comeau MJ, Potteiger JA. The effects of supplemental carbohydrate ingestion on intermittent isokinetic leg exercise. *J Sports Med Phys Fitness.* 2001;41:216–222.

28. Haff GG, Koch AJ, Potteiger JA, Kuphal KE, Magee LM, Green SB, Jakicic JJ. Carbohydrate supplementation attenuates muscle glycogen loss during acute bouts of resistance exercise. *Int J Sport Nutr Exerc Metab.* 2000;10:326–339.

29. Dalton RA, Walberg Rankin J, Sebolt D, Gwazdauskas F. Acute carbohydrate consumption does not influence resistance exercise performance during energy restriction. *Int J Sport Nutr.* 1999;9:319–332.

30. Langfort J, Zarzeczny R, Pilis W, Nazar K. The effect of a low-carbohydrate diet on performance, hormonal and metabolic responses to a 30-s bout of supramaximal exercise. *Eur J Appl Physiol.* 1997;76:128–133.

31. Lamb DR, Rinehardt K, Bartels RL, Sherman WM, Snook JT. Dietary carbohydrate and intensity of interval swim training. *Am J Clin Nutr.* 1990;52:1058–1063.

32. Vandenberghe K, Hespel P, Vanden Eynde B, Lysens R, Richter EA. No effect of glycogen level on glycogen metabolism during high intensity exercise. *Med Sci Sports Exerc.* 1995;27:1278–1283.

33. Pascoe DD, Costill DL, Fink WJ, Roberts RA, Zachwieja JJ. Glycogen resynthesis in skeletal muscle following resistance exercise. *Med Sci Sports Exerc.* 1993;25:349–354.

34. Haub MD, Potteiger JA, Jacobsen DJ, Nau KL, Magee LA, Comeau MJ. Glycogen replenishment and repeated maximal effort exercise: effect of liquid carbohydrate. *Int J Sport Nutr.* 1999;9:406–415.

35. Haub MD, Haff GG, Potteiger JA. The effect of liquid carbohydrate ingestion on repeated maximal effort exercise in competitive cyclists. *J Strength Cond Res.* 2003;17:20–25.

36. Houtkooper L, Abbot JM, Nimmo M. Nutrition for throwers, jumpers, and combined events. *J Sports Sci.* 2007:25(suppl):S39–S47.

37. Walberg Rankin J. Role of protein in exercise. *Clin Sports Med.* 1999;18:499–512.

38. Tipton KD. Role of protein and hydrolysates before exercise. *Int J Sport Nutr Exerc Metab.* 2007;17(suppl):S77–S86.

39. Tipton KD, Jeukendrup AE, Hespel P. Nutrition for the sprinter. *J Sport Sci.* 2007;25(suppl):S5–S15.

40. Tipton KD, Elliott TA, Cree MG, Wolf SE, Sanford AP, Wolfe RR. Ingestion of casein and whey proteins result in muscle anabolism after resistance exercise. *Med Sci Sports Exerc.* 2004;36:2073–2081.

41. Anthony TG, McDaniel BJ, Knoll P, Bunpo P, Paul GL, McNurlan MA. Feeding meals containing soy or whey protein after exercise stimulates protein synthesis and translation initiation in the skeletal muscle of male rats. *J Nutr.* 2007;137:357–362.

42. Tang JE, Moore DR, Kujbida GW, Tarnopolsky AM, Phillips SM. Ingestion of whey hydrolysate, casein, or soy protein isolate: effects on mixed muscle protein synthesis at rest and following resistance exercise in young men. *J Appl Physiol.* 2009;107:987–992.

43. Wilkinson SB, Tarnopolsky MA, MacDonald MJ, MacDonald JR, Armstrong D, Phillips SM. Consumption of fluid skim milk promotes greater muscle protein accretion after resistance exercise than does consumption of an isonitrogenous and isoenergetic soy-protein beverage. *Am J Clin Nutr.* 2007;85:1031–1040.

44. Moore DR, Robinson MJ, Fry JL, Tang JE, Glover EI, Wilkinson SB, Prior T, Tarnopolsky MA, Phillips SM. Ingested protein dose response of muscle and albumin protein synthesis after resistance exercise in young men. *Am J Clin Nutr.* 2009;89:161–168.

45. Rankin JW, Goldman LP, Puglisi MJ, Nickols-Richardson S, Earthman CP, Gwazdauskas FC. Effect of post-exercise supplement consumption on adaptations to resistance training. *J Am Coll Nutr.* 2004;23:322–330.

46. Chromiak JA, Smedley B, Carpenter W, Brown R, Koh YS, Lamberth JG, Joe LA, Abadie BR, Altorfer G. Effect of a 10-week strength training program and recovery drink on body composition, muscular strength and endurance, and anaerobic power and capacity. *Nutrition.* 2004;20:420–427.

47. Hartman JW, Tang JE, Wilkinson SB, Tarnopolsky MA, Lawrence RL, Fullerton AV, Phillips SM. Consumption of fat-free milk after resistance exercise promotes greater lean mass accretion than does consumption of soy or carbohydrate in young, male weightlifters. *Am J Clin Nutr.* 2007;86:373–381.

48. Anderson LL, Tufekovic G, Zebis MK, Crameri RM, Verlaan G, Kjaer M, Suetta C, Magnusson P, Aagaard P. The effect of resistance training combined with timed ingestion of protein on muscle fiber size and muscle strength. *Metab Clin Exper.* 2005;54:151–156.

49. Hoffman JR, Ratamess NA, Tranchina CP, Rashti S, Kang J, Faigenbaum AD. Effects of protein-supplement timing on strength, power, and body-composition changes in resistance-trained men. *Int J Sport Nutr Exerc Metab.* 2009;19:172–185.

50. Cribb PJ, Hayes A. Effects of supplement timing and resistance exercise on skeletal muscle hypertrophy. *Med Sci Sports Exerc.* 2006;38:1918–1925.

51. Spriet LL, Perry CG, Talanian JL. Legal pre-event nutritional supplements to assist energy metabolism. *Essays Biochem.* 2008;44:27–43.

52. Branch JD. Effect of creatine supplementation on body composition and performance: a meta-analysis. *Int J Sport Nutr Exerc Metab.* 2003;13:198–226.

53. Parise G, Mihic S, MacLennan D, Yarasheski KE, Tarnopolsky MA. Effects of acute creatine monohydrate supplementation on leucine kinetics and mixed-muscle protein synthesis. *J Appl Physiol.* 2001;91:1041–1047.

54. Pritchard NR, Kalra PA. Renal dysfunction accompanying oral creatine supplements. *Lancet.* 1998;351:1252–1253.

55. Clarkson PM, Rawson ES. Nutritional supplements to increase muscle mass. *Crit Rev Food Sci Nutr.* 1999;39:317–328.

56. Kreider RB. Dietary supplements and the promotion of muscle growth with resistance exercise. *Sports Med.* 1999; 27:97–110.

57. Nissen SL, Sharp RL. Effect of dietary supplements on lean mass and strength gains with resistance exercise: a meta-analysis. *J Appl Physiol.* 2003;94:651–659.

58. Institute of Medicine. *Use of Dietary Supplements by Military Personnel.* Washington, DC: National Academies Press; 2008:100–109,160–191,270–277.

59. Graham TE. Caffeine, coffee, and ephedrine: impact on exercise performance and metabolism. *Can J Appl Physiol.* 2001;26(suppl):S103–S119.

60. Davis JK, Green JM. Caffeine and anaerobic performance: ergogenic value and mechanism of action. *Sports Med.* 2009;39:813–832.

61. Anderson ME, Bruce CR, Fraser SF, Stepto NK, Klein R, Hopkins WG, Hawley JA. Improved 2000-meter rowing performance in competitive oarswoman after caffeine ingestion. *Int J Sport Nutr Exerc Metab.* 2000;10:464–475.

62. Bruce CR, Anderson ME, Fraser SF, Stepto NK, Klein R, Hopkins WG, Hawley JA. Enhancement of 2000-m rowing performance after caffeine ingestion. *Med Sci Sports Exerc.* 2000;32:1958–1963.

63. Skinner TL, Jenkins DG, Coombes JS, Taaffe DR, Leveritt MD. Dose response of caffeine on 2000-m rowing performance. *Med Sci Sports Exerc.* 2010;42:571–576.

64. McNaughton LR, Siegler J, Midgley A. Ergogenic effects of sodium bicarbonate. *Curr Sports Med Rep.* 2008;7: 230–236.

65. Derave W, Everaerl I, Beeckman S, Baguel A. Muscle carnosine metabolism and β-alanine supplementation in relation to exercise and training. *Sports Med.* 2010;40:247–263.

66. Van Thienen R, Van Proeyen K, Eynde BV, Puype J, Lefere T, Hespel P. β-alanine improves sprint performance in endurance cycling. *Med Sci Sports Exerc.* 2009;41:898–903.

67. Hofffman JR, Ratamess NA, Faigenbaum AD, Ross R, Kang J, Stout JR, Wise JA. Short-duration β-alanine supplementation increases training volume and reduces subjective feelings of fatigue in college football players. *Nutr Res.* 2008;28:31–35.

68. Derave W, Ozdemir MS, Harris RC, Pottier A, Reyngoudt H, Koppo K, Wise JA, Achten E. β-alanine supplementation augments muscle carnosine content and attenuates fatigue during repeated isokinetic contraction bouts in trained sprinters. *J Appl Physiol.* 2007;103:1736–1743.

69. Kendrick IP, Harris RC, Kim HJ, Kim CK, Dang VH, Lam TQ, Gui TT, Smith M, Wise JA. The effects of 10 weeks of resistance training combined with β-alanine supplementation on whole body strength, force production, muscular endurance and body composition. *Amino Acids.* 2008;34:547–554.

Chapter 21

NUTRITION FOR INTERMITTENT, HIGH-INTENSITY SPORTS

MICHELE A. MACEDONIO, MS, RD, CSSD

Introduction

The term *high-intensity intermittent exercise* (HIIE) refers to activities that require short periods of all-out effort (eg, sprints of up to 2 to 7 seconds), punctuated with periods of less-intense effort (eg, jogging sustained over 5 to 10 minutes), and low-intensity effort (eg, walking and standing still). Team sports such as soccer, football, basketball, field hockey, ice hockey, rugby, volleyball, as well as individual sports, such as tennis and squash are classified as HIIE sports. The stop-and-go nature of these sports often results in impaired performance after periods of intense effort and near the end of the competition. HIIE sports require a range of exercise intensity from low to very high in varying durations during which all of the major energy systems are tapped.

Soccer has been studied extensively (1–12), providing a good base for understanding the physiological demands and nutritional implications of HIIE. Other HIIE sports also have been studied (13–29), although each one not as extensively as soccer.

Nutrient needs of athletes performing HIIE can be high, but these needs can generally be met with a diet that provides sufficient energy to meet the demands of training and competition. Careful food and fluid selection is the key to meeting the additional nutrient demands. Observations of the dietary practices of athletes engaged in HIIE suggest that many athletes' diets are inadequate.

Physiological Demands of High-Intensity Intermittent Exercise

Energy Systems

Athletes engaged in HIIE train to improve endurance capacity as well as muscle strength and conditioning. Both anaerobic and aerobic energy production are important. Anaerobic energy production is essential for high-intensity exercise when the demand for adenosine triphosphate (ATP) exceeds the body's ability to produce it aerobically. At the onset of high-intensity exercise, anaerobically produced ATP provides the

TABLE 21.1 Approximate Relative Energy Contribution During 3 Minutes of High-Intensity Exercise

Duration, sec	Anaerobic, %	Aerobic, %
30	80	20
60–90	45	55
120–180	30	70

majority of the energy used because of the short supply of oxygen. Anaerobic production of ATP continues to play a key role in sustained high-intensity exercise because the demand for ATP is more than can be provided aerobically (see Table 21.1).

Both the intensity and the duration of exercise increase energy demands during vigorous, stop-and-go exercise that lasts for 60 minutes or more (4). For example, soccer encompasses a 90-minute game plus 15 to 30 minutes of warm-up activities prior to match play. Total energy expended during a soccer match is directly related to the distance covered during the 90 minutes of the game, usually 8 to 12 km (5 to 7 miles) (1,3,30). The total distance covered by any one player during a game varies due to many factors, including individual style of play and level of fitness. On average, midfielders cover the most distance, between 9 and 11 km. Generally, midfielders are the most active players on the field, traveling farther than either defenders or attackers and covering a greater percentage of distance at a jog. They are expected to play both defense and offense and are the key to continuity between defenders and the forwards. Attackers may cover much of their distance as a sprint. Center backs cover the least distance and a greater proportion of their distance is covered moving sideways and backwards. Over the course of a soccer game, players are required to sprint, jog, stride, walk, and move sideways and backwards while tackling, jumping, accelerating, and turning. Regardless of position, the greatest percentage of distance is covered at slower speeds.

The relative exercise intensity plays a major factor in determining the fuel mixture during exercise, and is expressed as percentage of maximum oxygen consumption (VO_{2max}), which is influenced by age, sex, genetic makeup, and level of aerobic training (see Table 21.2) (31,32).

The nature of the activity in stop-and-go team sports requires use of both types of muscle fibers (33,34). Fast twitch (FT) fibers exhibit the greatest degree of glycogen depletion after sprint-type activities (35). Costill and colleagues (36) showed that in distance running, glycogen was selectively depleted in slow twitch (ST) fibers but that FT fibers also bore some of the load. From these studies, it seems that ST fibers

TABLE 21.2 Muscle Energy Pathways During Activity of Varying Intensity

	Muscle Energy Pathways	Duration of Activity	Type of Activity (% MHR)
Immediate	ATP in muscles	1–6 sec	Surges and sprints (≥ 80–90)
	ATP + PCr	7–20 sec	
	ATP +PCr + Muscle glycogen	20–45 sec	
Short-term	Muscle glycogen	45–120 sec	Moderate-intensity running (70–80)
	Muscle glycogen + Lactic acid	120–180 sec	
Long-term	Muscle glycogen + Free fatty acids	> 30 min, limited by O_2	Low-moderate-intensity running (< 69)

Abbreviations: ATP, adenosine triphosphate; MHR, maximum heart rate; PCr, phosphocreatine.

are activated at lower workloads and that FT fibers are used during two conditions, when ST fibers are depleted of glycogen (37,38) and during high-intensity output (35).

Green et al (25) examined glycogen utilization in the muscle fibers of ice hockey players. Muscle glycogen depletion averaged 60% and this depletion indicated the utilization of both ST and FT fibers, with the greatest decline occurring in ST fibers. There was no apparent difference in glycogen depletion between forwards and defensemen. Krustrup et al (39) found that muscle glycogen was reduced to 150 to 350 mmol/kg by the end of a soccer match, with half of the fibers of both types depleted or almost depleted. The authors theorized that the pattern of glycogen depletion in some fibers may limit maximal sprint effort.

Effects of High-Intensity Intermittent Exercise on Substrate Utilization

The relative contribution of fat and carbohydrate depends on the intensity and duration of exercise (38,40). Endurance exercise training triggers metabolic adaptations that lead to a marked sparing of carbohydrate as a result of a slower utilization of glucose and muscle and liver glycogen during sustained exercise of the same intensity (41,42). Consequently, endurance training leads to a relatively smaller reliance on carbohydrates than on fatty acids during prolonged steady-state exercise. The reduced reliance on blood glucose and muscle glycogen during exercise in a trained state is part of the mechanisms by which exercise enhances endurance. In essence, endurance training helps spare muscle glycogen.

In addition to a relative shift in substrate, the absolute amount of fat used decreases as work rate increases (31,43). Plasma glucose and muscle glycogen utilization both increase in response to an increase in exercise intensity. Plasma glucose contributes approximately 10% to 15% of total energy at all work rates, whereas muscle glycogen supplies approximately 60% of the energy requirement in strenuous exercise at approximately 80% of VO_{2max} (31,32).

Studies have shown that blood free fatty acid (FFA) concentration increases during a soccer match, with more increase in the second half than the first and after the game (5,39). Blood FFA concentration during soccer is the net result of the uptake of FFA in various tissues and the release from adipose tissue. Trapp et al (44) examined the metabolic response to two forms of HIIE, short sprint and long sprint, in 16 trained and untrained females. The observed increase in glycerol concentration suggests an increased reliance on fats as fuel despite increased lactate concentrations. This pattern is attributed to periods of rest and a slower pace during the second half, which allows more blood flow to adipose tissue and possibly promotes a higher FFA release; this process, when coupled with hormonal changes, specifically decreased insulin and increased catecholamines, stimulates lipolysis and a release of FFA into the blood. These changes cause a greater uptake of FFA and utilization of triglycerides by contracting muscles. Such adaptations favor high blood glucose concentrations and may be compensatory mechanisms for progressively decreasing muscle glycogen levels. Based on these observations, a high uptake of glycerol in various tissues, primarily the liver, is presumed, indicating that glycerol might be an important gluconeogenic precursor. Ketone bodies may also function as a minor fat source during exercise.

Glycogen, an essential fuel during prolonged vigorous exercise, is required by athletes engaged in HIIE sports. With increasing energy intensity, the percentage of carbohydrate used as an energy substrate increases to meet most of the energy demands of muscle contraction at an intensity near an individual's VO_{2max}. From 40% to 85% VO_{2max}, the relative contribution of fat decreases with a concomitant increase in carbohydrate oxidation. At moderate- and high-intensity exercise (50% to 85% VO_{2max}), plasma fatty acids and muscle triglycerides supply the fats that are oxidized (31,43,45,46).

In trained athletes, during vigorous exercise there is an initial burst of glycogenolysis and a resulting lactic acid production, which is followed by a slowing of the rate of glycogenolysis and a reduction in muscle and blood lactate levels. During match play in stop-and-go sports, intermittent bursts of high-intensity exertion are followed by periods of relative rest and moderate-intensity effort. Aerobic fitness enhances recovery from high-intensity intermittent exercise through increased aerobic capacity, improved lactate removal, and enhanced phosphocreatine (PCr) regulation (47).

Skeletal muscle contraction and the central nervous system depend on carbohydrate as a fuel substrate, but the body's stores of carbohydrate are limited and often the fuel requirements of training and competition for HIIE team sports substantially exceed carbohydrate availability. When muscle glycogen stores are depleted, fatigue, both physical and mental, sets in and performance is compromised (48–50). Winnick et al (51) examined the effect of carbohydrate feedings on physical and central nervous system (CNS) function during HIIE trials comprised of four 15-minute quarters of shuttle running with variable intensities ranging from walking (30% VO_{2max}), to running (120% VO_{2max}), to maximal sprinting, and 40 jumps at a target hanging at 80% of their maximum vertical jump height (ie, activity similar to basketball) and found that participants who consumed a 6% carbohydrate solution during breaks resulted in fourth quarter improvements, including faster 20-meter sprint times, higher average jump height, enhanced motor skills, and improved mood, as compared with performance of participants who drank a placebo. Bangsbo (30) estimated the relative levels of aerobic and anaerobic energy turnover and substrate utilization during soccer based on the cumulative results of various studies (refer to Figure 21.1).

Aerobic Energy System

Attempts have been made to determine the aerobic energy contribution during soccer by measuring oxygen uptake; however, the procedure interferes with normal play and results are most likely imprecise. Heart rate

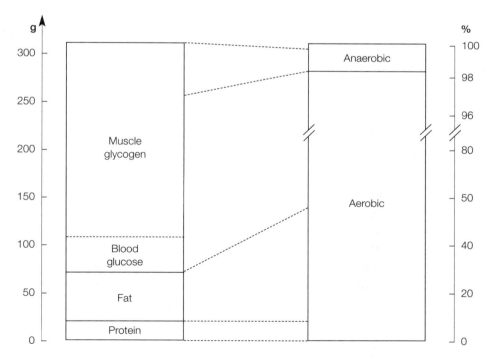

FIGURE 21.1 Estimated relative aerobic and anaerobic energy turnover and corresponding substrate utilization during a soccer match. Reprinted from Bangsbo J. Energy demands in competitive soccer. *J Sports Sci*. 1994;12(suppl):S10. Used by permission of Taylor & Francis Ltd (http://www.informaworld.com).

TABLE 21.3   Heart Rate Patterns of Athletes in High-Intensity Intermittent Sports

Sport (References)	Maximum Heart Rate, %
Basketball (14,19)	> 85
Ice hockey (23)	85–90
Racquet sports including squash, badminton (55)	80–85
Rugby (16,17)	> 85
Soccer (3,4,8)	80–100
Tennis (28,54)	80–85[a]

[a]Maximum heart rate reported in reference 54. In reference 28, heart rate averaged 144 beats/min.

is used to estimate oxygen uptake, but it does not always reflect the actual oxygen uptake. Aside from its use in predicting oxygen uptake, heart rate provides a useful index of the overall physiological demands of soccer (4).

During a match, soccer players spend a considerable amount of time working at heart rates estimated to be more than 160 beats/minute, with mean and peak heart rates around 85% and 98% of maximal values and heart rates rarely below 65% of maximum (3,8,52). Intermittent exercise has an effect on oxygen consumption similar to submaximal continuous running (5). Factors such as dehydration, hyperthermia, and mental stress elevate heart rate without affecting oxygen uptake. Although anaerobic activity is an important component of soccer, the greater demand is on aerobic metabolism. Considering total distance covered, the ratio of low-intensity to high-intensity activity is 2:1 and the relative time ratio is 7:1 (1). Sprinting occurs no more than 1.5% of total playing time (11,53). Considering all factors, relative work rates during soccer have been estimated between 70% and 80% of VO_{2max} (3–5,8). Estimates of VO_{2max} based on many studies of soccer players over the years suggest an average of 60 mL/kg/min (34). As shown in Table 21.3, similar heart rate patterns among athletes in other intermittent, high-intensity sports have been found (3,4,8,14,16,17,19,23,28,54,55).

Anaerobic Energy System

Adenosine Triphosphate and Phosphocreatine

Considerable energy fluctuations occur when playing HIIE team sports. Although the majority of the exercise in soccer is done at submaximal intensities, high-intensity or all-out exercise plays a crucial role, and players' ability to successfully carry out these high-intensity activities affects the result of the game. PCr concentration fluctuates throughout a soccer match because of the intermittent nature of the game and may decrease below resting values if a number of intense bouts of exercise are accompanied by short recovery time (39). Despite a small net utilization, PCr plays an important role as an energy buffer, providing phosphate for the resynthesis of ATP during the rapid increases in exercise intensity (5,30). Aerobic fitness enhances recovery from HIIE through increased aerobic response, improved lactate removal, and enhanced PCr regeneration (47).

Blood Lactate

Blood lactate concentrations have been used as indicators of anaerobic energy production in soccer (3,5). The concentration of blood lactate fluctuates throughout a soccer match. Lactate is metabolized within the active muscle after high-intensity exercise. When high-intensity exercise is coupled with low-intensity exercise, lactate metabolism increases. Furthermore, lactate released into the blood is taken up by the heart, liver, kidney, and other tissues. Evidence suggests that lactate is an important metabolic intermediate as a substrate for oxidative metabolism in cardiac and skeletal muscle and a precursor for gluconeogenesis (56). Thus, measurements of blood lactate concentration represent the balance of lactate released by muscle and taken up by blood and will not fully reflect lactate production during a soccer match. During HIIE, blood lactate may be high whereas muscle lactate may be relatively low (8).

It is reasonable to conclude that lactate production may be very high at points throughout a soccer game (3,5) with mean blood lactate concentrations of 2 to10 mmol/L during a match (39). During a tennis match, blood lactate levels were shown to have increased 50% to near, but not beyond, the anabolic threshold (28). The authors attribute this finding to several factors, including a highly trained aerobic system and variations in play that allow blood lactate levels to clear. McInnes et al (19) reported blood lactate levels averaging 6.8 mmol/L during basketball, indicating that glycolysis is involved in energy production.

Energy and Macronutrient Needs

Energy

Energy demands are high due to the intermittent nature of stop-and-go sports, and energy intake must be adequate to support training and competition (57). Several reports suggest that some players may not be meeting optimal nutrient intakes (57–62). Clark reports that professional male soccer players consume between 2,033 and 3,923 kcal/d (58). Data from a Major Indoor Soccer League team revealed that daily energy intakes of male players averaged 2,662 kcal and ranged from 1,618 to 4,394 kcal (59). More recent data examining the diet of soccer players support these findings (60–66).

It is estimated that a 75-kg male soccer player expends approximately 1,530 kcal per game. Bangsbo et al (8) estimated that soccer players expended 1,608 kcal on average during each training session in the 2 weeks leading up to the men's World Cup. Female soccer players experience similar exercise intensity during a match, but they expend less energy than males because women have smaller body mass. Brewer (60) reported that at 70% VO_{2max}, energy expenditure during a game is approximately 1,100 kcal. There are reports of insufficient energy intake among female and adolescent soccer players (62–65,67).

Data reported in 2003 about collegiate female soccer players indicate that their intakes met the Dietary Reference Intakes (DRIs) for total energy (37 kcal per kg of body weight), protein, and fat during the pre-season and were substantially higher than DRI intakes during the playing season (62). Although protein and fat intakes during the preseason were more than minimum recommendations, carbohydrate intakes were not sufficient to promote glycogen repletion. In this study, protein and fat displaced carbohydrate-rich, nutrient-dense foods, and supplied the energy requirements during training, but the diet failed to meet carbohydrate and micronutrient recommendations. It is important to note that total energy, carbohydrate, and micronutrient intakes during the season may not have been sufficient to support energy demands and recommended intakes.

An examination of female field hockey players (67) reveals an energy intake less than expenditure, with eight of the nine players attempting to lose weight. Several other observational studies reviewed by Brewer (60) suggest similar trends in the diets of female athletes. Papadopoulou et al (68) assessed the macro- and micronutrient intakes of two Greek national teams of adolescent female volleyball players and found that protein intake was satisfactory (approximately16% total kcal), but fat intake was generally higher than desired (approximately 37.5% total kcal) at the expense of carbohydrate consumption (45.9% total kcal), with mean energy intakes at less-than-optimal levels (2,013 kcal and 1,529 kcal, respectively).

Carbohydrate

Maughan et al (69), in a review of studies of cyclists, compared the effects of low-carbohydrate diets vs high-carbohydrate diets on high-intensity exercise. A low-carbohydrate diet (< 10% of total energy from carbohydrate) resulted in reduced endurance time. Conversely, diets that provided 65% to 84% carbohydrate were associated with increased performance, more consistently so with carbohydrate intakes at the higher end. Maughan et al (69) also noted that a high-protein diet, particularly in conjunction with a low-carbohydrate diet, resulted in metabolic acidosis, which is associated with fatigue. Although many questions about the causal mechanisms remain unanswered, the authors concluded the review with two distinct messages. The first is that it is possible to improve performance of short-duration, high-intensity exercise with a high-carbohydrate, low-protein diet for a few days before competition. Second, performance of this type may be impaired by a high-protein diet with insufficient carbohydrate or an energy-restricted diet in the precompetition period. In a review of the effects of nutritional interventions on molecular and cellular processes during exercise and recovery, Hawley et al (70) recommend that to maintain adequate muscle glycogen stores, the diet of athletes approach 7 g carbohydrate per kg of body mass during intense training. These considerations are important for athletes who compete in HIIE because of the periods of strenuous demands during competition.

Muscle Glycogen

The demands on muscle glycogen are great and performance is improved when carbohydrate is supplied before and during HIIE. Bangsbo et al (71) report that by increasing the carbohydrate content of the diet from 39% to 65% prior to a soccer match, muscle glycogen levels increased and resulted in a higher work rate and improved intermittent endurance. Akermark et al (23) compared the performance of ice hockey players given a carbohydrate-enriched diet vs a mixed diet. During a 3-day period between two games, players were fed a mixed diet of approximately 40% carbohydrate or a diet of approximately 60% carbohydrate. Distance skated, number of shifts skated, amount of time skated within shifts, and skating speed improved with the higher carbohydrate intake.

Glycogen depletion may seriously limit players' ability to maintain high-intensity work output, particularly during the later stages of the game. The glycogen utilization in leg muscle is markedly increased during bouts of intense exercise. During periods of rest and low-intensity play, glycogen is resynthesized (72). A study of Swedish elite ice hockey players (23) showed that distance and number of shifts skated, the skating speed, and the amount of time skated during shifts, improved with carbohydrate loading prior to activity.

In two separate studies, investigators found low levels of muscle glycogen after completion of a soccer match (33,73) and more use of glycogen in the first half compared with the second half (73). Furthermore, muscle glycogen concentration was only 50% of the prematch values 2 days after the match (33). The difference in muscle glycogen measured before and after a match represents the net glycogen utilization and does not fully reflect total glycogen turnover during play (5,30). Toward the end of a match, players experience fatigue and a decrease in performance. Although an exact mechanism for this phenomenon has not been identified, low levels of muscle glycogen are likely a major factor. Saltin (73) observed that players with low levels of glycogen covered 24% less distance, 50% of which was covered by walking. Without sufficient muscle glycogen, exercise is fueled by fat and the intensity of that exercise is typically less than 50% of capacity (31,74).

Blood Glucose

The stored glycogen in exercising muscle provides a major portion of carbohydrate used during a soccer match, but blood glucose also may be utilized by exercising muscles (5,75) and may, in fact, spare muscle glycogen. As exercise duration increases, the carbohydrate from muscle glycogen decreases while that from blood glucose increases (31). Blood glucose concentrations increase during HIIE as long as there is sufficient liver glycogen and glucose precursors (3,5,75).

Hypoglycemia and depletion of glycogen are associated with fatigue and reduced performance. Ferrauti and colleagues (76) assessed the incidence of hypoglycemia in tennis players during repeated tournament and practice matches by examining the change in glucose concentrations over the test period. The results indicate that glucose homeostasis is disrupted several times during tennis tournaments, leading to a decrease in glucose concentration and an increased risk of hypoglycemia, especially after a long match with only short breaks. In the absence of carbohydrate supplementation during extended play, blood glucose can decrease. To reduce the risk of hypoglycemia, a continuous intake of a low–glycemic index carbohydrate is recommended beginning with the third set through the end of the match and during changeovers.

Carbohydrate Recommendations

A 1994 review by Hargreaves (77) presents an overview of the most relevant research results about the role of carbohydrate in the performance of soccer players before, during, and after games and intensive training. Hargreaves concluded that a prematch diet of at least 55% of total energy as carbohydrate accompanied by additional carbohydrate consumed during and after a match maximizes liver and muscle glycogen stores and enhances the performance of athletes. The effects of consuming carbohydrate during HIIE have been researched (78–82). Davison et al (83) demonstrated that 8 mL/kg of a 6% carbohydrate-electrolyte solution consumed 15 minutes prior to HIIE helps maintain higher blood glucose as compared to a placebo or no fluid, resulting in delayed fatigue and improved performance.

Carbohydrate recommendations are more precisely expressed on a gram per kilogram basis (79,84,85). The current recommendations for athletes engaged in HIIE are summarized in Table 21.4 (58,85–93). Specific recommendations should be tailored to the needs of the individual athlete. Before adopting any eating and drinking strategies for immediately before or during a match, players should be cautioned to experiment on training days to establish a comfortable routine to avoid any untoward consequences.

Glycogen Repletion

In spite of measures to minimize glycogen losses, match play drastically reduces glycogen stores. Glycogen depletion is associated with fatigue and a decrease in exercise intensity. Resynthesis of depleted glycogen stores is both an important consideration and a challenge in postexercise recovery. When enough carbohydrate is supplemented immediately after exercise with sufficient recovery time, the rate of glycogen

TABLE 21.4 Carbohydrate Guidelines for High-Intensity Intermittent Exercise

	Carbohydrate	Conditions
Training diet	7–12 g/kg (60%–70% total energy)	Adequate energy
Pregame meal	1–4g/kg; > 200 g	1–4 h prior to competition; low–glycemic index solid carbohydrate may be beneficial
Before exercise	30–60 g	15 min to 1 h before competition
During exercise	0.5–1.0g/kg/h; 30–60 g/h	6%–8% carbohydrate solution
After exercise	1.0–1.67 g/kg	15- to 30-min intervals for 0–4 h postexercise

Source: Data are from references 58 and 85–93.

synthesis and the amount stored is optimal (94,95), increasing muscle glycogen up to seven-fold (93). Several studies suggest that the consumption of moderate– to high–glycemic index foods after exercise may be beneficial (93,96–98). There is a large body of research supporting the need for dietary carbohydrate before, during, and after exercise to fuel muscle glycogen stores and replenish liver glycogen content to help delay fatigue and maximize performance (see Chapter 2).

Protein

Studies have shown that amino acids can be oxidized for energy during endurance exercise (99) and that amino acid oxidation is inversely related to muscle glycogen availability (100). During team sports of intermittent exercise, muscle glycogen can be depleted depending on the intensity and duration of exercise and pregame glycogen stores. The higher the intensity of exercise, the greater is the glycogen utilization and amino acid oxidation. If the amino acids are not replaced via diet, a net loss in amino acids can occur over time, with losses in muscle strength and possibly performance.

Protein recommendations for soccer players are based on research that shows the strength component of soccer and the use of protein as an energy source. Lemon (101) concludes that soccer players need more dietary protein than sedentary individuals and suggests a protein intake of 1.4 to 1.7 g/kg/d for competitive soccer players. In a study of eleven 15-year-old soccer players by Boisseau et al (63), in which the mean daily energy intake of the athletes (2,345 kcal and 38.9 kcal/kg) was less than the Recommended Dietary Allowance [RDA] for nonactive 15 year olds), a protein intake of 1.57 g/kg was necessary to achieve nitrogen balance. A later study of 14-year-old male soccer players (64) demonstrated that both protein intakes and energy balance were important determinants of nitrogen balance and recommended a protein intake of 1.4 g/kg/d for adolescent males. Lemon cautions against extremely high protein intakes (> 2 g/kg/d) because of the lack of evidence of performance advantage (101). A review by Wolfe (102) addresses the use of protein supplements in exercise training and issues the same cautionary note that excessive protein intake may increase the potential for dehydration because of high urea excretion.

Attention has been given to the possible benefits of combining protein with carbohydrate during exercise to delay fatigue and immediately after exercise to maximize muscle glycogen synthesis (86,103–105). The results have been mixed, with inconclusive evidence to support the addition of protein in the presence of adequate carbohydrate intake. However, for glycogen repletion when energy intake does not provide sufficient carbohydrate, the addition of protein to carbohydrate during recovery may enhance overall glycogen recovery as well as assist with muscle repair.

Fat

Of the three macronutrients, dietary fat plays the smallest role in energy distribution. Fat is certainly an important component of a balanced diet, but the absolute quantity and the percentage of energy distribution contributed by fat should be limited. It is generally recommended that fat should contribute 35% or less of total energy. However, no performance benefits for any sports have been associated with diets with less than 20% total energy from fat.

To achieve energy intake levels that support weight and weight-training goals, athletes often consume diets high in fat. In a review of the role of dietary macronutrients in optimizing performance, Stellingwerff (106) observed reduced glycogenolysis during sprint exercise after 5 days of a high-fat diet followed by 1 day of carbohydrate restoration, and postulated that muscle glycogen "sparing" observed in studies of high-fat diets followed by carbohydrate restoration might be an impairment of glycogenolysis. In a review of the training adaptations via nutritional interventions, Hawley et al (70) caution against high-fat, low-carbohydrate diets as a strategy for HIIE.

Among the factors that contribute to less-than-optimal dietary intakes of athletes are: travel; all-you-can-eat buffet meals; limited time and ability to cook; and insufficient nutrition knowledge. Athletes benefit from instruction about choosing foods that support both their training and performance goals and their goals for fitness and long-term health.

Registered dietitians (RDs) working with athletes who participate in HIIE should observe the following guidelines on fat intake:

- Determine carbohydrate and protein intakes and then aim for 20% to 35% of energy from fat.
- Limit saturated fat to less than 7% of energy.
- Emphasize heart-healthy fats.
- Give practical guidelines for food selections that will control the contribution from fat, especially sources of "hidden" fats, such as full-fat dairy products, meats, processed foods, and foods prepared with fat, including restaurant and fast foods.
- Focus on selecting lean protein sources.
- Include tips for choosing foods away from home.

Micronutrient Needs

The energy demand of HIIE training and competition is considerable and requires adequate intake of all nutrients involved in energy production. There are no known micronutrient needs specific to athletes engaged in HIIE. The DRIs are appropriate goals for micronutrient intakes (107–111). Fogelholm (112) presents data on micronutrient status and the effects of micronutrient supplementation on exercise performance related to soccer and other team sports. In an effort to understand micronutrient needs and intakes of athletes and whether there is any performance benefit to micronutrient supplementation, data were reported from nine studies examining dietary intakes of athletes involved in soccer, football, basketball, hockey, volleyball, and handball, as well as three studies assessing the effect of micronutrient supplementation. The data from these studies suggest that, overall, micronutrient intakes correlate with energy intake. Male intakes of micronutrients were mostly in line with RDAs. Female athletes with energy intakes less than 2,400 kcal were more likely to have lower intakes than the RDAs for minerals and trace elements such as calcium, magnesium, iron, and zinc. The data also suggest that vitamin B-6 intake was less than the RDAs for all groups studied, but this may be due to incomplete data from vitamin B-6 nutrient databases.

With regard to supplementation, there was no clear evidence that micronutrient supplementation improved performance of athletes, but the number of subjects studied was small (112). There are two exceptions to this conclusion. First, female athletes with infrequent or irregular menstruation may benefit from calcium and vitamin D supplementation to help stem the loss of bone density. In the presence of estrogen deficiency, calcium and vitamin D supplementation alone will not improve bone density. Second, iron-depleted females (serum ferritin < 12 mcg/L), may benefit from daily supplementation with 100 mg elemental iron for 3 months or longer. The iron status of female athletes should be assessed annually. Those who are symptomatic (serum ferritin <35 mcg/L) or at high risk for iron deficiency should be rescreened 3 to 4 months after the initial assessment (113).

In general, the micronutrient status of an athlete is directly related to the quality of the dietary intake, especially energy intake. Among the athletes studied by Nutter (67,113), iron and calcium intakes were 30% less than the RDAs. Similarly, data collected from male and female team athletes identify some nutrients of concern (114). Low intakes of thiamin were observed in the diets of male athletes. Among female athletes whose daily energy intakes were less than 2,390 kcal, mineral and trace elements, such as calcium, magnesium, iron, and zinc, were suboptimal. More recently, concerns have been raised about the vitamin D status of athletes, especially athletes who train and compete indoors and those whose exposure to ultraviolet light and intakes of vitamin D–rich foods are limited (115,116).

Clark et al's 2003 investigation of collegiate female soccer players showed that, along with insufficient carbohydrate intake, several micronutrient intakes were less than 75% of the DRI pre- and postseason (62). Among these athletes, a greater consumption of protein- and fat-rich foods displaced more nutrient-dense complex carbohydrates. This diet becomes particularly troublesome when athletes focus on weight reduction or the maintenance of a low body weight. Fogelholm (112) recommends that nutrition education for soccer players start at an early age and focus on foods and macronutrients. Additionally, periodic dietary evaluation from an RD can detect early trouble signs, help prevent serious nutritional deficiencies, and screen for possible disordered eating.

Fluid Requirements

The major causes of fatigue in endurance sports are depletion of muscle glycogen and problems associated with thermoregulation and fluid loss. HIIE requires that players exercise at high intensities for a prolonged period of time, often at elevated ambient temperatures and high humidity. The added factor of clothing and equipment make heat dissipation, and thus thermoregulation, more difficult as can be exemplified in the sports of American football (114) and ice hockey. Palmer and Spriet (117) studied the hydration status and habits of elite ice hockey players and found that more than 50% of players arrived at practice in various degrees of hypohydration. In general, of players who drank sport drinks before practice and replaced 60% of lost fluid with water during practice, 30% still had a greater than 1% body mass loss. All players had high sweat rates during practice, with substantial loss of sodium in sweat that was not replaced by either the sport drink consumed before practice or the water during practice.

The energy demands of stop-and-go sports greatly reduce muscle glycogen stores and fluid reserves, which must be replenished before the next competition. Repletion of muscle glycogen depends not only on carbohydrate intake but also on fluid intake as well because each gram of muscle glycogen is stored with 2.7 g water.

Studies examining the effects of carbohydrate-electrolyte solutions on performance during high-intensity intermittent exercise found that muscle glycogen utilization was reduced (118), endurance running capacity was improved (78,119), time to fatigue was delayed, and mental function was improved (48,51) when a carbohydrate-electrolyte solution was consumed. Under moderate temperatures (10°C or 50°F), the sweat losses of soccer players during a match may be as much as 2 liters (98), and in high temperatures, a mean loss of 3 liters or more (4). When the ambient temperature is more than skin temperature, the body builds up additional heat and this reduces the capacity to perform prolonged exercise. Players who sweat profusely are likely to become dehydrated and fatigued toward the end of the exercise. Fluid ingestion in the heat should focus on maintenance of hydration status. Tennis players have been shown to sweat more than 2.5 L/h and replace fluids at a slower rate during competition than in practice (120). In warm and hot environments, it is recommended that tennis players consume a carbohydrate-electrolyte beverage at greater than >200 mL per changeover and ideally closer to 400 mL per changeover to maintain physiologic homeostasis and performance.

Full rehydration after exercise requires replacement of fluid and electrolytes, primarily sodium, lost in sweat. A study by Shirreffs et al (121) suggests that full rehydration after intense exercise is best achieved when the replacement fluid contains sufficient sodium and is consumed at 150% of the fluid lost through exercise. An investigation examined the effect on gastric emptying of intermittent exercise at varying intensities to simulate a soccer match. The results revealed that a greater volume of carbohydrate-electrolyte solution emptied during the lower-intensity walking trial than during the high-intensity soccer

---

BOX 21.1   Hydration Goals in High-Intensity Intermittent Exercise

Before Exercise
- Maximize fluid intake during the 24 hours preceding training or competition.
- Drink extra fluid during the last 10–15 minutes before the game begins.
- A carbohydrate-electrolyte solution consumed 15 minutes prior to exercise improves endurance.

During Exercise
- Consume fluid early and at regular intervals during exercise.
- Choose cool, flavored beverages that are more palatable and contain 4% to 8% carbohydrate (30–60 g carbohydrate per hour) and electrolytes (0.5–0.7 g sodium per liter of water)

After Exercise
- Achieve rapid and complete repletion of fluid, electrolyte, and carbohydrates lost during training and exercise. Each pound lost is about 480 mL (about 16 oz) of fluid.
- Drink at least 150% or 2.5 cups of fluid for every pound lost through exercise to cover obligatory urine loss.

General Precaution: Alcohol is dehydrating. Avoid alcohol within 72 hours before or after training.

Source: Data are from references 121 and 123–128.

---

trial, demonstrating that the intensity of activity during this type of stop-and-go team sports is sufficient to slow gastric emptying (122). More information on hydration and fluids is found in Chapter 6 and in Box 21.1 (121,123–128).

Special consideration and care should be given to the fluid needs of young athletes, particularly prepubescent youth (129). During exercise, children produce more heat than adults yet have a greater surface area-to-body mass ratio, thus increasing their influx of heat when ambient temperatures are more than skin temperature. In addition, they have less capacity for sweating and take longer to acclimatize to warm weather (129,130). These factors increase young athletes' risk for dehydration and heat illness. When children become dehydrated, their core temperatures increase faster than it does in dehydrated adults, underscoring the need for strict enforcement of hydration practices. Given the heightened risk of hyperthermia in children, the following precautions and practical measures should be taken:

- Five to 8 oz of fluid should be consumed at least every 15 to 20 minutes during training and exercise in the heat.
- Fluids should be cool and palatable to encourage drinking. In one study, grape was the preferred flavor and the one that encouraged the greatest rehydration following mild dehydration (131).
- In warm weather, avoid unnecessary layers of clothing. For example, soccer goalkeepers should remove the team jersey when wearing the goalkeeper shirt.
- Sweat-drenched clothing should be replaced with dry clothing when possible.
- Reduce the intensity of exercise when the relative humidity and ambient temperature are high.
- Allow frequent breaks.
- Provide shelter from direct sunlight during hot weather when the player is on the sidelines.

Summary

The stop-and-go nature of HIIE places a great physiological and metabolic demand on the body and involves all three energy systems. These sports require bursts of all-out effort interspersed with periods of moderate- and low-intensity effort.

The primary goals of nutrition in such sports is to support peak performance by ensuring adequate amounts of energy and nutrients, the right blend of fuel for a given effort, adequate hydration, and a plan for the rapid replacement of fluids and muscle glycogen. Coaches and trainers must take precautions to avoid or minimize some of the pitfalls of high-intensity intermittent exercise, such as fatigue, hypoglycemia, impaired performance, and dehydration and its consequences.

Carbohydrate is the preferred fuel for much of the work in stop-and-go sports and it is crucial to ensure adequate intakes of carbohydrate before, during, and after exercise. The general carbohydrate recommendation is 7 g/kg/d with 7 to 12 g/kg/d during training and competition. The timing of ingestion, as well as the amount of carbohydrate, helps fuel the athlete and enhances endurance and power. Recommended daily protein intake is 1.4 to 1.7 g/kg. Fat should comprise approximately 20% to 35% of total energy intake. When selecting foods, it is important to carefully choose nutrient-rich foods that also provide ample vitamins and minerals, an essential part of fuel production and good health. Fluid intake is critical, especially because many intermittent, high-intensity sports are played in hot and humid conditions.

References

1. Reilly T, Thomas V. A motion analysis of work rate in different positional roles in professional football match play. *J Hum Movement Stud.* 1976;2:87–97.
2. Withers R, Maricic Z, Wasilewski S, Kelly L. Match analysis of Australian professional soccer players. *J Hum Movement Stud.* 1982;8:159–176.
3. Ekblom B. Applied physiology of soccer. *Sports Med.* 1986;3:50–60.
4. Reilly T. Energetics of high-intensity exercise (soccer) with particular reference to fatigue. *J Sports Sci.* 1997;15:257–263.
5. Bangsbo J. The physiology of soccer—with special reference to intense intermittent exercise. *Acta Physiol Scand Suppl.* 1994;619:1–155.
6. Drust B, Reilly T, Rienzi E. Analysis of work rate in soccer. *Sports Exerc Injury.* 1988;4:151–155.
7. Shephard RJ. Biology and medicine of soccer: an update. *J Sport Sci.* 1999;117:757–786.
8. Bangsbo J, Mohr M, Krustrup P. Physical and metabolic demands of training and match-play in the elite football player. *J Sports Sci.* 2006;24:665–674.
9. Bradley P, Mascio M, Peart D, Olsen P, Sheldon B. High-intensity activity profiles of elite soccer players at different performance levels. *J Strength Cond Res.* 2010;24:2343–2551.
10. Kalapotharakos V, Strimpakos N, Vithoulka I, Karyounidis C, Diamantopoulos K, Kapreli E. Physiological characterisics of elite professional soccer teams of different ranking. *J Sports Med Phys Fitness.* 2006;46:515–519.
11. Orendurff M, Walker J, Jovanovic M, Tulchin K, Levy M, Hoffmann D. Intensity and duration of intermittent exercise and recovery during a soccer match. *J Strength Cond Res.* 2010;24:2683–2692.
12. Carling C, Orhant E. Variation in body composition in professional soccer players: interseasonal and intraseasonal changes and the effects of exposure time and player position. *J Strength Cond Res.* 2010;24:1332–1339.
13. Pincivero D, Bompa T. A physiological review of American football. *Sports Med.* 1997;4:247–260.
14. Abdelkrim N, Chaouachi A, Chamari K, Chtara M, Castagna C. Positional role and competitive-level differences in elite-level men's basketball players. *J Strength Cond Res.* 2010;2:1346–1355.
15. Ostojic S, Mazic S, Dikic N. Profiling in basketball: physical and physiological characteristics of elite players. *J Strength Cond.* 2006;20:740–744.
16. Gabbett T, King T, Jenkins D. Applied physiology of rugby league. *Sports Med.* 2008;38:119–138.

17. Sirotic A, Coutts A, Knowles H, Catterick C. A comparison of match demands between elite and semi-elite rugby league competition. *J Sports Sci*. 2009;27:203–211.

18. Gray A, Jenkins D. Match analysis and the physiological demands of Australian football. *Sports Med*. 2010;40:347–360.

19. McInnes S, Carlson J, Jones C, McKenna M. The physiological load imposed on basketball players during competition. *J Sports Sci*. 1995;13:387–397.

20. Montgomery D. Physiology of ice hockey. *Sports Med*. 1988;5:99–126.

21. Montgomery D. Physiological profile of professional hockey players—a longitudinal comparison. *Appl Physiol Nutr Metab*. 2006;31:181–185.

22. Durocher J, Leetun D, Carter J. Sport-specific assessment of lactate threshold and aerobic capacity throughout a collegiate hockey season. *Appl Physiol Nutr Metab*. 2008;33:1165–1171.

23. Akermark C, Jacobs I, Rasmusson M, Karlsson J. Diet and muscle glycogen concentration in relation to physical performance in Swedish elite ice hockey players. *Int J Sport Nutr*. 1996;6:272–284.

24. Houston M. Nutrition and ice hockey performance. *Can J Appl Sport Sci*. 1979;4:98–99.

25. Green H, Daub B, Painter D, Thomson J. Glycogen depletion patterns during ice hockey performance. *Med Sci Sports*. 1978;10:289–293.

26. Green H. Metabolic aspects of intermittent work with specific regard to ice hockey. *Can J Appl Sport Sci*. 1979;4:29–34.

27. Konig D, Huonker M, Schmid A, Halle M, Berg A, Keul J. Cardiovascular, metabolic, and hormonal parameters in professional tennis players. *Med Sci Sports Exerc*. 2001;33:654–658.

28. Bergeron M, Maresh C, Kraemer W, Abraham A, Conroy B, Gabaree C. Tennis: a physiological profile during match play. *Int J Sports Med*. 1991;12:474–479.

29. Smekal G, von Duvillard S, Rihacek C, Pokan R, Hofmann P, Baron R, Tschan H, Bachl N. A physiological profile of tennis match play. *Med Sci Sports Exerc*. 2001;33:999–1005.

30. Bangsbo J. Energy demands in competitive soccer. *J Sports Sci*. 1994;12(suppl):S5–S12.

31. Romijn J, Coyle E, Sidossis L, Gastaldelli A, Horowitz J, Endert E, Wolfe RR, Regulation of endogenous fat and carbohydrate metabolism in relation to exercise intensity and duration. *Am J Physiol*. 1993;265:E380–E391.

32. Roberts TJ, Weber JM, Hoppeler H, Weibel E, Taylor C. Design of the oxygen and substrate pathways. II. Defining the upper limits of carbohydrate and fat oxidation. *J Exp Biol*. 1996;199:1651–1658.

33. Jacobs I, Westin N, Karlsson J, Rasmusson M, Houghton B. Muscle glycogen and diet in elite soccer players. *Eur J Appl Physiol*. 1982;48:297–302.

34. Tumilty D. Physiological characteristics of elite soccer players. *Sports Med*. 1993;16:80–96.

35. Gollnick PD, Armstrong RB, Sembrowich WL, Shepherd RE, Saltin B. Glycogen depletion pattern in human skeletal muscle fibers after heavy exercise. *J Appl Physiol*. 1973;34:615–618.

36. Costill D, Gollnick P, Jansson E, Saltin B, Stein EM. Glycogen depletion pattern in human muscle fibers during distance running. *Acta Physiol Scand*. 1973;89:374–384.

37. Gollnick PD, Piehl K, Saubert CW 4th, Armstrong RB, Saltin B. Diet, exercise, and glycogen changes in human muscle fibers. *J Appl Physiol*. 1972;33:421–425.

38. Brooks G, Mercier J. Balance of carbohydrate and lipid utilization during exercise: the "crossover" concept. *J Appl Physiol*. 1994;76:2253–2261.

39. Krustrup P, Mohr M, Steensberg A, Bencke J, Kjaer M, Bangsbo J. Muscle and blood metabolites during a soccer game: implications for sprint performance. *Med Sci Sports Exerc*. 2006;38:1165–1174.

40. Brooks G. Importance of the "crossover" concept in exercise metabolism. *Clin Exp Pharmacol Physiol*. 1997;24:889–895.

41. Coggan A, Kohrt W, Spina R, Bier D, Holloszy J. Endurance training decreases plasma glucose turnover and oxidation during moderate-intensity exercise in men. *J Appl Physiol*. 1990;68:990–996.

42. Hurley B, Nemeth P, Martin WI, Hagberg J, Dalsky G, Holloszy J. Muscle triglyceride utilization during exercise: effect of training. *J Appl Physiol*. 1986;60:562–567.

43. Sidossis L, Gastaldelli A, Klein S, Wolfe R. Regulation of plasma fatty acid oxidation during low- and high-intensity exercise. *Am J Physiol*. 1997;272:E1065–E1070.

44. Trapp G, Chisholm D, Boutcher S. Metabolic response of trained and untrained women during high-intensity intermittent cycle exercise. *Am J Physiol Regul Integr Comp Physiol.* 2007;293:R2370–R2375.

45. Martin WH 3rd, Dalsky G, Hurley B, Matthews D, Bier D, Hagberg J, Rogers M, King D, Holloszy J. Effect of endurance-training on plasma free fatty acid turnover and oxidation during exercise. *Am J Physiol.* 1993;265:E708–E714.

46. Weber J, Brichon G, Zwingelstein G, McClelland G, Saucedo C, Weibel E, Taylor C. Design of the oxygen and substrate pathways: partitioning energy provision from fatty acids. *J Exp Biol.* 1996;199:1667–1674.

47. Tomlin D, Wenger H. The relationship between aerobic fitness and recovery from high-intensity intermittent exercise. *Sports Med.* 2001;31:1–11.

48. Welsh R, Davis J, Burke J, Williams H. Carbohydrates and physical/mental performance during intermittent exercise to fatigue. *Med Sci Sports Exerc.* 2002;34:723–731.

49. Newsholme E, Blomstrand E, Ekblom B. Physical and mental fatigue: metabolic mechanisms and importance of plasma amino acids. *Br Med Bull.* 1992;48:477–495.

50. Bergström J, Hermansen L, Hultman E, Saltin B. Diet, muscle glycogen and physical performance. *Acta Physiol Scand.* 1967;71:140–150.

51. Winnick J, Davis J, Welsh R, Carmichael M, Murphy E, Blackmon J. Carbohydrate feedings during team sport exercise preserve physical and CNS function. *Med Sci Sports Exerc.* 2005;37:306–315.

52. Smodlaka V. Cardiovascular aspect of soccer. *Phys Sportsmed.* 1978;6:66–70.

53. Bangsbo J, Norregaard L, Thorsoe F. Activity profile of competition soccer. *Can J Sport Sci.* 1991;16:110–116.

54. Therminarias A, Dansou P, Chirpaz-Oddou M, Gharib C, Quirion A. Hormonal and metabolic changes during a strenuous match. Effect of aging. *Int J Sports Med.* 1991;12:10–16.

55. Docherty D. A comparison of heart rate responses in racquet games. *Br J Sports Med.* 1982;6:96–100.

56. Brooks G. Current concepts in lactate exchange. *Med Sci Sports Exerc.* 1991;23:895–906.

57. Williams C, Nicholas C. Nutrition needs for team sport. *Sport Sci Exch.* 1998;11:70.

58. Clark K. Nutritional guidance to soccer players for training and competition. *J Sports Sci.* 1994;12(suppl):S43–S50.

59. Macedonio M. Nutrition management of the Cleveland Force soccer team. Summary report. Unpublished data. 1987.

60. Brewer J. Aspects of women's soccer. *J Sports Sci.* 1994;12(suppl):S35–S38.

61. Economos C, Bortz S, Nelson M. Nutrition practices of elite athletes. *Sports Med.* 1993;16:381–399.

62. Clark M, Reed D, Crouse S, Armstrong R. Pre- and post-season dietary intake, body composition, and performance indices of NCAA division I female soccer players. *Int J Sport Nutr Exerc Metab.* 2003;13:303–319.

63. Boisseau N, Le Creff C, Loyens M, Poortmans J. Protein intake and nitrogen balance in male non-active adolescents and soccer players. *Eur J Appl Physiol.* 2002;88:288–293.

64. Boisseau N, Vermorel M, Rance M, Duché P, Patureau-Mirand P. Protein requirements in male adolescent soccer players. *Eur J Appl Physiol.* 2007;100:27–33.

65. Iglesias-Gutierrez E, García-Roves P, García A, Patterson A. Food preferences do not influence adolescent high-level athletes' dietary intake. *Appetite.* 2008;50:536–543.

66. Noda Y, Iide K, Masuda R, Kishida R, Nagata A, Hirakawa F, Yoshimura Y, Imamura H. Nutrient intake and blood iron status of male collegiate soccer players. *Asia Pac J Clin Nutr.* 2009;18:344–350.

67. Nutter J. Seasonal changes in female athletes' diets. *Int J Sport Nutr.* 1991;1:395–407.

68. Papadopoulou S, Papadopoulou S, Gallos G. Macro- and micro-nutrient intake of adolescent Greek female volleyball players. *Int J Sport Nutr Exerc Metab.* 2002;12:73–80.

69. Maughan R, Greenhaff P, Leiper J, Ball D, Lambert C, Gleeson M. Diet composition on the performance of high-intensity exercise. *J Sports Sci.* 1997;15:265–275.

70. Hawley J, Tipton K, Millard-Stafford M. Promoting training adaptations through nutritional interventions. *J Sports Sci.* 2006;24:709–721.

71. Bangsbo J, Norregaard L, Thorsoe F. The effect of carbohydrate diet on intermittent exercise performance. *Int J Sports Med.* 1992;13:152–157.

72. Nordheim K, Vollestad N. Glycogen and lactate metabolism during low-intensity exercise in man. *Acta Physiol Scand.* 1990;139:475–484.

73. Saltin B. Metabolic fundamental in exercise. *Med Sci Sports Exerc.* 1973;5:137–146.
74. Kirkendall D. Effects of nutrition on performance in soccer. *Med Sci Sports Exerc.* 1993;25:1370–1374.
75. Coyle E. Substrate utilization during exercise in active people. *Am J Clin Nutr.* 1995;61(4 Suppl):968S–979S.
76. Ferrauti A, Pluim B, Busch T, Weber K. Blood glucose responses and incidence of hypoglycaemia in elite tennis under practice and tournament conditions. *J Sci Med Sport.* 2003;6:28–39.
77. Hargreaves M. Carbohydrate and lipid requirements of soccer. *J Sports Sci.* 1994;12(suppl):S13–S16.
78. Phillips S, Turner A, Gray S, Sanderson M, Sproule J. Ingesting a 6% carbohydrate-electrolyte solution improves endurance capacity, but not sprint performance, during intermittent, high-intensity shuttle running in adolescent team games players aged 12–14 years. *Eur J Appl Physiol.* 2010;109:811–821.
79. Ali A, Williams C, Nicholas C, Foskett A. The influence of carbohydrate-electrolyte ingestion on soccer skill performance. *Med Sci Sports Exerc.* 2007;39:1969–1976.
80. Backhouse S, Ali A, Biddle S, Williams C. Carbohydrate ingestion during prolonged high-intensity intermittent exercise: impact on affect and perceived exertion. *Scand J Med Sci Sports.* 2007;17:605–610.
81. Carter J, Jeukendrup A, Mundel T, Jones D. Carbohydrate supplementation improves moderate and high-intensity exercise in the heat. *Eur J Physiol.* 2003;446:211–219.
82. de Sousa M, Simões H, Oshiiwa M, Rogero M, Tirapegui J. Effects of acute carbohydrate supplementation during sessions of high-intensity intermittent exercise. *Eur J Appl Physiol.* 2007;99:57–63.
83. Davison G, McClean C, Brown J, Madigan S, Gamble D, Trinick T, Duly E. The effects of ingesting a carbohydrate-electrolyte beverage 15 minutes prior to high-intensity exercise performance. *Res Sports Med.* 2008;16:155–166.
84. Burke L, Cox G, Cummings N, Desbrow B. Guidelines for daily carbohydrate intake: do athletes achieve them? *Sports Med.* 2001;31:267–299.
85. Burke L. Strategies to optimize performance: training high or training low? *Scand J Med Sci Sports.* 2010;20 (Suppl 2):48–58.
86. Lambert E, Goedecke J. The role of dietary macronutrients in optimizing endurance performance. *Curr Sports Med Rep.* 2003;2:194–201.
87. Costill D, Hargreaves M. Carbohydrate nutrition and fatigue. *Sports Med.* 1992;13:86–92.
88. Wright D, Sherman W, Dernbach A. Carbohydrate feedings before, during, or in combination improve cycling performance. *J Appl Physiol.* 1991;71:1082–1088.
89. Maffucci D, McMurray R. Towards optimizing the timing of the pre-exercise meal. *Int J Sport Nutr Exerc Metab.* 2000;10:103–113.
90. Coleman E. Update on carbohydrate: solid versus liquid. *Int J Sport Nutr Exerc Metab.* 1994;8:80–88.
91. Kirwan J, Cyr-Campbell D, Campbell W, Scheiber J, Evans W. Effects of moderate and high glycemic index meals on metabolism and exercise performance. *Metabolism.* 2001;50:849–855.
92. Williams M, Raven P, Fogt D, Ivy J. Effects of recovery beverages on glycogen restoration and endurance exercise performance. *J Strength Cond Res.* 2003;17:12–19.
93. Burke L, Collier G, Davis P, Fricker P, Sanigorski A, Hargreaves M. Muscle glycogen storage after prolonged exercise: effect of the frequency of carbohydrate feedings. *Am J Clin Nutr.* 1996;64:115–119.
94. Ivy J. Optimization of glycogen stores. In: Maughan R, ed. *Nutrition in Sport.* Vol VII, Encyclopaedia of Sports Medicine. Malden, MA: Blackwell Science; 2000:97–111.
95. Mondazzi L, Arcelli E. Glycemic index in sport nutrition. *J Am Coll Nutr.* 2009;28(suppl):455S–463S.
96. Rankin J. Glycemic index and exercise metabolism. *Sports Sci Exch.* 1997;10:1.
97. Burke L, Hargreaves M, Collier G. Muscle glycogen storage after prolonged exercise. *J Appl Physiol.* 1993;74:1019–1023.
98. Coyle E. Timing and method of increased carbohydrate intake to cope with heavy training, competition and recovery. *J Sports Sci.* 1991;9:29–51.
99. Evans W, Fisher E, Hoerr R, Young V. Protein metabolism and endurance exercise. *Phys Sportsmed.* 1983;11:63–72.
100. Lemon P, Mullin J. Effect of initial muscle glycogen levels on protein catabolism during exercise. *J Appl Physiol.* 1992;48:624–629.

101. Lemon P. Protein requirements of soccer. *J Sports Sci.* 1994;12(suppl):S17–S22.

102. Wolfe R. Protein supplements and exercise. *Am J Clin Nutr.* 2000;72(suppl):551S–557S.

103. Ivy J, Goforth H Jr, Damon B, McCauley T, Parsons E, Price T. Early postexercise muscle glycogen recovery is enhanced with a carbohydrate-protein supplement. *J Appl Physiol.* 2002;93:1337–1344.

104. Davis J, Welsh R, De Volve K, Alderson N. Effects of branched-chain amino acids and carbohydrate on fatigue during intermittent, high-intensity running. *Int J Sports Med.* 1999;20:309–314.

105. Lemon P. Beyond the zone: protein needs of active individuals. *J Am Coll Nutr.* 2000;19(suppl):513S–521S.

106. Stellingwerff T, Spriet L, Watt M, Kimber N, Hargreaves M, Hawley J, Burke L. Decreased PDH activation and glycogenolysis during exercise following fat adaptation with carbohydrate restoration. *Am J Physiol Endocrinol Metab.* 2006;290:E380–E388.

107. Institute of Medicine. *Dietary Reference Intakes for Vitamin A, Vitamin K, Arsenic, Boron, Chromium, Copper, Iodine, Iron, Molybdenum, Nickel, Silicon, Vanadium, and Zinc.* Washington, DC: National Academies Press; 2001.

108. Institute of Medicine. *Dietary Reference Intakes for Calcium, Phosphorus, Magnesium, Vitamin D, and Fluoride.* Washington, DC: National Academies Press; 1997.

109. Institute of Medicine. *Dietary Reference Intakes for Calcium and Vitamin D.* Washington, DC: National Academies Press; 2010.

110. Institute of Medicine. *Dietary Reference Intakes for Thiamin, Riboflavin, Niacin, Vitamin B6, Folate, Vitamin B12, Pantothenic Acid, Biotin, and Choline.* Washington, DC: National Academies Press; 1998.

111. Institute of Medicine. *Dietary Reference Intakes for Vitamin C, Vitamin E, Selenium, and Carotenoids.* Washington, DC: National Academies Press; 2000.

112. Fogelholm M. Vitamins, minerals and supplementation in soccer. *J Sports Sci.* 1994;12(suppl):S23–S27.

113. Nielsen P, Nachtigall D. Iron supplementation in athletes: current recommendations. *Sports Med.* 1998;26:207–216.

114. Kulka T, Kenney L. Heat balance limits in football uniforms: how different uniform ensembles alter the equation. *Phys Sportsmed.* 2002;30:29–39.

115. Willis K, Peterson N, Larson-Meyer D. Should we be concerned about the vitamin D status of athletes? *Int J Sport Nutr Exerc Metab.* 2008;18:204–224.

116. Cannell J, Hollis B, Sorenson M, Taft T, Anderson J. Athletic performance and vitamin D. *Med Sci Sports Exerc.* 2009;41:1102–1110.

117. Palmer M, Spriet L. Sweat rate, salt loss, and fluid intake during an intense on-ice practice in elite Canadian male junior hockey players. *Appl Physiol Nutr Metab.* 2008;33:263–271.

118. Nicholas C, Tsintzas K, Boobis L, Williams C. Carbohydrate-electrolyte ingestion during intermittent high-intensity running. *Med Sci Sports Exerc.* 1999;31:1280–1286.

119. Nicholas C, Williams C, Lakomy H, Phillips G, Nowitz A. Influence of ingesting a carbohydrate-electrolyte solution on endurance capacity during intermittent, high-intensity shuttle running. *J Sports Sci.* 1995;13:283–290.

120. Kovacs M. A review of fluid and hydration in competitive tennis. *Int J Sports Physiol Perform.* 2008;3:413–423.

121. Shirreffs S, Taylor A, Leiper J, Maughan R. Post-exercise rehydration in man: effects of volume consumed and drink sodium content. *Med Sci Sports Exerc.* 1996;28:1260–1271.

122. Leiper J, Prentice A, Wrightson C, Maughan R. Gastric emptying of a carbohydrate-electrolyte drink during a soccer match. *Med Sci Sports Exerc.* 2000;33:1932–1938.

123. American College of Sports Medicine. Position stand on exercise and fluid replacement. *Med Sci Sports Exerc.* 1996;28:i–vii.

124. Greenleaf J, Castle B. Exercise temperature regulation in man during hypohydration and hyperthermia. *J Appl Physiol.* 1971;30:847–853.

125. Maughan R, Leiper J. Fluid replacement requirements in soccer. *J Sports Sci.* 1994;12(suppl):S29–S34.

126. Shi X, Gisolfi C. Fluid and carbohydrate replacement during intermittent exercise. *Sports Med.* 1998;25:157–172.

127. Horswill C. Effective fluid replacement. *Int J Sport Nutr Exerc Metab.* 1998;8:175–195.

128. Burke L, Hurley J. Fluid balance in team sports. *Sports Med.* 1997;24:38–54.

129. Petrie H, Stover E, Horswill C. Nutrition concerns for the child and adolescent competitor. *Nutrition.* 2004;20:620–631.

130. American Academy of Pediatrics. Committee on Sports Medicine and Fitness. Climatic heat stress and the exercising child and adolescent. *Pediatrics.* 2000;106:158–159.

131. Meyer F, Bar-Or O, Salsberg A, Passe D. Hypohydration during exercise in children: effect of thirst, drink preferences, and rehydration. *Int J Sport Nutr Exerc Metab.* 1994;4:22–35.

Chapter 22

NUTRITION FOR ENDURANCE AND ULTRA-ENDURANCE SPORTS

Ellen J. Coleman, MA, MPH, RD, CSSD

Introduction

Endurance events encompass a wide range of competitions, including 10-km and marathon runs, Olympic distance triathlons, cross-country skiing races, and road and mountain cycling events. Ultra-endurance events involve races that last from 4 to 24 hours and include running 31 to 100 miles, cycling 100-plus miles, and triathlons ranging from half-Ironman events to the full Ironman distance of a 2.4-mile swim, 112-mile bike ride, and 26.2-mile marathon run. Multistage ultra-endurance events entail competing over consecutive days, such as the Tour de France bicycle race (~2,500 miles over 22 days), the Race Across America (RAAM) cycling event (3,000 miles), the Australian Sydney to Melbourne foot race (628 miles), and adventure races.

Endurance athletes have unique nutrient demands because of their high energy expenditures, and they must cope with a variety of challenges to achieve their fuel and fluid replacement goals.

Energy Systems and Fuel Usage

The predominant energy system for endurance athletes is the aerobic energy system with brief, intermittent involvement of the anaerobic energy systems. During prolonged exercise, the oxidative metabolism of carbohydrate (muscle glycogen and plasma glucose) and fat (intramuscular triglycerides and plasma fatty acids) provide the vast majority of adenosine triphosphate (ATP) for muscle contraction. Although amino acid oxidation occurs to a limited extent during endurance exercise, carbohydrate and fat are the most important oxidative substrates (1,2).

During a high-intensity endurance event, the exercise intensity is often 85% of VO_{2max} or more, and carbohydrate (primarily muscle glycogen) is the primary fuel source. An endurance athlete can sustain exercise at 85% of VO_{2max} for approximately 90 minutes. During an ultra-endurance event, the exercise intensity averages about 65% of VO_{2max} or less and fat is the primary fuel source. An ultra-endurance athlete can sustain exercise at 65% of VO_{2max} for approximately 8 hours (2).

446

Fat oxidation reaches its peak during prolonged exercise at approximately 65% of VO_{2max}. Plasma fatty acids and intramuscular triglycerides contribute equally to fat oxidation during exercise at 65% of VO_{2max} in endurance-trained individuals (2,3).

Energy Intake

Endurance athletes should consume adequate energy and carbohydrate during training to maintain a desirable training intensity and thus maximize training adaptations. As shown in Table 22.1, these athletes have high energy requirements (4–8).

To meet energy demands, endurance athletes often need to eat meals and snacks continuously throughout the day. They should fine-tune their fueling strategies based on exercise intensity, duration, and mode, and environmental conditions. Testing specific foods and fluids before, during, and after training sessions also allows the athlete to determine effective fueling strategies for competition (9–11).

Failure to match energy intake to energy expenditure during training impairs endurance performance because of muscle and liver glycogen depletion (11). Compared to male endurance athletes, female endurance athletes are more likely to consume insufficient energy (11). However, Martin and associates reported that most elite female cyclists modulated energy intake based on energy expenditure (8).

Energy requirements for competition are often higher than during training, especially for ultra-endurance events (eg, Ironman triathlon, 100-mile runs) and multiple-day events, as shown in Table 22.2 (12–22). In ultra-endurance events lasting up to 24 hours, it is not necessary or practical to meet total energy expenditure (23).

Kimber et al determined that the average energy expenditure of triathletes in the New Zealand Ironman triathlon was much greater than their average energy intake, creating a substantial energy deficit for both men (5,973 kcal) and women (5,213 kcal) (12). This finding indicates that the triathletes obtained a large amount (59%) of their energy during the Ironman from endogenous fuel stores. The authors noted that total energy expenditure was similar between sexes when adjusted for fat-free mass (12).

TABLE 22.1   Energy Intakes of Endurance and Ultra-endurance Athletes

Type of Athlete (Reference)	Energy Intake, kcal/d
Male elite ultra-endurance triathletes[a] (4)	Training: 4,079
Male marathon runners[b] (4)	Training: 3,570
Male elite Kenyan distance runners (5)	Training: 3,478
Male Japanese distance runners[c] (6)	Training: 3,784
Male elite road cyclists (7)	Training: 5,333 Racing: 5,452
Female elite road cyclists (8)	Training: 3,261 Racing: 3,540

[a]8.1 miles swimming, 202 miles cycling, 47 miles running per week.
[b]91.6 miles/wk.
[c]405 miles/mo.

TABLE 22.2 Energy Intake and Energy Expenditure of Endurance and Ultra-endurance Athletes

Type of Athlete (Reference)	Energy Intake and Expenditure During Competition, kcal/d
Male New Zealand Ironman triathletes (12)	Intake: 3,940 Expenditure: 10,036
Female New Zealand Ironman triathletes (12)	Intake: 3,115 Expenditure: 8,570
Male ultra-runners[a] (13)	Intake: 6,047 Expenditure: 13,560
Male and female ultra-runners[b] (14)	Intake: 7,022 Expenditure: 9,538
Male Tour de France cyclists (15)	Intake: 5,785 Expenditure: 6,069
Male Pony Express Trail cyclists[c] (16)	Intake: 7,125 Expenditure: Not reported
Male Tour de Spain cyclists (17)	Intake: 5,595 Expenditure: Not reported
Male Run Around Australia runner[d] (12,18)	Intake: ~6,000 (12) Expenditure: 6,321 (19)
Male Sydney to Melbourne runner[e] (19)	Intake: 5,952 Expenditure: Not reported
Male RAAM cyclist[f] (20)	Intake: 8,429 Expenditure: Not reported
Male RAAM cyclist (4th place finish)[g] (21)	Intake: 9,612 Expenditure: Not reported
Female RAAM cyclist (1st place finish)[h] (22)	Intake: 7,950 Expenditure: Not reported

Abbreviation: RAAM, Race Across America.
[a] 100-mile run; 24.3 hours.
[b] 100-mile run; 26.2 hours.
[c] 2,050 miles in 10 days.
[d] 9,053 miles in 191 days.
[e] 628 miles in 8.5 days.
[f] 10 days, 7 hours, and 53 minutes.
[g] 9 days, 16 hours, and 45 minutes.
[h] 12 days, 6 hours, and 21 minutes.

Glace et al found that male ultra-runners incurred an energy deficit of 7,513 kcal in 24.3 hours during a 100-mile run (13). In another study, Glace et al found that male and female ultra-runners incurred an energy deficit of 2,516 kcal in 26.2 hours during a 100-mile run (14).

During multiple-day events (eg, Tour de France, RAAM), energy intake should match energy expenditure as much as possible to promote glycogen restoration, preservation of lean tissue, and an adequate intake of macro- and micronutrients (6). Saris et al found that mean daily energy intake (5,785 kcal) closely matched energy expenditure (6,069 kcal) and maintained body weight and composition for five male cyclists competing in the Tour de France (15). Two case studies, the one involving a runner (16) and the other involving two cyclists (19), found that the athletes maintained their body weight and composition over 9 to 10 days of ultra-endurance exercise, suggesting that energy intake was adequate to meet energy demands.

Remarkably, an athlete who ran around Australia only lost about 5 kg after averaging approximately 47 miles/d for 191 days. O'Connor noted that a typical day's intake provided about 100 g of protein, more than 1,000 g of carbohydrate, and 120 g of fat (23).

Practical suggestions to increase energy and carbohydrate intake are provided in subsequent sections of this chapter.

Nutrients

Carbohydrate

Adequate carbohydrate stores (muscle and liver glycogen and blood glucose) are critical for optimum endurance performance. Fatigue during endurance exercise is often associated with muscle glycogen depletion and/or hypoglycemia. Thus, nutritional strategies that optimize carbohydrate availability before, during, and after exercise are recommended to improve endurance performance (1).

Nutrient-dense carbohydrate foods and fluids should be emphasized during training because they contain other nutrients such as vitamins and minerals that are important for the overall diet as well as recovery from exercise (11).

The athlete's carbohydrate and energy intake should be adjusted or "periodized" to meet the requirements of the particular training cycle or phase for his or her sport. Excessive energy intake during light training can cause an increase in body fat, which may have a negative effect on performance. Conversely, inadequate carbohydrate and energy intake during heavy training can cause loss of lean tissue, depleted carbohydrate stores, and impaired performance. Ideally, the athlete should lose excess body fat in the off-season or early in the training cycle (24). The recommended daily carbohydrate intake for endurance athletes is found in Box 22.1.

BOX 22.1   Daily Carbohydrate Intake Recommendations for Endurance and Ultra-endurance Athletes

- Daily carbohydrate intake should be in the range of 5–12 g/kg. Adjust intake goals with consideration of the athlete's total energy needs, specific training needs, and feedback from training performance.
- Carbohydrate intake should be spread over the day (before, during, and after exercise) to promote fuel availability for key training sessions.
- The following are examples of daily guidelines for various activity levels:
  - 5–7 g/kg: moderate-intensity training programs for 1 h/d.
  - 6–10 g/kg: moderate- to high-intensity endurance exercise for 1–3 h/d.
  - 8–12 g/kg: moderate- to high-intensity exercise for 4–5 h/d.

TABLE 22.3 Average Daily Macronutrient Intake in Endurance and Ultra-endurance Athletes

Type of Athlete (Reference)	Carbohydrate, g/kg	Protein, g/kg	Fat, g/kg (Percentage of Energy Intake)
Male elite ultra-endurance triathletes, training (4)	9	2	1.8 (27%)
Male marathon runners (4)	8	2	2 (32%)
Male elite Kenyan distance runners (5)	9	2.1	1 (17%)
Male elite road cyclists (7)	Training: 11 Racing: 12	Training: 2.9 Racing: 2.6	Training: 2.8 (29.9%) Racing: 2.2 (25.3%)
Female elite road cyclists (8)	Training: 9 Racing: 9.9	Training: 2.6 Racing: 2.2	Training and racing: 1 (17%)
Male Tour de France cyclists (15)	12	3.1	2.1 (23%)
Male Pony Express Trail cyclists,[a] racing (16)	18	2.7	3.5 (27%)
Male Tour de Spain cyclists, racing (17)	12.6	3.0	2.3 (25.5)
Male Sydney to Melbourne runner,[b] racing (19)	17	2.9	3.2 (27%)
Male RAAM cyclist,[c] racing (20)	22.6	3.6	1.0 (9%)
Male RAAM cyclist (4th place finish),[d] racing (21)	24.8	2.8	2.3 (16.2%)

Abbreviation: RAAM, Race Across America.
[a] 2,050 miles in 10 days.
[b] 628 miles in 8.5 days.
[c] 10 days, 7 hours, and 53 minutes.
[d] 9 days, 16 hours, and 45 minutes.

Results of dietary surveys of male endurance athletes published between 1990 and 1999 suggest that they consume an appropriate amount of carbohydrate (7.6 g/kg/d). Results of dietary surveys of female endurance athletes published between 1990 and 1999 suggest they are less likely to consume adequate dietary carbohydrate because of lower energy intakes (5.7 g/kg/d) (11). Table 22.3 provides average daily macronutrient intake in endurance athletes (4,5,7,8,15–17,19–21).

Training for endurance events involves hours of prolonged exercise that may include multiple daily training sessions. The stress of such rigorous training can decrease appetite, resulting in reduced consumption of energy and carbohydrate (11,25). As discussed in Chapter 2, athletes who train heavily and have difficulty eating enough can consume a high-carbohydrate liquid supplement.

Brouns et al evaluated the effect of a simulated Tour de France on food and fluid intake, energy balance, and substrate oxidation (25). Although the cyclists consumed 630 g of carbohydrate (8.6 g/kg/d), they oxidized 850 g carbohydrate per day (11.6 g/kg/d). In spite of ad libitum intake of conventional foods, the cyclists were unable to ingest sufficient carbohydrate and calories to compensate for their increased energy expenditure. When the diet was supplemented with a 20% carbohydrate beverage, carbohydrate intake increased to 16 g/kg/d and carbohydrate oxidation rose to 13 g/kg/d (25).

Lindeman (20) reported that a male cyclist who competed in the RAAM obtained most of his total energy intake from a high-carbohydrate liquid supplement (23% carbohydrate). Saris et al (15) reported that approximately 30% of the total carbohydrate consumed by Tour de France cyclists came from high-carbohydrate beverages (eg, sport drinks, soft drinks, and liquid meals).

Athletes who have extremely high carbohydrate requirements and suppressed appetites due to heavy endurance training or competition should include compact, low-fiber forms of carbohydrate, such as pasta, white rice, sport bars and gels, baked goods (cake, tarts, biscuits), and sugar-rich foods (eg, candy). Carbohydrate-rich fluids such as sport drinks, juices, high-carbohydrate liquid supplements, low-fat chocolate milk, soft drinks, commercial liquid meals, milkshakes, yogurt drinks, and fruit smoothies may also be appealing to athletes who are very tired and dehydrated (11,23).

In addition to high-carbohydrate beverages, the Tour de France cyclists consumed sweet cakes, bread, macaroni, spaghetti, sugar, margarine/butter, meat, muesli, cheese, and yogurt. O'Connor and Cox (23) noted that the athlete who completed the run around Australia consumed pancakes, toast, porridge, sandwiches with protein fillings, rice/pasta, "instant" noodle meals, muffins, cereal bars, fruit, sweets/pastries, canned vegetables, cheese, tofu, eggs, nuts, fish, and pasta in addition to carbohydrate-rich fluids. A large range of sport foods (ie, liquid meals, sport bars, sport gels, high-carbohydrate supplements, and sport drinks) were used because they are easy to consume, portable, and easy to store (23).

Protein

Although acute endurance exercise results in the oxidation of several amino acids, the total amount of amino acid oxidation amounts to only 1% to 6% of the total energy cost of exercise. A low-energy and/or low-carbohydrate intake will increase amino acid oxidation and total protein requirements (26,27).

During low- to moderate-intensity endurance activity, protein intake of 1.2 g/kg/d is sufficient when energy and carbohydrate intake are adequate (27). Elite endurance athletes may require 1.6 g/kg/d (twice the recommended dietary allowance of protein for sedentary people) (27–30). In a simulated Tour de France cycling study, Brouns et al found that well-trained male cyclists required protein intake of 1.5 to 1.8 g/kg/d to maintain nitrogen balance (28). Tarnopolsky et al found that elite male endurance athletes required 1.6 g/kg/d to maintain nitrogen balance (29), and Friedman and Lemon found that well-trained endurance runners required 1.5 g/kg/d to maintain nitrogen balance (30).

Studies of male endurance athletes suggest that they are consuming an appropriate amount of protein. The data on female endurance athletes are extremely limited, as shown in Table 22.3.

The athlete's sex may affect protein metabolism. During endurance exercise, women oxidize more lipids and less carbohydrate and protein compared to equally trained and nourished men. Female endurance athletes may have a 10% to 20% lower protein requirement compared to male endurance athletes (26). This seems to be due to sex-based hormonal responses that promote fat metabolism in women and carbohydrate-protein metabolism in men (26). Endurance athletes can meet their higher protein requirements by consuming a mixed diet that provides adequate energy and 15% of energy from protein (26).

Although most endurance athletes get sufficient protein, those with low-energy and/or reduced-carbohydrate intakes may require nutrition counseling to optimize dietary protein intake (26).

Fat

The Food and Nutrition Board of the Institute of Medicine established an Acceptable Macronutrient Distribution Range (AMDR) for fat at 20% to 35% of total energy intake (31). Endurance athletes should consume at least 1 g/kg/d. Studies of male endurance athletes suggest they are consuming an appropriate amount of fat. The data on female endurance athletes is extremely limited, as shown in Table 22.3.

Micronutrients

Endurance athletes who consume adequate total energy usually meet or exceed population reference values such as the Dietary Reference Intakes (DRIs) for vitamins and minerals. Consuming a nutrient-dense diet containing fruits, vegetables, whole grains, legumes, lean meat, and dairy foods during training also helps to ensure adequate micronutrient intake (32).

Endurance athletes who regularly restrict energy intake or eat a limited variety of foods may be at risk for suboptimal micronutrient intakes. Some endurance and ultra-endurance athletes may have increased requirements due to excessive losses in sweat and or urine (32).

Supplementation may be necessary when intake is inadequate. However, athletes should not exceed the Tolerable Upper Intake Level (UL) for any nutrient to prevent possible adverse effects on health and performance. Supplementation with single micronutrients is not recommended (32) unless there is a medical necessity (eg, iron to treat iron-deficiency anemia).

The dietary antioxidant vitamins C and E play an important role in protecting cell membranes from oxidative damage. Although endurance exercise is associated with increased oxidative stress, it also increases the body's enzymatic and nonenzymatic antioxidant defenses as an adaptation to training (33). In fact, there may be negative effects from the routine consumption of antioxidant supplements during endurance training. Several studies have found that suppression of free radical generation during exercise can attenuate some of the signals for endogenous adaptation to endurance training (34,35). Until research suggests otherwise, it is prudent to recommend that endurance and ultra-endurance athletes consume an antioxidant-rich diet, rather than supplements, to protect against oxidative damage (33–35).

Endurance training can increase iron requirements (due to increases in hemoglobin, myoglobin, and iron-containing proteins involved in aerobic metabolism) and iron losses (through sweating, gastrointestinal bleeding, and mechanical trauma such as foot strike hemolysis). The debilitating effects of iron-deficiency anemia on endurance performance are well established. Anemia impairs erythropoiesis (red blood cell formation), thereby limiting oxygen delivery to the muscles, VO_{2max}, and endurance performance (36–38).

The effects of iron depletion (stage 1 iron deficiency) on endurance performance are less clear. At the very least, iron depletion can progress to iron-deficiency anemia if untreated. Endurance and ultra-endurance athletes, especially female athletes and runners of both sexes, are at risk for depleting their iron stores (37). Although depleted iron stores should not affect VO_{2max} because hemoglobin levels are not compromised, inadequate tissue iron stores may reduce oxidative metabolism in the muscle and impair endurance performance (39,40).

Recent research, using a new indicator for tissue iron deficiency known as serum transferrin receptor, suggests that even stage 1 iron deficiency (depleted iron stores) may compromise aerobic and endurance capacity (39). Hinton et al found that iron supplementation in iron-depleted, nonanemic women significantly improved endurance capacity and serum ferritin and serum transferrin receptor concentrations, but the supplementation did not affect hemoglobin concentrations (39). Further analysis of this data showed that tissue iron deficiency impaired adaptations to endurance training (40). Subjects with the most tissue iron depletion also showed the greatest improvement in endurance capacity after supplementation (41).

Athletes at risk for iron deficiency should have routine checks of their iron status. A low plasma ferritin level (< 20 mcg/dL) may indicate tissue iron deficiency, which can impair endurance. The athlete's iron stores can be increased through diet and/or iron supplementation to prevent the negative consequences of iron deficiency (36).

Inadequate dietary calcium and vitamin D increase the risk of low bone mineral density and stress fractures. Female endurance and ultra-endurance athletes who have low energy intakes, eliminate dairy products, or have menstrual dysfunction are at high risk for low bone mineral density. Supplementation with calcium and vitamin D should be determined after nutrition assessment (38).

There are limited data on the micronutrient intake of endurance athletes. Data on the micronutrient intake of female endurance athletes are virtually nonexistent. Burke et al found that male ultra-endurance triathletes and marathoners had adequate intakes of the major micronutrients during training (7). Singh et al reported that ultra-marathoners had adequate pre-race intakes of vitamins and minerals from both food and supplements (42). The biochemical indexes of the ultra-marathoners' vitamin and mineral status were also normal (42). Lindeman noted that a male cyclist had an adequate intake of micronutrients during training for the RAAM (20). García-Rovés et al reported that all of the vitamin and mineral intakes for elite male cyclists during training and competition were more than the Recommended Dietary Allowances (RDAs) (17).

O'Connor and Cox reported that the male ultra-distance runner who completed the run around Australia consumed two to three times the RDA for micronutrients (23). Eden and Abernathy found that all of the micronutrients except riboflavin were met in the diet of a male ultra-distance runner competing in the Australian Sydney to Melbourne foot race (19).

Gabel et al found that vitamin and mineral intakes were two to three times the RDA for most vitamins and minerals for two male cyclists during a 10-day, 2,050-mile ride (16). Saris et al found that Tour de France cyclists had low intakes of thiamin (in spite of very high energy intakes) due to their high consumption of refined carbohydrate foods such as sweet cakes and soft drinks (15). The researchers conceded that any questions and concerns about food quality and nutrient density became immaterial after the consideration of micronutrients from supplements, whether from pills or injections (15).

Water and Sodium

Drinking or hydration during endurance exercise is necessary to prevent the detrimental effects of excessive dehydration (> 2% body weight loss) and electrolyte loss on exercise performance and health. Dehydration increases physiologic stress as measured by core temperature, heart rate, and perceived exertion, and these effects are accentuated during exercise in warm to hot weather. The greater the body-water shortage, the greater the physiologic strain and greater the impairment of endurance performance (43).

It is not possible to propose a one-size-fits-all fluid and electrolyte replacement schedule because of the multiple factors that influence sweating rate and sweat electrolyte concentration (43). Endurance and ultra-endurance athletes who have high sweat rates and a high sweat-sodium concentration ("salty sweat") can sustain substantial losses of sodium (44).

Symptomatic exercise-associated hyponatremia (plasma sodium concentration < 135 mmol/L) can occur in prolonged endurance exercise lasting more than 4 hours. Contributing factors to exercise-associated hyponatremia include drinking an amount of fluid that exceeds sweat and urinary water losses and excessive loss of total body sodium (43).

In events that last less than 4 hours, hyponatremia is primarily caused by overdrinking before, during, and after the event (44,45). During a marathon, symptomatic hyponatremia is more likely to occur in smaller and less lean individuals who run slowly, sweat less, and drink excessively before, during, and after the race (44,45).

During prolonged ultra-endurance exercise (eg, Ironman triathlon), total sodium losses can induce symptomatic hyponatremia if the athlete is drinking too little or too much fluid (43). High sweat rates and a high sweat-sodium concentration confer a greater risk of developing hyponatremia because less fluid intake is required to produce dangerously low blood sodium levels (44).

TABLE 22.4 Fluid and Sodium Intake and Weight Loss in Endurance and Ultra-Endurance Athletes

Type of Athlete (Reference)	Fluid Intake	Sodium Intake	Weight Loss
Male elite Kenyan distance runners (5)	4.2 L/d	n/a	n/a
Male and female New Zealand Ironman triathletes (12)	Biking: 889 mL/h Running: 632 mL/h	n/a	Males: 3% Females: 4%
Male ultra-runners[a] (13)	18 L (0.7 L/h)	12 g (0.5 g/h)	2%
Male and female ultra-runners[b] (14)	19.4 L (0.7 L/h)	16.4 g (0.6 g/h)	0.5%
Male Tour de France cyclists (15)	6.7 L/d	n/a	n/a
Male Pony Express Trail cyclists[c] (16)	620 mL/h	n/a	n/a
Male Tour de Spain cyclists (17)	3.29 L/d	n/a	n/a
Male Run around Australia runner[d] (18)	6 L/d	n/a	n/a
Male Sydney to Melbourne runners[e] (19)	11 L/d	n/a	n/a
Male RAAM cyclist[f] (20)	15.7 L/d (~ 677 mL per hour of exercise)	n/a	n/a
Male 24-hour mountain bike racer (23)	13.5 L	12.3 g	n/a

Abbreviations: RAAM, Race Across America; n/a, not available.
[a] 100-mile run; 24.3 hours.
[b] 100-mile run; 26.2 hours.
[c] 2,050 miles in 10 days.
[d] 9,053 miles in 191 days; fluid intake assessed during 14-day period on the temperate eastern coast.
[e] 628 miles in 8.5 days.
[f] 10 days, 7 hours, and 53 minutes.

Endurance athletes can experience health problems from either dehydration or overdrinking. Dehydration is more common and can impair exercise performance and contribute to serious heat illness. However, symptomatic hyponatremia is more dangerous and can cause grave illness or death. Because of the considerable variability among individuals in sweat rates and sweat electrolyte content, athletes should customize their fluid replacement plans (43). More information on hydration and exercise is found in Chapter 6.

There are limited data on fluid and sodium intakes and body-weight changes during endurance events, as shown Table 22.4 (5,12–20,23).

Fueling and Fluid Replacement

Before Exercise

Carbohydrate loading can improve performance in endurance competitions exceeding 90 minutes. The regimen can be viewed as an extended period of "fueling up" to prepare for competition. Carbohydrate-loading guidelines are provided in Chapter 2.

Consuming carbohydrate prior to an endurance event may help to maintain blood glucose levels during prolonged exercise. The athlete should consume 1.0 to 4.0 g carbohydrate per kg of body weight, 1 to 4 hours before exercise. García-Rovés et al noted that the Tour de Spain cyclists consumed 4.5 g/kg approximately 3 hours before competition (17).

Foods typically consumed prior to endurance and ultra-endurance events include liquid meals, muesli, porridge, milk, yogurt, fruit and fruit juice, toast, jam, pancakes, and biscuits and jam or honey (15,17,19,23). Additional information on the pre-exercise meal is provided in Chapter 2.

Endurance athletes should also begin exercise with normal hydration and plasma electrolyte levels. Prior to exercise, the athlete should drink approximately 5 to 7 mL of fluid per kg of body weight about 4 hours before exercise; 7 mL/kg is equivalent to approximately 1 oz for every 10 lb of body weight. Drinking several hours before exercise allows adequate time for the urine output to return toward normal (40). Additional pre-exercise hydration guidelines are provided in Chapter 6.

Athletes should experiment with different pre-exercise foods and fluids during training. Before competition, the athlete should choose familiar, well-tolerated, and palatable foods and fluids (9).

During Exercise

Consuming carbohydrate is neither practical nor necessary during endurance exercise lasting less than 45 minutes (46). Small amounts of carbohydrate from sport drinks or foods may enhance performance during sustained high-intensity endurance exercise lasting 45 to 75 minutes (46). Athletes should consume 30 to 60 g of carbohydrate per hour from carbohydrate-rich fluids or foods during endurance sports and exercise lasting 1 to 2.5 hours (46). As the duration of the event increases, so does the amount of carbohydrate required to enhance performance (7). During endurance and ultra-endurance exercise lasting 2.5 to 3 hours and longer, athletes should consume up to 80 to 90 g carbohydrate per hour from products that provide multiple transportable carbohydrates (46).

Consuming carbohydrate in workouts enables the athlete to maintain a desirable training pace (and therefore maximize training adaptations) as well as practice fueling strategies for competition. Athletes should individually determine a refueling plan that meets their nutritional goals (including hydration) and minimizes gastrointestinal distress. Additional information on fueling during exercise is provided in Chapter 2. Table 22.5 shows the carbohydrate intake during various ultra-endurance events (12–17,19,23).

Kimber et al found that New Zealand Ironman triathletes consumed substantially more energy during the bike segment (2,233 kcal for women; 2,896 kcal for men) than during the run (883 kcal for women; 1,049 kcal for men). Energy intake during cycling provided 73% of the total energy intake. This is not surprising because foods and fluid are easier to consume and digest while on the bike, and the cycling portion was approximately 54% of the total race time. The bike portion of an Ironman also provides the opportunity to obtain energy and fluid in preparation for the marathon run (12).

Saris et al (15) found that Tour de France male cyclists consumed nearly half of their daily energy during the race, and (as noted previously in this chapter) about 30% of the total carbohydrate consumed came from high-carbohydrate beverages. Gabel et al found that two male cyclists consumed about 24% of their total energy intake from high-carbohydrate beverages (eg, sport drinks, fruit juices) during a 10-day, 2,050-mile ride (16). Eden and Abernathy reported that the male ultra-distance runner in the Sydney to Melbourne race utilized a combination of high-carbohydrate solid foods and a sport drink during running to meet his energy requirements (19).

Although high-carbohydrate beverages help increase carbohydrate and energy intake during endurance and ultra-endurance events, they may also cause gastrointestinal distress when consumed in large volumes.

TABLE 22.5 Carbohydrate Intake During Ultra-endurance Events

Type of Athlete (Reference)	Carbohydrate Intake, g/h
Male and female New Zealand Ironman triathletes (12)	Males: 82 Females: 62
Male ultra-runners[a] (13)	44
Male and female ultra-runners[b] (14)	54
Male Tour de France cyclists (15)	94
Male Pony Express Trail cyclists[c] (16)	60–75
Male Tour de Spain cyclists (17)	25
Male Sydney to Melbourne runner[d] (19)	39
Male 24-hour mountain bike racer (23)	75

[a] 100-mile run, 24.3 hours.
[b] 100-mile run, 26.2 hours.
[c] 2,050 miles in 10 days.
[d] 628 miles in 8.5 days.

Lindeman noted that a male RAAM cyclist's reliance on a 23% carbohydrate solution to meet the majority of his energy needs contributed to gastrointestinal distress during the race despite consistent dilution (20).

It is essential to have a variety of carbohydrate-rich foods and fluids available during ultra-endurance and multiday events to prevent "flavor fatigue" and an associated decrease in energy intake (23). Alternating between sweet choices (eg, gels, sodas, candy) and savory/salty choices (eg, vegetable soup, pretzels, baked chips) helps to maintain the athlete's desire to eat (23). Consuming solid food with small amounts of protein and fat (eg, a turkey, cheese, or peanut butter sandwich) also helps provide satiety and variety (23).

Consuming a small amount of protein during prolonged exercise improves protein balance. Koopman et al found that the combined ingestion of protein (0.25 g/kg/h) and carbohydrate (0.7 g/kg/h) before, during, and after prolonged moderate-intensity exercise (6 hours at 50% of VO_{2max}) improved net protein balance at rest, during exercise, and during subsequent recovery in endurance athletes (47).

Gabel et al reported that the two men who cycled 2,050 miles in 10 days achieved an optimal intake because of the variety and palatability of foods that were available during the event (16). The cyclists consumed sport drinks, fruit juices, sodas, potato chips, crackers, fruit, cookies, sandwiches, and candy. Eden and Abernathy noted that the foods eaten during the Sydney to Melbourne race were based on what the male runner had enjoyed eating during training and what he could tolerate while competing (19). The runner consumed a sport drink, pasta with meat sauce, rice, bread, biscuits, cheese, vegetable soup, muffin with egg and cheese, fruit, and fruit juice (19). O'Connor noted that the athlete who completed the run around Australia consumed sport drinks, fruit juice, soft drinks, high-carbohydrate supplements, milkshakes, and liquid meals during the run itself (23).

High-fiber foods should be limited during competition (10) to avoid gut distress such as abdominal bloating, cramping, and diarrhea. Lindeman noted that a male RAAM cyclist's high fiber intake (57 g/d) from consuming fiber-rich sports bars and fruit may have contributed to his gastrointestinal distress during the race (20).

Athletes should determine their hourly sweat rate and drink only enough to closely match fluid loss from sweating (43). The athlete should drink sufficient fluid to limit weight loss to 2% of initial body weight

(43). During endurance exercise, a loss of 1% to 2% of body weight is likely to occur from factors unrelated to sweat losses (substrate oxidation) and is acceptable (10). A weight loss of up to 3% may be tolerable and not impair performance in cool weather (43). Glace et al estimated that body fat loss (according to skinfold measurements) accounted for about 1.13 kg of the 1.6 kg lost (2% of body weight) during a 100-mile run (13). In a second study, Glace et al found that high fluid intakes during a 100-mile run were associated with decreased serum sodium levels and increased risk of mental status change, suggesting possible fluid overload (14).

To prevent hyponatremia, endurance athletes should avoid overconsumption of fluids and associated weight gain (43). Consuming a sodium-containing sport drink helps to maintain plasma sodium levels and may reduce the risk of hyponatremia during prolonged exercise (48,49).

Athletes participating in endurance exercise lasting longer than 3 hours should be particularly meticulous about establishing their fluid replacement schedule. As the exercise duration increases, the cumulative effects of slight disparities between fluid intake and loss can cause extreme dehydration or hyponatremia (43).

During training, athletes should experiment with different fluid replacement drinks and adjust their drinking strategies based on the workout intensity, duration, and environmental conditions. Drinking appropriately in workouts enables the athlete to maintain a desirable training pace (and maximize training adaptations), protects against heat illness, and allows the athlete to practice proper drinking strategies for competition (5). Additional information on fluid replacement during exercise is provided in Chapter 6.

When the athlete's gut blood flow is low (eg, during intense cycling or running), the athlete should emphasize carbohydrate-rich fluids (sport drinks, liquid meals, high-carbohydrate liquid supplements, fruit juices, and carbohydrate gels) to promote rapid gastric emptying and intestinal absorption. When the athlete's gut blood flow is moderate (eg, during moderate-paced cycling or slow running), the athlete may be able to consume easily digested carbohydrate-rich foods such as sport bars, fruit, and grain products (fig bars, bagels, graham crackers) in addition to liquid foods and fluids (50).

Athletes can generally consume more calories per hour cycling than running (10). Ironman triathlon competitors often decrease their calorie intake toward the end of the bike segment to start the run with a fairly empty gut. During the run segment of a triathlon, the athletes usually consume only sport drinks, gels, and water to reduce the risk of gut distress.

The athlete should develop and refine a fueling and hydration plan weeks and even months ahead of the priority race by experimenting in workouts and in lower-priority races (10). The athlete should test this fueling plan while exercising at race pace and in environmental conditions that simulate the race conditions (10). Athletes should not consume untested foods or fluids during the race because the result may be severe indigestion and poor performance.

Endurance athletes should consume liquid or solid fuel before feeling hungry or tired, usually within the first hour of exercise. Consuming small amounts at frequent intervals (every 15 to 20 minutes) helps prevent gastrointestinal upset, maintain blood glucose levels, and promote hydration (10,19). The athlete's foods and fluids should be easily digestible, familiar (tested in training), and enjoyable (to encourage eating and drinking) (10,16,19,23).

After Exercise

Restoring muscle and liver glycogen stores, replacing fluid and electrolyte losses, and promoting muscle repair are important for recovery after strenuous endurance training and multiday events.

When there is less than 8 hours between workouts or competitions that deplete muscle glycogen stores, the athlete should start consuming carbohydrate immediately after the first exercise session to maximize the effective recovery time between sessions (46). The athlete should consume carbohydrate at a rate of

1 to 1.2 g/kg/h for the first 4 hours after glycogen-depleting exercise (46). Consuming small amounts of carbohydrate frequently (every 15 to 30 minutes) further enhances muscle glycogen synthesis (46). During longer periods of recovery (24 hours), it does not matter how carbohydrate intake is spaced throughout the day as long as the athlete consumes adequate carbohydrate and energy (46). Liquid forms of carbohydrate may be desirable when athletes have decreased appetites due to fatigue and/or dehydration.

The athlete's initial recovery snack/meal should include 15 to 25 g high-quality protein in addition to carbohydrate (46). Consuming protein with recovery snacks and meals helps to increase net muscle protein balance, promote muscle tissue repair, and enhance adaptations involving synthesis of new proteins (51). Adding a small amount of protein (~ 0.3 g/kg/h) to a suboptimal carbohydrate intake (< 1 g/kg/h) also accelerates muscle glycogen restoration (52). Recovery meals and snacks contribute toward the athlete's daily protein and carbohydrate requirements (11). Additional information on recovery is found in Chapters 2 and 3. García-Rovés et al noted that the Tour of Spain cyclists consumed carbohydrate at a rate of 1.1 g/kg/h and protein at a rate of 0.35 g/kg/h for the first 6 hours after the race (17). This combined dose of carbohydrate and protein helped promote muscle glycogen restoration and muscle tissue repair.

The foods consumed during recovery meals and snacks should contribute to the athlete's overall nutrient intake. Nutritious carbohydrate-rich foods and lean sources of protein and dairy also contain vitamins and minerals that are essential for health and performance. These micronutrients are important for postexercise recovery processes. Athletes should avoid consuming large amounts of foods high in fat or protein when total energy requirements or gastrointestinal distress limits food intake during recovery. These foods can displace carbohydrate-rich foods and reduce muscle glycogen storage (11).

Ideally, the athlete should fully restore fluid and electrolyte losses between exercise sessions (43). Consuming sodium during recovery promotes fluid retention and stimulates thirst (53). Sodium losses are harder to determine than water losses because athletes have vastly different rates of sweat electrolyte losses (43). Although drinks containing sodium (eg, sport drinks) may be beneficial, many foods can supply the needed electrolytes (43). Extra salt can be added to meals and recovery fluids when sweat sodium losses are high; ½ tsp (2.5 g) salt supplies 1,000 mg sodium (43).

Athletes should drink 24 oz of fluid for each pound lost to achieve rapid and total recovery from dehydration (54). The additional volume (150% of sweat losses) is required to compensate for the increased urine production that goes along with the rapid intake of large volumes of fluid (43,54). Additional information on fluid replacement after exercise is provided in Chapter 6.

Ultra-endurance and Multiday Events

The importance of proper fueling and hydration during ultra-endurance and multiday events cannot be overemphasized. The athlete's fueling and fluid replacement strategies can mean the difference between completing the event and dropping out of the race (23).

During the event, the athlete's primary nutritional requirements are water, carbohydrate, and sodium (10,23). Athletes should limit foods that are high in fat, protein, and fiber during exercise to decrease the risk of gastrointestinal distress (10). The following pointers are also helpful:

- The food plan should be built around the athlete's food preferences and include a variety of foods (savory/salty and sweet) rather than a restricted assortment (16,19,22,23).
- Food and fluid intake should be closely monitored during multiday events (16,19,20,23). The crew should be prepared to enforce an eating and drinking schedule. If necessary, separate timers can be set for both liquid and solid feedings (22).

- Food records and body weight should be assessed daily during multiple-day events. By tracking the athlete's food and fluid intake and body weight, the crew can take immediate corrective action, without overfeeding or causing GI distress, if the athlete starts to fall behind on fluid or energy intake (16,22).
- Solid food should be easy to handle, chew, and digest (23). Beverages should promote rapid absorption of fluids and nutrients (43). Concentrated nutrition such as high-carbohydrate supplements or liquid meals may be offered immediately before scheduled rest (20,22,44).

The advice of a registered dietitian with expertise in sports nutrition, such as a Board Certified Specialist in Sports Dietetics (CSSD), is recommended to determine the ultra-endurance athlete's nutritional requirements and develop an individualized dietary plan. The sports dietitian can also help monitor the athlete's nutrition during multiple-day events and help enforce food and fluid intake when necessary (16,19,20,23).

Summary

Endurance athletes should consume adequate energy and carbohydrate (5 to 12 g/kg/d) during training to maintain a desirable training intensity and thus maximize training adaptations. Their increased protein requirements (~1.2 to 1.6 g/kg/d) can be met by consuming a mixed diet that provides adequate energy and 15% of the calories from protein. Endurance athletes should consume at least 1 g of fat per kg of body weight (~20% to 35% of calories from fat).

Endurance athletes who consume adequate total energy usually meet or exceed population reference values such as the DRI for vitamins and minerals. Consuming a nutrient-dense diet containing fruits, vegetables, whole grains, legumes, lean meat, and dairy foods during training and competition also helps to ensure adequate micronutrient intake. Endurance training can increase iron requirements as well as iron losses.

Drinking during endurance exercise is necessary to prevent the detrimental effects of excessive dehydration (> 2% body weight loss) and electrolyte loss on exercise performance and health. Athletes should customize their fluid replacement plans because of the considerable variability in sweating rates and sweat electrolyte content between individuals.

Carbohydrate loading can improve performance in endurance events exceeding 90 minutes. For most athletes, a carbohydrate loading regimen will involve 3 days of a high-carbohydrate intake (10 to 12 g of carbohydrate per kg) and tapered training. Consuming carbohydrate prior to exercise can help performance by "topping off" muscle and liver glycogen stores. The pre-exercise meal should contain approximately 1 to 4 g of carbohydrate per kg, consumed 1 to 4 hours before exercise. The athlete should also slowly drink about 5 to 7 mL/kg at least 4 hours before activity.

Consuming carbohydrate during exercise can improve performance by maintaining blood glucose levels and carbohydrate oxidation. Small amounts of carbohydrate from sport drinks or foods may enhance performance during sustained high-intensity endurance exercise lasting 45 to 75 minutes. Athletes should consume 30 to 60 g of carbohydrate per hour from carbohydrate-rich fluids or foods during endurance sports and exercise lasting 1 to 2.5 hours. During endurance and ultra-endurance exercise lasting 2.5 to 3 hours and longer beyond, athletes should consume up to 80 to 90 g of carbohydrate per hour.

Consuming carbohydrate following exercise facilitates rapid refilling of carbohydrate stores. During the early period of recovery (0 to 4 hours), the endurance athlete should consume 1 to 1.2 g/kg/h. The athlete's initial recovery snack/meal should also include 15 to 25 g high-quality protein to promote muscle tissue repair. Endurance athletes should drink 24 oz of fluid for each pound lost and consume adequate sodium to achieve rapid and total recovery from dehydration.

Endurance athletes should practice adjusting their fueling strategies based on workout intensity, duration, and environmental conditions. Testing specific foods and fluids before, during, and after training sessions also allows the athlete to determine effective fueling strategies for competition.

References

1. Hargreaves M. Exercise physiology and metabolism. In: Burke L, Deakin V, eds. *Clinical Sports Nutrition*. 3rd ed. Sydney, Australia: McGraw-Hill; 2006:1–20.
2. Coyle EF. Substrate utilization during exercise in active people. *Am J Clin Nutr*. 61(suppl):1995;968S–979S.
3. Hawley J, Burke L. Nutritional strategies to enhance fat oxidation during aerobic exercise. In: Burke L, Deakin V, eds. *Clinical Sports Nutrition*. 3rd ed. Sydney, Australia: McGraw-Hill; 2006:455–483.
4. Burke LM, Gollan RA, Reed RSD. Dietary intakes and food use of groups of elite Australian male athletes. *Int J Sport Nutr Exerc Metab*. 1991;1:378–394.
5. Fudge BW, Westerterp KR, Kiplamai FK, Onywera VO, Boit MK, Kayser B, Pitsiladis YP. Evidence of negative energy balance using doubly labeled water in elite Kenyan endurance runners prior to competition. *Br J Nutr*. 2006;95:59–66.
6. Motonaga K, Yoshida S, Yamagami F, Kawano T, Takeda E. Estimation of total daily energy expenditure and its components by monitoring the heart rate of Japanese endurance athletes. *J Nutr Sci Vitaminol* (Tokyo). 2006;52:360–367.
7. García-Rovés PM, Terrados N, Fernández S, Patterson AM. Comparison of dietary intake and eating behavior of professional road cyclists during training and competition. *Int J Sport Nutr Exerc Metab*. 2000;10:82–98.
8. Martin MK, Martin DT, Collier GR, Burke LM. Voluntary food intake by elite female cyclists during training and racing: influence of daily energy expenditure and body composition. *Int J Sport Nutr Exerc Metab*. 2002;12:249–267.
9. Burke L. Preparation for competition. In: Burke L, Deakin V, eds. *Clinical Sports Nutrition*. 3rd ed. Sydney, Australia: McGraw-Hill; 2006:355–384.
10. Maughan R. Fluid and carbohydrate intake during exercise. In: Burke L, Deakin V, eds. *Clinical Sports Nutrition*. 3rd ed. Sydney Australia: McGraw-Hill; 2006:385–414.
11. Burke L. Nutrition for recovery after training and competition. In: Burke L, Deakin V, eds. *Clinical Sports Nutrition*. 3rd ed. Sydney, Australia: McGraw-Hill; 2006:415–453.
12. Kimber NE, Ross JJ, Mason SL, Speedy DB. Energy balance during an ironman triathlon in male and female triathletes. *Int J Sport Nutr Exerc Metab*. 2002;12:47–62.
13. Glace B, Murphy C, McHugh M. Food and fluid intake and disturbances in gastrointestinal and mental function during an ultramarathon. *Int J Sport Nutr Exerc Metab*. 2002;2:414–427.
14. Glace BW, Murphy CA, McHugh MP. Food intake and electrolyte status of ultramarathoners competing in extreme heat. *J Am Coll Nutr*. 2002;21:553–559.
15. Saris WHM, van Erp-Baart MA, Brouns F, Westerterp KR, ten Hoor F. Study of food intake and energy expenditure during extreme sustained exercise: the Tour de France. *Int J Sport Med*. 1989;10(Suppl 1):S26–S31.
16. Gabel KA, Aldous A, Edgington C. Dietary intake of two elite male cyclists during a 10 day, 2,050 mile ride. *Int J Sport Nutr*. 1995;5:56–61.
17. García-Rovés PM, Terrados N, Fernández S, Patterson AM. Macronutrient intake of top level cyclists during continuous competition—change in the feeding pattern. *Int J Sports Med*. 1998;19:61–67.
18. Hill RJ, Davies PS. Energy expenditure during 2 wk of an ultra-endurance run around Australia. *Med Sci Sports Exerc*. 2001;33:148–151.
19. Eden BD, Abernathy PJ. Nutritional intake during an ultra-endurance running race. *Int J Sport Nutr*. 1994;4:166–174.
20. Lindeman AK. Nutrient intake of an ultra-endurance cyclist. *Int J Sport Nutr*. 1991;1:79–85.
21. Knechtle B, Enggist A, Jehle T. Energy turnover at the Race Across America (RAAM): a case report. *Int J Sports Med*. 2005;26:499–503.

22. Clark N, Tobin J, Ellis C. Feeding the ultra-endurance athlete: practical tips and a case study. *J Am Diet Assoc.* 1992;92:1258–1262.

23. O'Connor H, Cox G. Feeding ultra-endurance athletes: an interview with Dr. Helen O'Connor and Gregory Cox. Interview by Louise M Burke. *Int J Sport Nutr Exerc Metab.* 2002;12:490–494.

24. O'Connor H, Caterson I. Weight loss and the athlete. In: Burke L, Deakin V, eds. *Clinical Sports Nutrition.* 3rd ed. Sydney, Australia: McGraw-Hill; 2006.

25. Brouns F, Saris WH, Stroecken J, Beckers E, Thijssen R, Rehrer NJ, ten Hoor F. Eating, drinking, and cycling: a controlled Tour de France simulation study, part II. Effect of diet manipulation. *Int J Sport Med.* 1989;10(Suppl 1): S41–S48.

26. Tarnopolsky M. Protein and amino acid needs for bulking up. In: Burke L, Deakin V, eds. *Clinical Sports Nutrition.* 3rd ed. Sydney, Australia: McGraw-Hill; 2006:73–111.

27. Tarnopolsky M. Protein requirements for endurance athletes. *Nutrition.* 2004;20:662–668.

28. Brouns F, Saris WH, Stroecken J, Beckers E, Thijssen R, Rehrer NJ, ten Hoor F. Eating, drinking, and cycling. A controlled Tour de France simulation study. Part I. *Int J Sports Med.* 1989;10(Suppl 1):S32–S40.

29. Tarnopolsky MA, MacDougall JD, Atkinson SA. Influence of protein intake and training status on nitrogen balance and lean body mass. *J Appl Physiol.* 1988;64:187–193.

30. Friedman JE, Lemon PW. Effect of chronic endurance exercise on retention of dietary protein. *Int J Sports Med.* 1989;10:118–123.

31. Institute of Medicine. Dietary Reference Intakes for Energy, Carbohydrate, Fiber, Fat, Fatty Acids, Cholesterol, Protein, and Amino Acids. Washington, DC: National Academies Press; 2005.

32. Fogelholm M. Vitamin, mineral, and antioxidant needs of athletes. In: Burke L, Deakin V, eds. *Clinical Sports Nutrition.* 3rd ed. Sydney, Australia: McGraw-Hill; 2006.

33. Watson T. The science of anti-oxidants and exercise performance. In: Burke L, Deakin V, eds. *Clinical Sports Nutrition.* 3rd ed. Sydney, Australia: McGraw-Hill; 2006.

34. Gomez-Cabrera MC, Domenech E, Romagnoli M, Arduini A, Borras C, Pallardo FV, Sastre J, Viña J. Oral administration of vitamin C decreases muscle mitochondrial biogenesis and hampers training-induced adaptations in endurance performance. *Am J Clin Nutr.* 2008;87:142–149.

35. Ristow M, Zarse K, Oberbach A, Klöting N, Birringer M, Kiehntopf M, Stumvoll M, Kahn CR, Blüher M. Antioxidants prevent health-promoting effects of physical exercise in humans. *Proc Natl Acad Sci U S A.* 2009;106: 8665–8670.

36. Deakin V. Iron depletion in athletes. In: Burke L, Deakin V, eds. *Clinical Sports Nutrition.* 3rd ed. Sydney, Australia: McGraw-Hill; 2006:263–312.

37. Schumacher YO, Schmid A, Grathwohl D, Bültermann D, Berg A. Hematological indices and iron status in athletes of various sports and performances. *Med Sci Sports Exerc.* 2002;34:869–875.

38. Rodriguez NR, Di Marco NM, Langley S; American Dietetic Association; Dietitians of Canada; American College of Sports Medicine. Position of the American Dietetic Association, Dietitians of Canada, and the American College of Sports Medicine: nutrition and athletic performance. *J Am Diet Assoc.* 2009;109:509–527.

39. Hinton PS, Giordano C, Brownlie T, Haas JD. Iron supplementation improves endurance after training in iron-depleted, nonanemic women. *J Appl Physiol.* 2000;88:1103–1111.

40. Brownlie T, Utermohlen V, Hinton PS, Giordano C, Haas JD. Marginal iron deficiency without anemia impairs aerobic adaptation among previously untrained women. *Am J Clin Nutr.* 2002;75:734–742.

41. Brownlie T, Utermohlen V, Hinton PS, Haas JD. Tissue iron deficiency without anemia impairs adaptation in endurance capacity after aerobic training in previously untrained women. *Am J Clin Nutr.* 2004;79:437–443.

42. Singh A, Evans P, Gallagher KL, Deuster PA. Dietary intakes and biochemical profiles of nutritional status of ultramarathoners. *Med Sci Sports Exerc.* 1993;25:328–334.

43. Sawka MN, Burke LM, Eichner ER, Maughan RJ, Montain SJ, Stachenfeld NS. American College of Sports Medicine. Position stand: exercise and fluid replacement. *Med Sci Sports Exerc.* 2007;39:377–390.

44. Montain SJ, Cheuvront SN, Sawka NM. Exercise associated hyponatremia: quantitative analysis for understanding the aetiology. *Br J Sports Med.* 2006;40:98–106.

45. Hew TD, Chorley JN, Cianca JC, Divine JG. The incidence, risk factors, and clinical manifestations of hyponatremia in marathon runners. *Clin J Sports Med.* 2003;13:41–47.

46. Burke LM, Hawley JA, Wong S, Jeukendrup AE. Carbohydrates for training and competition. *J Sports Sci.* 2011 Jun 8:1–11. Epub ahead of print.

47. Koopman R, Pannemans DL, Jeukendrup AE, Gijsen AP, Senden JM, Halliday D. Combined ingestion of protein and carbohydrate improves protein balance during ultra-endurance exercise. *Am J Physiol Endocrinol Metab.* 2004;87:E712–E720.

48. Vrijens DM, Rehrer NJ. Sodium-free fluid ingestion decreases plasma sodium during exercise in the heat. *J Appl Physiol.* 1999;86:1847–1851.

49. Twerenbold R, Knechtle B, Kakebeeke TH, Eser P, Müller G, von Arx P, Knecht H. Effects of different sodium concentrations in replacement fluids during prolonged exercise in women. *Br J Sports Med.* 2004;37:300–303.

50. Laursen PB, Rhodes EC. Physiological analysis of a high-intensity ultra-endurance event. *J Strength Cond Res.* 1999;21:26–38.

51. Phillips SM, Moore DR, Tang JE. A critical examination of dietary protein requirements, benefits and excesses in athletes. *Int J Sport Nutr Exerc Metab.* 2007;17(Suppl):S58–S76.

52. Betts JA, Williams C. Short-term recovery from prolonged exercise: exploring the potential for protein ingestion to accentuate the benefits of carbohydrate supplements. *Sports Med.* 2010;40:941–959.

53. Nose HG, Mack W, Shi XR, Nadel ER. Involvement of sodium retention hormones during rehydration in humans. *J Appl Physiol.* 1988;65:332–336.

54. Shirreffs SM, Maughan RJ. Volume repletion after exercise-induced volume depletion in humans: replacement of water and sodium losses. *Am J Physiol.* 1998;274:F868–F875.

At A Glance

The preceding chapters help professionals understand the physiological and nutritional demands of related sports, but sports dietitians may find that they need a quick and easy reference for a specific sport. The At A Glance section features summaries for 18 sports. The summaries include brief descriptions of the sports and the URLs for Web sites where more information is available. General nutrition guidelines are included and can serve as a basis for an individualized plan. Common nutritional concerns are highlighted and briefly explained. These summaries may be helpful when preparing sports nutrition presentations for teams or as a topical guideline for an individual counseling session with an athlete.

BASEBALL AT A GLANCE

Baseball is a skill sport requiring fine-motor control, superb coordination, quick reaction time, as well as anaerobic power and general fitness conditioning. Baseball is not a high–energy demand sport because it is not a game of continuous activity. Professional baseball players begin spring training in February. The regular season is from April to September, followed by postseason play in October and then the off-season. Collegiate and youth baseball is a spring sport in school, and some players continue throughout the summer in recreational leagues. Learn more about the sport at the Major League Baseball Web site (http://www.mlb.com).

General Nutrition Guidelines

- Energy: Relatively low–energy expenditure sport.
- Carbohydrate: 3–5 g/kg/d.
- Protein: 1.2–1.7 g/kg/d.
- Fat: ~ 1.0 g/kg/d.

Common Nutritional Concerns

Weight Gain

Professional players may skip meals and then overeat, consume excess alcohol, and eat high-calorie snacks such as sunflower seeds during the game, all habits that can contribute to weight gain. Many overeat and reduce activity during the off-season.

Fluid Intake

Baseball is often played in hot and humid conditions and it is one of the only sports without a time limit. Dehydration is a daily concern.

Pregame Meal

Players often arrive for games having not eaten and must eat the food that is accessible, which is often high in calories, fat, sugar, and/or salt. Minor league players have a limited budget and seek out inexpensive food, which is often low in nutritional quality.

Postgame Meal

Late-night eating, large postgame meals, and alcohol intake often result in weight gain. Minor league and collegiate players typically eat fast food to break up a long bus ride.

Frequent Travel

Frequent travel makes it difficult to maintain a routine and increases exposure to high-calorie foods that are low in nutritional quality.

BASKETBALL AT A GLANCE

Basketball is an intermittent, high-intensity sport requiring strength, power, cardiovascular fitness, agility, and skill. It is usually played in four quarters with a break at halftime, although overtime periods are necessary if the game is tied. All of the body's energy systems are used to fuel the sport: adenosine triphosphate-creatine phosphate (ATP-CP) to jump and pass, the lactic acid system for multiple sprints, and the aerobic system to support several hours of play. The game may be played casually or with great intensity and duration and in a variety of venues, from the playground to the National Basketball Association (NBA) arena. Learn more about the sport at the NBA's Web site (http://www.nba.com).

General Nutrition Guidelines

- Energy: Energy needs of basketball players differ, depending on body size, intensity of training, cross-training, and playing time, but in general basketball is a high–energy expenditure sport.
- Carbohydrate: > 5 g/kg/d; 7–12 g/kg/d during heavy training/competition.
- Protein: 1.4–1.7 g/kg/d.
- Fat: Remainder of kcal as fat with an emphasis on heart-healthy fats.

Common Nutritional Concerns

Energy Intake

NBA players may need 6,000 to 7,000 kcal/d whereas other players, such as high school or recreational players, need considerably less. Low energy and nutrient intakes over the long season may contribute to fatigue, especially during playoffs, and to weight loss.

Carbohydrate Intake

Basketball players need a large amount of carbohydrate daily to replenish glycogen that is used during demanding training sessions and games.

Fluid Intake

Training and games are often held in hot environments. Dehydration can lead to early fatigue and heat illness. Fluid intake should balance fluid losses.

Restoration of Glycogen, Fluids, and Electrolytes

Basketball seasons are long and intense. A good nutrition plan can prevent the staleness that many athletes report as the season wears on. Demanding practices, games, and training sessions deplete glycogen, fluids, and electrolytes. Glycogen stores and fluid and electrolyte losses must be replenished beginning immediately after competition or training. Some postexercise protein consumption is also encouraged. Appetite may be depressed, so liquid meal replacements may become an important option.

BODYBUILDING AT A GLANCE

Bodybuilding is a subjectively judged sport based on muscular development and body presentation. Males and females participate in contests at the amateur and professional levels. Training and nutrition must be well matched and will vary depending on the demands of the training period—maintaining muscle mass, building muscle mass, tapering (precontest dieting), or cutting weight immediately before competition. Learn more about the sport at the International Federation of Bodybuilding and Fitness Web site (http://www.ifbb.com).

General Nutrition Guidelines

Bodybuilders are a variety of weights and sizes, and training and nutrient intakes change as they prepare for contests. Competitive bodybuilders spend about 1½ hours in the gym each day during the off-season and 2 to 3 hours per day during precompetition. Energy needs will vary with the phase and amount of training. A "muscle-building phase" begins after rest from the previous competitive season. A "tapering phase" is started approximately 12 weeks before competition with the goal of decreasing body fat and defining muscle mass, and a "cutting phase" is used if the tapering phase did not meet all of the goals for body composition. A maintenance phase should be used during the off-season. Sufficient carbohydrate is needed to meet the demands of training. Protein intakes generally increase during the muscle-building, tapering, and cutting periods. As energy and protein intakes change, the relative contributions of carbohydrates and fats change. These general guidelines must be highly individualized:

- Energy: Energy intake and expenditure must be individually determined. Estimated energy needs are as low as 30 kcal/kg/d for females trying to lose fat weight and maintain muscle mass and as high as 60 kcal/kg/d for males trying to build muscle mass.
- Carbohydrate: 5–7 g/kg/d.
- Protein: 1.4–1.7 g/kg/d (low energy intakes or individual preferences may result in higher intakes— 2g/kg/d during lowest energy intake).
- Fat: Remainder of kcal with an emphasis on heart-healthy fats.

Common Nutritional Concerns

Energy Intake

Baseline energy intake varies tremendously, and energy needs change as contests approach. Bodybuilders need personalized meal plans that reflect various energy (kcal) levels.

Other Macronutrients

Excessive intake of any one macronutrient may result in a low intake of another. The focus must be macronutrient balance (not just protein intake) with the understanding that the demands of training and competition change the relative balance. Emphasize the importance of carbohydrate and healthful fats for health and performance as well as an appropriate protein and energy intake.

Fluid Intake

Fluid loss must be balanced with fluid intake. Voluntary dehydration is one method that is used prior to competition and may be dangerous or life-threatening.

Lack of Variety

Diets tend to be repetitive and lack variety. Meal plans or suggestions for foods that contain similar energy and nutrient profiles are helpful.

Body Image and Disordered Eating

Due to the nature of the sport, there is a risk for distorted body image and disordered eating.

CYCLING AT A GLANCE

Cycling is a sport of various intensities and durations, from sprinters, whose races last only seconds, to endurance cyclists, such as Tour de France riders, who traverse more than 2,000 miles, much of it over mountainous terrain. Energy and nutrient needs vary according to the type of cycling (eg, track, road racing, mountain biking, and bicycle motocross [BMX]), the demands of training, and the intensity and duration of the race. Learn more about the sport at the USA Cycling Web site (http://www.usacycling.org).

General Nutrition Guidelines

Endurance cycling guidelines can be found under Endurance and Ultra-endurance sports in this At a Glance section. Sprint cycling is a very high-intensity, short-duration sport, and the general guidelines include the following:

- Energy: Calculate individual needs based on demands of training.
- Carbohydrate: 7–12 g/kg/d.
- Protein: 1.2–1.7 g/kg/d.
- Fat: Remainder of kcal with an emphasis on heart-healthy fats.

Many cyclists are between the two extremes of sprinting and endurance, and energy and macronutrient requirements must be adjusted accordingly to reflect the demands of training and competition.

Common Nutritional Concerns

Energy and Carbohydrate Intake

Nutrient needs are often high, and a well-balanced diet is important. Distance cyclists need carbohydrate during the ride and must learn to consume food on the bike. Carbohydrate/electrolyte drinks, energy bars, gels, and bananas are some foods that work well, but individual preferences and tolerances must be determined by trial and error.

Fluid Intake

Meeting fluids needs is challenging—road cyclists can carry only two water bottles and can get additional fluids only at special "feed zones" along the course. In road cycling and mountain biking, taking one hand off the bike to drink can lead to crashes.

Dehydration is a daily concern. Sweat rates should be calculated and an individualized hydration plan should be developed. Take precautions to prevent hyponatremia, especially in hot, humid environments.

Restoration of Glycogen, Fluids, and Electrolytes

Glycogen stores and fluid and electrolyte losses must be replenished beginning immediately after competition or training. Some postexercise protein consumption is also encouraged. Appetite may be depressed, so liquid meal replacements may become an important option.

ENDURANCE AND ULTRA-ENDURANCE SPORTS (DISTANCE RUNNING, CYCLING, AND SWIMMING) AT A GLANCE

Endurance and ultra-endurance sports include marathons, triathlons, and distance cycling and swimming events. All require year-round training and nutrition support. Training and nutrition must be well matched and will vary depending on the training period—preparation, pre-race, race, or active recovery. Reducing body fat or weight should be attempted during active recovery or early in the preparation period so that high-volume training or competition is not compromised. Learn more about these sports at the following Web sites: USA Track and Field (http://www.usatf.org/groups/roadrunning), USA Triathlon (http://www.usatriathlon.org), United States Masters Swimming: Long-Distance Swimming (http://www.usms.org/longdist), and Ultramarathon Cycling Association (http://www.ultracycling.com).

General Nutrition Guidelines

- Energy: High–energy expenditure sports.
- Carbohydrate: 5–7 g/kg/d when training is reduced and as high as 10–12 g/kg/d during heavy training and racing season. Carbohydrate loading (glycogen supercompensation) for competition is common.
- Protein: 1.2–1.7 g/kg/d, with higher levels consumed during pre-race and racing seasons.
- Fat: 0.8–2.0 g/kg/d to match energy expenditure, with emphasis on heart-healthy fats.

Common Nutritional Concerns

Energy and Macronutrient Intake

Needs are high and proper food intake must be an integral part of training. A structured eating plan must be developed to support training throughout the year.

Weight Gain

After the racing season is over, energy intake must be adjusted to reflect the decreased volume and intensity of training to prevent unwanted weight gain.

Body Composition

Leanness and low body weight is advantageous in sports in which the body must be moved. Excess body fat can be detrimental because, unlike muscle, it is non–force-producing mass. Rapid weight or fat loss can be detrimental to training and performance, so changes to body composition must be slow. Small reductions in daily energy intake and some increase in activities of daily living will promote slow weight loss. Weight loss is best attempted during the recovery period or early in the preparation period.

Fluid and Sodium Intake

Fluids to an endurance athlete are like water to a car's radiator—without it both will overheat and stall. Fluid intake must be balanced to avoid dehydration and prevent hyponatremia. Sodium needs must be individually established. The inclusion of sodium in products taken during training and racing is recommended.

Lack of Variety

Variety and balance can be difficult day after day. Athletes must avoid getting into a rut. Focus on whole foods, especially on "off" days.

Food Intolerances

Some foods are not tolerated well during competition. Practice using various race foods and beverages during training to prevent problems during competition.

FIELD EVENTS AT A GLANCE

Indoor field events include high jump, pole vault, long jump, triple jump, and shot put. Outdoor field events also include discus, hammer, and javelin throws. Both males and females compete in these events. The necessary athletic skills and body composition differ between jumpers and throwers. Jumpers tend to be leaner because they must move their body through space, whereas throwers depend on their strength and body mass to propel an object through space. Jumpers consume less energy than throwers. Learn more about the sports at the USA Track and Field Web site (http://www.usatf.org).

General Nutrition Guidelines

- Energy: Varies depending on the individual and the event.
- Carbohydrate: 5–7 g/kg/d.
- Protein: 1.2–1.7 g/kg/d.
- Fat: Remainder of kcal with an emphasis on heart-healthy fats.

Common Nutritional Concerns

Body Composition and Weight Loss

Jumpers are encouraged to have a low percentage of body fat. There is a performance disadvantage to having excess body fat because fat represents non–force-producing mass. A weight-loss plan must allow for sufficient amounts of carbohydrate and protein to support training as well as weight (fat) loss.

High-Fat Diets

Throwers have a tendency to have high-fat diets. Such diets may also be high in saturated fat. All athletes should be aware of the advantages of consuming heart-healthy fats, and substituting such fats for saturated fats should be encouraged. If weight loss is desired, reducing dietary fat would be appropriate.

Fluid Intake

Several factors unique to track and field contribute to dehydration, including unsupervised workouts (which places the responsibility for hydration on the athletes), limited availability of fluids at the training facility, frequent travel from cool environments to hot climates with little time to acclimate to the change in temperature, increased fluid loss during air travel due to the low humidity in an airplane cabin, and the competitive nature of the sport, which might push an athlete to exercise even when dehydrated. Fluid loss must be balanced with fluid intake.

FIGURE SKATING AT A GLANCE

Figure skating requires strength, power, and endurance. Individual competitions are held for men and women. Couples compete in pairs and ice dancing, and there are team skating competitions. Training starts very early, sometimes at age 3 years, and many world champions are in their teens. Technique and speed are important, and the degree of skating difficulty increases as skaters become more elite. An elite figure skater's training includes learning new skills, like jumping and spinning, and repeated practice of those skills. High-intensity work coupled with lower-intensity skating and training 6 days a week in two sessions per day is a usual routine. Artistry plays a critical role, and there are many subjective elements considered in scoring. Competitions at the elite level include a short program that is 2 minutes and 40 seconds and a long program that is 4 minutes (females) or 4.5 minutes (males and pairs). Learn more about the sport at the US Figure Skating Web site (http://www.usfsa.org).

General Nutrition Guidelines

- Energy: Individualize based on body composition goals.
- Carbohydrate: 3–7 g/kg/d.
- Protein: 1.2–1.7 g/kg/d.
- Fat: Remainder of kcal with an emphasis on heart-healthy fats.

Common Nutritional Concerns

Energy Restriction

Despite the high energy demands of training, many female figure skaters limit energy intake in an effort to attain or maintain a low percentage of body fat. Weight loss must be slow, with small restrictions of energy so that muscle mass can be protected and training will not be negatively impacted.

Body Composition

A low percentage of body fat, particularly for females, is considered necessary for success because of the physical demands of the sport and appearance, which is part of the subjective scoring system. The potential for disordered eating or eating disorders is great, and early intervention is imperative.

Nutrient Intake

The consumption of nutrient-dense foods is important, especially if energy intake is restricted. Many figure skaters are children and adolescents and need adequate nutrition to support growth and development.

FOOTBALL AT A GLANCE

American football is played by two teams of 11 players each. Each play involves some high-intensity, short-duration activity, and there is a short rest period between each play. Professional football games are four 15-minute quarters with a halftime break, but the clock is frequently stopped so the game takes about 4 hours to complete. Body composition varies by position, with receivers being lean and fast, whereas linemen depend on their strength and body mass to block. College football players usually have a smaller body mass than professional players and must increase size if they move into the professional ranks. Learn more about the sport at the National Football League Web site (http://www.nfl.com) or Football.com (http://www.football.com).

General Nutrition Guidelines

- Energy: Energy expenditure varies depending on the level of the sport (professional, college, high school, or youth), level of training, amount of muscle mass, growth, etc, and must be individually determined.
- Carbohydrate: > 5 g/kg/d; 7–12 g/kg/d may be needed during rigorous training.
- Protein: 1.4–1.7 g/kg/d.
- Fat: Remainder of kcal as fat with an emphasis on heart-healthy fats.

Common Nutritional Concerns

Energy Intake

Energy intake goals vary among athletes but can be more than 5,000 kcal/d. Many wish to change body composition by increasing muscle mass (which may require a higher energy intake) or decreasing body fat.

Off-season Weight Gain

Players need to match their off-season energy intake with energy expenditure. Some football players arrive at training camp or spring football practice overweight and out of shape. When this is the case they often look for quick weight-loss methods. Some of these methods may be dangerous, such as voluntary dehydration, use of drugs thought to reduce body fat, and severe restriction of food intake. A nutrition and training plan during the off-season can help athletes prevent unwanted off-season weight gain.

High Fat Intake

Some football players eat out frequently and consume a high-fat, high–saturated fat diet.

Fluid and Electrolyte Intake

Football players may play in hot and humid conditions, often early in the season, before they are acclimated to the heat. Dehydration is a serious and potentially life-threatening problem. Sweating rates can be as high as 10 L/d, and a football player can lose 12 pounds in practice. Hydration can be challenging because the weight of the uniform and pads are an additional burden when exercising in the heat. If heat illness occurs, it is most likely to happen on the first day or two of preseason practice when players are not used to the heat. Fluid and electrolyte intakes must be balanced with losses. Approximately 10% of players may be "cramp prone" due to large losses of sodium in sweat. They may need additional sodium in addition to fluids to prevent heat cramps.

GOLF AT A GLANCE

Golf is a low-endurance, precision-skill sport. It requires fine-motor control and coordination. Swinging a club requires power, and walking the course (especially if the golfer is carrying clubs) requires general fitness. Golf courses vary in length, but championship courses are approximately 6,000 to 7,000 yards, and an 18-hole course takes several hours to play. Women play shorter distances because of the location of the tees. Professional tournaments include four rounds (72 holes over 4 days) with additional holes played on the last day in case of ties. Learn more about the sport at the Web sites for the Professional Golfers' Association of America (http://www.pga.com) or the Ladies Professional Golf Association (http://www.lpga.com).

General Nutrition Guidelines

Golfers do not have significantly increased demands for energy or nutrients; thus, general nutrient guidelines are used and adjusted on an individual basis.

- Energy: Relatively low–energy expenditure sport.
- Carbohydrate: 3–5 g/kg/d.
- Protein: 1.2 –1.7 g/kg/d (often nearer the lower end of the range).
- Fat: ~ 1.0 g/kg/d or remainder of kcal with an emphasis on heart-healthy fats.

Common Nutritional Concerns

Energy Intake

The focus is typically on energy balance, although some players may wish to reduce energy intake to lose body fat. Slow weight loss should not affect performance, but severe restriction could lead to inadequate total energy intake and/or low blood glucose, which could negatively affect performance.

Fluid Intake

Golf often takes place in hot and humid conditions. Dehydration is a daily concern and golfers are encouraged to consume fluids between holes.

Precompetition Meal

Players need to eat a meal prior to play because they will be on the course for many hours. Start times vary and may be changed due to weather delays. Breakfast is vital because golfers often start early in the morning. Golfers should have a plan for a pregame meal that considers volume, macronutrient composition, and timing of intake that can be adjusted if the start time changes. Avoid the high-fat and high-sugar foods at the halfway house or in the club house. Golfers usually carry snacks, such as energy bars or sport drinks, to prevent hunger while playing.

Frequent Travel

Frequent travel makes it difficult to maintain a routine and increases exposure to high-calorie, low–nutrient dense foods.

GYMNASTICS AT A GLANCE

Gymnastics involves activities that are typically characterized as high to very high intensity and short duration. In competition, athletes perform and then rest before beginning a new event. Gymnastics requires strength, power, and flexibility. Training is demanding, often involving many repetitions of individual skills or routines, but athletes can rest when it is not their turn to perform. Female gymnasts tend to be shorter and lighter than most other athletes and other females their age. A high percentage of lean body mass and a low percentage of body fat are desirable, not only to perform the skills, but also because such bodies are aesthetically appealing. It is biologically easier for males to attain the currently held "ideal" body type than for females. Learn more about the sport at the USA Gymnastics Web site (http://www.usa-gymnastics.org).

General Nutrition Guidelines

- Energy: Individualize based on body composition goals.
- Carbohydrate: 3–7 g/kg/d.
- Protein: 1.2–1.7 g/kg/d.
- Fat: Remainder of kcal with an emphasis on heart-healthy fats.

Common Nutritional Concerns

Energy Restriction

Despite the high energy demands of training, surveys suggest that many female gymnasts limit energy intake. If body fat loss is an appropriate goal, it must be slow, with small restrictions of energy so that muscle mass can be protected and training will not be negatively affected.

Body Composition

A low percentage of body fat, which may be difficult for females to attain or maintain, is considered necessary for success because of the physical demands of the sport and appearance. Amenorrhea may be present and is a warning sign associated with excessive energy restriction and/or anorexia. The potential for disordered eating and eating disorders is great and early intervention is imperative.

Nutrient Intake

The consumption of nutrient-dense foods is important, especially if energy intake is restricted. Many gymnasts are children and adolescents and need adequate nutrition to support growth and development.

ICE HOCKEY AT A GLANCE

Ice hockey requires anaerobic power, aerobic conditioning, strength, agility, and speed. Similar to other intermittent, high-intensity sports, there are constant changes in speed and direction, but ice hockey differs from soccer or basketball in that there is full body contact. A game consists of three 16-minute periods, but frequent player substitutions reduce playing time to at least half of the game time. Learn more about the sport at the Web sites for the National Hockey League (http://www.nhl.com) and USA Hockey (http://www.usahockey.com).

General Nutrition Guidelines

- Energy: Varies based on level of training, but generally a high–energy expenditure sport.
- Carbohydrate: Daily intake > 5 g/kg/d; 8–10 g/kg/d during training and competition to ensure adequate glycogen in quadriceps.
- Protein: 1.4–1.7 g/kg/d.
- Fat: Remainder of kcal with an emphasis on heart-healthy fats.

Common Nutritional Concerns

Carbohydrate and Protein Intake

Hockey players need a large amount of carbohydrate daily to replenish glycogen that is used during demanding training sessions and games. Protein is important to repair the wear and tear on muscles that occurs in hockey. Constant body-checking can take its toll on muscles, bones, tendons, and teeth.

Hydration During Exercise

Hydration during training and competition is important because players can sweat profusely under all of their gear even though they are on ice. Many hockey players spit out fluids instead of swallowing them. Sipping on fluids between shifts can help prevent dehydration and improve performance.

Restoration of Glycogen, Fluids, and Electrolytes

Demanding practices, games, and training sessions deplete glycogen, fluids, and electrolytes. Glycogen stores and fluid and electrolyte losses must be replenished beginning immediately after competition or training. Some postexercise protein consumption is also encouraged. Appetite may be depressed. Liquid meal replacements may be beneficial.

MARTIAL ARTS AT A GLANCE

Martial arts is a broad term that describes combat activities. Boxing, fencing, judo, and tae kwon do may be the best known because they are Olympic sports, but there are hundreds of different types of martial arts. Each art is different, but most involve strength, flexibility, agility, and some also include explosive movements. Each art requires a strong level of mental and physical fitness. Many have weight classes and some martial artists use a variety of methods to "make weight." Participants in some competitions, such as judo or tae kwon do, compete several times over the course of a day. Learn more about the sports at the USA Dojo Web site (http://www.usadojo.com).

General Nutrition Guidelines

- Energy: Individualize based on body composition and weight goals.
- Carbohydrate: 5–7 g/kg/d.
- Protein: 1.2–1.7 g/kg/d.
- Fat: Remainder of kcal with an emphasis on heart-healthy fats.

Common Nutritional Concerns

Making Weight

As with any sport that has weight categories, rapid reduction of body weight, including extreme methods such as fasting, fluid restriction, or semistarvation, may be an issue. Rapid weight loss is more likely to be detrimental to performance than gradual weight loss. A weight-loss plan must allow for sufficient amounts of carbohydrate and protein to support training.

Nutrient Intake

The consumption of nutrient-dense foods is important, especially if energy intake is restricted. Meal timing and adequacy of intake during meets (multiple bouts during one day) should be addressed.

Fluid Intake

Dehydration is a daily concern. Fluid loss should be balanced with fluid intake. If an athlete uses dehydration to lose weight, restoration of fluid and electrolyte balance is critical.

ROWING (CREW) AT A GLANCE

A typical crew race is 2,000 meters lasting 5½ to 8 minutes and requiring strength, power, and endurance. The crew season begins in the fall with preseason training. Winter is a time of intense training and building muscle, whereas the spring racing season is known for its long daily practices leading up to a rest day and weekend competition. Summer is the off-season. There are lightweight and open (heavy) weight categories. Learn more about the sport at the US Rowing Web site (http://www.usrowing.org).

General Nutrition Guidelines

- Energy: Relatively high–energy expenditure sport.
- Carbohydrate: 5–7 g/kg/d.
- Protein: 1.2–1.7 g/kg/d.
- Fat: ~ 1.0 g/kg/d. Fat, in the form of heart-healthy fats, may be increased to meet high energy needs while training but decreased during the off-season.

Common Nutritional Concerns

Energy Intake

Fatigue and lack of appetite may result in involuntary underconsumption of energy. Lightweight rowers may voluntarily restrict energy to make weight.

Making Weight

Lightweight rowers who are genetically lean and biologically small can comfortably meet the requirements for lightweight rowing. Problems with disordered eating and eating disorders occur when extraordinary efforts must be made to attain and maintain a low body weight. Voluntary dehydration may also be an issue. Learning to manage weight in the off-season is preferred to cutting weight in-season. Dangerous weight-cutting practices and disordered eating are found in both male and female rowers.

Consumption of Foods with Low Nutrient Density

Rowers have high energy needs, and both male and female heavyweight rowers quickly discover that they must eat a lot of food to maintain energy balance. High-fat, high-sugar snack foods and beverages can provide the energy needed but not the nutrients.

Balancing Fluid Intake with Fluid Losses

Dehydration is a daily concern. Rowers have water bottles in the boat during training, but they do not have access to them during long training pieces (approximately 30 to 45 minutes each). It is unlikely that rowers can maintain fluid balance during training. Therefore, they should pay special attention to drinking sufficient fluid before and after training.

SOCCER AT A GLANCE

Soccer involves short, intense bursts of activity combined with moderately intense exercise and occasional rest periods. When played outdoors, the field is larger than a football field and the average soccer player will cover between 8 and 12 km (5 to 7 miles). The game consists of two 45-minute halves with a 15-minute halftime, although the game is shorter for younger players. Learn more about the sport at the Web sites for US Soccer (http://www.ussoccer.com) and international soccer (http://www.fifa.com).

General Nutrition Guidelines

- Energy: Relatively high–energy expenditure sport.
- Carbohydrate: > 5 g/kg/d; 7–12 g/kg/d during training and competition.
- Protein: 1.4–1.7 g/kg/d.
- Fat: Remainder of kcal with an emphasis on heart-healthy fats.

Common Nutritional Concerns

Energy Intake

Energy expenditure is high during training and games. A 75-kg male soccer player may expend more than 1,500 kcal in a game. Many players, both male and female, do not consume an adequate energy intake and this can lead to early onset of fatigue and poor nutrient intake.

Fluid Intake

Players should consume fluid early and at regular intervals during the game. Needs are especially high in hot and humid conditions. Carbohydrate/electrolyte solutions are beneficial during the game. Special attention should be paid to youth soccer players because they do not sweat as much as adults and the risk for dehydration and heat illness is high. Youth players should consume fluid at least every 15 to 20 minutes during practice and frequently during games.

Restoration of Glycogen, Fluids, and Electrolytes

Glycogen stores and fluid and electrolyte losses must be replenished beginning immediately after competition or training. Soccer games are often scheduled close to each other with little time between games to replace muscle glycogen. Recovery nutrition helps soccer players make it through the season without fatigue. Some postexercise protein consumption is also encouraged. Appetite may be depressed, so liquid meal replacements may become an important option.

Frequent Travel

Frequent travel makes it difficult to maintain a routine and increases exposure to high-energy, low–nutrient dense foods.

SWIMMING AT A GLANCE

Swimming is a sport of various intensities and durations. Swimming events can range from 50 and 100 meters (sprints), 200 and 400 meters (middle distances), and 800 and 1,500 meters (distance). Long-distance swimming includes the swim portion of the full triathlon (2.4 miles) and ultra-endurance events, such as swimming the English Channel (~ 24 miles). All swimmers have demanding training, so adequate daily energy and nutrient intake is important. Learn more about the sport at the USA Swimming Web site (http://www.usaswimming.org).

General Nutrition Guidelines

Recommendations must be tailored to the individual based on the level of training and the distance. For swimming events ranging from 50 to 1,500 meters, the general guidelines include the following:

- Energy: Calculate individual needs based on demands of training.
- Carbohydrate: 7–12 g/kg/d.
- Protein: 1.2–1.7 g/kg/d.
- Fat: ~ 1.0 g/kg/d or remainder of kcal with an emphasis on heart-healthy fats.

Long-distance swimming guidelines can be found under Endurance and Ultra-endurance Sports in this At a Glance section.

Common Nutritional Concerns

Energy and Carbohydrate Intake

Energy and nutrient needs are high, and a well-balanced diet is important. Chronic undereating can be a problem. Swimmers often complain of chronic fatigue; hard training coupled with poor nutrition leads to fatigue. Aim for a minimum of 500 g of carbohydrate each day during the competitive season. Frequent meals or snacks are important.

Fluid Intake

Dehydration is a daily concern and can occur within 30 minutes of swimming. Many swimmers ignore fluid intake because they are surrounded by water, but the environmental conditions of swimming (warm pool water, warm air temperatures, and high humidity) can lead to dehydration.

Restoration of Glycogen, Fluids, and Electrolytes

Glycogen stores and fluid and electrolyte losses must be replenished beginning immediately after competition or training. Some postexercise protein consumption is also encouraged. Two-a-day swim practices are often conducted and rapid replenishment of glycogen and fluid balance is critical.

Body Composition

Appropriate percentage of body fat varies depending on the distance. Reducing body fat should be a slow process because too great a reduction in energy, carbohydrate, and protein intakes can negatively affect training and performance.

Risk for Disordered Eating and Eating Disorders

Swimmers are at risk for developing disordered eating and eating disorders. Refer to qualified health professionals when necessary.

TENNIS AT A GLANCE

Tennis requires anaerobic power, aerobic conditioning, strength, and agility. The game may be played casually or with great intensity and duration; thus, training and nutrient requirements vary tremendously. One (singles) or two (doubles) players are on each side. Male professional singles players must win three of five sets, and singles matches typically last 2 to 4 hours. Females play the best of three sets. Most singles players hit from the baseline and long rallies require excellent fitness. Most tournaments are 1 week in length but major tournaments are 2 weeks long. Most points in tennis last less than 10 seconds, but there are only 25 seconds of rest between points and 90 seconds between games, so endurance is needed for long matches. Tennis requires about 300 to 500 bursts of energy over the course of a match, so energy levels must be maintained and hydration is critical for success. Recreational players play at a variety of intensities and some do not have significantly increased demands for energy or nutrients. Learn more about the sport at the US Tennis Association Web site (http://www.usta.com).

General Nutrition Guidelines

- Energy: Varies depending on the level of training and the intensity and duration of play. Professional and collegiate players have high energy expenditures.
- Carbohydrate: 7–12 g/kg/d.
- Protein: 1.2–1.7 g/kg/d.
- Fat: ~ 1.0 g/kg/d or the remainder of kcal as fat with an emphasis on heart-healthy fats.

Common Nutritional Concerns

Fluid and Electrolyte Intake

Practice and play typically take place in hot and/or humid conditions. Dehydration is a daily concern. Some players may be "cramp prone" due to large losses of sodium in sweat. They may need additional sodium in addition to fluids to prevent heat cramps. Tennis players who are prone to cramp can try adding ½ tsp of table salt to 32 oz of sport drink or choose an "endurance" formula sport drink that contains more sodium than regular sport drinks.

Restoration of Glycogen, Fluids, and Electrolytes

Demanding practices, training sessions, and match play deplete glycogen, fluids, and electrolytes. Glycogen stores and fluid and electrolyte losses must be replenished beginning immediately after competition or training. Some postexercise protein consumption is also encouraged. Near the end of the tournament, replenishment is especially important for peak performance.

Prematch Meal

Players, especially males, will be on the court for many hours and they need to eat a meal prior to play. Start time may not be known (due to the length of other matches) and play may be stopped and restarted with short notice due to rain. Tennis players should have a plan for a prematch meal that considers volume, macronutrient composition, and timing of intake. The meal can then be adjusted based on start time.

Multiple Matches in One Day

Tennis players may play more than one match in a day. This is especially true for younger athletes who compete in tournaments. "Mini-meals" or snacks may be needed, because sport drinks alone may not be substantial enough.

Frequent Travel

Frequent travel makes it difficult to maintain a routine and increases exposure to high-calorie, low–nutrient dense foods.

TRACK EVENTS AT A GLANCE

Track events range from the very fast 100-m race to the much longer 10,000-meter run or 20,000-meter walking events. Nutrition recommendations must consider the distance involved. Daily workouts are intense. Athletes may compete several times during the course of a day. For most very high-intensity, brief events, diet has less of an impact than other factors such as genetics and training. Compared with distance runners, middle-distance runners have more moderate carbohydrate needs. Learn more about the various track events and the demands of training at the USA Track and Field Web site (http://www.usatf.org).

General Nutrition Guidelines

- Energy: Individualize based on body composition goals.
- Carbohydrate:
  - Very high-intensity, brief events (100–400 meters): 5–7 g/kg/d.
  - High-intensity, short-duration events (800–10,000 meters): 5–7 g/kg/d.
- Protein: 1.2–1.7 g/kg/d.
- Fat: ~ 1.0 g/kg/d or remainder of calories after carbohydrate and protein needs are met.

Common Nutritional Concerns

Energy Intake

In general, daily energy expenditure is high due to demanding training. Reported daily intakes are often less than estimated needs.

Weight Loss

High muscularity is valued so many track athletes are attempting to lose body fat. Rapid weight loss is more likely to be detrimental to performance than gradual weight loss. A weight-loss plan must allow for sufficient amounts of carbohydrate and protein to support training.

Potential for Disordered Eating or Eating Disorders

Pressure to attain or maintain a low percentage body fat and an undue focus on body appearance increase the risk for athletes, particularly female middle-distance runners, to develop disordered eating or eating disorders.

WRESTLING AT A GLANCE

Wrestling involves hand-to-hand combat and requires strength and stamina. A high strength (power)-to-weight ratio is desirable. The sport features weight divisions and some wrestlers "make weight" using drastic measures. Deaths have resulted through the combined use of a variety of techniques, including voluntary dehydration and starvation. Rule changes have been instituted to reduce excessive weight loss, including assessing body fat at the beginning of the season, determining a minimum competitive weight, and holding weigh-ins close to the start of competition. No longer just a men's sport, women's wrestling became an Olympic sport in 2004, and the number of high school and collegiate female wrestlers is expected to grow. Learn more about the sport at the Web sites for USA Wrestling (http://themat.com), National Collegiate Athletic Association (http://www.ncaa.com/sports/wrestling), and Federation of State High School Associations (http://www.nfhs.org).

General Nutrition Guidelines

- Energy: Individualize based on body composition and weight goals.
- Carbohydrate: 5–7 g/kg/d.
- Protein: 1.2–1.7 g/kg/d protein requirements may increase to 2 g/kg/d during periods of lowest energy intake to achieve weight loss).
- Fat: Remainder of kcal with an emphasis on heart-healthy fats.

Common Nutritional Concerns

Energy Intake

Appropriate energy intake must be individually determined. A focus on performance and health, not just weight, can help wrestlers view energy intake from a positive perspective.

Cutting Weight or Making Weight

Weight-cutting practices can be severe and life-threatening, although new rules have resulted in less extreme weight-cutting behaviors than in the past. Collegiate wrestlers use more extreme methods than high school wrestlers. Wrestlers in lower weight classes have relatively larger weight changes than those in heavier weight classes. Fasting, fluid restriction, and semistarvation are popular methods to make weight at all levels. Saunas, sweat suits (although banned), and diuretics may also be used. Nutrition counseling across the season is important to develop individualized plans, discuss weight loss methods, and monitor weight changes.

Nutrient Intake

The consumption of nutrient-dense foods is important, especially if energy intake is restricted. Wrestlers have demanding training programs, and sufficient macro- and micronutrient intakes are important to support training, performance, and health. Many wrestlers are adolescents and need adequate nutrition to support growth and development as well.

Fluid Intake

Dehydration is a daily concern. Fluid loss should be balanced with fluid intake. If dehydration is used as a weight-loss method, restoration of fluid and electrolyte balance is critical. Some wrestlers believe they can lose weight for the weigh-in and then rehydrate before a match. That is a false belief because it takes up to 6 hours to reach normal hydration.

Appendix A

CLINICAL EATING DISORDER CRITERIA

Anorexia Nervosa

Individuals with anorexia nervosa are obsessed with the desire to be thinner and intensely fear gaining weight. No matter how thin the individual with anorexia becomes, she or he always "feels fat" and longs to be thinner. The diagnostic criteria for anorexia nervosa as described in the DSM-IV are as follows:

- A significant loss of body weight and/or the maintenance of an extremely low body weight (85% of "normal" weight for height)
- An intense fear of gaining weight or "becoming fat"
- Severe body dissatisfaction and body image distortion
- Amenorrhea (absence of three or more consecutive menstrual periods)

Two subtypes of anorexia nervosa have been identified: the "restricting type" and the "binge-eating/purging type." An individual with "restricting type" anorexia nervosa loses weight and/or maintains an abnormally low body weight by means of severe energy restriction and excessive exercise. An individual with "bingeing/purging type" anorexia nervosa also severely restricts energy intake and excessively exercises, but will occasionally binge and subsequently engage in compensatory purging behaviors, such as self-induced vomiting or laxative or diuretic abuse, to control his or her weight.

Bulimia Nervosa

Individuals with bulimia nervosa engage in regular cycles of bingeing and purging. The diagnostic criteria for bulimia nervosa as described in the DSM-IV are as follows:

- Episodes of binge eating (ie, consuming a large amount of food in a short period of time) followed by purging (via laxatives, diuretics, enemas, self-induced vomiting, and/or excessive exercise) that have occurred at least twice a week for 3 months

Note: The criteria in this appendix are from the *Diagnostic and Statistical Manual of Mental Disorders IV* (DSM-IV) (1). A draft of the fifth edition of the DSM has been released, with the final release scheduled for May 2013. For more information, go to www .dsm5.org.

- A sense of lack of control during the bingeing and/or purging episodes
- Severe body image dissatisfaction and undue influence of body image on self-evaluation

As with anorexia nervosa, two subtypes of bulimia nervosa have been identified: purging type and nonpurging type. The individual with purging type bulimia nervosa regularly engages in self-induced vomiting, or the misuse of laxatives, diuretics, and/or enemas to compensate for his or her bingeing behaviors, whereas the individual with nonpurging bulimia nervosa uses other inappropriate compensatory behaviors, such as fasting or excessive exercise, to compensate for episodes of overeating (but does not regularly engage in self-induced vomiting, or the misuse of laxatives, diuretics, and/or enemas).

Binge-Eating Disorder

Binge-eating disorder has only recently been recognized as a clinical eating disorder (it is sometimes referred to as compulsive overeating). Similar to bulimia nervosa, those with binge eating disorder frequently consume large amounts of food while feeling a lack of control over their eating. However, individuals with binge-eating disorder generally do not engage in purging behaviors (ie, vomiting, laxatives, excessive exercise, etc). The diagnostic criteria for binge-eating disorder as described in the DSM-IV include the following:

- Recurrent episodes of binge eating. An episode is characterized by eating a larger amount of food than normal during a short period of time (within any 2-hour period) and lack of control over eating during the binge episode.
- Binge-eating episodes are associated with three or more of the following: (*a*) eating until feeling uncomfortably full; (*b*) eating large amounts of food when not physically hungry; (*c*) eating much more rapidly than normal; (*d*) eating alone because you are embarrassed by how much you are eating; (*e*) feeling disgusted, depressed, or guilty after overeating.
- Marked distress regarding binge eating is present.
- Binge eating occurs, on average, at least 2 days a week for 6 months.
- The binge eating is not associated with the regular use of inappropriate compensatory behavior (ie, purging, excessive exercise, etc) and does not occur exclusively during the course of bulimia nervosa or anorexia nervosa.

Eating Disorders Not Otherwise Specified

Eating disorders not otherwise specified (EDNOS) is a clinical eating disorder category that was recently added to the DSM-IV to describe individuals who meet some but not all of the criteria for anorexia nervosa and/or bulimia nervosa. The characteristic features of EDNOS are as follows:

- All of the criteria for anorexia nervosa are met except amenorrhea.
- All of the criteria for anorexia nervosa are met except that, despite significant weight loss, the individual's current weight is within the normal range.
- All of the criteria for bulimia nervosa are met except that the binge and purge cycles occur at a frequency of less than twice per week for a duration of less than 3 months.
- The regular use of purging behaviors by an individual of normal body weight after eating small amounts of food (eg, self-induced vomiting after consuming only two cookies).
- Repeatedly chewing and spitting out, but not swallowing, large amounts of food.

Reference

American Psychiatric Association. *Diagnostic and Statistical Manual of Mental Disorders.* 4th ed. Washington, DC: American Psychiatric Association; 1994.

Appendix B

SELECTED SPORTS NUTRITION–RELATED POSITION PAPERS

Academy of Nutrition and Dietetics (formerly American Dietetic Association) Positions

The following are available at *http://www.eatright.org/positions:*

- Nutrition and Athletic Performance (joint position statement of the American Dietetic Association, Dietitians of Canada, and the American College of Sports Medicine)
- Food and Nutrition Misinformation
- Functional Foods
- Nutrient Supplementation
- Nutrition Intervention in the Treatment of Anorexia Nervosa, Bulimia Nervosa and Other Eating Disorders
- Total Diet Approach to Communicating Food and Nutrition Information
- Vegetarian Diets
- Weight Management

American College of Sports Medicine Positions

The following are available at *http://journals.lww.com/acsm-msse/pages/collectiondetails.aspx?Topical CollectionId=1:*

- Exercise and Type 2 Diabetes
- Exercise and Physical Activity for Older Adults
- The Female Athlete Triad
- Appropriate Intervention Strategies for Weight Loss and Prevention of Weight Regain for Adults
- Exertional Heat Illness During Training and Competition
- Exercise and Fluid Replacement
- Physical Activity and Bone Health
- Exercise and Hypertension

National Athletic Trainers' Association Positions

The following are available at *http://www.nata.org/position-statements:*

- Preventing, Detecting, and Managing Eating Disorders in Athletes
- Management of the Athlete with Type 1 Diabetes Mellitus
- Safe Weight Loss and Maintenance Practices in Sport and Exercise

Appendix C

SPORTS NUTRITION–RELATED WEB SITES

- Academy of Nutrition and Dietetics (formerly American Dietetic Association): *www.eatright.org*
- Aerobics and Fitness Association of America: *www.afaa.com*
- Amateur Athletic Union: *http://aausports.org*
- America on the Move: *www.americaonthemove.org*
- American Alliance for Health, Physical Education, Recreation and Dance: *www.aahperd.org*
- American College of Sports Medicine: *www.acsm.org*
- American Council on Exercise: *www.acefitness.org*
- American Diabetes Association: *www.diabetes.org*
- American Running Association: *www.americanrunning.org*
- American Sport Education Program: *www.asep.com*
- Australian Institute of Sport: *www.ausport.gov.au/ais*
- Body Positive: *www.bodypositive.com*
- Crucible Fitness: *www.endurancenation.us/blog/tag/crucible-fitness*
- Dietitians of Canada: *www.dietitians.ca*
- Gatorade Sports Science Institute: *www.gssiweb.com*
- IDEA Health and Fitness Association: *http://ideafit.com*
- Korey Stringer Institute at University of Connecticut: *http://ksi.uconn.edu*
- Lollylegs—Masters Athletics: *www.lollylegs.com*
- MomsTeam.com: *www.MomsTeam.com*
- National Athletic Trainers Association: *www.nata.org*
- National Eating Disorders Association: *www.nationaleatingdisorders.org*
- National Recreation and Park Association: *www.nrpa.org*
- Nicholas Institute of Sports Medicine and Athletic Trauma: *www.nismat.org*
- Physical Activity Guidelines for Americans: *http://www.health.gov/paguidelines*
- The Physician and Sports Medicine: *https://physsportsmed.org*
- Runners World: *www.runnersworld.com*
- Special Olympics: *www.specialolympics.org*
- Sports, Cardiovascular and Wellness Nutrition (Dietetic Practice Group of the Academy of Nutrition and Dietetics): *www.scandpg.org*
- Sports Dietitians Australia: *www.sportsdietitians.com.au*
- Sports Oracle: *www.sportsoracle.com*
- SportScience: *www.sportsci.org*

- Sports Science Insights: *http://sportsscienceinsights.com*
- UltraMarathon Cycling Association: *www.ultracycling.com*
- The Vegetarian Resource Group: *www.vrg.org*

Note: This list includes Web sites that may be valuable to sports dietitians and other health professionals. The inclusion of a Web site does not constitute an endorsement of that site. At the time of publication, all URLs were correct.

Appendix D

UNIQUE ROLES: SPORTS DIETITIANS IN THE MILITARY

Sports dietitians work with active people at all stages of life—from youth soccer to masters competitors—and in all of these situations nutrition and hydration needs are crucial for good health and optimal performance. Although sports dietitians are employed in a variety of settings, an especially critical role is working with the US military. Registered dietitians (RDs) serve the military in active duty, Reserves, and civilian positions. Military service by RDs has been long-standing, but RDs are increasingly being recognized for their contributions in enhancing the human performance of men and women in the armed forces.

Men and women in the armed services work under extreme conditions. Combat soldiers are termed tactical athletes because their training and work is very demanding, with unique challenges for fueling and hydration that are akin to the demands of athletic performance. Much of the research on sports nutrition can be, and has been, applied to the military arena. In turn, research conducted by the military on hydration and dietary supplements has been applied to recreational and elite athletes. Brief descriptions of the roles of RDs in the Army, Navy, and Air Force are provided here.

US Army

Many active-duty and reserve Army dietitians hold the Certified Specialist in Sports Dietetics (CSSD) credential. A nutrition residency course in sports nutrition is offered every year for Army RDs who want to obtain the CSSD credential. The course also prepares RDs to take the Certified Strength and Conditioning Specialist (CSCS) exam hosted by the National Strength and Conditioning Association. At the end of the seminar, participants take the CSCS exam. RDs take the CSSD exam after completing the residency course and achieving 1,500 practice hours.

Although active-duty RDs primarily serve in clinical dietetics and foodservice positions, they use the CSSD credential in various ways, from basic sports and supplement nutrition to human performance optimization through specialized nutrition and training:

- CSSDs in the Army serve on nutrition- and supplement-related committees that address Department of Defense (DOD) policy issues, plan and develop nutrition programs and policies affecting the DOD, and speak at various fitness-related workshops and seminars.
- As the Army moves toward Human Performance Programs (HPP), the demand for sports dietitians is increasing. Commonly referred to as performance dietitians, these professionals are filling the gap between the traditional roles of clinical and foodservice dietitians and that of sports- and performance-based education and services.

- In the realm of tactical athletes, performance dietitians are educating, counseling, and advising soldiers and their leadership on fueling for high-tempo operations, recovering from training/missions and injury/illness, establishing strong immune systems, achieving and maintaining mission-specific body composition, optimizing mental function, and preparing for arduous environments.
- One element of the Army's move toward HPP is the Soldier Fueling initiative. This initiative is designed to improve new soldiers' nutritional status and lifestyle habits. The goal is to fuel soldiers like athletes, change nutritional habits, and apply specific nutrition, product, and menu standards so that nutrient-dense foods are more readily available and identifiable to soldiers. This initiative includes the "Go for Green" labeling system throughout the dining facility to identify foods that will optimize performance, replace nonnutritive high-calorie foods with performance-focused foods, and provide more healthful beverage options.

US Navy

Navy RDs do everything from basic sports and supplement nutrition education to designing individualized programs for US sailors and marines and their families as well as retirees, including competitive athletes while at their home station and while deployed.

- The Navy employs RDs with the CSSD credential to work with the midshipmen at the Naval Academy, and with special operations units such as Navy SEALS, Explosive Ordinance Disposal units, Individual Augmentees, and the Marine Corps' Performance and Resiliency Program, which focuses on human performance encompassing physical, mental, and spiritual aspects of health care.
- CSSDs in the Navy (active duty, Reserves, and civilian) serve on nutrition- and supplement-related committees that address DOD policy issues, plan and develop nutrition programs and policies affecting the entire Navy, and speak at various fitness related workshops and seminars.
- The Navy Operational Fitness and Fueling Series (NOFFS) is designed to provide the Navy with a world-class performance training resource for fleet sailors as well as Navy health and fitness professionals. Developed as a complete fitness package, the fueling aspect of this resource provides sailors with the tools required to make healthful nutrition choices in both shore-based and operational environments. Using the latest sports science methodologies, the logic engine for NOFFS combines both human performance and injury-prevention strategies.

US Air Force

The Air Force recognizes the value of credible experts in the field of human performance and encourages RDs working with airmen in the health and wellness centers at each installation to earn the CSSD credential. As the Air Force continues to improve and enhance performance of all airmen, the expectations for specialty certification may grow. Those working in headquarters positions rely on CSSDs for input to DOD and Air Force policy and programs and for technical expertise to Air Force–wide initiatives and aircrew specific issues.

Acknowledgment: The following military officers are acknowledged for their contributions to this appendix: MAJ Reva Rogers, MHA, RD, CSSD, CSCS (US Army); LTC Lori Sigrist, PhD, RD, CSSD, CSCS (US Army); CDR Kim A. Zuzelski, MPH, MS, RD, CSSD, CDE (US Navy); and Lt Col Dana Whelan, USAF, MS, MA, RD, CHES (US Air Force). Thank you as well to Patti Steinmuller, MS, RD, CSSD, and Nancy DiMarco, PhD, RD, CSSD, FACSM, for coordinating this appendix.

INDEX

Page number followed by a *b* indicates box; *f*, figure; *t*, table.